The Companion to Specialist Surgical

Series edited by

O. James Garden and Simon Paterson-Brown

The content of all eight volumes of the Fifth Edition of the **Companion to Specialist Surgical Practice** is now available both in print and as part of an electronic library. Your purchase of this book allows you to download the fully searchable contents to your desktop, laptop, tablet or smartphone.

Your **Companion to Specialist Surgical Practice eLibrary** is portable: the titles in the series download to you whenever you need them.

DATE DUE

Your eBook is much more than just 'pictures of pages':

- customize your page views
- search in single books that you have purchased or across any volumes in the series in your collection
- highlight and take searchable notes, and even print and copy-and-paste with bibliographic support
- utilize reference lists linked where available to Medline citations (including authors, title, source, and often an abstract) to journal articles and an indication of free electronic full-text availability.

To purchase other eBooks in the **Companion to Specialist Surgical Practice eLibrary** please visit www.elsevierhealth.com/companionseries

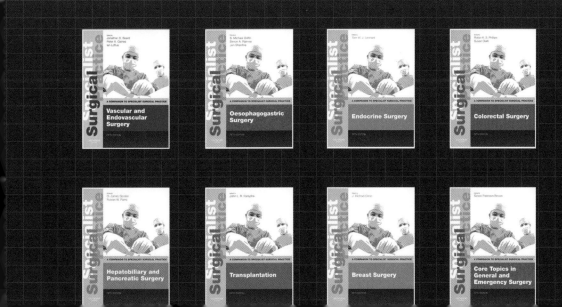

Core Topics in General and Emergency Surgery

A COMPANION TO SPECIALIST SURGICAL PRACTICE

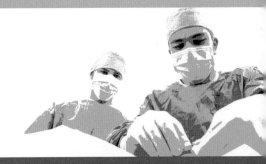

Series Editors
O. James Garden
Simon Paterson-Brown

Core Topics in General and Emergency Surgery

FIFTH EDITION

Edited by
Simon Paterson-Brown
MBBS MPhil MS FRCS(Ed) FRCS(Engl) FCS(HK)
Honorary Senior Lecturer,
Clinical Surgery School of Clinical Sciences,
The University of Edinburgh;
Consultant General and Upper Gastrointestinal Surgeon,
Royal Infirmary of Edinburgh,
Edinburgh, UK

SAUNDERS

ELSEVIER

Edinburgh   London   New York   Oxford   Philadelphia   St Louis   Sydney   Toronto   2014

SAUNDERS
ELSEVIER

First edition 1997
Second edition 2001
Third edition 2005
Fourth edition 2009
Fifth edition 2014

ISBN 978-0-7020-4964-4
e-ISBN 978-0-7020-4972-9

British Library Cataloguing in Publication Data
A catalogue record for this book is available from the British Library

Library of Congress Cataloging in Publication Data
A catalog record for this book is available from the Library of Congress

Notice

Knowledge and best practice in this field are constantly changing. As new research and experience broaden our understanding, changes in research methods, professional practices, or medical treatment may become necessary.

Practitioners and researchers must always rely on their own experience and knowledge in evaluating and using any information, methods, compounds, or experiments described herein. In using such information or methods they should be mindful of their own safety and the safety of others, including parties for whom they have a professional responsibility.

With respect to any drug or pharmaceutical products identified, readers are advised to check the most current information provided (i) on procedures featured or (ii) by the manufacturer of each product to be administered, to verify the recommended dose or formula, the method and duration of administration, and contraindications. It is the responsibility of practitioners, relying on their own experience and knowledge of their patients, to make diagnoses, to determine dosages and the best treatment for each individual patient, and to take all appropriate safety precautions.

To the fullest extent of the law, neither the Publisher nor the authors, contributors, or editors, assume any liability for any injury and/or damage to persons or property as a matter of products liability, negligence or otherwise, or from any use or operation of any methods, products, instructions, or ideas contained in the material herein.

Printed in China

Commissioning Editor: Laurence Hunter
Development Editor: Lynn Watt
Project Manager: Vinod Kumar Iyyappan
Designer/Design Direction: Miles Hitchen
Illustration Manager: Jennifer Rose
Illustrator: Antbits Ltd

Contents

Contents

Contributors

Iain D. Anderson, BSc, MD, FRCS(Eng), FRCS(Gen), FRCS(Glas)
Consultant Surgeon, Intestinal Failure Unit, Salford Royal Hospital, Manchester, UK

Emma Barrow, MBChB, MD, FRCS(Gen)
Specialist Registrar, Intestinal Failure Unit, Salford Royal Hospital, Manchester, UK

Paul Baskerville, MA, DM, BMBCh, FRCS
Consultant Vascular and General Surgeon and Director of Surgical Practice, King's College Hospital, London, UK

Andrew C. de Beaux, MBChB, FRCS, MD
Honorary Senior Lecturer, Clinical Surgery School of Clinical Sciences, The University of Edinburgh; Consultant General and Upper Gastrointestinal Surgeon, Royal Infirmary of Edinburgh, Edinburgh, UK

David E. Beck, MD, FACS, FASCRS
Professor and Chairman, Department of Colon and Rectal Surgery, Ochsner Clinic, New Orleans, LA, USA; Ochsner Clinical School, University of Queensland School of Medicine, Brisbane, Australia

Kenneth D. Boffard, MBBCh, FRCS, FRCS(Edin), FRCPS(Glas), FCS(SA), FACS
Professor and Head, Department of Surgery, Charlotte Maxeke Johannesburg Academic Hospital, University of the Witwatersrand, Johannesburg, South Africa

Felicity J. Creamer, BSc(Hons), MBChB, MRCSEd
Specialty Registrar, Colorectal Surgery, Western General Hospital, Edinburgh, UK

Dafydd A. Davies, MD, MPhil, FRCSC
Fellow, Division of Paediatric and Thoracic Surgery, The Hospital for Sick Children, Toronto, Ontario, Canada

Chris Deans, MBChB (Hons), FRCS, MD
Part-time Senior Lecturer, Clinical Surgery School of Clinical Sciences, The University of Edinburgh; Consultant General and Upper Gastrointestinal Surgeon, Royal Infirmary of Edinburgh, Edinburgh, UK

Mark Duxbury, MA, DM, FRCSEd(Gen Surg)
Consultant Hepatopancreaticobiliary and General Surgeon, Glasgow Royal Infirmary, Glasgow, UK

R. Michael Grounds, MD, FRCA, FFICM
Professor of Critical Care Medicine, St George's University of London; Consultant in Anaesthesia and Intensive Care Medicine, St George's Hospital, London, UK

Steven D. Heys, BMedBiol, MD, PhD, FRCS, FRCS(Ed), FRCS(Glasg)
Deputy Head of the School of Medicine and Dentistry and Head of Division, University of Aberdeen; Honorary Consultant Surgeon, Grampian University Hospitals Trust, Aberdeen, UK

Peter Lamb, MBBS, MD, FRCS(Gen), FRCS(Ed)
Honorary Senior Lecturer, Clinical Surgery School of Clinical Sciences, The University of Edinburgh; Consultant General and Upper Gastrointestinal Surgeon, Royal Infirmary of Edinburgh, Edinburgh, UK

Jacob C. Langer, MD
Professor of Surgery, University of Toronto, Robert M. Filler Chair and Chief, Paediatric General and Thoracic Surgery, The Hospital for Sick Children, Toronto, Ontario, Canada

James Lau, MD
Professor of Surgery, Department of Surgery, Prince of Wales Hospital, Shatin, Hong Kong, China

Contributors

Rhona M. Maclean, MBChB, FRCP, FRCPath
Consultant Haematologist, Royal Hallamshire
Hospital, Sheffield, UK

Colin J. McKay, MBChB, MD, FRCS
Consultant Surgeon, West of Scotland Pancreatic
Unit, Glasgow Royal Infirmary, Glasgow, UK

**B. James Mander, MBBS, BSc, FRCS, MS,
FRCS(Gen)**
Consultant Colorectal Surgeon and Honorary Senior
Lecturer, Colorectal Unit, Western General Hospital,
Edinburgh, UK

Jonathan A. Michaels, MChir, FRCS
Honorary Professor of Clinical Decision Science,
School of Health and Related Research, Sheffield
University, Sheffield, UK

Enders K.W. Ng, MD, FRCSEd, MBChB
Head, Upper GI Division, Department of Surgery,
Prince of Wales Hospital, The Chinese University of
Hong Kong, Hong Kong, China

Sharath C.V. Paravastu, MBBS, MRCS, PGDip, MD
Clinical Lecturer in Vascular Surgery, Academic
Vascular Unit, University of Sheffield, Sheffield, UK

**Simon Paterson-Brown, MBBS, MPhil, MS,
FRCS(Ed), FRCS(Engl), FCS(HK)**
Honorary Senior Lecturer, Clinical Surgery School
of Clinical Sciences, The University of Edinburgh;
Consultant General and Upper Gastrointestinal
Surgeon, Royal Infirmary of Edinburgh, Edinburgh, UK

Andrew Rhodes, FRCP, FRCA, FFICM
Reader in Critical Care Medicine, St George's
University of London; Consultant in Anaesthesia
and Intensive Care Medicine, St George's Hospital,
London, UK

Kathryn A. Rigby, MBChB, MSc, FRCS(GEN)
Locum Consultant Oncoplastic Breast Surgeon,
York Teaching Hospitals NHS Trust, York, UK

William G. Simpson, MBChB
Consultant Chemical Pathologist, Clinical
Biochemistry, Aberdeen Royal Infirmary,
Aberdeen, UK

Bruce R. Tulloh, MB, MS
Honorary Senior Lecturer, Clinical Surgery School
of Clinical Sciences, The University of Edinburgh;
Consultant General and Upper Gastrointestinal
Surgeon, Royal Infirmary of Edinburgh, Edinburgh, UK

Series Editors' preface

It is now some 17 years since the first edition of the *Companion to Specialist Surgical Practice* series was published. We set ourselves the task of meeting the educational needs of surgeons in the later years of specialist surgical training, as well as consultant surgeons in independent practice who wished for contemporary, evidence-based information on the subspecialist areas relevant to their general surgical practice. The series was never intended to replace the large reference surgical textbooks which, although valuable in their own way, struggle to keep pace with changing surgical practice. This Fifth Edition has also had to take due account of the increasing specialisation in 'general' surgery. The rise of minimal access surgery and therapy, and the desire of some subspecialties such as breast and vascular surgery to separate away from 'general surgery', may have proved challenging in some countries, but has also served to emphasise the importance of all surgeons being aware of current developments in their surgical field. As in previous editions, there has been increasing emphasis on evidence-based practice and contributors have endeavoured to provide key recommendations within each chapter. The eBook versions of the textbook have also allowed the technophile improved access to key data and content within each chapter.

We remain indebted to the volume editors and all the contributors of this Fifth Edition. We have endeavoured where possible to bring in new blood to freshen content. We are impressed by the enthusiasm, commitment and hard work that our contributors and editorial team have shown and this has ensured a short turnover between editions while maintaining as accurate and up-to-date content as is possible. We remain grateful for the support and encouragement of Laurence Hunter and Lynn Watt at Elsevier Ltd. We trust that our original vision of delivering an up-to-date affordable text has been met and that readers, whether in training or independent practice, will find this Fifth Edition an invaluable resource.

O. James Garden, BSc, MBChB, MD, FRCS(Glas), FRCS(Ed), FRCP(Ed), FRACS(Hon), FRCSC(Hon), FRSE
Regius Professor of Clinical Surgery, Clinical Surgery School of Clinical Sciences, The University of Edinburgh and Honorary Consultant Surgeon, Royal Infirmary of Edinburgh

Simon Paterson-Brown, MBBS, MPhil, MS, FRCS(Ed), FRCS(Engl), FCS(HK)
Honorary Senior Lecturer, Clinical Surgery School of Clinical Sciences, The University of Edinburgh and Consultant General and Upper Gastrointestinal Surgeon, Royal Infirmary of Edinburgh

Editor's preface

Although surgical sub-specialisation within the specialty of 'General Surgery' has progressed rapidly over the last decade or so, most general surgeons on-call, irrespective of their sub-specialty interest, require a core knowledge in both elective and emergency 'general' surgery in order to be able to see and treat undifferentiated referrals and conditions outwith their normal everyday elective 'specialist' practice. This volume of the *Companion to Specialist Surgical Practice* provides the background information on these key areas of 'general surgery' for all practising general surgeons in both the elective and emergency situation. It is the only volume in this series which provides detailed descriptions of evidence-based medicine and how surgical outcomes can be measured, in addition to other important areas common to all of 'general surgical practice'. These include an overview of day case surgery, abdominal hernias, thromboembolic prophylaxis, the management of sepsis and the intensive care patient, the use of scoring systems in patient assessment and surgical nutrition. This volume should be considered complementary to the other more specialist volumes in the series by including all the emergency areas which remain within the remit of the general surgeon on-call. As in everyday practice, there remain emergency patients who, having been resuscitated and a diagnosis reached, might be better served by referral to a colleague or unit with the relevant sub-specialist interest. This volume discusses those conditions which the general surgeon might be expected to deal with and, where appropriate, identifies those which might be better managed by a 'specialist'. In these cases the reader will be referred on to the relevant specialist volume of this series.

Acknowledgements

Once again I remain grateful to my long-suffering wife and family for their ongoing support and understanding in the time taken for me to complete the Fifth Edition of this volume of *Core Topics in General and Emergency Surgery*. The success of this volume, as for previous editions, very much lies in the quality of the chapters produced by my co-authors and I am grateful to all of them for the hard work that has obviously gone into writing, or re-writing, each chapter and their timely delivery. The additional workload required in the writing of concise, well-referenced and up-to-date chapters for a book such as this, by busy practising surgeons, should never be under-estimated. I would also like to recognise the support of Elsevier Ltd, as well as the help, enthusiasm and friendship of my co-editor of all five editions of the *Companion to Specialist Surgical Practice* series, James Garden.

Simon Paterson-Brown
Edinburgh

Evidence-based practice in surgery

Critical appraisal for developing evidence-based practice can be obtained from a number of sources, the most reliable being randomised controlled clinical trials, systematic literature reviews, meta-analyses and observational studies. For practical purposes three grades of evidence can be used, analogous to the levels of 'proof' required in a court of law:

1. **Beyond all reasonable doubt.** Such evidence is likely to have arisen from high-quality randomised controlled trials, systematic reviews or high-quality synthesised evidence such as decision analysis, cost-effectiveness analysis or large observational datasets. The studies need to be directly applicable to the population of concern and have clear results. The grade is analogous to burden of proof within a criminal court and may be thought of as corresponding to the usual standard of 'proof' within the medical literature (i.e. $P<0.05$).

2. **On the balance of probabilities.** In many cases a high-quality review of literature may fail to reach firm conclusions due to conflicting or inconclusive results, trials of poor methodological quality or the lack of evidence in the population to which the guidelines apply. In such cases it may still be possible to make a statement as to the best treatment on the 'balance of probabilities'. This is analogous to the decision in a civil court where all the available evidence will be weighed up and the verdict will depend upon the balance of probabilities.

3. **Not proven.** Insufficient evidence upon which to base a decision, or contradictory evidence.

Depending on the information available, three grades of recommendation can be used:

a. Strong recommendation, which should be followed unless there are compelling reasons to act otherwise.

b. A recommendation based on evidence of effectiveness, but where there may be other factors to take into account in decision-making, for example the user of the guidelines may be expected to take into account patient preferences, local facilities, local audit results or available resources.

c. A recommendation made where there is no adequate evidence as to the most effective practice, although there may be reasons for making a recommendation in order to minimise cost or reduce the chance of error through a locally agreed protocol.

✔✔ Evidence where a conclusion can be reached 'beyond all reasonable doubt' and therefore where a strong recommendation can be given.
  This will normally be based on evidence levels:
- Ia. Meta-analysis of randomised controlled trials
- Ib. Evidence from at least one randomised controlled trial
- IIa. Evidence from at least one controlled study without randomisation
- IIb. Evidence from at least one other type of quasi-experimental study.

✔ Evidence where a conclusion might be reached 'on the balance of probabilities' and where there may be other factors involved which influence the recommendation given. This will normally be based on less conclusive evidence than that represented by the double tick icons:
- III. Evidence from non-experimental descriptive studies, such as comparative studies and case–control studies
- IV. Evidence from expert committee reports or opinions or clinical experience of respected authorities, or both.

Evidence which is associated with either a **strong recommendation** or **expert opinion** is highlighted in the text in panels such as those shown above, and is distinguished by either a double or single tick icon, respectively. The references associated with double-tick evidence are highlighted in the reference lists at the end of each chapter along with a short summary of the paper's conclusions where applicable.

The reader is referred to Chapter 1, 'Evidence-based practice in surgery', in this volume for a more detailed description of this topic.

Evidence-based practice in surgery

Kathryn A. Rigby
Jonathan A. Michaels

Introduction

> ✔ Evidence-based medicine is the conscientious, explicit and judicious use of current best evidence in making decisions about the care of individual patients. The practice of evidence-based medicine means integrating individual clinical expertise with the best external clinical evidence from systematic research.[1]

The concept of evidence-based medicine (EBM) was introduced in the 19th century but has only flourished in the last few decades. Historically, its application to surgical practice can be traced back to the likes of John Hunter and the American Ernest Amory Codman, who both recognised the need for research into surgical outcomes in an attempt to improve patient care.

In mid-19th century Paris, Pierre-Charles-Alexander Louis used statistics to measure the effectiveness of bloodletting, the results of which helped put an end to the practice of leeching. Ernest A. Codman began work as a surgeon in 1895 in Massachusetts. His main area of interest was the shoulder and he became a leading expert in this topic as well as being instrumental in the founding of the American College of Surgeons. He developed his 'End Result Idea', a notion that all hospitals should follow up every patient it treats 'long enough to determine whether or not its treatment is successful and if not, why not?' in order to prevent similar failures in the future.[2] Codman also developed the first registry of bone sarcomas.

In the UK, one of the most important advocates of EBM was Archie Cochrane. His experiences in the prisoner of war camps, where he conducted trials in the use of yeast supplements to treat nutritional oedema, influenced his belief in reliable and scientifically proven medical treatment. In 1972 he published his book *Effectiveness and Efficiency*. Cochrane advocated the use of the randomised controlled trial (RCT) as the gold standard in the research of all medical treatment and, where possible, systematic reviews of these trials. One of the first systematic reviews of RCTs was of the use of corticosteroid therapy to improve lung function in threatened premature birth. Although RCTs had been conducted in this area, the message of the results was not clear from the individual studies, until the review overwhelmingly showed that corticosteroids reduced both neonatal morbidity and mortality. Had a systematic review been conducted earlier, then the lives of many babies could have been saved, as the review clearly showed that this inexpensive treatment reduced the chance of these babies dying from complications of immaturity by 30–50%.[3] In 1992, as part of the UK National Health Service (NHS) Research and Development (R&D) Programme, the Cochrane Collaboration was founded.

Subsequently, in 1995, the first centre for EBM in the UK was established at the Nuffield Department of Clinical Medicine, University of Oxford. The driving force behind this was the American David Sackett, who had moved to a new Chair in Clinical Epidemiology in 1994 from McMaster University in Canada, where he had pioneered self-directed teaching for medical students.

From these roots, interest in EBM has exploded. The Cochrane Collaboration is rapidly expanding, with review groups in many fields of medicine and surgery. EBM is not limited only to hospital-based medicine but is increasingly seen in nursing, general practice and dentistry, and there are many new evidence-based journals appearing.

While clinical experience is invaluable, the rapidly changing world of medicine means that clinicians must keep abreast of new advances and, where appropriate, integrate research findings into everyday clinical practice. Neither research nor clinical experience alone is enough to ensure high-quality patient care; the two must complement each other. Sackett et al. identified five steps that should become part of day-to-day practice and in which a competent practitioner should be proficient:[4]

1. to convert information needs into answerable questions;
2. to be able to track down efficiently the best evidence with which to answer them (be it evidence from clinical examination, the diagnostic laboratory, research evidence or other sources);
3. to be able to appraise that evidence critically for its validity and usefulness;
4. to apply the results of this appraisal in clinical practice;
5. to evaluate performance.

This chapter discusses the steps that are necessary to identify, critically appraise and combine evidence, to incorporate the findings into clinical guidance, and to implement and audit any necessary changes in order to move towards EBM in surgery. Many of the organisations and information sources that are relevant to EBM are specific to a particular setting. Therefore, the emphasis in this chapter is on the health services within the UK, although there are comparable arrangements and bodies in many other countries. Links to a number of these are given in the Internet resources described at the end of the chapter.

The need for evidence-based medicine

In 1991, there was still a widely held belief that only a small proportion of medical interventions were supported by solid scientific evidence.[5] Jonathan Ellis and colleagues, on behalf of the Nuffield Department of Clinical Medicine, conducted a review of treatments given to 109 patients on a medical ward.[6] The treatments were then examined to assess the degree of evidence supporting their use.

The authors concluded that 82% of these treatments were in fact evidence based. However, they did suggest that similar studies should be conducted in other specialities. The importance of evidence-based health care in the NHS was formally acknowledged in two government papers, *The new NHS*[7] and *A first class service*.[8] These led to the development of the National Service Frameworks and the National Institute of Clinical Excellence (NICE).

In surgery there is a limited body of evidence from high-quality RCTs. For an RCT to be ethical there needs to be a clinical equipoise. That is, there needs to be a sufficient level of uncertainty about an intervention before a trial can be considered. For example, it would be unethical to conduct an RCT in the use of burr holes for extradural haematomas, because the observational data alone are so overwhelming as to the high degree of effectiveness that it would be unethical to deny someone a burr hole to prove the point.

Many surgeons feel unhappy with having to explain to a patient that there is clinical uncertainty about a treatment, as patients have historically put their trust in surgeons' hands. This reluctance to perform RCTs and the belief that they would be difficult to carry out has led to practices that are poorly supported by high-quality evidence. For example, there is widespread use of radical prostatectomy to treat localised prostatic carcinoma in the USA, despite a distinct lack of evidence to support this procedure.[9]

New technologies in surgery may be driven into widespread use by market forces, patients' expectations and clinicians' desire to improve treatment options. For example, with laparoscopic surgery, many assumed that it must be 'better' because it made smaller holes, there was less pain involved and therefore patients left hospital sooner. It was only after many hospitals had instituted its use that concerns were raised about its real benefits and the adequacy of training in the new technology. In 1996, a group of surgeons from Sheffield published a randomised, prospective, single-blind study that compared small-incision open cholecystectomy with laparoscopic cholecystectomy.[10] They demonstrated that in their hands the laparosopic technique offered no real benefit over a mini-cholecystectomy in terms of the postoperative recovery period, hospital stay and time off work, but it took longer to perform and was more expensive.[10] There were, however, other factors that may have influenced the results from this study, including surgeon experience, and mini-cholecystectomy has not been widely adopted.

The MRC Laparoscopic Groin and Hernia Trial Group undertook a large multicentre randomised comparison between laparoscopic and open repair of groin hernias.[11] The results demonstrated that the laparoscopic procedure was associated with an earlier return to activities and less groin pain 1 year after surgery but it was also associated with more serious surgical complications, an increased recurrence rate and a higher cost to the health service. They suggested that laparoscopic hernia surgery should be confined to specialist surgical centres. NICE have since published guidelines which recommend that laparoscopic surgery is now one of the treatment options for the repair of inguinal hernias.

Some would argue that surgery, unlike drug trials, is operator dependent and that operating experience and skill can affect the outcome of an RCT, and cite this as a reason for not undertaking surgical trials. Although operator factors can introduce bias into a trial, the North American Symptomatic Carotid Endarterectomy Trial has shown that such problems can largely be overcome through appropriate trial design.[12] Only surgeons who had been fully trained in the procedure, and who already had a proven low complication rate, were accepted as participants in the trial.

These examples illustrate a clear need for high-quality research to be undertaken into any new technology to assess both its efficacy and its cost-effectiveness before it is introduced into the healthcare system.

However, concerns have been raised about EBM. Sceptics have suggested that it may undermine clinical experience and instinct and replace it with 'cookbook medicine' or that it may ignore the elements of basic medical training such as history-taking, physical examination, laboratory investigations and a sound grounding in pathophysiology. Another fear is that purchasers and managers will use it as a means to cut costs and manage budgets.

Nevertheless, EBM can formalise our everyday procedures and highlight problems. It can provide answers by ensuring that the best use is made of existing evidence or it can identify areas in which new research is needed. Although it has a role in assessing the cost-effectiveness of an intervention, it is not a substitute for rationing and often results in practice that, despite being more cost-effective, has greater overall cost.[13]

The process of evidence-based medicine

EBM requires a structured approach to ensure that clinical interventions are based upon best available evidence. The first stage is always to pose a clinically relevant question for which an answer is required. Such a question should be clear, specific, important and answerable. One way of formulating questions is to think of them as having four key elements (PICO):

- the population to whom the question applies;
- the intervention of interest (and any other interventions with which it is to be compared);
- the comparison (the main alternative);
- the outcome of interest.

Therefore, the question 'What is the best treatment for cholecystitis?' needs to be much more clearly formulated if an adequate, evidence-based approach is to be used. A much better question would be 'For adult patients admitted to hospital with acute cholecystitis (the **population**), does early open cholecystectomy, laparoscopic cholecystectomy (the **interventions**) or best medical management (the **comparison**) produce the lowest mortality, morbidity and total length of stay in hospital (the **outcomes**)?' Even this may require more refinement to define further the exact interventions and outcomes of interest.

Once such a question has been clearly defined, a number of further stages of the process can follow:

1. Relevant sources of information must be searched to identify all available literature that will help in answering the question.
2. Published trials must be critically appraised to assess whether they possess internal and external validity in answering the question posed (**internal validity** is where the effects within the study are free from bias and confounding; **external validity** is where the effects within the study apply outside the study and the results are therefore generalisable to the population in question).
3. Where relevant, a systematic review and meta-analysis may be required to provide a clear answer from a number of disparate sources.
4. The answers to the question need to be incorporated into clinical practice through the use of guidelines or through other methods of implementation.
5. Adherence to 'best practice' needs to be monitored through audit, and the process needs to be kept under review in order to take account of new evidence or clinical developments.

Sources of evidence

Once a question has been formulated, the next step in undertaking EBM is the identification of all the relevant evidence. The first line for most practitioners is the use of journals. Many clinicians will subscribe to specific journals in their own specialist area and have access to many others through local libraries. However, the vast increase in the number of such publications makes it impossible for an individual to access or read all the relevant papers, even in a highly specialist area.

There has been a huge expansion in the resources that are available for identifying relevant material from other publications, including indexing and abstracting services such as MEDLINE (computerised database compiled by the US National Library of Medicine) and EMBASE. There is also a rapidly expanding set of journals and other services that provide access to selected, appraised and combined results from primary information sources.

As a result, the information sources that provide the evidence to support EBM are vast and include the following:

- Media – journals, online databases, CD-ROMs and the Internet.
- Independent organisations – research bodies and the pharmaceutical industry.
- Health services – purchasers and providers at local, regional and national levels.
- Academic units.

Some of these are described in more detail below and the Appendix to this chapter provides a list of contact details for further information.

Journals

The following are a selection of journals that act as secondary sources, identifying and reviewing other research that is felt to be of key importance to evidence-based practice.

Evidence-based Medicine
This was first launched in October 1995, by the *British Medical Journal* (BMJ) Publishing Group. It systematically searches high-quality international journals and provides summaries of the most clinically relevant research articles. The validity of the research is critically appraised by experts and assessed for its clinical applicability. This consequently allows the reader to keep up with the latest advances in clinical practice. It also publishes articles relating to the study and practice of EBM.

Evidence-based Nursing
This follows similar lines to *Evidence-based Medicine*, but contains articles more relevant to the nursing field.

Evidence-based Mental Health
This is produced by the BMJ Publishing Group in collaboration with the Royal College of Psychiatrists and British Pyschological Society.

Internet resources

The Internet is becoming an increasingly useful source of medical information and evidence. Details of Internet addresses for many of the sources referred to below are given in the Appendix to this chapter, although this is a rapidly progressing and changing area. There are many journals and databases that are available either free or through subscription, and dedicated search engines such as Google Scholar. This medium also provides a number of advantages over printed material, including ease of searching, hyperlinks to other sources, access to additional supporting materials or raw data and the provision of discussion groups. There are, however, potential problems with the Internet in that there is no quality control and much of the available material is of dubious quality, or published by those with particular commercial or other interests.

NHS Evidence
This is a new service that provides online access to evidence-based information. It is managed by NICE and is free to use. It has access to NICE pathways, journals and databases, ebooks and the Cochrane library.

BMJ Evidence Centre
This provides information, resources and tools that aid evidence-based practice. It has access to sites that target EBM in relation to patient care, research and patient information, and has updates on current evidence and treatment options.

Academic units

Cochrane Collaboration
As described above, the British epidemiologist who inspired this collaboration realised that in order to make informed decisions about healthcare, reliable evidence must be accessible and kept up to date with any new evidence. It was felt that failure to achieve this might result in important developments in healthcare being overlooked. This was to be a key aspect in providing the best healthcare possible for patients. It was also hoped that by making clear the result of an intervention, then work would not be duplicated.

The Cochrane library is the electronic publication of the Cochrane Collaboration and it includes six databases:

- The Cochrane Database of Systematic Reviews contains systematic reviews and protocols of reviews in preparation. These are regularly updated and there are facilities for comments and criticisms along with authors' responses.
- The Cochrane Central Register of Controlled Trials is the largest database of RCTs.

Information about trials is obtained from several sources including searches of other databases and hand searching of medical journals. It includes many RCTs not currently listed in databases such as MEDLINE or EMBASE.

- The Database of Abstracts of Reviews of Effectiveness (DARE) contains abstracts of reviews that have been critically appraised by peer reviewers. These reviews evaluate the effects of healthcare interventions and the delivery and organisations of health services.
- The Cochrane Review Methodology Register is a bibliography of articles on the science of research synthesis.
- Health Technology Assessment Database (HTA) – see below.
- NHS Economic Evaluation Database (NHS EED) – see below.

The Reviewers' Handbook includes information on the science of reviewing research and details of the review groups. It is also available in hard copy.[14]

The Cochrane library is regularly updated and amended as new evidence is acquired. It is distributed on disk, CD-ROM and the Internet.[3] In order to allow the results of the reviews to be widely used, no one contributor has exclusive copyright of the review.

Centre for Evidence-based Medicine

The Centre for Evidence-based Medicine was established in Oxford. Its chief remit is to promote EBM and Evidence-Based Practice (EBP) in healthcare. It runs workshops and courses in both the practice and teaching of EBM. It also conducts research and development on improving EBP and its website also has many free EBM resources and tools.

Review Body for Interventional Procedures (ReBIP)

This is a joint venture between the Health Services Research Unit at Sheffield University and Aberdeen University. It works under the auspices of NICE's Interventional Procedures Programme (IPP). When there is doubt about the safety and efficacy of any procedure they will be commissioned to provide a systematic review or gather additional data.

NHS agencies

Centre for Reviews and Dissemination (CRD)

The CRD was established in January 1994 at the University of York and is now also part of the National Institute for Health Research (NIHR). It is funded by NIHR England, the Department of Health, Public Health Agency, Northern Ireland, and the National Institute for Social Care and Health Research, Welsh Assembly Government. The CRD concentrates specifically on areas of priority to the NHS. It is designed to raise the standards of reviews within the NHS and to encourage research by working with healthcare professionals. It undertakes and disseminates systematic reviews and maintains three databases:

- NHS EED contains mainly abstracts of economic evaluations of healthcare interventions and assesses the quality of the studies, stating any practical implications to the NHS.
- DARE (see above).
- The Health Technology Assessment (HTA) database details completed and ongoing HTAs from around the world. The contents of this database have not been critically appraised.

NIHR Health Technology Assessment Programme

The HTA is now part of National Institute for Health Research (NIHR). It commissions independent research into high-priority areas. This includes many systematic reviews and primary research in key areas. The programme publishes details of ongoing HTA projects and monographs of completed research.

Critical appraisal

✔ This is the process by which we assess the evidence presented to us in a paper. We need to be critical of it in terms of its validity and clinical applicability.

From reading the literature, it is evident that there may be many trials on the same subject, which may all draw different conclusions. Which one should be believed and allowed to influence clinical practice? We owe a duty to our patients to be able to assess accurately all the available information and judge each paper on its own merits before changing our clinical practice accordingly.

Randomised controlled trials

The RCT is a comparative evaluation in which the interventions being compared are allocated to the units being studied purely by chance. It is the 'gold standard' method of comparing the effectiveness of different interventions.[15] Randomisation is the only way to allow valid inferences of cause and effect,[16] and no other study design can potentially protect as well against bias.

Unfortunately, not all clinical trials are done well, and even fewer are well reported. Their results may therefore be confusing and misleading, and it is necessary to consider several elements of a trial's design, conduct and conclusions before accepting the results. The first requirement is that there must be sufficient detail available to make such an assessment.

It became clear that there was a need for the presentation of clinical trials to be standardised. The CONSORT (Consolidated Standards of Reporting Trials) statement was developed. The most recent version is CONSORT 2010 (Table 1.1).[17,18]

Table 1.1 • CONSORT 2010 checklist of information to include when reporting a randomised trial*

Section/topic	Item no.	Checklist item
Title and abstract		
	1a	Identification as a randomised trial in the title
	1b	Structured summary of trial design, methods, results, and conclusions (for specific guidance see CONSORT for abstracts)
Introduction		
Background and objectives	2a	Scientific background and explanation of rationale
	2b	Specific objectives or hypotheses
Methods		
Trial design	3a	Description of trial design (such as parallel, factorial) including allocation ratio
	3b	Important changes to methods after trial commencement (such as eligibility criteria), with reasons
Participants	4a	Eligibility criteria for participants
	4b	Settings and locations where the data were collected
Interventions	5	The interventions for each group with sufficient details to allow replication, including how and when they were actually administered
Outcomes	6a	Completely defined pre-specified primary and secondary outcome measures, including how and when they were assessed
	6b	Any changes to trial outcomes after the trial commenced, with reasons
Sample size	7a	How sample size was determined
	7b	When applicable, explanation of any interim analyses and stopping guidelines
Randomisation:		
Sequence generation	8a	Method used to generate the random allocation sequence
	8b	Type of randomisation; details of any restriction (such as blocking and block size)
Allocation concealment mechanism	9	Mechanism used to implement the random allocation sequence (such as sequentially numbered containers), describing any steps taken to conceal the sequence until interventions were assigned
Implementation	10	Who generated the random allocation sequence, who enrolled participants, and who assigned participants to interventions
Blinding	11a	If done, who was blinded after assignment to interventions (for example, participants, care providers, those assessing outcomes) and how
	11b	If relevant, description of the similarity of interventions
Statistical methods	12a	Statistical methods used to compare groups for primary and secondary outcomes
	12b	Methods for additional analyses, such as subgroup analyses and adjusted analyses
Results		
Participant flow (a diagram is strongly recommended)	13a	For each group, the numbers of participants who were randomly assigned, received intended treatment, and were analysed for the primary outcome
	13b	For each group, losses and exclusions after randomisation, together with reasons
Recruitment	14a	Dates defining the periods of recruitment and follow-up
	14b	Why the trial ended or was stopped

Table 1.1 • *(Cont.)* CONSORT 2010 checklist of information to include when reporting a randomised trial

Section/topic	Item no.	Checklist item
Baseline data	15	A table showing baseline demographic and clinical characteristics for each group
Numbers analysed	16	For each group, number of participants (denominator) included in each analysis and whether the analysis was by original assigned groups
Outcomes and estimation	17a	For each primary and secondary outcome, results for each group, and the estimated effect size and its precision (such as 95% confidence interval)
	17b	For binary outcomes, presentation of both absolute and relative effect sizes is recommended
Ancillary analyses	18	Results of any other analyses performed, including subgroup analyses and adjusted analyses, distinguishing pre-specified from exploratory
Harms	19	All important harms or unintended effects in each group (for specific guidance see CONSORT for harms)
Discussion		
Limitations	20	Trial limitations, addressing sources of potential bias, imprecision, and, if relevant, multiplicity of analyses
Generalisability	21	Generalisability (external validity, applicability) of the trial findings
Interpretation	22	Interpretation consistent with results, balancing benefits and harms, and considering other relevant evidence
Other information		
Registration	23	Registration number and name of trial registry
Protocol	24	Where the full trial protocol can be accessed, if available
Funding	25	Sources of funding and other support (such as supply of drugs), role of funders

*We strongly recommend reading this statement in conjunction with the CONSORT 2010 Explanation and Elaboration for important clarifications on all the items. If relevant, we also recommend reading CONSORT extensions for cluster randomised trials, non-inferiority and equivalence trials, non-pharmacological treatments, herbal interventions, and pragmatic trials. Additional extensions are forthcoming: for those and for up-to-date references relevant to this checklist, see www.consort-statement.org.
Reproduced from Schulz KF, Altman DG, Moher D et al. Br Med J 2010; 340:c332 and Moher D, Hopewell S, Schulz KF et al. Br Med J 2010;340:c869. With permission from the BMJ Publishing Group Ltd.

✔✔ The CONSORT 2010 statement lists 25 items that should be included in any trial report, along with a flow chart.[17,18]

Many journals now encourage authors to submit a copy of the CONSORT statement relating to their paper. A similar checklist has been proposed for the reporting of observational studies (cohort, case–control and cross-sectional). This is called the Strengthening the Reporting of Observational Studies in Epidemiology (STROBE) statement.[19] The QUORUM statement is a similar checklist that has been developed to improve the quality of reporting relating to systematic reviews of RCTs.[20]

✔✔ The STROBE statement provides a recommended checklist for the reporting of observational studies[19] and the QUORUM statement provides similar recommendations for systematic reviews of RCTs.[20]

The Critical Appraisal Skills Programme (CASP) is a UK-based project designed to develop appraisal skills about effectiveness. It provides half-day workshops and has developed appraisal frameworks based on 10 or 11 questions for RCTs, qualitative research and systematic reviews.

Assuming that the relevant information is available, critical appraisal is required to ensure that the methodology of the trial is such that it will minimise effects on outcome other than true treatment effects, i.e. those owing to **chance**, **bias** and **confounding**:

• Chance – random variation, leading to imprecision.

• Bias – systematic variation leading to inaccuracy.

• Confounding – systematic variation resulting from the existence of extraneous factors that affect the outcome and have distributions that are not taken into account, leading to bias and invalid inferences.

All good study designs will reduce the effects of chance, eliminate bias and take confounding into account. This requires consideration of many aspects of trial design, including methods of randomisation, blinding and masking, analysis methods and sample size. It also requires the reviewer to consider aspects such as sponsorship and vested interests that may introduce sources of bias. Discussion of methodology for the critical appraisal of RCTs and other forms of study is readily available elsewhere.[21]

Systematic literature reviews

✅ A systematic review is an overview of primary studies carried out to an exhaustive, defined and repeatable protocol.

There has been an explosion in the published medical literature, with over two million articles a year published in 20 000 journals. The task of keeping up with new advances in medical research has become quite overwhelming. We have also seen that the results of trials in the same subject may be contradictory, and that the underlying message can be masked. Systematic reviews are designed to search out meticulously all relevant studies on a subject, evaluate the quality of each study and assimilate the information to produce a balanced and unbiased conclusion.[22]

One advantage of a systematic review with a meta-analysis over a traditional subjective narrative review is that by synthesising the results of many smaller studies, the original lack of statistical power of each study may be overcome by cumulative size, and any treatment effect is more clearly demonstrated. This, in turn, can lead to a reduction in delay between research advances and clinical implementation. For example, it has been demonstrated that if the original studies done on the use of anticoagulants after myocardial infarction had been reviewed, their benefits would have been apparent much earlier.[23,24] It is obviously essential that both the benefit or any harm caused by an intervention becomes apparent as soon as possible.

Unfortunately, as in reported trials, not all reviews are as rigorously researched and synthesised as one would hope and are open to similar pitfalls as RCTs. The Cochrane Collaboration has sought to rectify this and has worked upon refining the methods used for systematic reviews. It has consequently produced some of the most reliable and useful reviews, and its methods have been widely adopted by other reviewers. The Cochrane Collaboration advises that each review must be based on an explicit protocol, which sets out the objectives and methods so that a second party could reproduce the review at a later date if required.

Because of the increasing importance of systematic reviews as a method of providing the evidence base for a variety of clinical activities, the methods are discussed in some detail below. There are several key elements in producing a systematic review.

1. Develop a protocol for a clearly defined question

Within a protocol:

- the objectives of the review of the RCTs must be stated;
- eligibility criteria must be included (e.g. relevant patient groups, types of intervention and trial design);
- appropriate outcome measures should be defined.

In the Cochrane Collaboration, each systematic review is preceded by a published protocol that is subjected to a process of peer review. This helps to ensure high quality, avoids duplication of effort and is designed to reduce bias by setting standards for inclusion criteria before the results from identified studies have been assessed.

2. Literature search

All published and unpublished material should be sought. This includes examining studies in non-English journals, grey literature, conference reports, company reports (drug companies can hold a lot of vital information from their own research) and any personal contacts, for personal studies or information. The details of the search methodology and search terms used should be specified in order to make the review reproducible and allow readers to repeat the search to identify further relevant information published after the review. The most frequently used initial source of information is MEDLINE but this does have limitations. It only indexes about one-third of all medical articles that exist in libraries (over 10 million in total),[25] and an average search by a regular user would only yield about one-fifth of the trials that can be identified by more rigorous techniques for literature searching.[26] It also has a bias towards articles published in English. Other electronic and indexed databases should also be searched, but often the only way to ensure that the maximum number of relevant trials are found, wherever published and in whatever language, is to hand search the journals. This is one of the tasks of the Cochrane Collaboration through a database maintained at the Baltimore Cochrane Centre.

One must also be aware, however, that there is a potential for 'publication bias'. Trials that are more likely to get published are those with a positive result rather than a negative or no-effect result,[27] and are also more likely to be cited in other articles.[28]

3. Evaluating the studies

Each trial should be assessed to see if it meets the inclusion criteria set out in the protocol (eligibility). If it meets the required standards, then the trial is subjected to a critical appraisal, ideally by two independent reviewers, to ascertain its validity, relevance and reliability. Any exclusions should be reported and justified; if there is missing information from the published article, it may be necessary to attempt to contact the author of the primary research. Reviewers should also, if possible, be 'blinded' to the authors and journals of publication, etc. in order to minimise any personal bias.

The Cochrane reviewers are assisted in all these tasks by instructions in the Cochrane Handbook[14] and through workshops at the Cochrane Centres.[29]

4. Synthesis of the results

Once the studies have been graded according to quality and relevance, their results may be combined in an interpretative or a statistical fashion. It must be decided if it is appropriate to combine some studies and which comparisons to make. Subgroup or sensitivity analyses may also be appropriate. The statistical analysis is called a meta-analysis and is discussed below.

5. Discussion

The review should be summarised. The aims, methods and reported results should be discussed and the following issues considered:

- quality of the studies;
- possible sources of heterogeneity (reasons for inconsistency between studies, e.g. patient selection, methods of randomisation, duration of follow-up or differences in statistical analysis);
- bias;
- chance;
- applicability of the findings.

As with any study, a review can be done badly, and the reader must critically appraise a review to assess its quality. Systematic errors may be introduced by omitting some relevant studies, by selection bias (such as excluding foreign language journals) or by including inappropriate studies (such as those considering different patient groups or irrelevant outcomes). Despite all precautions, the findings of a systematic review may differ from those of a large-scale, high-quality RCT. This will be discussed below in relation to meta-analysis.

Meta-analysis

> ✔ A meta-analysis is a specific statistical strategy for assembling the results of several studies into a single estimate, which may be incorporated into a systematic literature review.[30]

Here we must make the distinction that the term 'meta-analysis' refers to the statistical techniques used to combine the results of several studies and is not synonymous with systematic review, as it is sometimes used.

A common problem in clinical trials is that the results are not clear-cut, either because of size or because of the design of the trial. The systematic review is designed to eliminate some of these problems and give appropriate weightings to the best- and worst-quality studies, regardless of size. Meta-analysis is the statistical tool used to combine the results and give 'power' to the estimates of effect.

Meta-analyses use a variety of statistical techniques according to the type of data being analysed (dichotomous, continuous or individual patient data).[14] There are two main models used to analyse the results: the fixed-effect model (logistic regression, Mantel–Haenszel test and Peto's method) and the random-effect model. The major concern with fixed-effect methods is that they assume no clinical heterogeneity between the individual trials, and this may be unrealistic.[31] The random-effect method takes into consideration random variation and clinical heterogeneity between trials. In the presentation of meta-analysis, a consistent scale should be chosen for measuring treatment effects and to cope with the possible large scale of difference in proportions, risk ratios or odds ratios that can be used.

Heterogeneity

Trials can have many different components[21] and therefore a meta-analysis is only valid if the trials that it seeks to summarise are homogeneous: you cannot add apples and oranges.[32] If trials are not comparable and any heterogeneity is ignored, the analysis can produce misleading results.

Figure 1.1 shows an example of this from a meta-analysis of 19 RCTs investigating the use of endoscopic sclerotherapy to reduce mortality from

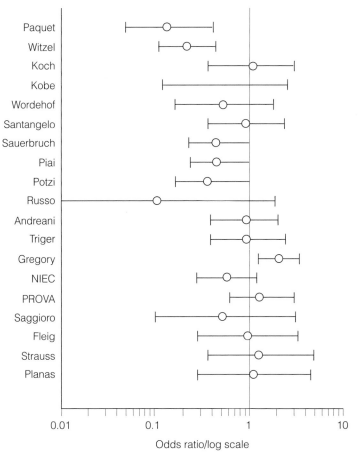

Figure 1.1 • An example of a meta-analysis of 19 randomised controlled trials investigating the use of endoscopic sclerotherapy to reduce mortality from oesophageal varices in the primary treatment of cirrhotic patients. Reproduced from Chalmer I, Altman DG. Systematic reviews. London: BMJ Publishing, 1995; p. 119. With permission from Blackwell Publishing Ltd.

oesophageal varices in the primary treatment of cirrhotic patients.[33] Each trial is represented by a 'point estimate' of the difference between the groups, and a horizontal line showing the 95% confidence interval (CI). If the line does not cross the line of no effect, then there is a 95% chance that there is a real difference between the groups. It can be seen that in this case the trials are not homogeneous as some of the lower limits of the CIs are above the highest limits of CIs in other trials. Such a lack of homogeneity may have a variety of causes, relating to clinical heterogeneity (differences in patient mix, setting, etc.) or differences in methods. The degree of statistical heterogeneity can be measured to see if it is greater than is compatible with the play of chance.[34] Such a statistical tool may lack statistical power; consequently, results that do not show significant heterogeneity do not necessarily mean that the trials are truly homogeneous and one must look beyond them to assess the degree of heterogeneity.

✓ 'Meta-analysis is on the strongest ground when the methods employed in the primary studies are sufficiently similar that any differences in their results are due to the play of chance.'[30]

Views on the usefulness of meta-analyses are divided. On the one hand, they may provide conclusions that could not be reached from other trials because of the small numbers involved. However, on the other hand, they have some limitations and cannot produce a single simple answer to all complex clinical problems. They may give misleading results if used inappropriately where there is a biased body of literature or clinical or methodological heterogeneity. If used with caution, however, they may be a useful tool in providing information to help in decision-making.

Figure 1.2 shows a funnel plot of a meta-analysis relating to the use of magnesium following myocardial infarction.[35] The result of each study in the

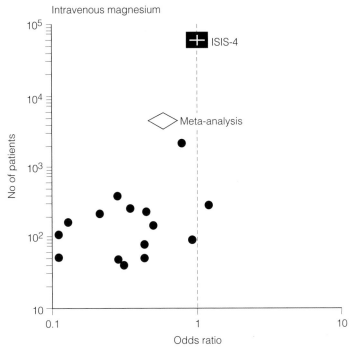

Figure 1.2 • A funnel plot of a meta-analysis relating to the use of magnesium following myocardial infarction. Points indicate values from small and medium-sized trials; the diamond is the combined odds ratio with 95% confidence interval from the meta-analysis of these trials and the square is that for a mega trial. Reproduced from Egger M, Smith GD. Misleading meta-analysis. Br Med J 1995; 310:752–4. With permission from the BMJ Publishing Group Ltd.

analysis is represented by a circle plotting the odds ratio (with the vertical line being at 1, the 'line of no effect') against the trial size. The diamond represents the overall results of the meta-analysis with its pooled data from all the smaller studies shown. This study[36] was published in 1993 and showed that it was beneficial and safe to give intravenous magnesium in patients with acute myocardial infarction. The majority of the studies involved show a positive effect of the treatment, as does the meta-analysis. However, the results from this study were contradicted in 1995 by ISIS-4, a very large RCT involving 58 050 patients.[37] It had three arms, in one of which intravenous magnesium was given to patients suspected of an acute myocardial infarction. The results are marked on the funnel plot and show that there is no clear benefit for this treatment, contrary to the results of the earlier meta-analysis.

Some would say that this is one of the major problems with using statistical synthesis. An alternative viewpoint is that it is an example of the importance of ensuring that the material fed into a meta-analysis from a systematic review is researched and critically appraised to the highest possible standard. Explanations for the contradictory findings in this review have been given as:[32,35]

- publication bias, since only trials with positive results were included (see funnel plot);
- methodological weakness in the small trials;
- clinical heterogeneity.

Clinical guidelines

> ✔ Clinical guidelines are systematically developed statements to assist practitioner and patient decisions about appropriate healthcare for specific clinical circumstances.[38]

EBM is increasingly advocated in healthcare, and evidence-based guidelines are being developed in many areas of primary healthcare such as asthma,[39] stable angina[40] and vascular disease.[41] Over 2000 guidelines or protocols have been developed from audit programmes in the UK alone. An observational study in general practice has also shown that recommendations that are evidence based are more widely adopted than those that are not.[42] The UK Department of Health has also endorsed the policy of using evidence-based guidelines.[43]

Guidelines may have a number of different purposes:

- to provide an answer to a specific clinical question using evidence-based methods;
- to aid a clinician in decision-making;
- to standardise aspects of care throughout the country, providing improved equality of access to services and enabling easier comparisons to be made for audit and professional assessment (a reduction in medical practice variation);
- to help to make the most cost-effective use of limited resources;
- to facilitate education of patients and healthcare professionals.

For clinical policies to be evidence based and clinically useful, there must be a balance between the strengths and limitations of relevant research and the practical realities of the healthcare and clinical settings.[44]

There are, however, commonly expressed concerns about the use of guidelines:

- There is a worry that the evidence used may be spurious or not relevant, especially in areas where there is a paucity of published evidence.
- Guidelines may not be applicable to every patient and are therefore only useful in treating diseases and not patients.
- Clinicians may feel that they take away their autonomy in decision-making.
- A standardised clinical approach may risk suffocating any clinical flair and innovation.
- There may be geographic or demographic limitations to the applicability of guidelines; for instance, a policy developed for use in a city district may not be transferable to a rural area.

The effectiveness of a guideline depends on three areas, as identified by Grimshaw and Russell:[45]

1. How and where the guidelines are produced (development strategy) – at a local, regional or national level or by a group internal or external to the area.
2. How the guidelines have been disseminated, e.g. a specific education package, group work, publication in a journal or a mailed leaflet.
3. How the guidelines are implemented (put into use).

In the UK, there are a number of bodies that produce guidelines and summaries of evidence-based advice.

The National Institute for Clinical Excellence (NICE)

NICE is a special health authority formed on 1 April 1999 by the UK government. The board comprises executive and non-executive members. It is designed to work with the NHS in appraising healthcare interventions and offering guidance on the best treatment methods for patients. It assesses all the evidence on the clinical benefit of an intervention, including quality of life, mortality and cost-effectiveness. It will then decide, using this information if the intervention should be recommended to the NHS.

It produces guidance in three main areas:

- public health;
- health technologies – including the newly developed Medical Technologies Evaluation Programme (MTEP) and Diagnostic Assessment Programme (DAP);
- clinical practice.

Its role was further expanded in 2010 following the NHS White Paper, Equity and Excellence – Liberating the NHS and was tasked with developing 150 quality standards in key areas in order to improve patient outcomes. It is now linked in with NHS Evidence and manages the online search engine that allows easy access to an extensive evidence base and examples of best practice.

Scottish Intercollegiate Guidelines Network (SIGN)

The SIGN was formed in 1993. Its objective is to improve the effectiveness and efficiency of clinical care for patients in Scotland by developing, publishing and disseminating guidelines that identify and promote good clinical practice. SIGN is a network of clinicians from all the medical specialities, nurses, other professionals allied to medicine, managers, social services and researchers. Patients and carers are also represented on the council. Since 2005, SIGN has been part of NHS Quality Improvement Scotland.

Effective Practice and Organisation of Care (EPOC)

EPOC is a subgroup of the Cochrane Collaboration that reviews and summarises research about the use of guidelines.

Guidelines also need to be critically appraised and a framework has been developed for this[46] that uses

37 questions to appraise three different areas of a clinical guideline:

1. rigour of development;
2. content and context;
3. application.

Integrated care pathways (ICPs)

ICPs are known by a number of names, including integrated care plans, collaborative care plans, critical care pathways and clinical algorithms. ICPs are a development of clinical practice guidelines and have emerged over recent years as a strategy for delivering consistent high-quality care for a range of diagnostic groups or procedures. They are usually multidisciplinary, patient-focused pathways of care that provide a framework for the management of a clinical condition or procedure and are based upon best available evidence.

The advantage of ICPs over most conventional guidelines is that they provide a complete package of protocols relating to the likely events for all healthcare personnel involved with the patient during a single episode of care. By covering each possible contingency with advice based upon best evidence, they provide a means of both identifying and implementing optimum practice.

Grading the evidence

There is a traditional hierarchy of evidence, which lists the primary studies in order of perceived scientific merit. This allows one to give an appropriate level of significance to each type of study and is useful

Box 1.1 • Hierarchy of evidence

1. Systematic reviews and meta-analyses
2. Randomised controlled trials with definitive results (the results are clinically significant)
3. Randomised controlled trials with non-definitive results (the results have a point estimate that suggests a clinically significant effect)
4. Cohort studies
5. Case–control studies
6. Cross-sectional studies
7. Case reports

From Greenhalgh T. How to read a paper: the basics of evidence based medicine. London: BMJ Publications, 1997; Vol. xvii, p. 196. With permission from the BMJ Publishing Group Ltd.

when weighing up the evidence in order to make a clinical decision. One version of the hierarchy is given in Box 1.1.[21] It must be remembered, however, that this is only a rough guide and that one needs to assess each study on its own merits. Although a meta-analysis comes above an RCT in the hierarchy, a good-quality RCT is far better than a poorly performed meta-analysis. Similarly, a seriously flawed RCT may not merit the same degree of importance as a well-designed cohort study. Checklists have been published that may assist in assessing the methodological quality of each type of study.[21]

Similar checklists are available for systematic reviews.[21,47,48] As already discussed, the preparation of a systematic review is a complex process involving a number of steps, each of which is open to bias and inaccuracies that can distort the results. Such lists can be used as a guide when preparing a review as well as in assessing one. One checklist used to assess the validity of a review does so by identifying potential sources of bias in each step (Table 1.2).[49]

Table 1.2 • Checklist for assessing sources of bias and methods of protecting against bias

Source	Check
Problem formulation	Is the question clearly focused?
Study identification	Is the search for relevant studies thorough?
Study selection	Are the inclusion criteria appropriate?
Appraisal of the studies	Is the validity of the studies included adequately assessed?
Data collection	Is missing information obtained from investigators?
Data synthesis	How sensitive are the results to changes in the way the review is done?
Interpretation of results	Do the conclusions flow from the evidence that is reviewed? Are recommendations linked to the strength of the evidence?
	Are judgments about preferences (values) explicit?
	If there is 'no evidence of effect', is care taken not to interpret this as 'evidence of no effect'?
	Are subgroup analyses interpreted cautiously?

From Oxman A. Checklists for review articles. Br Med J 1994; 309:648–51. With permission from the BMJ Publishing Group Ltd.

It is hoped that the results of a systematic review will be precise, valid and statistically powerful in order to provide the highest quality information on which to base clinical decisions or to produce clinical guidelines. The strength of the evidence provided by a study also needs to be assessed before making any clinical recommendations. A grading system is required to specify the levels of evidence, and several have previously been reported (e.g. those of the Antithrombotic Therapy Consensus Conference[50] or that shown in Table 1.3).

The grading of evidence and recommendations within textbooks, clinical guidelines or ICPs should allow users easily to identify those elements of evidence that may be subject to interpretation or modification in the light of new published data or local information. It should identify those aspects of recommendations that are less securely based upon evidence and therefore may appropriately be modified in the light of patient preferences or local circumstances. This raises different issues to the grading of evidence for critical appraisal and for systematic reviews.

In 1979, the Canadian Task Force on the Periodic Health Examination was one of the first groups to propose grading the strength of recommendations.[51] Since then there have been several published systems for rating the quality of evidence, although most were not designed specifically to be translated into guideline development. The Agency for Health Care Policy and Research has published such a system, although this body considered that its level of classification may be too complex to allow clinical practice guideline development.[52] Nevertheless, the Agency advocated evidence-linked guideline development, requiring the explicit linkage of recommendations to the quality of the supporting evidence. The Centre for Evidence-based Medicine has developed a more comprehensive grading system, which incorporates dimensions such as prognosis, diagnosis and economic analysis.[53]

These systems are complex; for textbooks, care pathways and guidelines, such grading systems need to be clear and easily understood by the relevant audience as well as taking into account all the different forms of evidence that may be appropriate to such documents.

Determining strength of evidence

There are three main factors that need to be taken into account in determining the strength of evidence:

- the type and quality of the reported study;
- the robustness of the findings;
- the applicability of the study to the population or subgroup to which the guidelines are directed.

Type and quality of study

Meta-analyses, systematic reviews and RCTs are generally considered to be the highest quality evidence that is available. However, in some situations these may not be appropriate or feasible. Recommendations may depend upon evidence from other kinds of study, such as observational studies of epidemiology or natural history, or synthesised evidence, such as decision analyses and cost-effectiveness modelling.

For each type of evidence, there are sets of criteria as to the methodological quality, and descriptions of techniques for critical appraisal are widely available.[21] Inevitably, there is some degree of subjectivity in determining whether particular flaws or a lack of suitable information invalidates an individual study.

Table 1.3 • Agency for Health Care Policy and Research grading system for evidence and recommendations

Category	Description
Evidence	
Ia	Evidence from meta-analysis of randomised controlled trials
Ib	Evidence from at least one randomised controlled trial
IIa	Evidence from at least one controlled study without randomisation
IIb	Evidence from at least one other type of quasi-experimental study
III	Evidence from non-experimental descriptive studies, such as comparative studies and case–control studies
IV	Evidence from expert committee reports or opinions or clinical experience of respected authorities, or both
Recommendation strength	
A	Directly based on category I evidence
B	Directly based on category II evidence or extrapolated recommendation from category I evidence
C	Directly based on category III evidence or extrapolated recommendation from category I or II evidence
D	Directly based on category IV evidence or extrapolated recommendation from category I, II or III evidence

From Hadorn DC, Baker D, Hodges JS et al. Rating the quality of evidence for clinical practice guidelines. J Clin Epidemiol 1996 49:749–54. With permission from Elsevier.

Robustness of findings

The strength of evidence from a published study would depend not only upon the type and quality of a particular study but also upon the magnitude of any differences and the homogeneity of results. High-quality research may report findings with wide confidence intervals, conflicting results or contradictory findings for different outcome measures or patient subgroups. Conversely, sensitivity analysis within a cost-effectiveness or decision analysis may indicate that uncertainty regarding the exact value of a particular parameter does not detract from the strength of the conclusion.

Applicability

Strong evidence in a set of guidelines must be wholly applicable to the situation in which the guidelines are to be used. For example, a finding from high-quality research based upon a hospital population may provide good evidence for guidelines intended for a similar setting but a lower quality of evidence for guidelines intended for primary care.

Grading system for evidence

The following is a simple pragmatic grading system for the strength of a statement of evidence, which will be used to grade the evidence in this book (and the other volumes in the Companion series).

Details of the definitions are given in Table 1.4. For practical purposes, only the following three grades are required, which are analogous to the levels of proof required in a court of law:

I. **'Beyond reasonable doubt'**. Analogous to the burden of proof required in a criminal court case and may be thought of as corresponding to the usual standard of 'proof' within the medical literature (i.e. $P < 0.05$).

II. **'On the balance of probabilities'**. In many cases, a high-quality review of literature may fail to reach firm conclusions because of conflicting evidence or inconclusive results, trials of poor methodological quality or the lack of evidence in the population to which the guidelines apply. Where such strong evidence does not exist, it may still be possible to make a statement as to the 'best' treatment on the 'balance of probabilities'. This is analogous to the decision in a civil court where all the available evidence will be weighed up and a verdict will depend upon the 'balance of probabilities'.

III. **'Unproven'**. Where the above levels of proof do not exist.

All evidence-based guidelines require regular review because of the constant stream of new information that becomes available. In some areas, there is more rapid development and the emergence of

Table 1.4 • Grading of evidence and recommendations

Category	Description
Evidence	
I	'Beyond reasonable doubt'. Evidence from high-quality randomised controlled trials, systematic reviews, high-quality synthesised evidence, such as decision analyses, cost-effectiveness analyses or large observational datasets, which is directly applicable to the population of concern and has clear results
II	'On the balance of probabilities'. Evidence of 'best practice' from a high-quality review of literature, which fails to reach the highest standard of 'proof' because of heterogeneity, questionable trial methodology or lack of evidence in a relevant population
III	'Unproven'. Insufficient evidence upon which to base a decision or contradictory evidence
Recommendations	
A	A strong recommendation, which should be followed unless there are compelling reasons against to act otherwise
B	Recommendations based on evidence of effectiveness that may need interpretation in the light of other factors (e.g. patient preferences, local facilities, local audit results or available resources)
C	Recommendation where there is inadequate evidence on effectiveness but pragmatic or financial reasons to institute an agreed policy
Other considerations	
	The evidence should be presented as clear and brief points, with reference to original source material
	Individual evidence requiring early review should be identified with reference to known sources of work in progress

new evidence; in these instances, relevant reference will be made to ongoing trials or systematic reviews in progress.

Grading of recommendations

Although recommendations should be based upon the evidence presented, it is necessary to grade the strength of recommendation separately from the evidence. For example, the lack of evidence regarding an expensive new technology may lead to a strong recommendation that it should only be undertaken as part of an adequately regulated clinical trial. Conversely, strong evidence for the effectiveness of a treatment may not lead to a strong recommendation for use if the magnitude of the benefit is small and the treatment very costly.

The following grades of recommendations are suggested and details of the definition are given in Table 1.4:

A. A strong recommendation, which should be followed.
B. A recommendation using evidence of effectiveness, but where there may be other factors to take into account in the decision-making process.
C. A recommendation where evidence as to the most effective practice is not adequate, but there may be reasons for making the recommendations in order to minimise cost or reduce the chance of error through a locally agreed protocol.

Implementation of evidence-based medicine

Healthcare professionals have always sought evidence on which to base their clinical practice. Unfortunately, the evidence has not always been available, reliable or explicit, and when it was available it has not been implemented immediately. James Lancaster in 1601 showed that lemon juice was effective in the treatment of scurvy, and in 1747 James Lind repeated the experiment. The British Navy did not utilise this information until 1795 and the Merchant Navy not until 1865. When implementation of research findings is delayed, ultimately the people who suffer are the patients.

A number of different groups of people may need to be committed to the changes before they can take place with any degree of success. These include:

• healthcare professionals (doctors, nurses, etc.);
• healthcare providers and purchasers;
• researchers;
• patients and the public;
• government (local, regional and national).

Each of these groups has a different set of priorities. To ensure that their own requirements are met by the proposal, negotiation is required, which takes time. There are many potential barriers to the implementation of recommendations, and clinicians may become so embroiled in tradition and dogma, that they are resistant to change. They may lack knowledge of new developments or the time and resources to keep up to date with the published literature. Lack of training in a new technology, such as laparoscopic surgery or interventional radiology, may thwart their use, even when shown to be effective. Researchers may become detached from the practicalities of clinical practice and the needs of the health service and concentrate on inappropriate questions or produce impractical guidelines. Managers are subject to changes in the political climate and can easily be driven by policies and budgets. The resources available to them may be limited and not allow for the purchase of new technology, and even potentially cost-saving developments may not be introduced because of the difficulties in releasing the savings from elsewhere in the service.

Patients and the general public can also influence the development of the healthcare offered. They are susceptible to the persuasion of the mass media and may demand the implementation of 'miracle cures' or fashionable investigations or treatments. Such interventions may not be practical or of any proven benefit. They can also determine the success or failure of a particular treatment. For instance, a treatment may be physically or morally unacceptable, or there may be poor compliance, especially with preventative measures such as diets, smoking cessation or exercise. All these aspects can lead to a delay in the implementation of research findings.

Potential ways of improving this situation include the following:

• Provision of easy and convenient access to summaries of the best evidence, electronic databases, systematic reviews and journals in a clinical setting.
• Development of better disease management systems through mechanisms such as clinical guidelines, ICPs and electronic reminders.
• Implementation of computerised decision-support systems.
• Improvement of educational programmes – practitioners must be regularly and actively apprised of new evidence rather than relying on the practitioner seeking it out; passive dissemination of evidence is ineffective.

Organisations specialising in evidence-based practice, systematic reviews, etc

Aggressive Research Intelligence Facility (ARIF)
http://www.arif.bham.ac.uk

BMJ Evidence Centre
http://group.bmj.com/products/evidence-centre

CASP (Critical Appraisal Skills Program)
http://www.casp-uk.net/

Centre for Evidence-based Child Health
http://www.ucl.ac.uk/ich/research-ich/mrc-cech/training/evidence-based-child-health

Centre for Evidence-based Medicine, established in Oxford.
http://www.cebm.net

Centre for Evidence-based Mental Health
http://www.cebmh.com

Centre for Health Evidence, University of Alberta.
http://www.cche.net/

Evidence Network – an initiative of the ESRC UK Centre for Evidence-Based Policy and Practice
http://www.kcl.ac.uk/schools/sspp/interdisciplinary/evidence

JAMA Evidence
http://www.jamaevidence.com/

McMaster University Health Information Research Unit
http://hiru.mcmaster.ca/hiru/

NIHR Health Technology Assessment Programme
http://www.hta.ac.uk/

NHS Centre for Reviews and Dissemination University of York.
http://www.york.ac.uk/inst/crd/

National Institute for Clinical Excellence (NICE)
http://www.nice.org.uk/

Intute: Health and Life Sciences – closed in July 2011 but website still open for next 3 years although will not be updated.
http://www.intute.ac.uk/medicine/

National Institute for Health and Research
http://www.nihr.ac.uk/Pages/default.aspx

NHS Evidence – web-based portal managed by NICE and linked with the National Electronic Library for Health (NeLH). Includes access to My Evidence.
https://www.evidence.nhs.uk/

UK Cochrane Centre
Summertown Pavilion, Middle Way, Oxford OX2 7LG
Tel. 01865 516300
email: general@cochrane.ac.uk
home page – http://ukcc.cochrane.org/

The Cochrane Collaboration
http://www.cochrane.org/

Internet access to the Cochrane library and databases:
http://www.thecochranelibrary.com/view/0/index.html

Cochrane Central Register of Controlled Trials
http://onlinelibrary.wiley.com/o/cochrane/cochrane_clcentral_articles_fs.html

EPOC – Effective Practice and Organisation of Care
http://epoc.cochrane.org/about-epoc

University of Alberta Evidence Based Practice Centre
http://www.ualberta.ca/ARCHE/epc.htm

Sources of reviews and abstracts relating to evidence-based practice

ACP Journal Club
http://acpjc.acponline.org/

Bandolier (now an electronic version, independently written by Oxford scientists)
http://www.medicine.ox.ac.uk/bandolier/

BMJ Clinical Evidence – a compendium of evidence for effective health care
http://clinicalevidence.bmj.com/ceweb/index.jsp

Centre for Evidence Based Purchasing
http://nhscep.useconnect.co.uk/Default.aspx

Cochrane Systematic Reviews (abstracts only)
http://www.cochrane.org/cochrane-reviews

Effective Health Care Bulletins
http://www.york.ac.uk/inst/crd/ehcb_em.htm

Evidence Based Nursing Practice
http://www.ebnp.co.uk/index.htm

Chapter 1

Evidence Based On-call
http://www.eboncall.org/

PROSPERO – worldwide prospective register of systematic reviews
http://www.crd.york.ac.uk/prospero/

Journals available on the internet

eBMJ (electronic version of the *British Medical Journal*)
http://www.bmj.com

Journal of the American Medical Association (JAMA)
http://jama.ama-assn.org/

Canadian Medical Association Journal (CMAJ)
http://www.cmaj.ca/

Evidence-based Medicine
http://ebm.bmj.com/

Evidence-based Mental Health
http://ebmh.bmj.com/

Evidence-based Nursing
http://ebn.bmj.com/

Databases, bibliographies and catalogues

PUBMED (the free version of MEDLINE)
http://www.ncbi.nlm.nih.gov/pubmed/

BestBets – best evidence topics
http://www.bestbets.org

Trip database – turning research into practice
http://www.tripdatabase.com/index.html

BMJ Best Health
http://besthealth.bmj.com/x/index.html

DUETs – The Database of Uncertainties about the Effects of Treatments publishes uncertainties that cannot currently be answered by referring to reliable up-to-date systematic reviews of existing research evidence
http://www.library.nhs.uk/DUETs/Default.aspx

Google Scholar
http://www scholar.google.co.uk

National Research Register Archive – a searchable copy of the archives held by the National Research Register (NRR) Projects Database, up to September 2007
http://www.nihr.ac.uk/Pages/NRRArchive.aspx

National Institute for Health Research (NIHR) Clinical Network Research Portfolio is a database of clinical research studies that it supports, undertaken in the NHS
http://public.ukcrn.org.uk/search/

Sources of guidelines and integrated care pathways

AHRQ (Agency for Healthcare Research and Quality) – provides practical healthcare information, research findings and data to help consumers
http://www.ahcpr.gov/

Evidence Based Practice Centres – developed in conjunction with the AHRQ
http://www.ahcpr.gov/clinic/epc/

Cedars – Sinai Medical Center, Health Services Research
Home page: http://www.csmc.edu/

National Guideline Clearinghouse
http://www.guideline.gov/

NICE Pathways
http://pathways.nice.org.uk/

Scottish Intercollegiate Guidelines Network (SIGN)
http://www.sign.ac.uk

Scottish Pathways Association
http://www.icpus.org.uk/

Towards Optimised Practice (TOP) Clinical Guidelines
http://www.topalbertadoctors.org/cpgs.php

Useful texts

Cochrane Collaboration Handbook
http://www.cochrane-handbook.org/

2

Outcomes and health economic issues in surgery

Sharath C.V. Paravastu
Jonathan A. Michaels

Introduction

Evidence-based medicine demands that all those making decisions regarding clinical management, either on an individual patient basis or at a policy level, consider existing evidence in order to maximise the chance of favourable outcomes and optimise the use of available resources. However, such evidence is rarely clear-cut and there may be conflicting advice because of differences in the way that outcomes are measured, the way in which costs are assessed or the perspective from which an economic evaluation is carried out.

This chapter deals with some of the issues around the measurement of outcomes, the calculation of costs and the methods of economic evaluation. The available outcome measures are considered, drawing the distinctions between disease-specific and generic measures and explaining concepts such as health-related quality of life, quality-adjusted life-years (QALYs) and utilities. The differences between costs, charges and resource use are highlighted, followed by a discussion of issues such as discounting, sensitivity analysis and marginal costing. Finally, a section on economic evaluation describes the different techniques available – cost minimisation, cost-effectiveness, cost–utility and cost–benefit analysis – and discusses the use of cost-effectiveness league tables. The intention is not to provide a full reference work on these subjects but to raise awareness of some of the important issues to be considered when evaluating evidence on specific interventions that may rely on differing outcome measurements or methods of economic evaluation.

Outcome measures

Clinicians tend routinely to consider health outcomes in terms of clinical or biomedical measures such as blood pressure levels, blood sugar levels or bone mineral density. Process-based outcomes such as readmission rates, reintervention or complications are readily considered alternatives. Data such as these are seen as readily available, easily measured, objective and comparable between differing settings. However, the present environment in medical services makes it necessary for the healthcare professional to consider more than just the treatment of the condition. A greater emphasis is now placed upon the consideration by the clinician of the actual status of the patient's quality of life. Now, considerations extend beyond assessing the value of an intervention and the effectiveness, or otherwise, of drug regimens. There should also be an assessment of the patient's physical, mental and social well-being. In line with such interests, there has been considerable research and a greater emphasis upon applying subjective non-biomedical measures and the development of such tools (or 'instruments') has been substantial since the early 1980s.

When considering which instrument of assessment to choose from the plethora now available, the user should carefully consider what parameter is to be measured before making a final selection of an outcome measure. Before applying this measure to a patient population, particular consideration needs to be given to deciding whether it will measure what we are interested in measuring and whether it will answer the questions that we wish to be answered.

All too often assessment tools may be applied to patients in the wrong circumstances or used when there is no realistic opportunity to measure what we wish to measure. These are important considerations because the administration and analysis of these measures can be costly, as well as taking up valuable time for both patients and clinicians. In addition, the use of unsuitable measures applied in the wrong context might yield results that are perhaps plausible but wrong, thus leading to erroneous conclusions. The implications of such findings for patients or the health service can be substantial.

Instruments should therefore be carefully selected for their appropriateness (able to answer the research question), acceptability (acceptable to patients), feasibility (ease of administering), reliability (reproducibility), validity (measures the outcome it is meant to), responsiveness (ability to respond to changes), precision (of scores) and interpretability (ease of understanding the results).[1] In particular, attention should be given to reliability and validity. **Reliability** refers to whether the instrument will be reproducible, such that if applied in different settings or circumstances to the same unchanged population then the same results should be achieved. This has particular implications for studies using instruments to derive longitudinal data on a particular sample of patients. In such circumstances, we need to be confident that observed changes over a given time period reflect actual change. Test–retest reliability is an important consideration and is assessed by making repeated assessments under the same circumstances at differing points in time and comparing the results using correlations or differences. Similarly, for instruments that require administration by interviewers, there needs to be a high level of agreement between different raters assessing the same patients but at different periods in time. For example, Collin et al. found a high level of agreement between the patients, a trained nurse and two skilled observers during applications of the Barthel Index (assesses patients' ability to carry out daily activities) to the same group of patients.[2] In another example, Aissaoui et al. found a high level of agreement between doctors and nurses during the application of Behavioural Pain Score (BPS) in the same group of critically ill patients.[3]

Another psychometric criterion for consideration is that of **validity**, which means that instruments measure precisely what they set out to do. It should be borne in mind that measures can be reliable without being valid, but they cannot be valid without being reliable. Three types of validity are described. First, **content validity**, which relates to the choice, appropriateness and representativeness of the content of the instrument. Judging content validity involves an assessment of whether all of the relevant concepts are represented. For example, a representative sample of asthmatic patients could be used to develop an asthma questionnaire in order to ensure that it captures all the domains of interest for such a patient population. Second, there is a requirement to consider **criterion validity**, which is the degree to which the measure obtains results that are comparable to some kind of 'gold standard'. While this is theoretically a simple concept, there are very few such gold standards for comparison. Finally, there is **construct validity**. This relates to observation of when expected patterns of given relationships are observed. For example, if a method of valuation of outcomes predicts that a patient prefers option A to option B, then one would expect this to be reflected by their behaviour when faced with genuine clinical choices. This is normally assessed through the use of multitrait–multimethod techniques,[4] which map the correlations between alternative approaches to measuring the same construct and between measures of different constructs.

As can be seen, the choice of an outcome measure is not always as straightforward as it may seem at first. In addition to considerations regarding the patient group, there are also important considerations regarding the psychometric properties of the instruments. Different outcome measures will have uses for differing patient groups. For example, a biomedical measure such as blood pressure alone might be considered suitable for comparing two similar drug regimens to assess 'best' control of blood pressure. However, a study that attempts to compare renal transplant with dialysis might also wish to consider a much broader picture and would be likely to require consideration of quality-of-life issues together with mortality as outcome measures.

It is extremely important to choose the right outcomes for the purpose in question, as different conclusions can be drawn from the application of different outcome measures in the same study. For example, a study of vascular patients compared exercise training with angioplasty for stable claudication with results expressed in terms of ankle–brachial pressure indices and walking distance.[5] In the short term, it was found that angioplasty improved the pressure but not the walking distance, while exercise improved the walking distance but not the pressure. This example shows that different outcome measures may not always change in the same direction and used in isolation could lead to opposite conclusions.

The following sections examine some of the issues involved in the evaluation and application of some common specific outcome measures.

Mortality

The mortality rate expresses the incidence of death in a population of interest over a given period of time. It is calculated by dividing the number of fatalities in the given population by the total population.

Mortality is often used as an outcome measure in studies as an indication of the effectiveness, or otherwise, of a treatment. It is often easily derived and as such represents a readily accessible outcome measure. While mortality can indeed provide much useful information, its use in reporting results should always be interpreted with caution. First, procedure- and diagnosis-related mortality rates often refer to inpatient deaths only or perhaps mortality over a given postoperative period, for example 30 days. Variations in short-term survival rates might simply reflect differing discharge practices between differing hospitals or settings. Longer-term survival rates are frequently reported for cancer and other chronic conditions. In interpreting these, it must be borne in mind that distortion may occur as a result of the starting point or choice of time frame. For example, survival may be longer in a screened population because there is an earlier starting point,[6] and comparisons between surgical and medical treatments may be very sensitive to follow-up periods because of early excess operative mortality in surgical treatments, which may be offset by better long-term survival. For these reasons, it is often necessary to compare survival curves rather than total survival at a specific time point. This may raise further issues regarding the possible need for discounting, to take account of a preference for survival in the earlier years after treatment (see below).

Second, mortality can only be a partial measure of quality, and it is often not the most appropriate outcome measure for use in most situations. Many studies report mortality and tend to ignore other important outcomes such as morbidity and quality of life. These are more complex to quantify and are not routinely collected. Mortality is particularly limited in usefulness for studies investigating low-risk procedures. Accurate assessment of the quality of such procedures requires more sensitive measures. For example, use of mortality alone as an outcome measure for parathyroidectomy would not be appropriate as it is associated with an extremely low mortality. A more appropriate measure would be to assess improvement in symptoms or quality of life.

It is also necessary to highlight the effect that differences in case mix can have on the mortality rate. For example, there is a tendency in studies relating workload to outcome for the results to be reported for the whole sample of patients. It is important to be aware that results reported in this way may be misleading as no account is taken of the diversity of patient characteristics that may be contained in such a sample. Both differences in severity of illness and in risk of adverse outcomes relating to comorbidity can significantly affect any interpretation of mortality

rates. This problem is illustrated by Sowden and Sheldon, who discuss examples from coronary artery bypass grafting and intensive care to demonstrate the importance of adjusting for case mix.[7] For coronary artery bypass grafting, they report that the strength of the relationship between low volume and increased mortality is reduced in studies that adjust for differences in risk among patients receiving treatment. With adult intensive care, they cite a study by Jones and Rowan[8] in which the apparent higher mortality associated with smaller intensive care units ceased to be significant once the data were adjusted to reflect the fact that severity of illness was on average higher among patients admitted to small units. These examples clearly demonstrate that, in order to minimise bias in such studies, account must be taken of all possible factors (beyond workload) that are likely to affect patient outcomes.

Condition-specific outcome measures

The term 'condition specific' describes instruments designed to measure health outcomes considered to be of specific interest to patients who incur health problems attributable to a particular disease or as the result of other processes. Such instruments are often referred to as 'disease specific', but this term is more general as it encompasses more diverse areas such as natural ageing, trauma and pregnancy, which are not diseases.[9]

The measurement of health status is not restricted to broad generic measures. There are many instances when researchers and clinicians are interested in assessing the health status of individuals with a certain condition or disease. As might be anticipated, many tools have been designed for this purpose and these are primarily aimed at measuring changes that are of importance to clinicians. For example, Spilker et al. identified over 300 such instruments in 1987 and many more are presently available.[10] Examples of such instruments include: measures for arthritis, such as the Arthritis Impact Measurement Scales;[11] measures for the heart, such as the Specific Activity Scale;[12] measures that assess pain, such as the McGill Pain Questionnaire;[13] and measures for varicose veins, such as the Aberdeen Varicose Vein Questionnaire.[14] These instruments have a varying number of dimensions, differing numbers of items and are generally self-completion or interview, though some methods include professional assessment and clinical interview. Such questionnaires are usually scored in a simplistic fashion. Most have simple numerical scaling, such as from 1 to 5, and these scores are usually summed across the items for each dimension, or across all items.

Advantages of condition-specific measures include their relevance and their greater responsiveness to health change.[15] Disadvantages are that they often exclude items relevant to potential complications of treatment and symptoms that do not easily fit the medical model of disease. Generic measures have tended to be used in preference because they can be used to assess benefits for differing treatments or conditions, in a common and exchangeable currency. This enables decisions to be made on allocative efficiency between healthcare programmes within the total healthcare budget, rather than helping to establish the technical efficiency of producing health benefits for a specific condition.[9]

Patient-reported outcome measures (PROMs)

Due to increasing need for assessing the effectiveness of care from a patient's perspective, a number of PROMs have been developed. For example, in the NHS patients undergoing primary hip or knee replacement, hernia surgery and varicose vein surgery are requested to fill questionnaires to assess their symptoms and disability before and after surgery. Some NHS trusts use electronic methods of recording outcome data, such as the Patient Assessment Questionnaires (ePAQ) in gynaecology. The advantage of PROM is that it minimises observer bias, wherein patient experience is directly assessed. These results can be useful in informing patients, redesigning the provision of services and quality improvement. One disadvantage can be the response rate and, in the case of electronic data collection, the access to and use of technology by patients to complete the questionnaires.

The measurement of pain

Pain is a common and important symptom of many medical conditions and deserves special consideration. While many generic and condition-specific instruments dedicate specific dimensions to the measurement of pain, there are also a number of instruments designed specifically to assess levels of pain. The measurement of pain cannot be directly assessed through clinical measures (e.g. blood samples) and, in the absence of such objective approaches, it is necessary to assess pain subjectively through the patient's own perceptions.

Subjective measures allow for reproducible results provided that the tools used to assess pain are measured appropriately. While subjective measures for the measurement of pain have many advantages over other instruments, there are problems in assessing subjects for whom communication is difficult. Examples include very young children and patients who are incapable of expressing how they feel. Those patients who are unconscious or who are terminally ill will continue to present particular difficulties for those attempting to assess levels of pain.

As with other outcome measures, options exist to use binary, categorical or visual analogue scales. Within this area, there are both pain-relief scales and pain-intensity scales to be considered. There are often occasions when it will be necessary to measure the state of the pain rather than the effect of a particular intervention or therapy, and in these circumstances pain-intensity scales will be appropriate. Pain-relief scales may well encompass more than an intensity scale, as any side-effects resulting from an intervention, such as dizziness, might be included in such measurements. Pain-relief scales also require the patient to make a judgment as to how the current pain compares with remembered pain, before the intervention. This might make such scales more complicated for patients to grasp compared with intensity scales and this may raise doubts about validity. In situations where both pain-relief and pain-intensity scales are appropriate, a decision is required regarding which one should be used.

Pain can manifest itself in a variety of qualities, and one of the most widely used tools is the McGill Pain Questionnaire.[13] This is a generic instrument, designed primarily for adults, which was developed to specify the qualities and intensities of pain; as such, it is intended to provide a quantifiable profile of pain. The questionnaire can be completed by the patient or administered in an interview. Completion takes roughly 15–20 minutes but becomes quicker on subsequent applications. The instrument contains 78 pain descriptor words, which are grouped into 20 subclasses, each of which contains two to five words that describe pain on an ordinal scale. These words are arranged to reflect three dimensions of pain: sensory, affective and evaluative. The questionnaire can yield three indices of pain: a pain-rating index based on the scale values of the words chosen by the patient; a rank score using the rank values within each subgroup chosen; and the total number of descriptions chosen by the patient.

The McGill Pain Questionnaire has been thoroughly investigated in recent years and the instrument has proved to be the most reliable in applications to patients with moderate-to-severe chronic or acute pain. It has been shown to be particularly useful in disaggregating explained pain from unexplained pain. When the instrument was used in a cohort of cancer patients with lymphoedema, it proved to be more sensitive than categorical or analogue scales.[16]

In those patients who are critically ill or unconscious, Behavioural Pain Score (BPS) was developed to assess response to pain. BPS is based on three items: facial expression, movement of upper limbs and compliance with mechanical ventilation. Each of these items is graded with values from 1 to 4, 1 being no response and 4 being full response, giving a minimal score of 3 and maximal score of 12.[17] Over the last decade BPS has been validated in a number of studies.[3,18]

Health-related quality of life

Recent years have witnessed quite an upsurge in interest in the measurement of health-related quality of life, much of which has no doubt been stimulated by the analytical demands of researchers and the need for outcome information as a basis for policy decisions.

Such health status measures are standardised questionnaires, or instruments, which are used to evaluate patient health across a broad range of areas. These areas include symptoms, physical functioning, mental well-being, work and social activities. Measures can be either generic or condition specific, and such measures can generate a profile of scores or a single index. These scores can be based upon people's preferences (e.g. EQ-5D) or, more usually, arbitrary scoring procedures (e.g. SF-36, assumes equal weighting for most items).[19] Four of the most frequently used instruments are discussed in more detail below.

EQ-5D

Of those instruments that generate a single index, EQ-5D has been rapidly adopted and widely used.[19] The measure was developed by a group of researchers from seven centres across five countries.[20] The present measure has five dimensions, whereas the original version had six. Patients are classified by the completion of a five-item questionnaire. The EuroQol is a brief, easy-to-use questionnaire of two pages. It can be made even simpler by using the one-page descriptive classification. Self-completion, or interview, usually only takes a matter of minutes and response rates tend to be extremely high.[19] The five dimensions of the EQ-5D comprise mobility, self-care, usual activities, pain/discomfort and anxiety/depression. Each of the five questions has three levels; therefore, combining the five questions defines 243 health states. In addition, the instrument contains a visual analogue scale: a thermometer scale calibrated from 0 (representing 'worst possible health state') to 100 (representing 'best imaginable health state').

> ✓ The EQ-5D is now one of the most widely adopted methods for measuring health-related quality of life and is the method favoured by the National Institute for Health and Clinical Excellence (NICE) for deriving utility weightings for cost-effectiveness analysis (see below). It has been used in a wide variety of clinical areas, many pharmaceutical companies now include it as a standard outcome measure in clinical research, and the questionnaire has been translated into many different languages and validated in a number of different countries.[21]

SF-36

The SF-36 is a self-administered questionnaire composed of 36 items. It measures health across eight multi-item dimensions, covering functional status, well-being and overall evaluation of health. Responses within each of the dimensions are combined in order to generate a score from 0 to 100, where 0 represents 'worst health' and 100 indicates 'best health'. Dimension scores should not be aggregated into a single index score. The questionnaire takes about 5 minutes to complete, attains good response rates and is suitable for completion by the patients themselves or for administration by trained interviewers on a face-to-face or telephone basis.[22]

The questionnaire has been used in a variety of settings, administered on differing populations and exhibits good psychometric properties. Detailed information regarding the scoring process and computation are readily available, as are published data for comparative norms. The question complexity can be a problem in situations where the sample comprises individuals with low education levels, but otherwise the instrument is suitable for administration in a wide range of settings.[22]

SF-6D

This is a newer health measure, which is derived from various items of SF-36 or SF-12 and provides a single index measure.[23] It comprises six multi-level dimensions and describes 18 000 health states. The SF-6D measure can be derived for any individual patient completing SF-36 or SF-12. A standard gamble technique has been used to obtain parametric and non-parametric preference weights from a sample of the general population who were asked to rate a variety of health states. These weights are modelled to predict health states obtained from SF-6D. This measure, however, may not be readily used in all countries as preferences vary between people living in different countries. Currently, SF-6D preference weights are available for the UK, Australia, Brazil, Hong Kong, Japan, Portugal and Singapore.

Nottingham Health Profile

The Nottingham Health Profile (NHP) measures levels of self-reported distress. The instrument consists of two parts, each of which can be used independent of the other. Part 1, the most frequently used component, comprises 38 statements that are grouped into six sections: physical mobility, pain, sleep, social isolation, emotional reaction, and energy. The number of statements in each of these sections varies from three for the energy dimension to nine for emotional reaction. The second part of the instrument asks respondents to indicate whether or not their state of health influences activity in seven areas of everyday life: work, looking after the home, social life, home life, sex life, interests and hobbies, and holidays. Responses for both parts 1 and 2 are yes/no responses.[24]

Scoring is straightforward, with 0 assigned to a 'no' response and 1 to a 'yes' response. Scores for each of the sections range between 0 ('worst health') and 100 ('best health'). The NHP was designed for self-completion and can readily be used in postal surveys, although it can also be administered by an interviewer. Generally, the instrument takes around 5 minutes to complete.

Quality-adjusted life-years

QALYs were developed as an outcome measure to incorporate effects on both the quality (morbidity) and quantity (mortality) of life. Each year of life is multiplied by a weighting factor reflecting quality of life.[25] An alternative to QALYs is healthy years equivalent (HYE), which is discussed below.

QALYs are estimated by assigning every life-year a weight between 0 and 1, where a weight of 0 reflects a health status that is valued as equal to being dead and a weight of 1 represents full health. For example, consider a patient with a colon cancer who has a health state of 0.9. Without surgery, he will die in 2 years. With surgery, his health state deteriorates slightly to 0.7, but he lives 5 more years (in total 7 years). Therefore, the QALY gained with surgery $= [(0.7 \times 7) - (0.9 \times 2)] = 4.9 - 1.8 = 3.1$. Another way of expressing QALY gained is from QALY charts. For example, a patient with a particular disease is expected to deteriorate and die at an estimate point 1. With intervention the patient would deteriorate slowly and die at an estimate point 2. The area between the two curves is the QALY gained by the intervention (**Fig. 2.1**).[26]

The QALY is frequently used by decision-makers or researchers to draw comparisons between differing types of health programme or intervention. The QALY can be used in economic evaluation: the number of additional QALYs that a new surgical

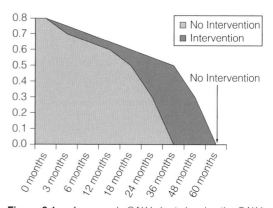

Figure 2.1 • An example QALY chart showing the QALY gained with intervention.

intervention might yield can be compared with the costs of the new procedure, thus enabling cost per QALY ratios to be generated.[27] Such ratios have been used in so-called QALY league tables, whereby procedures or interventions are ranked on this basis. These tables might be seen as useful within the decision-making process, but caution should be exercised in making quick decisions regarding the allocation of resources based upon these comparative tables (see below).[28–31]

HYEs were developed as an alternative in order to address some of the suggested shortcomings of QALYs.[32] HYEs produce a hypothetical combination of the number of years in full health that equates to the individual's utility of living a number of years at a health state rated at less than full health. In effect, this can be considered as a lifetime profile of health and is often referred to as a stream of health states. In order to produce the values for the HYEs, a two-stage gamble procedure is used. There has, however, been criticism of the use of HYEs and at present the use of QALYs remains the most common method of performing cost-effectiveness analysis.[33,34] For the QALY to be a useful measure of outcome, it should reflect patient or individual preferences, which means that if an individual has a choice between two or more treatments or interventions then they should choose the treatment option that yields the most QALYs.

> ✔ QALYs remains the most common measure of effectiveness used in cost-effectiveness analysis.[33,34]

Utilities

Quality weights for use in QALYs can be obtained directly using one of three main methods – visual analogue scales (VAS), standard gamble and time trade-off – which are described in turn below. In addition to these direct methods of measurement, it is possible to obtain utilities through the mapping of health states derived from other quality-of-life measures onto valuations obtained from members of the general population.[35] The method for obtaining utility weightings is currently the subject of considerable research, and there is evidence that different values are obtained depending on the method of evaluation and framing of questions. In addition, there is considerable controversy as to whether the most appropriate utility values for economic evaluation are those of the general population or of patients with the particular conditions.[36]

Rating scale or visual analogue scales

In this approach respondents are asked to rate their preference of outcomes or their present health state on a straight-line chart, often a thermometer with fixed points, where the bottom of the thermometer is represented by 0, which is a health state equivalent to being dead, and the top of the thermometer is 1, which indicates full health. If thermometers ranging between 0 and 100 are used, these values are equated to 0–1, and the same assumptions regarding the health states hold. If, by way of an example, we wanted to measure the quality weight for being an amputee, and the respondent selects the health state at 55 on the thermometer scale of 0–100, then for that health state their quality weight is equivalent to 0.55. Advantages of VAS include their simplicity, but this can be counterbalanced by the fact that there is no choice to be made between health states and therefore it is not possible to observe any trade-offs that the individual might have between health states. Another problem with VAS is that it is uncertain whether the responses lie on a linear interval scale: it is questionable whether moving from 20 to 30 is equivalent to moving from 70 to 80. Further, there is scope for end-of-scale bias, where respondents tend to avoid the extremes of scales, and spacing out bias, where respondents tend to space out the outcomes irrespective of the significance.[37] Given these reservations, it is difficult to use VAS methods to determine quality weights in a way that is consistent with the theoretical basis of utility measurement.[38]

Standard gamble

The second method routinely used to estimate quality weights is standard gamble. Under this approach, the quality weight of a health state (patients' feeling of being well or unwell) can be constructed by comparing a specific number of years in the health state to a gamble with a probability (P) of achieving full health for the same number of years and a complementary probability ($1-P$) of immediate death. The probability of full health is varied until the individual is indifferent between the alternatives, and the quality weight of the assessed health state is therefore equal to P. As an example, let us consider that we are comparing 10 years with heart disease with the gamble of full health for 10 years (probability P) or immediate death, with a complementary probability ($1-P$). Here, let us assume that the individual is indifferent at a probability of 0.6 of full health. In practical terms, this means that the individual would consider a certainty of living 10 years with the heart disease to be equivalent to taking a gamble that gives a 60% chance of living 10 years in full health and a 40% chance of immediate death. The quality weight here would be 0.6 for the heart disease health state. The advantages of standard gamble include the fact that it is based on expected utility theory;[38] however, one of the major disadvantages is that respondents might find the concept difficult to understand because of the probabilities associated with the method. Another drawback is that the hypothetical choices used in such an approach are not representative of 'real' life, since choices between large improvements in health status and large mortality risks are seldom encountered, especially with the assumption that we will live for a certain number of years for sure.

Time trade-off

A third approach to estimating quality weights is time trade-off.[39] This method compares D years duration in the health state with X years in full health. The number of years in full health is varied until the individual is indifferent between their options; at this point, the quality weight of the health state is calculated by X/D. As an example, consider that we wish to calculate the quality weight for heart disease and that we assess the measurement for 10 years of heart disease. If the individual considers that 10 years of living with heart disease ($D=10$) is equivalent to 6 years of full health ($X=6$), then the quality weight is equal to 0.6 (6/10).

Obtaining utilities from health-related quality of life

The direct methods of obtaining utilities have a number of drawbacks. In particular, the VAS has a poor theoretical basis, and standard gamble and time trade-off methods may be complex to administer.[40] An alternative approach is to derive single index measures from generic or disease-specific health-related quality-of-life measures.[41,42]

One of the most widely adopted methods is derived from the EQ-5D, as described above.[42] The questionnaire generates a limited number of discrete health states depending upon the grading of the responses to each of the questions and previous research has used direct measurement methods to obtain a utility tariff associated with each of these states.[43] These tariffs have been widely used for cost-effectiveness analysis and alternative tariffs for different populations have also been developed.[21] Another generic measure that has been used to generate utilities is the SF-6D, a measure derived from the SF-36 questionnaire.[44] This has been extensively validated and compared with EQ-5D in a number of studies.[45]

In cases where information from generic scores is not available, methods have been developed to derive utility weightings from disease-specific measures such as scoring systems for arthritis[46] or even from laboratory measures such as haemoglobin levels, used as a proxy for anaemia-related symptoms.[47] Disease-specific scores may be more sensitive to changes in symptoms for the condition in question, but suffer from the disadvantage that they may fail to capture adverse events or other outcomes of treatment that are outside the main domains that are of interest in the specific disease so that comparability with other diseases may be questionable. There remains considerable controversy about the relative benefits of the use of generic and disease-specific measures to generate utilities.[48,49]

Costs, charges and resource use

From the above discussion, it can be seen that, from a health economist's perspective, there are several methods for assessing the benefits that might be accrued from a healthcare intervention within the context of an economic evaluation. Whichever approach is adopted within the economic evaluation, the method of identifying either the costs or the benefits is essentially the same for each of the approaches. In order to identify the relevant costs, it will be necessary to categorise all items of resource that will be utilised within the healthcare programme. Therefore, we need to identify which resources are required and which are not. Measurement requires an estimation of the amount of resources used within the programmes, and these should be measured using natural units of measurement. For example, to look specifically at staffing time, one would use units of time (such as hours) that are spent on activities relating to the programme and the specific grades of staff. For other categories of resource use, different units would be appropriate. One might look at drug use in units such as doses of specific drugs. Other examples of resource use and their relevant methods of measurement are outlined in Table 2.1.

Many of the items in Table 2.1 are readily identifiable and straightforward to value. Of these, staffing

Table 2.1 • Resource use and methods for measurement

Resource	Measurement	Valuation
Health services		
Staff time	Time (e.g. hours/days worked)	Salary levels
General consumables	Units/quantities used	Market price
Capital	Units/quantities used	Market price
Overheads	Units/quantities used	Market price/salary levels
Other services		
Community services	Units/quantities used	Market price
Ambulance services	Units/quantities used	Market price
Voluntary services	Units/quantities used	Estimated values for staff costs
Patients and their families		
Personal time	Hours of input	Salary levels
Expenses	Units/quantities used	Market price or cost of actual expenses
Time off work	Duration of time	Salary levels plus other imputed values

costs usually have the greatest impact upon healthcare costs, and these can be readily costed provided that we are aware of the staffing scale and can use wage rates or salary levels attached to the staff level. For example, to cost consultant time one would multiply the number of hours of consultant time in the programme by their hourly pay, with added allowance to cover the costs of leave, sick pay and superannuation, etc. The majority of the other categories of resource use for health services identified in the table (consumables, overheads, capital, etc.) can be readily costed through the use of the market price.

Elsewhere, community services, ambulance services and the expenses incurred by patients and their families would usually be costed in the same manner as health service resources.

Within the above, certain components are notoriously difficult to cost. For example, using patient or family leisure time incurs an opportunity cost, which is complex to measure as there are differing types of activity that are forgone in such situations. It is also complex to attach monetary values to activity involving voluntary care or time lost from housework. No accessible market value exists for either of these areas; therefore, it is customary to use a comparable market value from another market. As an example, Gerard used the wage rate for auxiliary nursing staff in order to cost the inputs by volunteers assisting with respite services for mentally handicapped adults.[50] However, there are occasions when comparable proxy market values are not readily accessible. This is often the case for the costing of 'time off usual activities', such as housework, which by its nature is not of routine duration and is often irregular in its occurrence, making comparison with other occupations virtually impossible. One approach that is advocated in such circumstances is to use average female labour costs as a relatively accurate reflection of the opportunity cost of housework.[51]

While costing might appear to be rather simplistic and straightforward, there are a number of considerations that need to be taken into account before embarking upon such an exercise.

Counting costs in base year

First, we should consider whether healthcare costs should be counted during the base year. By this, we mean that the costs should be adjusted in order to take account of inflation. If we assume that the annual inflation rate is running at 6% then £1060 would be required to purchase an item of medical equipment in a year's time that would currently cost £1000. The two values (both now and in 1 year's time) are considered to be equivalent in real terms, although of course they represent two different amounts of money. This problem becomes more acute if we are considering a comparison of two or more health programmes that have their costs spread at differing proportions over a different number of years. To illustrate this point, let us consider the following example from Auld et al.[51] where surgical and drug treatment options are considered for the same hypothetical condition (Table 2.2). We assume that each option has the same effect, but the cost streams are different between the two options, and the inflation rate is 5% per annum. This rate means that a cost of £1050 in a year's time is equivalent to £1000

now (i.e. £1050/1.05), and likewise £1102.5 in 2 years' time is also equivalent to £1000 now (i.e. £102.5/1.05²). If we compare the costs between the different options in this example, we would conclude that surgery is the more efficient option when compared with the unadjusted drug option, since it is the least costly of the two but equally effective. However, it should be noted at this point that the drug therapy option is only greater in terms of cost owing to inflation. Therefore, if the costs are adjusted to take account of inflation, by adjusting costs to year 0 prices, then both therapies cost exactly the same, with the same effectiveness, and neither of the options can be considered superior to the other.

Discounting

Not all costs and benefits of healthcare programmes are observed to occur at the same point in time. For example, the costs associated with a vaccination programme are incurred very early in order to provide benefits to the individual, or society, in later life. In general, individuals prefer to reap the benefits sooner rather than later and prefer to incur the costs later rather than sooner. The most common method of allowing for such circumstances is to apply a discount rate to future costs and benefits.[26] This leads us to consider whether the costs (and benefits) occurring at differing time points should be allocated equal weighting. There is not a consensus amongst health economists over what the appropriate discount rates are, or whether costs and benefits should be discounted at the same rate. Choosing the appropriate discount rate can have significant implications for the results of evaluations; the current recommended rates in England and Scotland are 3.5%. Consequently, sensitivity analysis is essential to assess the implications of varying the discount rate. Recent convention dictates that costs should be discounted at the same rate as benefits,[52,53] though again this should be done in conjunction with sensitivity analysis to assess variations in such assumptions. Issues of discounting of costs and benefit may have a particularly dramatic effect on conclusions if different options have marked differences in the timing of expenditure or outcomes. This is

Table 2.2 • Adjusting costs to base year (assuming 5% inflation)

| Options | Costs arising (£/person/year) | | | |
	Year 0	Year 1	Year 2	Total
Surgery	3000			
Drug (unadjusted for inflation)	1000	1050	1102.5	3125.5
Drug (adjusted to year 0 prices)	1000	1000	1000	3000

particularly important when considering screening programmes and preventative treatments.

Marginal costing

The marginal cost is the cost incurred or saved from producing one unit more, or one unit less, of a healthcare programme. This is in contrast to the average cost, which is the total cost of a programme divided by the total units produced.

In calculating marginal costs the costs of treating an extra case, or moving from one programme to another, need to be assessed. For example, if there is currently a breast-screening programme for 50- to 65-year-old women and one wishes to consider whether breast screening is as cost-effective in women aged 40–50 years of age, this should be done by looking at the marginal costs and benefits of reducing the age at which screening is started rather than assessing average costs for the entire programme. The use of marginal rather than average costs has been found to be extremely important in screening programmes, where the marginal cost of screening an additional individual can be significantly lower than the average cost.[54]

Auld et al. illustrate this point with an example of hospital care.[51] Although it may well cost £25 000 per annum, on average, to care for an elderly person in hospital, it is extremely unlikely that this amount would be saved if one person less were admitted to the hospital. Similarly, this figure is unlikely to equate to an additional expense if one person more were admitted to the hospital. The reasoning behind this is that some costs, such as capital and overhead costs plus some staffing costs, will not differ with small incremental changes in the numbers of patients entering the hospital.

The use of full costs or marginal costs may depend upon the purpose of an economic evaluation and also the time scale of interest. For example, if one is considering making the most cost-effective use of limited resources then the issue may be one of opportunity costs in that a change in activity may be more or less cost-effective depending upon the activity that is displaced. Marginal costing depends upon an ability to distinguish between fixed and variable costs, and this can be difficult as it may depend upon time-scale and capacity issues. In the long term most resources can be altered in line with activity, although there may be issues of economies of scale. In general the assessment of whether a new technology is considered a cost-effective use of resources will depend upon an assessment of the full costs that would be incurred; however, there may be special considerations where a particular resource has limited availability that could not be influenced by additional expenditure due to capacity constraints.[55]

Another issue that arises in addressing costs is the difference between the true cost of providing care or treatment and the charge that may be made for that treatment by the providing authority. In the UK in recent years the costs of treatment have been classified according to health resource groups that may cover a range of related procedures and/or diagnostic groupings. For these procedures, reference costs have been determined that represent the average costs of treatment within the NHS and a set of tariffs has been developed that determines the level of funding available to providers that deliver the services. In some cases these tariff rates or reference costs are used for economic analysis; however, they frequently cover a wide of range of procedures and case mix and may not represent true costs.[56]

Summary of cost analysis

This section highlights the importance of adhering to the appropriate methods when undertaking the costing component of an evaluation. Failure to do so might well lead to incorrect conclusions and to recommendations based upon flawed analysis. Clearly, not all studies that are published will have fully adopted the principles underlying the methods outlined in this section, and it is important when assessing the results from evaluations to consider whether appropriate analyses have been undertaken.

Economic evaluation

Within the healthcare sector, there will never be enough resources to allow the sufficient provision of healthcare to satisfy the demands of society. Quite simply, resources are scarce and choices need to be made about how best to distribute such resources. Such problems are further increased by the fact that healthcare is a mercurial environment with changing technology and population structures. This leads on to the concept of opportunity cost. Because of the scarcity of resources, choices need to be made regarding the best method for their deployment. It is therefore inevitable that choosing to use resources for one activity requires that their use in other activities must be forsaken. The benefits, often referred to as utility, that would have resulted from these forsaken activities are referred to as opportunity costs. In healthcare, the opportunity costs of the use of resources for a particular healthcare programme or intervention are equivalent to the benefits forsaken in the best alternative use of these resources.

It is necessary to identify from whose perspective the economic evaluation is undertaken. The perspective can be that of the individual patient, the NHS, the individual hospital or service provider, the government or society as a whole. If we considered the societal perspective, then we would seek to include all costs and benefits, no matter where they occur. In the UK, the methods recommended by NICE consider that the base case for cost-effectiveness analysis should include health and personal social service costs, but not all societal or costs incurred by patients, although other issues may be taken into account in evaluating technologies.

Within healthcare, economic evaluation is used as a general term to describe a range of methods that look at the costs and consequences of different programmes or interventions.[54] Each of the methods involves identifying, measuring and, where necessary, valuing all of the relevant costs and consequences of the programme or intervention under review.

There are four main approaches for undertaking economic evaluation: cost-minimisation analysis, cost-effectiveness analysis, cost–utility analysis and cost–benefit analysis. A summary of the features of these is given in Table 2.3 and each is discussed below, outlining their appropriate use in healthcare.

Cost-minimisation analysis

Cost-minimisation analysis is often considered to be a form of cost-effectiveness analysis but is treated here as a separate method of economic evaluation. This particular form of economic evaluation is appropriate in circumstances where, prior to investigation, there is no reason to expect that there will be any therapeutic difference in the outcomes of the procedures under consideration. For example, we might wish to consider two different settings of treatment for varicose veins, such as day-case and inpatient treatment. Here, one might assume that

there would be no expected differences in outcome between the two forms of treatment, and therefore the preferred option would involve choosing the treatment method that was the least costly of the two. Care should be taken in applying cost minimisation and it should be borne in mind that the lack of evidence regarding differences in outcomes is not the same as evidence that such differences do not exist. If there is potential for such differences then a safer approach is to carry out cost-effectiveness analysis with a sensitivity analysis to examine the effect of possible differences in outcome (see below). It is not unusual to find that plausible but unsubstantiated differences in outcome would outweigh the cost differences, which might have led to incorrect conclusions had analysis been confined to cost-minimisation techniques.

Cost-effectiveness analysis

Cost-effectiveness analysis should be used when the outcomes from the different programmes or interventions are anticipated to vary. The outcomes are expressed in natural units, though the appropriate measure to be used in such studies depends ultimately upon the programmes that are being compared. For interventions that would be expected to extend life, natural units such as life-years gained would be an appropriate measure. However, there might be a programme, such as the surgical approach for a hernia repair, where other measures might be considered appropriate, in this case, for example, recurrence rates or time taken to return to work. Likewise, there might be a comparison of two different preventative treatments for coronary heart disease, where heart attacks avoided might be a suitable measure to use. In order to assess the cost-effectiveness, or otherwise, of the interventions, cost is expressed per unit of outcome (cost-effectiveness ratios). The outcome of interest in the appraisal of two or more interventions must be exactly the same

Table 2.3 • Methods of economic evaluation

Type of economic evaluation	Units of measurement
Cost-minimisation analysis	Outcomes are the same between the different options; evaluation based upon cost
Cost-effectiveness analysis	Benefits are quantity or quality of life, which are measured in natural units (e.g. life-years gained, cases avoided, etc.)
Cost–utility analysis	Benefits are quantity and quality of life, which are measured using QALYs or HYEs
Cost–benefit analysis	Benefits are quantity and quality of life, which are measured in monetary terms such as human capital or willingness to pay

HYE, healthy years equivalent; QALY, quality-adjusted life-year.

for each of the alternatives that are considered. Therefore, the results from cost-effectiveness studies cannot often be generalised in order to assess the impact of interventions for differing conditions unless a unified measure that reflects both quantity and quality of survival is used (see cost–utility analysis). In conclusion, cost-effectiveness analysis is a useful tool for informing choices between alternatives where common outcomes have been used for the analysis.

As an example, one might assess the cost per stroke avoided in comparing the cost-effectiveness of a drug treatment for stroke prevention with that of carotid endarterectomy. However, such figures would be of little help in comparing the value of these treatments with that of a treatment for a different condition, such as joint replacement.

Cost–utility analysis

As has been discussed above, one of the potential limitations of cost-effectiveness analysis is that it does not allow for decisions to be made regarding different treatments for differing diseases or conditions if the units of outcome differ between disease areas.

Cost–utility analysis can be thought of as a special case of cost-effectiveness analysis where the outcomes are expressed in generic units that are able to represent the outcome for different conditions and treatments. Therefore, the units of outcome combine both mortality and morbidity information into a single unit of measurement (such as QALYs or HYEs). This two-dimensional outcome measure allows comparisons to be drawn between treatments for different therapeutic areas. These units of measurement are often expressed in terms of a universal unit, usually cost per QALY gained. Such units have resulted in league tables that compare the outcomes for treatments in different areas, and these will be discussed below.

> ✔ Cost–utility analysis expressed in terms of cost per QALY gained has become the predominant form of cost-effectiveness analysis in recent years.

Incremental cost-effectiveness ratios

In comparing the results of cost-effectiveness analysis for different treatments it is usual to report the incremental cost-effectiveness ratio (ICER). The ICER is the ratio between the additional cost that is incurred and the additional benefit (frequently measured in QALYs). Thus, for example, if a treatment produces 0.5 of a quality-adjusted life-year more than the next best treatment but costs an additional £5000, the incremental cost-effectiveness ratio would be £5000 divided by 0.5 or £10 000 per QALY. If the treatment that produces greater clinical benefit is less costly than the alternative then the ICER is negative and the treatment with better outcomes is said to 'dominate', thus being the preferred option in that it produces greater benefit at lower cost.

Where the ICER is positive it reflects the fact that the additional benefit comes at an additional cost and the ICER can be compared with other alternative uses for the available resources. Such calculations have been used to produce league tables to compare the cost of providing benefits by treatment in different clinical settings.

Cost-effectiveness league tables

Decision-makers face difficult decisions when asked how to allocate resources in healthcare. Such decisions are increasingly influenced by the relative cost-effectiveness of different treatments and by comparisons between healthcare interventions in terms of their cost per life-year or per QALY gained. The first compilation of such league tables was undertaken by Williams, who calculated the cost per QALY of a range of interventions and divided them into strong candidates for expansion and less strong candidates for expansion.[27] Advocates of such analyses argue that if properly constructed, these tables provide comprehensive and valid information to aid decision-makers.

There are, however, problems with the use of such tables and these can make interpretation and comparison between studies problematical.[57] First, the year of origin for the studies varies and, because of technological changes and shifts in relative prices, the ranking might not be truly reflective of the intervention under current practice. Second, differing discount rates have been used in the studies, some appropriately and others inappropriately, which impacts upon the results. Third, there have been a variety of preference values for health states, and currently it is difficult to determine which measure of quality of life has been used to derive the estimates concealed within the statistics presented in the league table. Clearly, if there is a high degree of homogeneity between the methods used to derive such estimates then these statistics might well aid decision-makers. Fourth, there is a wide range of costs used within the studies, and often costs are presented at an insufficient level of detail to allow recalculation to reflect local circumstances. In addition, many studies used in such league tables are often compared with differing programmes from which the incremental cost per QALY has been assessed. For example, some might compare with a 'do nothing' or 'do minimum' alternative, while other programmes would compare with the incremental cost per QALY of expanding services to other groups of patients. Finally, the setting of the study will prove important in drawing comparisons between the statistics in such tables, especially in situations where the studies are undertaken in different countries, requiring adjustments for exchange rates.

There has been a substantial amount of literature on the topic,[28–31] and while these tables might aid the decision-maker they also need to be interpreted with extreme caution as there is ample opportunity to mislead the casual observer.

Willingness-to-pay thresholds

A more common practice in recent years has been to compare incremental cost-effectiveness ratios against a 'willingness-to-pay' (WTP) threshold rather than directly against the ICER of other specific treatments. The WTP threshold is a figure that represents the amount that those who fund the healthcare consider is the maximum that should be paid to generate one unit of benefit, usually one QALY. This figure may be specific to local circumstances, depending upon the population and funding arrangements. In the UK, there has been some discussion in recent years on the appropriate level of WTP thresholds and the theoretical basis for the figures.[58,59] On one hand it may be thought of as representing the amount that society is prepared to pay to generate additional healthcare benefit. An alternative interpretation is that if one assumes that the resources available to health are finite then additional expenditure on a new treatment will displace expenditure elsewhere. Assuming that healthcare provision was fully efficient, the WTP threshold would be the level of cost per additional QALY at which the activity displaced resulted in a net loss of health benefit that was equivalent to that produced by the new treatment. Thus, any treatments that fell below the threshold would displace activities that produced less overall benefit, providing a net gain in health, whilst any treatment that was purchased above the threshold would be displacing greater health gain than was provided by the new treatment.

At present there is active empirical research to try to establish a realistic WTP threshold. In the UK setting NICE works with a threshold of £20 000–30 000 per QALY,[60] although early empirical research suggests that this may be set rather high.[61,62]

Cost–benefit analysis

Whilst cost-effectiveness analysis and cost–utility analysis tell us whether a programme or intervention has better outcomes at additional costs or gains more QALYs, they cannot tell us whether the use of resources to achieve those outcomes is justified. Cost–benefit analysis is a type of evaluation that places a single value, usually in monetary terms, upon the benefits and outcomes from differing programmes of healthcare, i.e. it determines the absolute benefit of both quality and quantity, which is vital in resource allocation. In order to do this the health outcomes from treatment need to be measured in the same units as cost. This can be carried out as an extension to cost–utility analysis where the costs and benefits are converted to the same units. In the UK this is usually done with reference to the WTP threshold set by NICE. For example, if one were to consider a treatment that produces one additional QALY then at a WTP threshold of £20 000 this may be considered equivalent to a £20 000 benefit. If the cost of providing that treatment were £10 000 the treatment would result in a net benefit of £10 000. However, at a cost of £30 000 the net benefit would be –£10 000, implying that there would be a net loss from providing the treatment (as, for example, if it were to displace a more cost-effective use of the available resources). An alternative way of presenting such analysis is in terms of net health benefit rather than economic benefit, so that the result is presented in terms of QALY rather than monetary terms (0.5 or –0.5 QALY in the above example).[63]

Choosing an evaluation method

The appropriate method of economic evaluation depends upon which choices need to be made and the context within which those choices need to be reached (for example, refer to Table 2.4). If outcomes are expected to be the same then the choice is quite straightforward: cost-minimisation analysis may be used. The limitations of cost-effectiveness with disease-specific outcomes should be borne in mind. Cost–utility analysis has increased in popularity in an attempt to standardise and allow comparisons across different conditions and healthcare programmes. Cost–benefit analysis may offer decision-makers an alternative way of viewing such analysis but is dependent upon a predetermined WTP threshold.

Table 2.4 • An example of how to choose a type of economic evaluation based on the question

Question	Outcomes	Economic evaluation	What is assessed?
Is day-case open hernia repair better than inpatient repair?	Similar	Cost-minimisation analysis	Purely the cost difference
Is laparoscopic hernia repair better than open hernia repair?	Different	Cost-effectiveness analysis	Cost-difference in relation to varying outcomes
Is the quality of life better with laparoscopic hernia repair compared to open repair?	Different	Cost–utility analysis	Changes in quality of life with differing outcomes
Is laparoscopic hernia repair better compared to open repair in terms of willingness to pay threshold or the resources available?	Different	Cost–benefit analysis	Costs and quality together with the available resources

Sensitivity analysis

Evaluations will always be subject to elements of uncertainty, be it in terms of resource use, costs or effectiveness. Sensitivity analysis is essential in such circumstances as it allows us to assess how sensitive the study results are to variations in key parameters or assumptions that have been used in the analysis. This allows us to assess whether changes in key parameters will result in savings or costs.

It is possible to undertake sensitivity analysis using as few or as many variables as desired. Commonly, variables such as production variables or discount rates will be used, or if statistical analysis of the variables has been undertaken one can carry out sensitivity analysis around known confidence intervals. Although sensitivity analysis is advocated for evaluations, a review by Briggs and Sculpher[52] found that only 39% of articles reviewed had taken at least an adequate account of uncertainty, while only 14% were judged to have provided a good account of uncertainty. In addition, 24% had failed to consider uncertainty at all. There are differing methods of sensitivity analysis, which are discussed below.

Simple sensitivity analysis

Simple sensitivity analysis, in which one or more parameters contained within the evaluation are varied across a plausible range, is widely practised. With one-way analysis, each uncertain component of the evaluation is varied individually in order to assess the separate impact that each component will have upon the results of the analysis. Multi-way sensitivity analysis involves varying two or more of the components of the evaluation at the same time and assessing the impact upon the results. It should be noted that multi-way sensitivity analysis becomes

more difficult to interpret as progressively more variables are varied in the analysis.[52]

Threshold analysis

Threshold analysis involves the identification of the critical value of a parameter above or below which the conclusion of a study will change from one conclusion to another.[64] Threshold analysis is of greatest use when a particular parameter in the evaluation is indeterminate, for example a new drug with a price that has not yet been determined. A major limitation of threshold analysis is that it deals only with uncertainty in continuous variables, meaning that it is normally only useful for addressing uncertainty in analyses with data inputs.[52]

Analysis of extremes

In analysis of extremes, a base-case analysis is undertaken that incorporates the best estimates of the inputs and then further analyses consider extreme estimates of the relevant variables. For example, if two alternative treatment strategies are being compared, then both the high and low costs can be considered for both therapies and costs can be assessed for each of the options based upon combinations of these. Analysis of extremes can be particularly effective in situations where a base-case value is known together with a plausible range, but the actual distribution between the outer limits is unknown. However, a problem with this approach is that it does not consider how likely it is that the various scenarios will arise.[52]

Probabilistic sensitivity analysis

A final approach to dealing with uncertainty is through the use of probabilistic sensitivity analysis (PSA). This method allows ranges and distributions to be assigned to variables about which we are uncertain, thus allowing for combinations of items that are more likely to take place. For example, it is unlikely that all of the pessimistic factors regarding costs will occur in the evaluation. Techniques such as Monte Carlo simulations allow for the random simultaneous selection of items at designated values and undertake analysis based upon hypothetical patient cohorts. This approach allows the proportion of patients to be estimated for whom one of the options under evaluation is preferred; generally, proportions approaching 100% suggest that the intervention is nearly always preferable under a range of conditions. PSA is generally considered to be the most rigorous form of sensitivity analysis and is gaining widespread use.[65]

Value of information analysis

Value of information analysis is a recent development that is an extension of PSA. The method uses the results of PSA to consider the effect of reducing the uncertainty. Whilst PSA can provide a measure of the uncertainty around a prediction of cost-effectiveness, expected value of perfect information (EVPI) gives a measure that also incorporates the importance of such uncertainty.[66] Further developments of this may help to guide priorities for future research[67] or help to design studies and estimate required sample size.[68]

Ethical issues

Any formal method for determining the costs and benefits of different treatments that may be used to allocate resources is likely to raise complex ethical issues. In particular, certain methods may create apparent discrimination against certain groups, such as the elderly or disabled, due to reduced capacity to gain from a particular treatment. Such methods may also fail to take into account other issues that are seen by society as being important in allocating resources, such as preferences relating to the process of care and issues such as equity.[69] It is important that such economic methods should not be used without considering these wider implications of the decisions which stem from such analyses.

Recent advances

Most economic evaluations in healthcare use the above-mentioned methods looking at monetary value for new treatment options. There are, however, a number of complex issues in economic evaluation that remain controversial. These include whether to use patient or societal preferences, weighting of QALY to consider severity of disease, carer benefits and the incorporation of a value for innovation. Over the last decade, multi-criteria decision analysis (MCDA) has been suggested as a way to incorporate these complex and often conflicting values in economic evaluation. In MCDA, 'criteria' refers to the value taken into consideration. The process involves consideration of multiple criteria, each of which is given a weight in coming to an 'objective' decision.[70] Currently, NICE health technology appraisals predominantly use ICER provided by cost–utility analysis. This is considered, using informal methods for incorporating other issues that are not thought to be incorporated in the costs or QALY measures, often by adjusting the WTP threshold that is considered acceptable.[71]

Another major change in NICE economic evaluations evolved in appraisals for interventions involving 'end of life'. As mentioned in earlier sections, NICE considers interventions to be cost-effective if the cost per QALY gained is less than £20 000–30 000. However, in 2009, NICE issued guidance wherein some 'end-of-life' interventions or therapeutics that cost more than £30 000 per QALY gained may be given consideration if the treatment is indicated for conditions with a life expectancy of less than 24 months and if there is sufficient evidence that the new intervention improves life expectance by at least 3 months compared to the available NHS treatment and if the treatment if licensed for small population groups.[72]

Summary

Whether making individual or policy decisions regarding healthcare provision, it is becoming increasingly important for clinicians to take into account evidence about both the effectiveness and the cost-effectiveness of the treatment options. This requires that they examine the available evidence with particular attention to the appropriateness of the outcome measures used and of any techniques for economic analysis. In particular, there is a need for both clinicians and researchers to focus upon outcomes that are relevant to patients and truly represent their views about the relative values of the health states and events that they may encounter. Outcome research and economic evaluation are relatively new areas of healthcare research but they are progressing rapidly. An understanding of the methods used is a prerequisite for an adequate interpretation of the conclusions drawn from such work.

Key points

- The choice of outcome measure is important in assessing the results of surgical treatment and needs to be carefully considered.
- The measure used should be clinically relevant and preferably have been validated by previous research.
- Possible measures relevant to surgery include mortality, condition-specific measures, standard pain questionnaires and generic measures of health-related quality of life.
- Quality-adjusted life-years are a commonly used measure of outcome and there are several different ways to produce the weights (utilities) that are required to calculate these.
- The estimation of the cost of treatments should include a detailed analysis of the resources used and their valuation, and may require consideration of the timing of incurring various costs.
- There are several different methods of economic evaluation, including cost-minimisation, cost-effectiveness, cost–utility and cost–benefit analysis.
- The use of cost-effectiveness analysis may allow comparison of health benefits to be gained by expenditure on different treatments but is not without both technical and ethical problems in its application.

References

1. Fitzpatrick R, Davey C, Buxton MJ, et al. Evaluating patient-based outcome measures for use in clinical trials. Health Technol Assess 1998;2(14):i–iv, 1–74.

2. Collin C, Wade DT, Davies S, et al. The Barthel Index: a reliability study. Int Disabil Stud 1988;10(2):61–3.

3. Aissaoui Y, Zeggwagh AA, Zekraoui A, et al. Validation of a behavioral pain scale in critically ill, sedated, and mechanically ventilated patients. Anesth Analg 2005;101(5):1470–6.

4. Campbell DT, Fiske DW. Convergent and discriminant validation by the multitrait–multimethod matrix. Psychol Bull 1959;56(2):81–105.

5. Perkins JM, Collin J, Creasy TS, et al. Exercise training versus angioplasty for stable claudication. Long and medium term results of a prospective, randomised trial. Eur J Vasc Endovasc Surg 1996;11(4):409–13.

6. Stockton D, Davies T, Day N, et al. Retrospective study of reasons for improved survival in patients with breast cancer in east Anglia: earlier diagnosis or better treatment. Br Med J 1997;314(7079):472–5.

7. Sowden AJ, Sheldon TA. Does volume really affect outcome? Lessons from the evidence. J Health Serv Res Policy 1998;3(3):187–90.

8. Jones J, Rowan K. Is there a relationship between the volume of work carried out in intensive care and its outcome? Int J Technol Assess Health Care 1995;11(4):762–9.

9. Brazier J, Dixon S. The use of condition specific outcome measures in economic appraisal. Health Econ 1995;4(4):255–64.

10. Spilker B, Molinek Jr FR, Johnston KA, et al. Quality of life bibliography and indexes. Med Care 1990;28(12, Suppl):DS1–77.

11. Meenan RF, Mason JH, Anderson JJ, et al. AIMS2. The content and properties of a revised and expanded Arthritis Impact Measurement Scales Health Status Questionnaire. Arth Rheum 1992;35(1):1–10.

12. Goldman L, Hashimoto B, Cook EF, et al. Comparative reproducibility and validity of systems for assessing cardiovascular functional class: advantages of a new specific activity scale. Circulation 1981;64(6):1227–34.

13. Melzack R. The McGill Pain Questionnaire: major properties and scoring methods. Pain 1975;1(3):277–99.

14. Garratt AM, Macdonald LM, Ruta DA, et al. Towards measurement of outcome for patients with varicose veins. Qual Health Care 1993;2(1):5–10.

15. Guyatt GH, Berman LB, Townsend M, et al. A measure of quality of life for clinical trials in chronic lung disease. Thorax 1987;42(10):773–8.

16. Carroll D, Rose K. Treatment leads to significant improvement. Effect of conservative treatment on pain in lymphoedema. Prof Nurse 1992;8(1):32–3, 35–6.

17. Payen JF, Bru O, Bosson JL, et al. Assessing pain in critically ill sedated patients by using a behavioral pain scale. Crit Care Med 2001;29(12):2258–63.

18. Young J, Siffleet J, Nikoletti S, et al. Use of a Behavioural Pain Scale to assess pain in ventilated, unconscious and/or sedated patients. Intensive Crit Care Nurs 2006;22(1):32–9.

19. Brazier J, Deverill M, Green C, et al. A review of the use of health status measures in economic evaluation. Health Technol Assess 1999;3(9):i–iv, 1–164.

20. Group TE. EuroQol – a new facility for the measurement of health-related quality of life. The EuroQol Group. Health Policy 1990;16(3):199–208.

21. Rabin R, de Charro F. EQ-5D: a measure of health status from the EuroQol Group. Ann Med 2001;33(5):337–43.

22. Brazier JE, Harper R, Jones NM, et al. Validating the SF-36 health survey questionnaire: new outcome measure for primary care. Br Med J 1992;305(6846): 160–4.

23. Brazier JE, Roberts J. The estimation of a preference-based measure of health from the SF-12. Med Care 2004;42(9):851–9.

24. Hunt SM, McKenna SP. McEwen J. Measuring health status. London: Croom-Helm; 1986.

25. Torrance GW. Measurement of health state utilities for economic appraisal. J Health Econ 1986;5 (1): 1–30.

26. Drummond MF, Sculpher MJ, Torrance GW, et al. Methods for the economic evaluation of healthcare programmes. 3rd ed. Oxford: Oxford University Press; 2005.

27. Williams A. Economics of coronary artery bypass grafting. Br Med J (Clin Res Ed) 1985;291(6491): 326–9.

28. Birch S, Gafni A. Cost-effectiveness ratios: in a league of their own. Health Policy 1994;28(2):133–41.

29. Drummond M, Torrance G, Mason J. Cost-effectiveness league tables: more harm than good? Soc Sci Med 1993;37(1):33–40.

30. Mason J, Drummond M, Torrance G. Some guidelines on the use of cost effectiveness league tables. Br Med J 1993;306(6877):570–2.

31. Drummond M, Mason J, Torrance G. Cost-effectiveness league tables: think of the fans. Health Policy 1995;31(3):231–8.

32. Mehrez A, Gafni A. Healthy-years equivalents versus quality-adjusted life years: in pursuit of progress. Med Decis Making 1993;13(4):287–92.

33. Buckingham K. A note on HYE (healthy years equivalent). J Health Econ 1993;12(3):301–9.

34. Johannesson M, Jonsson B, Karlsson G. Outcome measurement in economic evaluation. Health Econ 1996;5(4):279–96.

35. Brazier J, Roberts J, Deverill M. The estimation of a preference-based measure of health from the SF-36. J Health Econ 2002;21(2):271–92.

36. Johannesson M, O'Conor RM. Cost–utility analysis from a societal perspective. Health Policy 1997;39(3):241–53.

37. Bleichrodt H, Johannesson M. Standard gamble, time trade-off and rating scale: experimental results on the ranking properties of QALYs. J Health Econ 1997;16(2):155–75.

38. von Neumann J, Morgenstern O. Theory of games and economic behaviour. New York: Wiley; 1967.

39. Torrance GW, Thomas WH, Sackett DL. A utility maximization model for evaluation of health care programs. Health Serv Res 1972; 7(2):118–33.

40. Hollingworth W, Deyo RA, Sullivan SD, et al. The practicality and validity of directly elicited and SF-36 derived health state preferences in patients with low back pain. Health Econ 2002;11(1):71–85.

41. Stein K, Fry A, Round A, et al. What value health? A review of health state values used in early technology assessments for NICE. Appl Health Econ Health Policy 2005;4(4):219–28.

42. Rasanen P, Roine E, Sintonen H, et al. Use of quality-adjusted life years for the estimation of effectiveness of health care: a systematic literature review. Int J Technol Assess Health Care 2006;22(2): 235–41.

43. Dolan P. Modeling valuations for EuroQol health states. Med Care 1997;35(11):1095–108.

44. Brazier J, Usherwood T, Harper R, et al. Deriving a preference-based single index from the UK SF-36 Health Survey. J Clin Epidemiol 1998;51(11):1115–28.

45. Brazier J, Roberts J, Tsuchiya A, et al. A comparison of the EQ-5D and SF-6D across seven patient groups. Health Econ 2004;13(9):873–84.

46. Bansback N, Marra C, Tsuchiya A, et al. Using the health assessment questionnaire to estimate preference-based single indices in patients with rheumatoid arthritis. Arth Rheum 2007;57(6):963–71.

47. Wilson J, Yao GL, Raftery J, et al. A systematic review and economic evaluation of epoetin alpha, epoetin beta and darbepoetin alpha in anaemia associated with cancer, especially that attributable to cancer treatment. Health Technol Assess 2007;11(13):iii–iv, 1–202.

48. Sculpher MJ, Price M. Measuring costs and consequences in economic evaluation in asthma. Respir Med 2003;97(5):508–20.

49. Stolk EA, Busschbach JJ. Validity and feasibility of the use of condition-specific outcome measures in economic evaluation. Qual Life Res 2003;12(4):363–71.

50. Gerard K. Determining the contribution of residential respite care to the quality of life of children with severe learning difficulties. Child Care Health Dev 1990;16(3):177–88.

51. Auld C, Donaldson C, Mitton C, et al. Economic evaluation. In: Detel R, et al., editors. Oxford textbook of public health, Vol. 2: The methods of public health. Oxford: Oxford University Press; 2002.

52. Briggs A, Sculpher M. Sensitivity analysis in economic evaluation: a review of published studies. Health Econ 1995;4(5):355–71.

53. Cairns J. Discounting and health benefits: another perspective. Health Econ 1992;1(1):76–9.

54. Drummond M, Maynard A. Purchasing and providing cost-effective health care. Edinburgh: Churchill Livingstone; 1993.

55. Hartwell D, Colquitt J, Loveman E, et al. Clinical effectiveness and cost-effectiveness of immediate angioplasty for acute myocardial infarction: systematic review and economic evaluation. Health Technol Assess 2005;9(17):iii–iv, 1–99.

56. Baboolal K, McEwan P, Sondhi S, et al. The cost of renal dialysis in a UK setting – a multicentre study. Nephrol Dial Transplant 2008;23(6):1982–9.

57. Mason J, Drummond M. Reporting guidelines for economic studies. Health Econ 1995;4(2):85–94.

58. Raftery J. Should NICE's threshold range for cost per QALY be raised? No. Br Med J 2009;338: b185.

59. Towse A. Should NICE's threshold range for cost per QALY be raised? Yes. Br Med J 2009;338: b181.

60. Rawlins MD, Culyer AJ. National Institute for Clinical Excellence and its value judgments. Br Med J 2004;329(7459):224–7.

61. Appleby J, Devlin N, Parkin D. NICE's cost effectiveness threshold. Br Med J 2007;335(7616): 358–9.

62. Martin S, Rice N, Smith P. The link between health care spending and health outcomes: evidence from English programme budgeting data. Centre for Health Economics Research Paper 24, University of York; 2007.

63. Stinnett AA, Mullahy J. Net health benefits: a new framework for the analysis of uncertainty in cost-effectiveness analysis. Med Decis Making 1998;18 (2, Suppl):S68–80.

64. Pauker SG, Kassirer JP. The threshold approach to clinical decision making. N Engl J Med 1980;302(20):1109–17.

65. Claxton K, Sculpher M, McCabe C, et al. Probabilistic sensitivity analysis for NICE technology assessment: not an optional extra. Health Econ 2005;14(4):339–47.

66. Felli JC, Hazen GB. Sensitivity analysis and the expected value of perfect information. Med Decis Making 1998;18(1):95–109.

67. Claxton KP, Sculpher MJ. Using value of information analysis to prioritise health research: some lessons from recent UK experience. Pharmacoeconomics 2006;24(11):1055–68.

68. Ades AE, Lu G, Claxton K. Expected value of sample information calculations in medical decision modeling. Med Decis Making 2004;24(2):207–27.

69. Ubel PA, DeKay ML, Baron J, et al. Cost-effectiveness analysis in a setting of budget constraints – is it equitable? N Engl J Med 1996;334(18):1174–7.

70. Belton V, Stewart TJ. Multi criteria decision analysis: an integrated approach. Dordrecht: Kluwer Academic; 2002.

71. Thokala P. Multiple criteria decision analysis for health technology assessment. Decision Support Unit, NICE; 2011.

72. (NICE) NIoCE. Appraising life-extending, end of life treatments 2009. Available at http://www.nice.org.uk/media/E4A/79/SupplementaryAdviceTACEoL.pdf [accessed 05.01.12].

3

Day case surgery

Paul Baskerville

Introduction

One of the main aims of surgery is to return the postoperative patient to their home environment, in a safe and timely fashion. If, following a surgical procedure, the patient does not spend a few days in hospital, but returns home the same day, we describe that process as day case surgery. Why should this obvious and rather banal variation in length of hospital stay deserve a chapter of its own in a surgical textbook? The reason is that the development of successful day surgery practice, and the knowledge gained from studying its component parts, have been instrumental in improving the delivery of all surgical care in the last 30 years. It has helped all parties responsible for that delivery to understand how to introduce, create and then manage surgical developments in a timely, safe, efficient and cost-effective manner.

Understanding how day surgery works, how traditional inpatient care can be successfully transferred to the day unit, and what is required to enable that to happen is a fundamental requirement for all those involved in the care of the surgical patient, be they surgeon or anaesthetist, nurse or manager, health purchaser or provider.

Day surgery has been described as the planned admission of a patient to hospital for a surgical procedure which, while requiring recovery from a bed or trolley, allows the patient to return home the same day. As a consequence, procedures not requiring full operating theatre facilities and/or general anaesthesia, procedures which can be performed in outpatient or endoscopic suites, are no longer called true 'day surgery'.

Successful and well-managed day surgery has the potential to improve the quality of care for patients by separating their elective treatment from the bustle of emergency surgical care, both of which are traditionally managed on the same wards. Most people would rather not stay in hospital longer than necessary, and short stays reduce the risks of hospital-acquired infections. Reducing length of stay also reduces costs and can improve efficiency, reasons that make day surgery attractive to all healthcare systems worldwide.

In the UK, the NHS plan proposed by the government in 2001 set the patient firmly at the centre of a framework for modernising the NHS.[1] The idea was to reduce waiting times, implement booking systems and introduce patient choice. However, the government was faced with capacity constraints and one solution to increase patient throughput was to reduce the length of patients' stay by focusing on increasing national day surgery rates by implementing a National Day Surgery Programme.

✓✓ The day surgery strategy was launched in 2002 with the broad aim of achieving 75% of all elective surgery in the UK to be performed on a day case basis by the year 2005.[2]

Day surgery now comprises over 70% of all elective surgery in the UK, over 80% in the USA and is likely to become the default method of treating most surgical patients in the next two decades. This growth has occurred over the last 30 years, most of it in the last 15. How has this come about? What are the main driving forces behind it? What are its strengths and weaknesses? This chapter covers those aspects of day surgery that are essential to good practice, and highlights some areas of current controversy.

The development of day surgery

The concept of day surgery is not new. In 1909, James Nicholl, a surgeon working at the Royal Hospital for Sick Children in Glasgow, reported on nearly 9000 children undergoing operations for conditions such as hernia and harelip, all of whom went home on the day of surgery.[3] He described the benefits for parent and child of returning home the same day, but stressed the importance of suitable home conditions in the success of day surgery. A decade later, in 1919, Ralph Waters, an anaesthetist in Sioux City, Iowa, reported on the 'downtown anaesthesia clinic' where adults underwent minor surgical procedures, returning home within a few hours.[4]

The modern era of day surgery began in the years following World War II with the realisation that prolonged bed rest was associated with high rates of postoperative complications such as deep vein thrombosis.[5] The move towards early ambulation led to earlier discharge and, for the first time, the economic benefits of day surgery were noted.[6] In 1955, Eric Farquharson of Edinburgh described a series of 458 consecutive inguinal hernia repairs performed on a day case basis at a time when the average length of postoperative stay was approximately 2 weeks.[7] The medical benefits of early ambulation were recorded and the potential impact on surgical waiting times was considered.

Further development of day surgery occurred not in the UK but in North America, where cost savings associated with day surgery in privately run healthcare systems led to the early development of day units within hospitals, and by 1969 the first free-standing ambulatory surgical centre in Phoenix, Arizona. The huge commercial success of such units led to a significant shift in surgical care out of hospital inpatient beds, and forced surgeons, anaesthetists and hospital managers to study and improve the safety and efficiency of surgical care.

The UK, with its state-run NHS, was much slower to introduce day surgery. The few existing units were poorly utilised and there was little support for the expansion seen in the USA. In 1980 Paul Jarrett, in the day unit at Kingston Hospital, demonstrated once again the benefits of dedicated day surgery lists for hernias, including the rapid reduction of waiting times from 3 years to 3 months.[8] This time the government was quick to see the advantages, and supported day surgery expansion throughout the UK for a decade. In 1985 the Royal College of Surgeons of England published a report (revised in 1992) entitled *Guidelines for day case surgery*.[9] At that time, it was estimated that only 15% of elective surgery

was performed on a day case basis and the report suggested 50% as an appropriate target. In 1989, the gathering momentum of day surgery demonstrated a need for a professional body to promote the speciality and set quality standards of care. The result was the British Association of Day Surgery (BADS) encompassing surgeons, anaesthetists, nurses and managers involved in day surgery. The same year the NHS Management Executive's value-for-money unit demonstrated that the cost of treating patients as day cases was significantly less than as inpatients.[10] By 1990, the Audit Commission had taken over the role of external auditors within the NHS and it introduced the concept of a 'basket' of 20 surgical procedures suitable for day case surgery to allow benchmarking between health authorities.[11] The audit figures also demonstrated wide variations between hospitals.

By 1991, the Audit Commission Report *Measuring quality: the patient's view of day surgery* found that 80% of day case patients preferred this mode of treatment to traditional inpatient treatment, adding further impetus to the development of day surgery.[12]

By the end of the decade, the introduction of newer surgical and anaesthetic techniques to the day unit and the loss of others to the outpatient department forced a reassessment of the surgical basket to reflect modern-day case activity, as many day units were already performing more complex procedures on a day surgery basis. In 1999, continuing the supermarket analogy, the BADS recommended an additional 20 operations to form a 'trolley' of procedures suitable for day surgery in the more experienced day unit (Box 3.1). The trolley included major operations such as laparoscopic cholecystectomy, thoracoscopic sympathectomy, partial thyroidectomy and laser prostatectomy. The concept of the trolley was that a target of 50% of these procedures on a day case basis would be realistic.

Following this lead by the professions, the Audit Commission updated its own basket of procedures (Box 3.2) and this was incorporated into the Department of Health's *Day surgery: operational guide* published to support the National Day Surgery Programme to achieve a 75% day case rate for elective surgery by 2005.[2] Although this tool is still used as a comparator in assessing output by Trusts and Health Authorities,[13] for development purposes it has now been superseded by the introduction of a regularly updated Directory of Procedures by the BADS.[14] The Directory, which was first introduced in 2007 and is regularly updated, lists over 200 procedures by speciality, including their OPCS and HRG codes, and provides a breakdown of how each procedure might be treated within four areas: procedure room, day surgery, 24-hour stay or under

Box 3.1 • British Association of Day Surgery 'trolley' of procedures 1999, of which 50% should be suitable for day case surgery

Laparoscopic hernia repair
Thoracoscopic sympathectomy
Submandibular gland excision
Partial thyroidectomy
Superficial parotidectomy
Wide excision of breast lump with axillary clearance
Haemorrhoidectomy
Urethrotomy
Bladder neck incision
Laser prostatectomy
Transcervical resection of endometrium
Eyelid surgery
Arthroscopic meniscectomy
Arthroscopic shoulder decompression
Subcutaneous mastectomy
Rhinoplasty
Dentoalveolar surgery
Tympanoplasty
Laparoscopic cholecystectomy
Bunion operations

Box 3.2 • Audit Commission basket of 25 procedures 2001

Orchidopexy
Circumcision
Inguinal hernia repair
Excision of breast lump
Anal fissure dilatation or excision
Haemorrhoidectomy
Laparoscopic cholecystectomy
Varicose vein stripping or ligation
Transurethral resection of bladder tumour
Excision of Dupuytren's contracture
Carpal tunnel decompression
Excision of ganglion
Arthroscopy
Bunion operations
Removal of metalware
Extraction of cataract with or without implant
Correction of squint
Myringotomy
Tonsillectomy
Submucous resection
Reduction of nasal fracture
Operation for bat ears
Dilatation and curettage/hysteroscopy
Laparoscopy
Termination of pregnancy

72-hour stay. It therefore allows for the planning and development of day surgery practice within a Unit or Trust.

How does it work for the patient?

Facilities for day surgery

The organisation of day surgery services differs from traditional inpatient surgery. Patients arrive at the hospital on the day of surgery, fully assessed, with the results of investigations already checked. Following operation, patients recover in the day unit and are discharged home, accompanied by their carer. The entire admission episode is pre-planned and the routine nature of the hospital visit ensures quality care. Any error in the system results in an unnecessary overnight admission and it is therefore not surprising that the facilities for day surgery differ from inpatient surgery.

Initially, day surgery was attempted from the inpatient ward, but this environment is a mixture of emergency admissions, unwell elective surgery patients and the 'well' elective day surgery patient. Quality of care for the day case patient suffered as busy ward staff naturally concentrated on the acutely ill. There was also no incentive to ensure the day

patient was able to go home the same evening. In the UK, the patient's procedure was often cancelled on the day of admission as their projected bed had been occupied overnight by an emergency admission.

Self-contained day units or dedicated day wards were therefore developed and unplanned overnight admission rates dropped dramatically from 14% on an inpatient ward to 2.4% in a dedicated day unit.[2] These units may be free-standing or integrated within the main hospital, where they benefit from the full range of available support services. The self-contained unit should have its own day surgery theatre within the day surgery suite, performing dedicated day case lists.

Dedicated lists require appropriate staffing levels to be allocated as there is a greater intensity of work for theatre staff if several day cases are to be treated rather than a single major case. Experience has shown that the most effective units unite all managerial as well as nursing and operative functions under the same roof. Further efficiencies are made if the day unit can be accessed directly from the street or car park, and if day patients have their own dedicated car parking facilities.

The day surgery cycle

In traditional inpatient surgery, the patient is admitted either from the waiting list or directly from the surgical outpatient clinic if the patient is classified as urgent. In day surgery, the processes are different (**Fig. 3.1**). In many hospitals the patient is seen in the outpatient clinic and then sent directly for pre-assessment. While this has the advantage of a single hospital visit, some patients become overwhelmed with the amount of information they are given in a short space of time. Therefore, some patients find it convenient to come back for pre-assessment at a later date.

A few hospitals accept fast tracking by general practitioners, who refer patients directly for pre-assessment to the day unit. In this case, the surgeon will not see the patient until the morning of operation and, for obvious reasons, the process is only suitable for the young, fit patient with a straightforward surgical problem.

Patient selection

Patient selection addresses the suitability of the patient for day surgery. The majority of patients will be suitable unless an overnight stay would be of particular benefit. Factors that may also influence selection include the risk of major complications, social conditions and medical fitness. There should be no upper limits on age or body mass index (BMI), although each patient is judged on an individual basis, and American Society of Anesthesiologists (ASA) class III patients are routinely accepted.

In any hospital, over 75% of traditional inpatient procedures can therefore be performed safely on a day case basis.[2] UK guidelines have recently been published by BADS and the Association of GB and Ireland.[15]

Social factors

The effects of general anaesthesia on cerebral function, affecting judgment and coordination, are well recognised. After day surgery, all patients must be accompanied home by a responsible and physically able adult, who should be available for the first 24 hours following operation. Patients themselves must not drive home and preferably should avoid public transport. Greater travelling times are associated with increased discomfort and nausea,[16] and patients should reside within an hour's journey from the hospital in case of emergency. The patient's home conditions should be sufficient to allow them to recover in comfort. In general, they should have access to a telephone in case of emergency, there should be adequate toilet facilities and household stairs should be minimal, but each set of circumstances requires individual judgment.

Age

Biological age is more important than chronological age, although some day units arbitrarily and illogically apply upper limits of 65 or 70 years of age. Whilst the older patient is more likely to suffer from respiratory and cardiovascular disease and the carer may also be in an elderly age group, with careful preoperative evaluation the elderly patient can

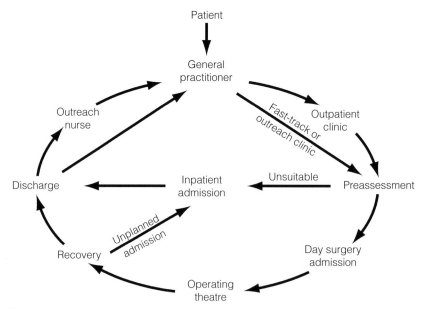

Figure 3.1 • The day surgery cycle.

benefit from day surgery through a rapid return to familiar home circumstances and less postoperative confusion.

Body mass index

Obesity is measured by BMI (in kg/m²) and height–weight charts are used as 'ready reckoners' to calculate it (**Fig. 3.2**). Obesity is defined as a BMI equal to or greater than 30.[17] The prevalence of obesity has doubled since the 1990s, with 24% of adults in England now fulfilling the definition.[18] The very obese were excluded from day surgery because of delayed recovery related to the absorption of volatile anaesthetic agents into body fat, but this is less of a problem with modern total intravenous anaesthetic agents such as propofol.[19] The problems that do occur with the obese patient are related to comorbidity, the surgical procedure and the anaesthetic. Obesity is associated with cardiac disease, diabetes mellitus, hiatus hernia, hypertension and sleep apnoea, and it may be the comorbidity factor that excludes an obese patient from day surgery rather than the obesity itself. Operating on the obese patient is often more technically demanding and the complication rate is often higher, with increased rates of postoperative haematoma formation and pain as a result of the need for greater surgical access. Anaesthetic problems include problems of venous access, intubation and airway control. Operating on patients early in the day is advisable to ensure that any minor postoperative complications can be corrected and do not prevent the patient from returning home.

✔ The upper safe BMI limit for day surgery remains controversial. While some day units still remain at a restrictive BMI of 30, others have safely increased this upper limit to 35, 37 and even 40.[20]

Smoking

Smokers undergoing surgery have increased intraoperative complications such as impaired gas exchange and increased secretions, with postoperative problems consisting of an increased incidence of bronchospasm, chest infection and wound complications.[21] Advice at pre-assessment regarding cessation of smoking depends on whether the patient would like to stop permanently or else temporarily suspend their habit in the perioperative period. For those attempting permanent cessation, this should commence 6–8 weeks before surgery since this is the minimum time required for lung function to improve significantly.[22] The least effective time of smoking cessation is in the week before surgery, when the effects of withdrawal are maximal.[23] For those who intend continuing their habit, temporary cessation 12 hours before surgery confers a reduction in circulating carboxyhaemoglobin, thereby improving perioperative lung function.

Medical factors

✔✔ In 1991 the ASA classified surgical patients into five classes of physical fitness (Table 3.1), which has provided a framework for patient selection in day surgery.[24]

While ASA class I or class II patients are generally accepted for day surgery, the suitability of patients in the ASA class III group is less clear. While hypertension,

✔ Stable ASA class III patients have the same risk of unplanned overnight admissions as lower ASA status patients,[25] and any increase in complications with ASA class III patients is related to the surgical procedure rather than comorbidity.

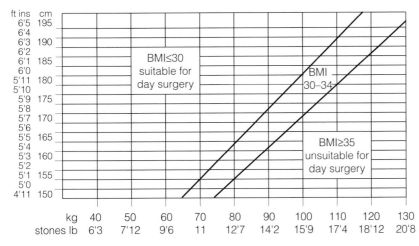

Figure 3.2 • Assessment chart for body mass index (BMI).

Table 3.1 • Adaptation of the American Society of Anesthesiologists' classification of physical status

Class I	A healthy patient
Class II	Mild-to-moderate systemic disease caused by the surgical condition to be treated or by another disease process, with no functional limitation, controlled hypertension, mild diabetes, mild asthma
Class III	Severe systemic disease with some functional limitation plus diabetes with complications, severe asthma, myocardial infarction >6 months
Class IV	Severe systemic disease that is a constant threat to life plus unstable angina, severe cardiac, pulmonary, renal, hepatic or endocrine insufficiency
Class V	Moribund patient not expected to survive 24 hours even with surgical intervention

chronic lung disease and symptomatic heart disease increase the risk of complications, this is not evident with asthma or insulin-dependent diabetes mellitus.

Diabetes mellitus

Patients with stable diabetes mellitus are usually best managed as day cases as this interferes least with their routine. Nevertheless, type I diabetic patients are more difficult to manage in the perioperative period than type II patients and are more liable to unplanned admission. Stability of the disease in the months before surgery is therefore central to success of the admission, especially in the type I patient. A glycosylated haemoglobin (HbA1c) result of less than 8% suggests that the patient is suitable for day surgery. Most intermediate surgical procedures, such as those in the Audit Commission basket of 25 (Box 3.2), can be safely undertaken in adult diabetic patients with the occasional exception of laparoscopic cholecystectomy due to the increased risk of postoperative nausea and vomiting.

Where possible, the patient should be managed with local or regional anaesthesia as this may remove the need for the patient to starve preoperatively. However, if general anaesthesia is required, diabetic medication is omitted on the morning of surgery, the procedure is scheduled as early as possible on the list and the normal regimen is resumed as soon as possible.[26] Well-controlled non-insulin-dependent diabetics present few problems but insulin-dependent diabetics require intensive monitoring throughout the day surgery process.

Cardiac disease

The risk of myocardial ischaemia during anaesthesia is increased in the hypertensive patient, and elevated blood pressure is one of the most common reasons for 'on the day' cancellation: the blood pressure has either not been accurately measured at preoperative assessment or it has not been adequately treated (see 'Preoperative assessment'). Preoperative sedation can lower a marginally elevated blood pressure but the underlying cause requires further investigation. Many patients with significant cardiovascular disease can still undergo day surgery procedures provided exercise tolerance is good.

✔✔ The specific blood pressure that is unsafe for the patient undergoing day surgery remains unclear, but a systematic review and meta-analysis of 30 observational studies found little evidence for an association between admission arterial pressure and perioperative complications if systolic and diastolic pressures are less than 180 and 110 mmHg, respectively.[27]

Asthma

The stable asthmatic using an inhaler and with good exercise tolerance is suitable for day surgery. Only those with unstable or steroid-controlled asthma require investigation before proceeding and may require exclusion. Non-steroidal anti-inflammatory drugs (NSAIDs) can be administered safely for pain relief to 95% of asthmatics.[28] A history of previous administration without bronchial spasm, usually from over-the-counter preparations, is often available.

Preoperative assessment

The admission, operation and discharge of a patient within a day requires accurate forward planning, with the procedure occurring on a scheduled day at a scheduled time. Day surgery pioneered the role of preoperative assessment, performed up to 6 weeks prior to surgery. As a result nursing, anaesthetic and surgical assessment on the day of admission is both rapid and minimal. Pre-assessment of patients also ensures that 'on the day' cancellation for clinical reasons is rare. Cancellations not only waste hospital resources but cause distress to patients and their families and often disrupt work commitments.

To maximise day surgery throughput, pre-assessment may be accomplished by:

- automatic assignment to day surgery of all patients undergoing a procedure included in the BADS's trolley of procedures (Box 3.1) or the Audit Commission's updated basket of procedures (Box 3.2);
- hospital-wide pre-assessment for all elective surgical procedures (with procedure-specific exclusions for major surgical procedures such as major bowel resection and aortic aneurysm repair).

Successful pre-assessment should focus on educating the patient and their carers about their condition, identifying any preoperative risk factors and optimising the patient's condition. All three aspects need to be performed well in order to maximise success on the day of surgery. Strict assessment criteria ensure patient safety, and identifying any anomalies at pre-assessment allows for timely correction of these factors. Day surgery pre-assessment is best performed by trained nurses in nurse-based pre-assessment clinics. The availability of a consultant anaesthetist to deal immediately with some queries and concerns further improves efficiency. The most common treatable exclusion factors are hypertension and identifying an overnight carer for patients living on their own.

Pre-assessment clinics use a patient questionnaire to screen for social and medical problems. Most questionnaires follow a standard format to screen and triage the suitability of patients for day surgery. Questionnaires should address the generic status of the health of the patient, but additional questions may be added for specific surgical specialities.

Patient information leaflets should also be available covering both general day surgery information and information specific to the proposed operation. These may have been issued at the outpatient consultation where first-stage consent is usually obtained. The later pre-assessment visit allows the patient to ask questions that may have arisen since their consultation, and subsequent discussion leads to better understanding by the patient and family, and may reduce anxiety levels.[29] Involvement of the patient at this stage permits flexibility and choice regarding their operating date and improves non-attendance rates.

Investigations

Routine investigations are unnecessary in the a symptomatic day surgery patient[30] and preoperative testing should be limited to circumstances in which the results will affect patient treatment and outcomes. Investigations should not be prescriptive but should be tailored to the individual's needs because most investigations required can be predicted from the history alone. Even when minor abnormalities are found they rarely entail cancellation. A full blood count is only required if there is a risk of anaemia, chronic renal disease, rectal bleeding or haemorrhage. Similarly, analysis for urea and electrolytes is only indicated if the patient has renal disease or is taking diuretics. Urinalysis is often routinely performed as part of the preoperative routine but, again, unsuspected disease is more likely to be picked up on history alone. In Oxford, routine urine testing of more than 30 000 day case admissions resulted in only one cancellation, caused by unsuspected diabetes mellitus.[19]

The incidence of electrocardiographic (ECG) abnormalities increases with age but minor preoperative ECG abnormalities do not predict adverse cardiovascular perioperative events in day surgery.[31] The only indications for preoperative ECG include chest pain, palpitations and dyspnoea, but these patients have often already been excluded from day surgery by other comorbidity. A chest X-ray examination is also unnecessary. If required, then the patient is probably unsuitable for day surgery in the first place.

Testing for sickle cell disease is more controversial. Patients with sickle cell disease usually present in childhood with chronic haemolytic anaemia. Preoperative screening in adults is unlikely to identify a patient with previously unknown sickle cell disease but will, of course, identify those with sickle cell trait. However, the 'at-risk' population (those of African, Asian and Mediterranean origin) is often difficult to define in Britain today as a result of ethnic mixing. Furthermore, those factors that precipitate sickling (hypotension, hypoxaemia and acidosis) are unlikely to occur during day case surgery.

Day of surgery admission

On arrival at the day unit on the prearranged day of operation, most documentation is already complete and bureaucracy is minimised. Any change of circumstance, either social or medical, should be noted since the time of pre-assessment, and the preoperative surgical visit by the person performing the operation need only consist of verification of the consent and marking the appropriate operation site. The final anaesthetic assessment is performed at this time and not in the anaesthetic room, where levels of anxiety are already high. Many day surgery units have successfully introduced staggered admission times for patients, which is more convenient for both patient and the day unit. In most centres, the 12-hour fasting ritual has now been replaced by regimens of no solids (including milk) within 4–6 hours and up to 300 mL of clear fluid within 2 hours of surgery.

Patient discharge

Discharge after inpatient surgery for procedures suitable for day surgery usually occurs at least 24 hours after its completion. By then, there is little concern regarding postoperative complications or the adverse effects of the anaesthetic. In contrast, discharge on the day of surgery must address strict discharge criteria if complications are to be avoided. Before returning home, patients may be seen by the surgeon and anaesthetist involved in their care, but the final decision to discharge is usually nurse initiated, based on clear and agreed discharge guidelines. Some units adhere to strict scoring systems

Box 3.3 • Discharge criteria

Vital signs stable for at least 1 hour
Correct orientation as to time, place and person
Adequate pain control and supply of oral analgesia
Understanding the use of oral analgesia supplied, supported by written information
Ability to dress, walk (if appropriate)
Minimal nausea, vomiting or dizziness
Oral fluids taken
Minimal bleeding (or wound drainage)
Has passed urine (if appropriate)
Has a responsible escort for the homeward journey
Has a carer at home for next 24 hours
Written and verbal instructions given about postoperative care
Knows when to return for follow-up (if appropriate)
Emergency contact number supplied

that address vital signs, patient activity, postoperative nausea and vomiting (PONV), pain and bleeding,[32] but whether such regimented protocols offer any advantage over the checklist of criteria outlined in Box 3.3 is debatable. Generic criteria have their limitations. For example, the criterion of being able to 'walk unaided' from the day unit may be inappropriate following orthopaedic surgery to the foot. Common sense in such situations is clearly required and the individual surgical procedure or type of surgery undertaken may prompt additional specific criteria.[33]

How do we do it?

Developing and maintaining good practice in day surgery requires attention to detail in all aspects of anaesthetic and surgical care. Special considerations apply to management of children in the day unit.

Anaesthesia

Day surgery may be performed under four basic anaesthetic techniques: sedation, local, regional or general anaesthesia, with or without premedication. Where local or regional anaesthetic techniques can be applied safely, advantages arise both for the patient and for the efficient running of the service.

Premedication

In day surgery, premedication relates to any drugs administered in the day unit before the patient leaves for surgery and they are usually administered orally or rectally. There is a widely held belief that premedication sedatives for anxiety are unnecessary

in day surgery and, if given, recovery time may be prolonged. In most cases this is true, but up to 19% of patients suffer significant anxiety and these may benefit from sedative premedication.[34]

Other premedication drugs commonly used in day surgery include oral ranitidine 150 mg for known acid reflux and NSAIDs for postoperative pain if the procedure is of short duration. In addition, the patient's normal drug therapy, including antihypertensive agents, should be given as normal.

Sedation

Sedation, commonly used in dental and endoscopy practice, may be defined as 'a technique in which the use of a drug or drugs produces a state of depression of the central nervous system enabling treatment to be carried out, but during which verbal contact with the patient is maintained'.[35] Standards of monitoring for sedation in gastrointestinal endoscopy were published in 1991 and address safety issues such as the availability of resuscitation equipment and the safe use and administration of benzodiazepines.[36] Patient responses to sedative agents vary considerably and they should be titrated to the desired clinical effect to minimise overdose. Ideally, the sedationist should be an experienced anaesthetist. Monitoring during the procedure is mandatory and consists of pulse oximetry to measure oxygen saturation, an assessment of the patient's level of consciousness, and ECG and blood pressure monitoring, especially for patients with a history of ischaemic heart disease or cardiac arrhythmias. Oxygen supplementation is provided by oxygen mask or nasal cannulae.

In surgical practice, intravenous sedation should be kept simple and consists in adults of midazolam at a titrated dose of 0.07 mg/kg. Dosage is reduced in the elderly patient because hypotension and respiratory depression can occur. It is a better amnesic drug than diazepam and its solubility has reduced the incidence of pain on injection or phlebitis. As it has a short half-life of 2–4 hours, 'hangover' effects are reduced. If overdose occurs, the competitive benzodiazepine antagonist flumazenil is given, but as its half-life is only approximately 1 hour, it is important to recognise that re-sedation may occur and premature discharge of the patient must be avoided.

Sedo-analgesia is a combination of a benzodiazepine and an analgesic agent such as pethidine (meperidine) or morphine. It is often used in the more painful endoscopic procedures such as colonoscopy. The longer-acting traditional opioids are often now replaced by the more rapid onset short-acting agents such as fentanyl (50–200 µg i.v.), alfentanil and remifentanil, which act within several minutes.

Local and regional anaesthesia

As with sedation, perioperative monitoring is required and should include pulse oximetry, with ECG and blood pressure monitoring in the elderly or cardiovascularly unfit. Several local anaesthetic agents are available (Table 3.2) but toxic reactions can occur in overdosage. Toxic blood levels lead to circumoral tingling, tinnitus and dizziness. Serious overdosage is reflected in loss of consciousness, convulsions or cardiac dysrhythmia. Dosage levels therefore need to be controlled. Higher dosage can be administered if it is given with adrenaline (epinephrine; 1:200000), which causes vasoconstriction. This assists haemostasis, slow absorption and prolongs anaesthesia. The administration of adrenaline is contraindicated, however, in end-artery procedures such as in the penis or in the digits of the hand or feet.

Local or regional anaesthesia may be used alone, with sedation or with general anaesthesia to prolong pain relief after completion of the procedure. Cocaine, which also has vasoconstrictor properties, may be topically applied to the nasal mucosa prior to nasal surgery. Amethocaine (tetracaine), which is systemically toxic, is mainly used for topical anaesthesia in ophthalmology. Prilocaine is short acting, has less toxic levels in the blood and is useful in intravenous regional anaesthesia such as Bier's block. Field infiltration with local anaesthetic and adrenaline may be used for the removal of minor 'lumps and bumps'. Bupivacaine (and the newer ropivacaine) has a long duration of action, lasting several hours, but can take up to 30 minutes to achieve simple nerve block. It is therefore a useful adjunct for wound infiltration or nerve block in association with general anaesthesia.

Spinal anaesthesia is not widespread in UK day surgery practice, in contrast to many other parts of the world. The main advantage of spinal anaesthesia is for operations below the waist such as arthroscopic surgery on the knee, foot surgery, haemorrhoidectomy or other rectal surgery, neurological surgery and inguinal hernia repair. The principal reasons for selecting spinal anaesthesia are in the obese or those with cardiorespiratory disease who would otherwise be excluded from day surgery.[37]

General anaesthesia

The techniques and drugs used in general anaesthesia today permit up to 90 minutes of anaesthetic time for day surgery. The use of the laryngeal mask rather than the endotracheal tube has changed anaesthetic practice in day surgery since its introduction in 1988. Muscle relaxants are not required with its insertion, which is quicker and easier, and it is tolerated in light anaesthesia, allowing rapid patient turnaround. The introduction of total intravenous anaesthesia using propofol for induction and maintenance of anaesthesia has major advantages over inhalation agents; these include reduced PONV, early recovery and rapid control of the depth of anaesthesia, making it ideal for day case surgery. PONV after surgery is best prevented rather than treated, but is likely if surgery lasts more than 1 hour or involves laparoscopy, dental procedures, squint surgery or correction of bat ears.

✔✔ Adequate hydration reduces PONV and intravenous fluid should be administered during longer procedures. Intravenous fluids at a dose of 20 mL/kg significantly reduce the incidence of postoperative drowsiness and dizziness.[38]

Pain management during anaesthesia is based on a concept of multimodal analgesia, which is a combination of two or more analgesic agents or analgesic techniques to minimise side-effects. A common strategy is to use an NSAID or short-acting opioid in combination with regional or local anaesthesia. The administration of stronger opiates such as morphine and pethidine at this stage is to be avoided as its longer-lasting effects may lead to unplanned overnight admission. Administration of analgesia in recovery and on the day ward before discharge should be given before 'breakthrough' pain occurs

Table 3.2 • Dosage and application of local anaesthetic agents

| Agent | Dose (mg/kg) | | Application |
	Alone	With adrenaline	
Cocaine	–	–	Topical
Amethocaine (tetracaine)	–	–	Topical
Prilocaine	5	7	Intravenous regional anaesthesia
Lidocaine	3	5	Infiltration nerve blocks
Bupivacaine	1–2	1–2	Infiltration nerve blocks, spinal/epidural
Ropivacaine	1–2	1–2	Infiltration nerve blocks, spinal/epidural

and is based on the accurate measurement of pain by the patients themselves.

Surgery

The safe, effective and efficient surgery required for a day case procedure demands the competence of a trained surgeon, a consultant or an experienced specialist registrar. In the past, the day surgery list of intermediate procedures was delegated to the most junior surgical trainee to perform without supervision. Not surprisingly, this led to prolonged operating times, patient cancellations, increased complications and an inevitable rise in the unplanned overnight admission rate. As surgical trainees may no longer work unsupervised, such poor-quality practices should be features of the past. Nevertheless, some consultant surgeons' attitudes towards day surgery remain lukewarm, mainly because many have never considered the importance of their role in the overall delivery of patient care and the need for them to be more actively involved in the process of care through the hospital system. A frequent excuse was that the surgery itself was mundane and lacked the technical challenge of complex major procedures. With the introduction of more major minimal access procedures into the field of day surgery, this excuse no longer holds true. Indeed, many day surgery experts would contend that any intermediate or major surgery performed on a day case basis is a true surgical challenge if morbidity is to be maintained at near zero levels.

Day surgery rates for specific procedures still vary between individual surgeons, between hospitals and even between regions. In November 2011, there was still a 17% variation in day case rates for inguinal hernia repair and varicose vein surgery between the best and the worst performing Strategic Health Authorities (SHAs) in England, whilst the rates for day case laparoscopic cholecystectomy in all SHAs ranged from 23% to 56%![13] The reasons for such variations are complex and remain largely unexplained, but often reflect an inability to organise healthcare effectively and follow guidelines.[39–42]

Whilst these variations were understandable in the development phase of day surgery, they become increasingly difficult to justify as we move to a genuine National Healthcare system, with equal access to treatment for all. A new generation of surgeons and anaesthetists who are more familiar with the skills and techniques necessary to provide high-quality day surgery should ensure that most of these extreme variations disappear over the next few years.

Surgical practice: controversies
Laparoscopic cholecystectomy
The day case rate for laparoscopic cholecystectomy in the UK is just under 40% and still shows large variations between surgeons, trusts and regions.[13] The reasons for this relate to fears about reactionary haemorrhage, delayed haemorrhage and bile leak. Reactionary haemorrhage occurs within 4–6 hours after surgery and can be addressed within the ordinary working day if the surgery is performed before noon. Delayed haemorrhage usually occurs 3–4 days after cholecystectomy and even if the patient had undergone their operation as an inpatient, they would still have gone home before the secondary haemorrhage was apparent. Bile leaks rarely become apparent before 48 hours after surgery: accessory duct injury is often insidious, diathermy injury to the biliary tree may take days to leak and cystic duct stump leakage likewise. Again, if the patient had undergone inpatient surgery the likelihood is that they would already have been discharged home. It is therefore more important to warn these patients of possible delayed complications and that they should seek medical review in the first few days after discharge if alarm symptoms such as abdominal pain, nausea and vomiting occur. The NHS Institute published a clinical pathway in 2007 which noted that 70% of laparoscopic cholecystectomies could be safely performed as day cases[40] and this target has been recommended to NHS commissioners as part of the 18-week programme.[43]

Successful day case laparoscopic cholecystectomy relies on rigorous patient selection, accepting only well-motivated and non-obese patients, and attention to detailed surgical technique. Patients require approximately 6 hours of recovery time and the procedure is best performed early in the operating day.

✔ Age greater than 50 and ASA class II and III are poor prognostic indicators.[44,45]

Good operative technique is also relevant when creating the pneumoperitoneum, as carbon dioxide inadvertently placed in the extraperitoneal space can cause considerable discomfort. Shoulder tip pain from diaphragmatic irritation has been related to the size of the gas bubble under the diaphragm[46] and attempts should therefore be made to expel as much gas as possible at the end of the procedure. Blood in the peritoneal cavity is an irritant, and liver bed haemostasis and peritoneal lavage before exiting the abdomen are worthwhile. While much of the postoperative pain in laparoscopic cholecystectomy is deep in nature, laparoscopy port sites should always be infiltrated with a long-acting local anaesthetic (such as bupivacaine). There appears to be little difference between infiltration at the beginning or the end of the procedure.[47]

Prostatectomy

For benign prostatic disease, the current national day case rate for laser ablation is 10% and for transurethral resection is just over 1%, although the rates are 30% in London and 10% in south central England.[13] Patients requiring prostatectomy tend to be older and less fit and many have previously been excluded from day surgery by their comorbidity. Conventional transurethral resection of the prostate (TURP) can be performed as a day case but postoperative haemorrhage remains a problem. Over the last decade, laser prostatectomy day case programmes have been developed,[48,49] with the patients discharged with a catheter in situ, returning to the day unit approximately 1 week later for trial without catheter. Some units now perform over 90% of prostatectomies as day cases.[50]

Head and neck

> ✅ In the UK, 6% of tonsillectomies are performed on a day case basis due to worries about reactionary haemorrhage. This risk is small and in a series of 668 adults and children undergoing day case tonsillectomy in Salisbury, the reactionary haemorrhage rate was 0.3%, each occurring within the first 6–8 hours after the operation while the patient was still on the day unit.[51]

Secondary haemorrhage occurs in approximately 1% of post-tonsillectomy patients and occurs several days after discharge, but may cause rapid airway obstruction at home with fatal consequences. The Salisbury Unit has a high readmission rate of 6% that reflects their policy of readmitting even minor bleeds for 24 hours in case they herald a more major bleed.

Similarly, parathyroid surgery has not been deemed suitable for day case surgery because of the risk of haemorrhage and hypocalcaemia. Nevertheless, McLaren and colleagues have demonstrated high and safe day surgery rates in patients with positive preoperative localisation.[52]

Bariatric and other surgery

Bariatric or weight loss surgery is increasingly performed in the UK, as a result of the growing number of morbidly obese in the population who fail to respond to dietary methods or exercise. Obesity is a risk factor for any surgery,[17] but shorter, minimal access procedures such as laparoscopic gastric banding have been performed successfully as day case procedures,[53] the limiting criteria being the 150-kg weight limit of most operating trolleys. Of greater significance is perhaps the implied message that BMI should no longer be seen as a limiting factor in the delivery of day surgery generally.

Other areas of surgery are developing fast-track or short-stay admissions as a preferred clinical pathway for their patients, for the same reasons surgeons applied day surgery techniques 30 years ago for hernia and paediatric surgery: when delivered to a high standard, safely and efficiently, patients and providers benefit. Kehlet described his experience in developing enhanced recovery programmes in colorectal surgery a decade ago and the principles have been extended to broader aspects of surgery.[54,55] Clinicians using techniques as diverse as abdominoplasty, colorectal cancer surgery, thoracic surgery and even endovascular aortic grafting are now using these techniques to shorten lengths of stay while enhancing patient care.[56–59]

Recovery

Upon completion of anaesthesia at the end of a surgical procedure, the patient is transferred to the operating theatre recovery area known as 'first-stage recovery'. Formerly, patients remained here for a predetermined period, commonly 30 or 60 minutes. However, the development of short-acting anaesthetic agents, the introduction of minimally invasive surgical techniques and individual patient variability meant that patients were often ready for transfer to 'second-stage recovery' before their predetermined time. Therefore, 'time-based recovery' is no longer necessary and has in many units been superseded by 'criteria-based recovery', where discharge is determined by the observations of stable vital signs, return of protective reflexes and the ability to obey commands.[60] 'Second-stage recovery' occurs back in the ward or trolley area of the day unit itself, where patients recover sufficiently to allow safe discharge home. Certain patients may be suitable for direct transfer to second-stage recovery from the operating theatre itself (**Fig. 3.3**) and include patients who have received local or regional anaesthesia with or without minimal sedation.

Postoperative instructions and discharge

Before leaving the day unit, patients require specific information regarding their medication, wound care and when they are able to bath or shower, arrangements for suture removal or dressing renewal, when they can resume normal activities and arrangements for follow-up (if appropriate). It is also important to offer a contact telephone number for emergency purposes on the night of discharge. In addition, patients must be clearly instructed not to drive a motor vehicle for at least 24 hours.[61] Appropriate preoperative information may also have a beneficial effect on return to work after surgery.[62]

Figure 3.3 • Staged patient recovery.

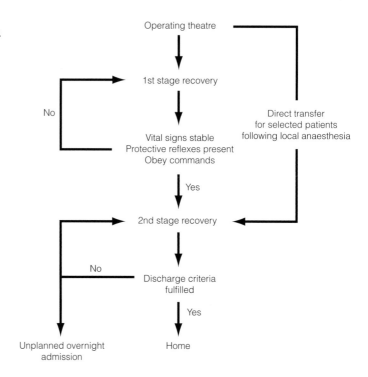

The most common reason for a patient visiting their general practitioner after day surgery is to obtain certification for time off work. The second commonest reason, usually in an unplanned manner, relates to worries about their wound. After discharge, many day surgery units therefore offer outreach or telephone follow-up for their patients 24 hours later. This can be an effective evaluation tool, where any identified actual or potential problems can be highlighted to the day surgery team for action. This may only be necessary after specialised surgery (e.g. cataract surgery, where a change of dressing can be combined with outreach follow-up) or after the introduction of an unfamiliar procedure to the unit.

Postoperative complications

Precise patient selection should ensure that postoperative morbidity is minimised, but complications do occur and can be classified into major and minor problems.[63] Major complications occur less often than anticipated in the day surgery patient population with an incidence of 1 in 1455[64] and are independent of ASA status. Mortality is low and varies between 1 in 66500 and 1 in 11273.

Minor complications are more common and may precipitate unplanned overnight admission; these range from 0.1% to 5% depending on case mix.[65] Postoperative morbidity is usually related to the procedure undertaken and the anaesthetic agent used rather than the ASA status, which predicts complications in major inpatient surgery but not in day surgery patients. Surgical causes account for 60–70% of unplanned admissions and are usually the result of the surgeon embarking on a more extensive procedure than planned rather than surgical misadventure. Day surgery lists require careful planning, with the more major surgical procedures performed earlier in the day to allow adequate recovery time. Failure to adhere to this policy often leads to unplanned admissions.[66] The more lengthy and invasive surgical procedures tend to increase postoperative pain, PONV and drowsiness, and preclude safe discharge. Even once the patient has returned home, PONV may return and last up to 5 days in 35% of patients[67] and is often severe. Readmission rates are similar to unplanned admission rates (0.7–3.1%) and again are most often from surgically related causes.

Paediatric day surgery

Children find surgery and hospital visits a daunting and stressful prospect, and are therefore treated both separately and differently from adults. In 1991, the National Association for the Welfare of Children in Hospital published quality standards for care of paediatric day cases and suggested that children should be managed by staff trained in their care, in a child-safe and child-friendly environment with open access to the conscious child for the parents.[68] As a result, excellent results have been reported from non-specialised District General Hospitals as long as regular auditing of quality is practised.[69]

Most children are fit and healthy ASA class I patients. ASA class II and III patients are not excluded but an anaesthetist with paediatric expertise is recommended.[15] Procedures for children with respiratory infections should be postponed for 2–4 weeks depending on severity, but after measles or whooping cough this should be extended to 6 weeks because of irritability of the respiratory tract.[70] In many units, children under the age of 6 months are considered unsuitable for day surgery, but if specialist facilities are available, full-term neonates are acceptable provided inpatient neonatal care is available. Premature babies are excluded up to 60 weeks after conception because of the risk of postoperative apnoea.[71] Many units also exclude children who are less than 5 kg because of the risk of hypothermia or hypoglycaemia associated with their physical status.

Psychosocial factors also determine a child's suitability for day surgery, and may limit access to day surgery especially in single parents with many children and little support, or very timid children with overly anxious parents.

Therefore, while the range of surgical procedures undertaken is similar to adult day surgery, in children it is often confined to a more restricted list (Box 3.4). In the anaesthetic room, venous access is obtained after the application of topical local anaesthetic 1 hour before; parental presence in the anaesthetic room is useful, especially in the preschool group. Postoperative pain relief is obtained first through adjunctive local or regional anaesthesia. NSAIDs cannot be given to children under 1 year of age or 10 kg in weight because of their immature kidneys, but paracetamol is effective if given in a premedication dose of 20 mg/kg. Before discharge, the parents require clear instructions regarding pain control, wound care, mobilisation and resumption of normal activities.

What will happen next?

The shift of elective surgery from the inpatient setting to short stay and eventually day care is now inexorable and will continue to be driven by three factors. The first and most important is the natural dislike in most people of in-hospital stays, accelerated by the growing fear of hospital-acquired infections; most people prefer to be at home, and as soon as a day surgery procedure can be shown to be performed as safely and effectively as in the traditional inpatient setting, most of us will opt for the former.

The second drive for change is the continued growth of minimal access techniques, including the use of robotics and the development of natural orifice transluminal endoscopic surgery (NOTES).[72] These techniques are associated with less surgical trauma and reduced postoperative pain both in the short and medium term, and have led to the concept of 'fast-track' surgery for inpatient procedures.[54] The concomitant development of better anaesthetic and pain-relieving techniques will further reduce the need for inpatient postoperative care.

The third and greatest factor currently driving change is that of healthcare costs. By dispensing with inpatient hotel costs including staffing, procedures performed as day cases offer significant cost savings to healthcare providers and purchasers, and the impact of this can be seen in many areas:

- **Emergency surgery.** There has been a significant growth in emergency and urgent surgery now being performed in the ambulatory setting, which reduces costs as well as avoiding the reported postponements that occur in the inpatient setting. Recent studies have shown that care of these patients in the day unit can be preferable to inpatient care.[73,74]
- **Short stay and enhanced recovery.** New research and developments in enhanced recovery are enabling the performance of more complex and advanced day surgery in patients who are anaesthetically more challenging.[54–59,75] This allows the high standards of care explicit in day surgery to be applied to early recovery and mobilisation, and discharge in these cases can usually take place in under 72 hours.

Box 3.4 • Paediatric day surgery procedures

General surgery
Herniotomy, hydrocele excision, examination under anaesthesia, anal stretch, excision of minor lumps and bumps, ingrowing toenail treatment, endoscopy, biopsy (rectal, skin, lymph node)

Urology
Circumcision and associated procedures, orchidopexy

ENT
Myringotomy/grommets, adenoidectomy, tonsillectomy

Dental
Extractions

Ophthalmology
Correction of squint

Orthopaedic
Change of plaster cast

- **Tariffs and commissioning.** We have seen how much variability in day case rates persists across the UK.[13] New funding rules are likely to have beneficial effects on this 'postcode lottery'. The impact of payment by results is already changing the way in which hospital trusts perceive day surgery, and its role in the delivery of elective care.[76] The added impact of both primary care commissioning[77] and tariffs that financially penalise organisations performing inpatient rather than day case procedures is accelerating the shift to day care.[78,79]

Key points

- The UK government targeted 75% of all elective surgery to be performed on a day case basis by the end of 2005.
- All elective surgical patients should be pre-assessed by a nurse-led pre-assessment team who make the decision to allocate the patient to 12-hour, 23-hour or inpatient surgery.
- Day surgery should be independent and separate from the inpatient infrastructure as successful day surgery depends on day of surgery admission, pre-assessment and nurse-led discharge.
- Regional and local anaesthetic block techniques are ideal for day surgery but are currently underutilised.
- Major surgical procedures, such as laparoscopic cholecystectomy, TURP, bilateral varicose vein surgery and arthroscopic procedures, can now be performed safely and routinely as day cases.

References

1. Department of Health. The NHS plan: a plan for investment, a plan for reform. London: Department of Health; 2000.

2. Department of Health. Day surgery: operational guide. London: Department of Health; 2002.
   The Department of Health operational guide for day surgery helps day surgery units achieve 75% elective surgery on a day case basis and covers aspects of patient selection, day surgery activity, day surgery accommodation, management and staffing.

3. Nicholl JH. The surgery of infancy. Br Med J 1909;ii:753–6.

4. Waters RM. The downtown anesthesia clinic. Am J Surg 1919;33(Suppl):71–3.

5. Asher RAJ. The dangers of going to bed. Br Med J 1947;ii:967–8.

6. Palumbo LT, Laul RE, Emery FB. Results of primary inguinal hernioplasty. Arch Surg 1952;64:384–94.

7. Farquharson EL. Early ambulation with special references to herniorrhaphy as an outpatient procedure. Lancet 1955;ii:517–9.

8. Baskerville PA, Jarrett PEM. Day case inguinal hernia repair under local anaesthetic. Ann R Coll Surg Engl 1983;65:224–5.

9. Royal College of Surgeons of England. Report of the working party for day case surgery. London: RCS; 1992.

10. NHS Management Executive. A study of the management and utilisation of operating departments. London: HMSO; 1989.

11. Audit Commission. A short cut to better services: day surgery in England and Wales. London: HMSO; 1990.

12. Audit Commission. Measuring quality: the patient's view of day surgery. London: HMSO; 1991.

13. NHS Institute for Innovation and Improvement. Website: www.productivity.nhs.uk/Dashboard/For/National/And/25th/Percentile [accessed 01.08.12].
    This section enables comparative assessments between health authority sites in England (not Scotland or Wales) for a large number of procedures.

14. British Association of Day Surgery. BADS directory of procedures. 3rd ed. London: BADS; 2009.

15. Verma R, Alladi R, Jackson I, et al. Day case and short stay surgery: 2. Anaesthesia 2011;66:417–34.

16. Fogg KJ, Saunders PRI. Folly! The long distance day surgery patient. Ambul Surg 1995;3:209–10.

17. National Institutes of Health. Clinical guidelines on the identification, evaluation, and treatment of overweight and obesity in adults – evidence report. Obesity Res 1998;6(Suppl. 2):51S–209S.

18. Department of Health. Annual health statistics. London: Department of Health; 2010.

19. Miller JM. Selection and investigation of adult day cases. In: Miller JM, Rudkin GE, Hitchcock M, editors. Practical anaesthesia and analgesia for day surgery. Oxford: BIOS Scientific; 1997. p. 5–16.

20. Davies KE, Houghton K, Montgomery J. Obesity and day case surgery. Anaesthesia 2001;56:1090–115.

21. Myles PS, Iacono GA, Hunt JO, et al. Risks of respiratory complications and wound infection in patients undergoing ambulatory surgery: smokers versus non-smokers. Anesthesiology 2002;97:842–7.

22. Buist AS, Sexton GJ, Magy JM, et al. The effect of smoking cessation and modification on lung function. Am Rev Respir Dis 1976;114:115–22.

23. Stechman MJ, Healy J, McMillan R, et al. Is current advice on smoking prior to day surgery in the UK appropriate? J One Day Surg 2004;14:5–8.

24. American Society of Anesthesiology. ASA classification of surgical patients. Chicago: American Society of Anesthesiology; 1991.
A definitive classification of comorbidity by the American Society of Anesthesiology that has become universally accepted to assess fitness for anaesthesia.

25. Ansel GL, Montgomery J. Outcome of ASA III patients undergoing day case surgery. Br J Anaesth 2004;92:71–4.

26. Watson B, Smith I, Jennings A, et al. Day surgery and the diabetic patient. London: British Association of Day Surgery; 2002.

27. Howell SJ, Sear JW, Foex P. Hypertension, hypertensive heart disease and perioperative cardiac risk. Br J Anaesth 2004;92:570–83.
A systematic review and meta-analysis of 30 observational studies demonstrated no association between admission arterial pressure when less than 180 mmHg systolic and 110 mmHg diastolic and perioperative complications. This evidence indicates that patients whose blood pressure is elevated within these limits can undergo routine safe surgery without cancellation.

28. Committee on Safety of Medicines. Avoid all NSAIDs in aspirin sensitive patients. Curr Prob Pharmacovig 1993;19:8.

29. Li JT. The quality of caring. Mayo Clin Proc 2006;81:294–6.

30. Carlisle J. Guidelines for pre-operative testing. J One Day Surg 2004;14:13–6.

31. Gold BS, Young ML, Kinman JL, et al. The utility of preoperative electrocardiograms in the ambulatory surgical patient. Arch Intern Med 1992;152:301–5.

32. Aldrete BA. The Post-anaesthesia Recovery Score revisited. J Clin Anesth 1995;7:89–91.

33. Cahill H, Jackson I, McWhinme D. Ready to go home? London: British Association of Day Surgery; 2000. p. 1–8.

34. Mackenzie JW. Day case anaesthesia and anxiety. Anaesthesia 1989;44:437–40.

35. Wylie report. Report of the Working Party on Training in Dental Anaesthesia. Br Dent J 1981;151:385–8.

36. Bell GD, McCloy RF, Charlton JE, et al. Recommendations for standards of sedation and patient monitoring during gastrointestinal endoscopy. Gut 1991;32:823–7.

37. Watson B, Allen J, Smith I. Spinal anaesthesia: a practical guide. London: British Association of Day Surgery; 2004.

38. Yogendran S, Asokumar B, Cheng DC, et al. A prospective randomised double blinded study of the effect of intravenous fluid therapy on adverse outcomes on outpatient surgery. Anaesth Analg 1995;80:682–6.
Two hundred ASA grade I–III ambulatory surgical patients were prospectively randomised into two groups to receive high (20 mL/kg) or low (2 mL/kg) prospective isotonic infusion over 30 minutes preoperatively. The incidence of thirst, drowsiness and dizziness was significantly lower in the high-infusion group 60 minutes after surgery, confirming an advantage to routine perioperative intravenous fluid administration.

39. Department of Health. 10 high impact changes for service improvement and delivery. NHS Modernisation Agency; 2004.

40. NHS Institute for Innovation and Improvement. Focus on: Cholecystectomy. 2007.

41. Association of Anaesthetists of Great Britain and Ireland. Preoperative assessment and patient preparation – the role of the anaesthetist 2. London: AAGBI; 2010.

42. Orchard M, Ellms J, McWhinnie D. What do we mean by 'theatre utilisation'? J One Day Surg 2010;20:4–6.

43. Department of Health. Tackling hospital waiting: the 18 week patient pathway. London: Department of Health; 2006.

44. Robinson TN, Biffl WL, Moore EE. Predicting failure of outpatient laparoscopic cholecystectomy. Am J Surg 2002;184:515–8.

45. Lau H, Brookes DC. Predictive factors for unanticipated admission after ambulatory laparoscopic cholecystectomy. Arch Surg 2001;136:1150–3.

46. Jackson SA, Lawrence AS, Hill JC. Does post laparoscopy pain relate to residual carbon dioxide? Anaesthesia 1996;51:485–7.

47. Mjaland O, Raeder J, Aasboe V, et al. Outpatient laparoscopic cholecystectomy. Br J Surg 1997;84:958–61.

48. Keoghane SR, Millar JM, Cranston DW. Is day case prostatectomy feasible? Br J Urol 1995;76:600–3.

49. Gomez Sancha F, Bachmann A, Choi BB, et al. Photoselective vaporization of the prostate (Greenlight PV): lessons learnt after 3500 procedures. Prostate Cancer Prostatic Dis 2007;10(4):316–22.

50. Urological recommended lengths of stay. BADS directory of procedures. 2nd ed. 2007. p. 16–7.

51. Dennis S, Georgallow M, Elcock L, et al. Day case tonsillectomy: the Salisbury experience. J One Day Surg 2004;14:17–22.

52. Parameswaram R, Allouni K, Varghese P, et al. Day case parathyroidectomy in a district hospital: safe and feasible. J One Day Surg 2010;20(1):20–2.

53. Dunsire MF, Patel AG, Awad N, et al. Laparoscopic gastric banding for morbid obesity in the day surgery setting. J One Day Surg 2007;17:1.

54. Kehlet H, Wilmore DW. Fast track surgery. Br J Surg 2005;92:3–4.

55. Houghton K. Enhanced recovery and ray surgery: the ultimate partners for elective surgery. J One Day Surg 2010;20:4–6.

56. Salman R, Salman A. Outpatient abdominoplasty: is it a safe practice? J One Day Surg 2009;(Suppl)28.

57. Wong T, Shekouh A, Wilkin R, et al. Day case colon and rectal cancer surgery: are we ready for take-off? J One Day Surg 2009;(Suppl.):A23.

58. Chieza JT, Found P, Rajagopal K, et al. Ambulatory thoracic surgery: setting up a service and the first 100 cases. J One Day Surg 2010;(Suppl.):A10.

59. Flindall IR, Ward S, Day A, et al. EVAR – reducing length of stay and costs. J One Day Surg 2009;(Suppl.):A21.

60. Association of Anaesthetists of Great Britain and Ireland. Immediate postanaesthetic recovery. London: AAGBI; 2002.

61. Chung F, Kayumov L, Sinclair DR, et al. What is the driving performance of ambulatory surgical patients after general anaesthesia? Anesthiology 2005;103:951–6.

62. Crook TB, Banerjee S, De Souza K, et al. Supplementary preoperative information encourages return to work after inguinal hernia repair. J One Day Surg 2005;15(1):18–20.

63. Natof HE. Complications. In: Wetcher BV, editor. Anaesthesia for ambulatory surgery. Philadelphia: Lippincott; 1985. p. 321.

64. Hitchcock M. Postoperative morbidity following day surgery. In: Millar JM, Rudkin GE, Hitchcock M, editors. Practical anaesthesia and analgesia for day surgery. Oxford: BIOS Scientific; 1997. p. 205–11.

65. Levy ML. Complications: prevention and quality assurance. Anesth Clin North Am 1987;5:137–66.

66. Twersky RS, Abiona M, Thorne AC, et al. Admissions following ambulatory surgery: outcome in seven urban hospitals. Ambul Surg 1995;3:141–6.

67. Carrol NV, Miederhoff P, Cox FM, et al. Postoperative nausea and vomiting after discharge from outpatient surgery centres. Anesth Analg 1995;80:903–9.

68. Thornes R. Just for the day. London: National Association for the Welfare of Children in Hospital; March 1991.

69. Rees S, Stocker M, Montgomery J. Paediatric outcomes in a District General Hospital Day Surgery Unit. J One Day Surg 2009;19:92–5.

70. McEwan AI, Birch M, Bingham R. The preoperative management of the child with a heart murmur. Paediatr Anaesth 1995;5:151–5.

71. Steward DJ. Preterm infants are more prone to complications following minor surgery than are term infants. Anesthesiology 1982;56:304–6.

72. Buyske J. Natural orifice transluminal endoscopic surgery. JAMA 2007;298:1560–1.

73. Conaghan PL, Figueira E, Griffin MA, et al. Randomised clinical trial of the effectiveness of emergency day surgery against standard inpatient treatment. Br J Surg 2002;89:423–7.

74. Mayall AC, Barnes SJ, Stocker ME. Introducing emergency surgery to the day case setting. J One Day Surg 2009;19:23–6.

75. Smith I, McWhinnie D, Jackson I, editors. Day case surgery. Oxford: Oxford Specialist Handbooks; 2011.

76. Department of Health. Payment by Results 2010/11. http://www.dh.gov.uk/en/Managingyourorganisation/Financeandplanning/NHSFinancialReforms/index.htm [accessed 01.08.12].

77. British Association of Day Surgery. Commissioning day surgery. London: BADS; 2003.

78. Howard D, Yao S, Wasey J, et al. Incentivising day-case laparoscopic surgery. J One Day Surg 2011;21:4–7.

79. Kreckler S, McWhinnie D, Khaira H, et al. Running a financially viable hernia service in the era of best practice tariffs. J One Day Surg 2012;22:20–2.

4

Abdominal hernias

Andrew C. de Beaux

Introduction

A hernia is defined as an abnormal protrusion of a cavity's contents, through a weakness in the wall of the cavity, taking with it all the linings of the cavity, although these may be markedly attenuated. The anterior abdominal wall can be divided into two structural/functional zones: the upper 'parachute area' aiding respiratory movement and a lower 'belly support' area. Functional failure in the abdomen may lead to epigastric and umbilical hernia in the upper zone and to inguinal and femoral hernia in the lower zone. The external abdominal hernia is the commonest form of hernia, the most frequent varieties being the inguinal (75%), umbilical (15%) and femoral (8.5%).

Hernias can be described as reducible, incarcerated or strangulated. A reducible hernia is one in which the contents of the hernial sac can be manually introduced back into the abdomen while, conversely, an irreducible or incarcerated hernia cannot be manipulated back into the abdomen. A strangulated hernia occurs when the vascular supply to the contents contained within the hernia is compromised, resulting in ischaemic and gangrenous tissue.

Aetiology

Multiple factors contribute to the development of hernias. Hernias are associated with a number of medical conditions, including connective tissue disorders such as Ehlers–Danlos syndrome, as well as a number of abnormal collagen-related disorders

such as varicose veins and arterial aneurysm. In essence, hernias can be considered design faults, either anatomical or through inherited collagen disorders, although these two aetiological factors probably work together in the majority of patients. Anatomical design faults can be considered at any site where structures within the cavity exit through an opening in the wall of the cavity, such as blood vessels, bowel or the spermatic cord. This is typical, for example, around the oesophagus and in the groin. However, not everyone develops a groin hernia so other factors must be important. The fascia and surrounding tissues that cover muscle, acting to hold the muscle bundles together, may appear relatively avascular, but it remains a complex and living structure. The genetic code for fascia is coded on DNA, and within fibroblasts the sequence is messenger RNA, transfer RNA, peptide formation, with fusion of peptides into approximately 1000-amino-acid polypeptides called alpha chains. The endoplasmic reticulum converts these to procollagen. Procollagen is the large building block of collagen, comprising triple-helix strands, stabilised by hydroxylation of proline and lysine, which is vitamin C dependent. These triple-helix strands form microfibrils, then fibrils, then fibres and finally bundles. These collagen bundles surrounded by extracellular matrix comprise fascia. The control of this process is mediated through matrix metalloproteinases, which in turn are controlled by tissue inhibitory metalloproteinases. If this is not complex enough, there is also control by collagen-interacting proteins and receptors such as fibronectin, tenasin and collagen receptor discoidin domain receptor 2.

Fascia and tendon are made up of type I and type III collagen (type II is found in cartilage and type IV in the basement membrane of cells). In cross-section, there is a bimodal distribution of bundle size. The larger bundles are type I collagen, imparting the strength to the fascia or tendon. The type III collagen bundles are smaller and are thought to provide elastic recoil following stretch when the tissues have been loaded. The type I to III collagen ratio varies between individuals but is constant in all the fascia of a particular individual.

A clinical observation was made by surgeons in the late 1960s that the anterior rectus sheath some distance from the hernial defect was thinner than normal, especially in those patients with direct hernias.[1] Since then, research has demonstrated a variety of defects in collagen synthesis in such patients.[2,3] The current notion is that the majority of hernias are a disease of collagen metabolism. One of the key factors in this is the type I to III collagen ratio. The lower this ratio, from an average of around 5, the more likely the individual is to develop a hernia. Currently, collagen typing is not used in clinical practice to help decide perhaps which patients merit a mesh as opposed to a suture repair, but this may well be a development in the near future.

✔ Hernias are a collagen disease, with reduced collagen type I to III ratio.[2,3]

Mesh

Much will be mentioned about mesh repairs of hernias in the remainder of this chapter, but this section gives a brief overview of mesh and its science.

Many companies produce a variety of mesh for hernia repair. These are either synthetic (man made) or biological (preparations from animal or human tissue). The majority of synthetic meshes are woven from either polypropylene or polyester. Biological meshes are typically animal collagen, either from skin or bowel, but there are also human preparations. Biological meshes tend to be much more expensive and are thus reserved for specialist use.

It goes without saying that any mesh should have the usual properties of any implant, including being non-allergenic, non-carcinogenic, have good incorporation into tissue and mimic the tissue it is replacing or reinforcing. The abdominal wall is not a rigid structure, but regularly copes with increases in abdominal pressure on coughing and sneezing, etc. of up to 200 mmHg. The abdominal wall elasticity is greater in women than in men and is greater in the craniocaudal direction than transversely or obliquely. The traditional standard weight polypropylene mesh, of around 100 g/m², is significantly over-engineered, with a burst strength at least an order of magnitude greater than the anterior abdominal wall and an elasticity of much less.[4] As a result there are now many polypropylene meshes on the market of lighter weight. There are no strict definitions of light weight and heavy weight but a reasonable guideline is that mesh of 40–80 g/m² is medium weight and <40 g/m² is light weight. However, it is not just the weight of the mesh that imparts elasticity and flexibility. The weave of the strands in the mesh may impart varying flexibility or elasticity to the mesh in different directions of pull, so-called anisotropy. Pore size or the size of the large holes in the mesh is also important. Mesh has a volume with length, breadth and thickness. The amount of empty space within the 'volume' of the mesh is the porosity and the effective porosity is the amount of empty space within the volume of the mesh made up of holes that are bigger than 1 mm diameter. It has recently been proposed that an effective porosity of a mesh for hernia repair should be at least 60%.[5] Fibrosis will occur around each strand of the mesh. If the strands are close together, the fibrosis around each strand will coalesce together, forming a solid scar plate. As the scar plate matures it will shrink, reducing the overall size of the mesh. The minimum pore size should be about 1 mm² but many meshes have pore sizes around 3–5 mm. Increasing the macroporosity of the mesh produces a scar net, rather than a scar plate, with normal tissue in between the fibre/scar complex, reducing mesh/scar shrinkage and improving flexibility (**Fig. 4.1**). In addition to the macropore size, mesh also has micropores within the mesh material itself. These should be at least 10 μm in size. If the micropore size is smaller, bacteria can harbour in the pores out of reach of the larger inflammatory cells.

The majority of synthetic meshes in the UK are polypropylene. Gore-tex and other polytetrafluoroethylene (PTFE)-based meshes also have some popularity. PTFE has no macropores so will be encapsulated by fibrous tissue with minimal tissue ingrowth. Polyester-based meshes are gaining popularity and have some advantages over polypropylene but are multifilament rather than monofilament. The multifilament arrangement increases the developed surface of the mesh (around 2000 mm² per cm² mesh as compared to 200 mm² per cm² for polypropylene) and thus improves tissue incorporation. As a result, the peel strength (the effort required to separate the mesh from the tissues once it is incorporated) is greater, in the region of 190 N as compared to 160 N for a polypropylene mesh (**Fig. 4.2**).

There is increasing evidence that lightweight, large pore mesh is of benefit to the patient.[6] Although there are some reports that suggest the recurrence

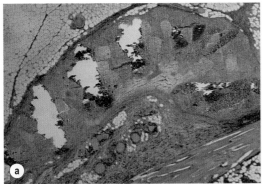

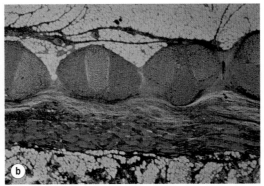

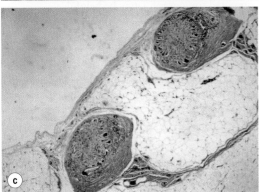

Figure 4.1 • **(a)** Micrograph of a macropore mesh of <0.5mm pore size showing scar plate formation and contraction/distortion of the mesh. **(b)** Micrograph of a macropore mesh of 0.8mm pore size showing minimal scar bridging and no distortion of the mesh. **(c)** Micrograph of a macropore mesh of 3mm pore size showing scar net formation and no contraction/distortion of the mesh. Micrographs used by permission of Covidien UK.

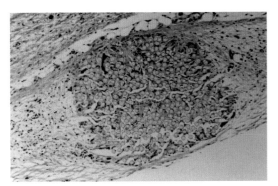

Figure 4.2 • Micrograph of a polyester mesh fibre. There is evidence of fibrosis around the fibre bundle as well as fibrous ingrowth around each strand. Micrograph used by permission of Covidien UK.

rate may be higher[7] when such mesh is used, it is likely that this is due to technical reasons. Fixation sutures on such mesh should be placed at least 1 cm in from the edge of the mesh and slightly larger meshes may need to be used.

✔ Preferred mesh should be lightweight (<80 g/m²), large pore (>1 mm) and macroporous (>10 µm).[6]

Traditional meshes placed within the abdominal cavity have a high rate of adhesions of the omentum and bowel to the mesh. This can result in bowel fistulation or make subsequent laparotomy more difficult, with increased risk of bowel perforation and thus the need for bowel resection during the process of re-entering the abdominal cavity.[8] A number of tissue-separating meshes are available, where the intra-abdominal side of the mesh is coated with a product to minimise adhesion formation. It would be fair to say that while such coatings do reduce adhesion formation, in the majority of patients significant adhesion to such coatings still occurs. The main points of adhesion appear to be the edge of the mesh and to the points of fixation, either sutures, tacks or staples. Nevertheless, it is likely that these products will improve in the future, as meshes become more physiological, perhaps impregnated with growth hormones and other biologically active molecules to improve the mesh/tissue integration.

Biological mesh (a slight misnomer as most biological meshes are really sheets of collagen) has gained popularity in hernia repair. It is, however, disappointing that, from the thousands of biological meshes that have been implanted worldwide (often at great expense as biological mesh is 10–100 times more expensive than polypropylene mesh), follow-up data on only just a few hundred patients have been published.

What is becoming evident, though, is that biological meshes are not all the same. The major difference, in addition to the animal and anatomical source of the mesh, is the degree of chemical processing, or crosslinking, of the biological product. The more the collagen is crosslinked, the more resistant it is to bacterial collagenase breakdown in the presence of infection. The downside to crosslinking is that the more the collagen is crosslinked, the less tissue ingrowth and integration occurs, with reduction in potential strength to the repair. It is becoming evident that most biological meshes have no role in dirty wounds, acting as little more than a very expensive dressing. They are too expensive for use in clean wounds as any benefit is not worth the huge price difference, and using them for bridging (mesh spanning the fascial gap as opposed to augmentation, where the mesh reinforces or augments the fascial closure) also results in a high percentage of failure. The author's opinion is that there is no good evidence available to suggest that biological mesh is superior or even as good as polypropylene in clean/contaminated operations. Similarly, there is a lack of comparative evidence in contaminated operations, although fortunately this is a very small part of hernia surgery.

Epigastric hernia

An epigastric hernia is defined as a fascial defect in the linea alba between the xiphoid process and the umbilicus. The true incidence is unknown but autopsy studies have suggested a prevalence of 0.5–10% in the general population. There is a male preponderance, with a male to female ratio of approximately 4:1, with the diagnosis usually being made in the third to fifth decades.

Aetiology

The aetiology is related to the functional anatomy of the 'parachute area'. The anterior abdominal wall aponeurosis consists of tendinous fibres that lie obliquely in aponeurotic sheets, allowing for changes in the shape of the abdominal wall, for example during respiration. However, the midline can change only in length and breadth, an increase in one necessitating a decrease in the other. During abdominal distension, the linea alba must increase in both dimensions, the resulting tearing of fibres possibly leading to the development of an epigastric hernia.

Clinical presentation

The majority of epigastric hernias (probably 75%) are asymptomatic. Typical symptoms, if present, include vague upper abdominal pain and nausea associated with epigastric tenderness. The symptoms tend to be more severe when the patient is lying down, attributed to traction on the hernial contents. Pain on exertion localised to the epigastrium is also a common symptom. Incarceration is common, and strangulation of pre-peritoneal fat or omentum results in localised pain and tenderness. Incarceration or strangulation of intra-abdominal viscera is extremely rare, the symptoms obviously depending on the incarcerated organ.

The presence of a midline mass on physical examination usually confirms the diagnosis. In obese patients, palpation of the mass may be difficult and confirmation of the diagnosis by ultrasound or computed tomography may be helpful.

Management

Epigastric hernias are rare in infants and children, and asymptomatic hernias in children under the age of 10 years may resolve spontaneously. The decision for surgical intervention depends on the presence and severity of symptoms.

Operative details

Small solitary defects may be approached with either a vertical or transverse incision in the midline, centred over the hernia. For larger hernias, if the defects are multiple or in the emergency setting when a strangulated viscus is suspected, a vertical incision is preferred. The hernia and its contents are dissected free of the surrounding tissues and, if present, the hernial contents examined and dealt with appropriately. If the defect is small (<2 cm), repair by primary suture closure using non-absorbable material is usually sufficient. The orientation of the suture closure remains controversial, some surgeons preferring a vertical closure and others a horizontal orientation. There are very few data to support one technique over the other and probably the direction resulting in the least tension is the most appropriate. If the defect is large (>6 cm²), or occurs within a divarification of the recti, the hernia should be repaired with prosthetic mesh. This technique is described later in the chapter when considering incisional hernias. The technique applied to intermediate-sized hernias is controversial and suture or mesh techniques are both currently deemed acceptable. Laparoscopic repair of epigastric hernias[9] was first described in 1993 and the technique has grown in popularity. The author prefers an open technique under local anaesthetic whenever possible for smaller hernias (defect <2 cm), suture or mesh depending on the quality of the tissues, and the laparoscopic approach for larger, multiple, recurrent hernias, or hernias in the obese. At laparoscopic repair, it is important to take down the falciform ligament and remove any pre-peritoneal fat above the linea alba, otherwise the 'hernia' may still be palpable following the alleged repair.

Complications

Complication rates are low and most are the usual complications associated with abdominal wall incisions (haematoma, infection). There are very few data on recurrence rates, historical series reporting rates around 7%.[10] In perhaps 50% of patients, however, the recurrence probably represents the persistence of a second hernia or area of weakness overlooked at the initial procedure. The laparoscopic technique avoids this problem because all fascial defects are visible laparoscopically if adequate dissection is carried out.

Umbilical and para-umbilical hernias

There are several distinct types of hernia that occur around the umbilicus: congenital (omphalocele), infantile, para-umbilical and adult umbilical hernias.

Congenital umbilical hernias

A congenital umbilical hernia occurs when the abdominal viscera herniate into the tissue of the umbilical cord. Normally, the gut returns to the abdominal cavity at 10 weeks of gestation. If this fails to occur, normal rotation and fixation of the intestine are prevented, the umbilicus is absent and a funnel-shaped defect in the abdominal wall is present through which viscera protrude into the umbilical cord. The abdominal wall defect may vary in size from no larger than an umbilical stump to a defect that appears to involve the entire abdominal wall. Congenital umbilical hernia occurs in 1 in 5000 births and is associated with other serious congenital anomalies.

Clinical presentation
Congenital umbilical hernia may be diagnosed in utero or at birth. On ultrasound examination, foetal abdominal wall defects are not subtle and may be visualised as early as 15 weeks of gestation. The management is surgical correction and one of the most important contributors to the morbidity and mortality of isolated abdominal wall defects is the delay between delivery and appropriate surgical repair. Antenatal knowledge of the existence of a congenital hernia can allow for the birth of the child at a tertiary care institution with the appropriate neonatal and paediatric surgical expertise (see also Chapter 12).

Management
Surgical correction should only be undertaken in specialised centres. If the diagnosis is made prenatally, the mother should be transferred to such a centre for delivery. If the diagnosis only becomes apparent at birth, the baby should be kept warm and hydrated, and the sac handled with care to avoid rupture or twisting of the sac. The sac should be wrapped in moist sterile gauze and covered with impervious plastic sheeting or aluminium foil. Mother and baby should then be transferred as soon as feasible to a tertiary centre for further management.

Infantile umbilical hernias

Infantile umbilical hernias occur when the umbilical vessels fail to fuse with the urachal remnant and umbilical ring. It presents with a protrusion of the umbilicus, usually at the superior margin of the ring. The infantile hernia, as opposed to the congenital type, is always covered by skin. It is the third most common surgical disorder in children, occurring in approximately one in five live births.

Clinical presentation
Clinically, the commonest presenting 'symptom' is the cosmetic appearance, the hernia resulting in a cone-like protrusion of the umbilicus that bulges every time the child cries or strains. Infantile umbilical hernias rarely enlarge over time and 90% disappear by the time the child is 2 years of age, although they are unlikely to close spontaneously if they persist to the age of 5 years.[11] Spontaneous resolution of umbilical hernias appears to be directly influenced by the size of the umbilical ring. If, at the age of 3 months, the hernia has a fascial ring of <0.5 cm, 96% heal spontaneously within 2 years. Defects that have a fascial diameter >1.5 cm are unlikely to heal spontaneously. Complications of umbilical hernias are rare, occurring in approximately 5%, and include strangulation of the omentum, strangulation of the intestine and evisceration.

Management
Management of the infant with an umbilical hernia is expectant. The majority will resolve spontaneously without surgical correction. The indications for surgery in children less than 2 years of age are the development of complications or tenderness over the site of the hernia. There is no consensus on the appropriate timing of herniorrhaphy in older children but generally repair is performed before school/nursery to avoid the child becoming self-conscious of the umbilical protrusion.

Operative details

Elective repair of infantile umbilical hernia is performed on an outpatient basis under general anaesthesia. A curvilinear incision is made within a skin fold on the inferior aspect of the hernia. The sac is then encircled by blunt dissection. If there is any concern regarding the contents of the sac, the sac should be opened on its caudal aspect, as abdominal contents usually adhere to the fundus of the sac. Once dealt with appropriately, the contents should be reduced and the incision continued to the cephalic aspect of the sac. If the sac is empty, the fundus may simply be disconnected from the umbilicus and reduced intact. Repair is by simple fascial apposition using horizontal mattress sutures of absorbable material. While the Mayo ('vest-over-pants') technique of umbilical hernioplasty is frequently taught, there is no evidence that the results are any better than simple apposition of the fascial edges. The umbilicus is refashioned by leaving a small button of the fundus of the sac attached to the inner surface of the cicatrix and tacking it down to the area of fascial repair.

Complications

Complications of umbilical hernioplasty are rare, but include seroma or haematoma formation and infection. Recurrence is possible if large defects are closed under tension or if an associated para-umbilical hernia is overlooked.

Para-umbilical hernias

Para-umbilical hernias are acquired hernias and occur in all age groups. They occur secondary to disruption of the linea alba and generally occur above the umbilical cicatrix. Aetiological factors include stretching of the abdominal wall by obesity, multiple pregnancy and ascites. Para-umbilical hernias are more common in patients over the age of 35 years and are five times more common in females.

Clinical presentation

Clinically, para-umbilical hernias are frequently symptomatic. Patients complain of intermittent abdominal pain (possibly caused by dragging on the fat and peritoneum of the falciform ligament) and, when the hernial sac contains bowel, colic resulting from intermittent intestinal obstruction. The hernia tends to progress over time and intertrigo and necrosis of the skin may occur in patients with large dependent hernias. Such symptoms are a good indication for surgery.

Management

It is important to distinguish para-umbilical hernias from true umbilical defects as the latter may resolve spontaneously in the young, whereas the former require surgical correction. Umbilical hernias classically

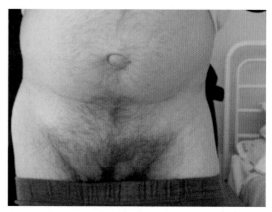

Figure 4.3 • Clinical photograph of a para-umbilical hernia. Note the swelling of the right groin of an associated right inguinal hernia – a common finding consistent with a generalised collagen disorder.

produce a symmetric bulge with the protrusion directly under the umbilicus. This is in contrast to para-umbilical hernias, where about half the fundus of the sac is covered by the umbilicus and the remainder is covered by the skin of the abdomen directly above or below the umbilicus(**Fig. 4.3**). Para-umbilical hernias do not resolve spontaneously and have a high incidence of incarceration and strangulation; therefore, surgical repair is nearly always indicated.

Operative details

For solitary hernias separated from the umbilicus, a transverse incision over the hernia produces the best exposure. In patients with a para-umbilical and umbilical hernia, a midline incision may provide better access. Similarly, if multiple fascial defects are present or there is concern about the integrity of visceral contents of the sac, a vertical incision may be better employed. If the defect simply contains pre-peritoneal fat, this may be reduced. In patients with strangulated or ischaemic pre-peritoneal fat, it is best excised. If there is a sac present, it should be dissected free from the fascial edges, opened and the contents examined. Once the contents have been dealt with appropriately, they may be reduced and redundant sac excised. There is no requirement to close the peritoneum but some authors recommend transfixing the neck of the sac once the contents have been reduced. Repair is performed by fascial apposition either transversely or longitudinally, depending on the defect and the direction of least tension. As this is an acquired defect, non-absorbable sutures are recommended. Indeed, the author usually creates a pre-peritoneal pocket, inserting a 5 cm × 5 cm square (minimum size – bigger if necessary) mesh and closing the fascia over this. The classic Mayo approach[12] overlaps the edges, but there has never been any demonstration that the bursting strength of the wound is improved by imbrications and may actually be impaired to a degree proportional to the amount of overlapping and tension. For larger para-umbilical hernias, with a neck size >3 cm (or smaller hernias in an obese patient), it is the author's preference to repair these laparoscopically and very large hernias with a neck size >8 cm by an open sublay technique (described later).

The overlying umbilical skin need not be excised unless it is macerated or infected, although the cosmetic appearance is often enhanced by judicious removal of excess skin and subcutaneous fat. All patients should be warned that it might be necessary to excise the umbilicus. If a new umbilicus is to be created, care should be taken as recurrences may occur at the point on the linea alba where the new umbilicus is fixed to the fascia.

Complications

Complications include the development of seromas, haematomas and infection. Sealed suction drains may be employed in the retromuscular and subcutaneous planes to avoid the development of large seromas. In addition to local problems, these patients may have respiratory and cardiovascular complications.

Adult umbilical hernias

Umbilical hernias in adults represent a spectrum of conditions from the partially unfolded cicatrix to huge dependent sacs. The umbilicus may become partially unfolded in patients with acute abdominal distension. Persistent elevation of intra-abdominal pressure eventually results in the umbilical cicatrix giving way and the development of an umbilical hernia. Although uncommon, causes include ascites from cirrhosis, congestive cardiac failure or nephrosis. Patients undergoing peritoneal dialysis also have a high incidence of these hernias. Management should be non-operative where possible, as the majority of these patients have serious underlying pathology. Operative repair is not indicated unless the hernia incarcerates or becomes extremely large and the overlying skin is thinned down to such an extent that spontaneous rupture is possible.

Umbilical hernias in adults do not represent persistence of infantile hernias but are indirect herniations through an umbilical canal, which is bordered by umbilical fascia posteriorly, the linea alba anteriorly and the medial edges of the two rectus sheaths on each side. They have a tendency to incarcerate and strangulate and do not resolve spontaneously.

Umbilical hernias in adults have a high morbidity and mortality. Over 90% occur in females and almost all patients are obese and multiparous.

The clinical presentation, management and complications of adult umbilical hernia are very similar to those of para-umbilical hernia, as described above.

Inguinal hernias

Anatomy

The anatomy of the inguinal region is complex. The inguinal canal is approximately 4 cm in length and is located just above the inguinal ligament between the internal and external rings. The inguinal canal allows passage of the spermatic cord into the scrotum, along with the testicular, deferential and cremasteric vessels. The superficial ring is a triangular aperture in the aponeurosis of the external oblique and lies about 1 cm above the pubic tubercle. The ring is bounded by a superomedial and an inferolateral crus joined by criss-cross intercrural fibres. Normally, the ring will not admit the tip of the little finger. The deep ring is a U-shaped condensation of the transversalis fascia and it lies about 1 cm above the inguinal ligament, midway between the pubic tubercle and the anterior superior iliac spine. The transversalis fascia is the fascial envelope of the abdomen and the competency of the deep inguinal ring depends on the integrity of this fascia.

The anterior boundary of the inguinal canal comprises mainly the external oblique aponeurosis with the conjoined muscle laterally. The posterior boundary is formed by the fascia transversalis and the conjoined tendon (internal oblique and transversus abdominus medially). The inferior epigastric vessels lie posteriorly and medially to the deep inguinal ring. The superior boundary is formed by the conjoined muscles (internal oblique and transversus) and the inferior boundary by the inguinal ligament.

Definition

An indirect hernia travels down the canal on the outer (lateral and anterior) side of the spermatic cord. A direct inguinal hernia comes out directly forwards through the posterior wall of the inguinal canal. While the neck of an indirect hernia is lateral to the epigastric vessels, the direct hernia usually emerges medial to these vessels, except in the saddle-bag or pantaloon type, which has both a lateral and a medial component (**Fig. 4.4**).

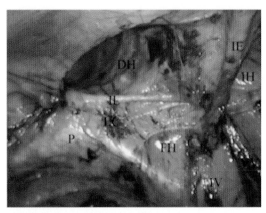

Figure 4.4 • Laparoscopic totally extraperitoneal (TEP) view of the right groin with a direct inguinal hernia (DH) lying medial to the inferior epigastric vessels (IE), above the inguinal (IL) and lacunar (LC) ligaments. The pubic bone (P), iliac vessels (IV), vas and vessels (VV) are also seen. The positions of a femoral hernia (FH) and indirect inguinal hernia (IH) are also marked.

Inguinal hernia in infants and children (see also Chapter 12)

Repair of congenital inguinal hernia is the most frequently performed operation in the paediatric age group. Although inguinal hernias can present at any age, the peak incidence is during infancy and childhood. About 3–5% of full-term infants may be born with a clinical inguinal hernia. Between 80% and 90% of paediatric hernias occur in boys, about one-third of the hernias presenting in the first 6 months of life. Congenital inguinal hernias have a 15% bilateral presentation.

Clinical presentation

Examination of the inguinal area for a hernia may show an obvious bulge at the site of the external ring or within the scrotum that can often be gently reduced. However, the bulge may only be seen during severe straining, such as with crying or defecation. If the infant is old enough to stand, he or she should be examined in both the supine and standing positions. If not, the parent can hold the infant upright so that the surgeon can closely observe the inguinoscrotal area. Sometimes, photographs taken by the parent when a swelling appears can aid in the diagnosis in the difficult case. It is essential to make sure that the testis is within the scrotal sac to avoid mistaking a retractile testis for a hernial bulge. The presence of an empty scrotum should alert the examining surgeon to a possible unde-scended or ectopic testis, which is associated with

an inguinal hernia in more than 90% of patients. Although routine orchidopexy is usually delayed until the child is 1 year of age, a coexisting symptomatic hernia should be promptly repaired and orchidopexy accomplished at the same time.

Inguinal hernias in infants and children are prone to incarcerate, with the overall rate being 12%.[13] Incarceration is most common in the first 6 months of life, when more than half of all instances are observed. An incarcerated hernia usually presents as an acute tender mass in the inguinal canal. The mass may protrude beyond the external inguinal ring or into the scrotum. The skin over the mass may be discoloured, oedematous, erythematous or blue. Strangulation, characterised by abdominal distension, vomiting, failure to pass faecal material, tachycardia and radiological evidence of small-bowel obstruction, demands emergency operative intervention for relief of obstruction, intestinal salvage and hernia repair. In contrast to the adult with an incarcerated hernia, in children testicular ischaemia is far more common than intestinal ischaemia, and it is therefore appropriate to be aggressive about reducing the hernia (see Chapter 12).

Management

In general, hernias in children and particularly infants should be managed by experienced paediatric surgeons (see also Chapter 12). However, this is not always possible depending on geography and availability. In these circumstances the general surgeon on call may be required to manage these patients. As most (80%) incarcerated hernias in children may be managed initially by non-operative measures, which include sedation, and then gentle reduction when the baby is quiet, exploration may be safely delayed for about 24–48 hours, allowing, if possible, a more experienced paediatric surgeon to become involved. However, if the hernia remains irreducible at this stage, emergency repair is indicated. The complication rate is approximately 20 times greater after emergency repair for incarcerated hernia than after elective procedures.[14] It is therefore worthwhile to reduce the hernia whenever possible and perform an elective procedure within 24–48 hours of the reduction. The high risk of incarceration in the paediatric age group makes the presence of an inguinal hernia an indication for surgical repair.

Operative details

Surgical access is achieved through a short (2–3 cm) transverse incision in the lowest inguinal skin crease. The superficial fascia (Scarpa's fascia) is incised and the external oblique fascia identified. The aponeurosis is traced laterally to identify the inguinal ligament and the exact location of the external inguinal ring identified. Although some surgeons advocate repair through the external ring (Mitchell Banks technique[15]), an alternative approach is to incise the external oblique fascia in the long axis of its fibres, perpendicular to the external inguinal ring. This exposes the cremasteric muscle and fascia, which envelop the cord structures.

The hernial sac is always located in an anteromedial position in relation to the cord and gentle blunt dissection of the cremasteric fibres usually brings the sac into view. The sac is elevated with a haemostat and the cremasteric fibres carefully freed from the anterior and lateral aspects. Retraction of the sac medially allows identification of the spermatic vessels and vas deferens, and these structures may be carefully teased away from the sac in a posterolateral direction. Injection of 1–2 mL of saline into the cord may help to define the planes of separation. The vas itself should not be grasped and the floor of the canal not disturbed. Once the end of the sac has been freed, the dissection of the sac is carried superiorly to the level of the deep inguinal ring. If the sac extends down into the scrotum, it may be divided once the cord structures are identified and protected. The base of the sac may then be gently twisted to reduce any fluid or viscera into the peritoneal cavity. The base of the sac should be suture ligated with an absorbable suture and, once the suture is cut, the peritoneal stump should retract proximally through the deep inguinal ring. Free ties should not be used because of the risk of them becoming dislodged if abdominal distension occurs. Absolute haemostasis is essential to prevent postoperative haematoma formation. The position of the testis within the scrotum should be confirmed to avoid iatrogenic entrapment within the inguinal canal. There is an increasing role for laparoscopic hernia repair in infants and young children.[14]

An emergency operation is required for patients with an incarcerated hernia, with toxicity and obvious intestinal obstruction or after failed attempts at reduction. As previously mentioned, a paediatric surgeon should be involved in all cases if possible as this can be a difficult undertaking. After appropriate resuscitation, prophylactic antibiotics and insertion of a nasogastric tube, the operation begins with preparation of the whole abdomen in case laparotomy is required. An inguinal incision is utilised and the incarcerated intestine carefully inspected for viability once the obstruction at the internal ring is relieved. A rapid return of pink colour, sheen, peristalsis and palpable or visible pulsations at the mesenteric border should be observed. If there is any question regarding intestinal viability, resection and anastomosis should be carried out and hernial repair accomplished.

In certain circumstances, the incarcerated intestine may reduce during surgical manipulation, before the intestine has been visualised. However, such spontaneous reduction of infarcted bowel is very rare. Laparoscopy through the hernial sac can be undertaken if there are serious concerns regarding bowel viability. Surgery for incarcerated hernia may be difficult because of oedema, tissue friability and the presence of the mass, which may obscure the anatomy. The gonad should be carefully inspected because it may become infarcted by vascular compression caused by the incarcerated intestine. The undescended testis is more vulnerable to this complication in the presence of incarcerated intestine.

Complications

Complications may be divided into intraoperative and postoperative categories. Intraoperative complications include: division of the ilioinguinal nerve, which can be avoided if the external oblique fascia is elevated before incision; division of the vas deferens, which should be repaired with interrupted 7–0 monofilament sutures; and bleeding, which is usually secondary to needle-hole injury and can usually be controlled with withdrawal of the suture and the application of pressure.

Postoperative complications include wound infection, scrotal haematoma, postoperative hydroceles and recurrence. The wound infection rate is low (1–2%) and recurrence rates of less than 1% are reported, 80% of recurrences being noted within the first postoperative year. The major causes of recurrence in infants and children include: (i) a missed hernial sac or an unrecognised tear in the peritoneum; (ii) a broken suture ligature at the neck of the sac; (iii) injury to the floor of the inguinal canal, resulting in the development of a direct inguinal hernia; (iv) severe infection in the inguinal canal; and (v) increased intra-abdominal pressure, as is noted in patients with ascites after ventriculoperitoneal shunts, in children with cystic fibrosis, after previous operation for incarceration and in patients with connective tissue disorders. Although failure to repair a large internal inguinal ring is a possible (and very occasional) cause of recurrence, attempts to tighten the internal ring at the time of the first repair by approximating the transversalis fascia medial to the inferior epigastric vessels risk compromising the blood supply to the testicle and should be avoided where possible. Simple excision of the sac is all that is required in most patients. Reoperations for recurrent inguinal hernia may be a technical challenge and a pre-peritoneal approach is an extremely useful alternative for recurrent hernias.

Adult inguinal hernias

Inguinal hernias are more frequent in males, with a male to female ratio of 12:1. The peak incidence is in the sixth decade and 65% are indirect in type. Right-sided inguinal hernias are slightly more common than left-sided, 55% occurring on the right. Bilateral hernias are four times more common in direct than indirect forms.

Aetiology

The pathogenesis of groin hernias is multifactorial. It was initially believed that persistence of a patent processus vaginalis into adult life was the predisposing factor for indirect inguinal hernia formation. However, post-mortem studies have shown that 15–30% of adult males without a clinically apparent inguinal hernia have a patent processus vaginalis.[16] Similarly, review of the contralateral side in infantile inguinal hernias reveals a patent processus vaginalis in 60% of neonates and a contralateral hernia in 10–20%. During 20 years of follow-up after infantile hernia repair, only 22% of men will develop a contralateral hernia.

It is therefore apparent that the problem of indirect inguinal hernia is not simply one of a congenital defect. The high frequency of indirect inguinal hernia in middle-aged and older people suggests a pathological change in connective tissue of the abdominal wall to be a contributory factor,[1] as discussed earlier.

Management

The essential goal of hernia repair is to restore the functional integrity of the laminar musculo-aponeurotic structure of the groin region and the musculo-aponeurotic fenestration, which allows the vessels to the genitalia to penetrate this structure. It is beyond the scope of this chapter to review the history of the various repair techniques that have been previously employed and are now mainly historical. However, **Fig. 4.5** illustrates how the popularity of suture and mesh techniques has changed in the Lothian region of Scotland in the last 20 years.

Only the latest techniques (i.e. prosthetic repairs) will be considered here.

Tension-free prosthetic mesh repair

Lichtenstein first described the technique of tension free repair of groin hernia, which now bears his name.[17] Tension-free repair of primary groin hernias may be performed as an outpatient procedure under local anaesthesia, although in the UK open mesh repair is still more commonly performed under general anaesthetic.

Once the local anaesthesia has been administered (typically a mixture of 0.5% bupivacaine and 1% lignocaine) along the line of the proposed incision, a cut is made in the groin-crease and a window established through the subcutaneous tissues including Scarpa's fascia at the lateral end of the wound, exposing the external oblique aponeurosis. The window is increased in size to expose the medial end of the external oblique aponeurosis, the inguinal ligament and the superficial ring. Additional anaesthetic is then injected under the external oblique aponeurosis, following which a small incision is made in the external oblique along the line of the fibres, approximately 2 cm above the inguinal ligament. The edges are carefully lifted with haemostatic forceps to avoid damage to the ilioinguinal nerve. The external oblique aponeurosis is then opened along a line from the incision to the superficial ring and the contents of the inguinal canal gently separated from it. After a self-retaining retractor has been inserted under the edges of the external oblique aponeurosis, the spermatic cord is mobilised utilising the avascular space between the pubic tubercle and the cord itself to avoid damage to the floor of the canal, injury to the testicular blood flow and crushing of the genital nerve, which always lies in juxtaposition to the external spermatic vessels (**Fig. 4.6**).

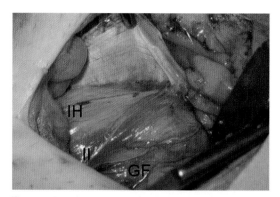

Figure 4.6 • Open right inguinal hernia repair. External oblique has been opened. Medial is to the right of the picture with superior at the top. Note the iliohypogastric (IH), ilioinguinal (II) that splits into two branches, and the small genitor-femoral nerve (GF) lying inferiorly. Clinical photograph used with permission of Mr Martin Kurzer, London, UK.

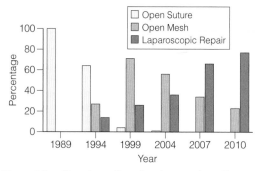

Figure 4.5 • Changing patterns in suture, mesh and laparoscopic inguinal hernia repair in the Lothian Region, Scotland.

In order to thin out the spermatic cord and remove any lipoma present, the cremaster fibres are incised longitudinally at the level of the deep ring. Complete excision of the cremaster fibres from the spermatic cord is unnecessary and may result in damage to the vas deferens, increasing the likelihood of post-operative neuralgia and ischaemic orchitis. Indirect hernial sacs are opened and digital exploration performed to detect any other defects or the presence of a femoral hernia. Lichtenstein states that the sac may be simply inverted into the abdomen without excision, suture or ligation, which he feels is unnecessary and may contribute to postoperative discomfort.[17] However, it is the author's practice to suture ligate any but the smallest hernial sacs at the level of the deep ring and excise any redundant peritoneum. To prevent postoperative hydrocele formation, complete scrotal sacs are transected at the midpoint of the canal, with the distal section left open and in situ. If performing the procedure under local anaesthetic, handling of the sac at this stage can cause pain and often further local anaesthetic to the sac area in the region of the deep ring is required.

In the event of a large direct hernia, the sac (transversalis fascia) is invaginated with an imbricating suture to achieve a flat surface over which to lay the prosthetic mesh. The external oblique aponeurosis is separated from the underlying internal oblique muscle at a point high enough to accommodate a mesh measuring around 11 cm×6 cm. This size will vary depending on the size of the patient and the size of the hernial defect.

The mesh is trimmed as appropriate so that the patch overlaps the internal oblique muscle and aponeurosis by at least 2 cm above the border of the Hesselbach triangle. The medial portion of the mesh is rounded to the shape of the medial corner of the inguinal canal. The mesh is sutured to the aponeurotic tissue over the pubic bone, overlapping the bone to prevent any tension or weakness at this critical point, but ensuring the periosteum is not caught in the suture as this is believed to be a good source of chronic pain. The medial part of the mesh should extend at least 2 cm medial to the pubic tubercle to reduce the risk of medial recurrence. The same suture is continued along the lower edge, attaching the mesh to the shelving portion of the inguinal ligament to a point just lateral to the deep ring with a continuous suture.

A slit is made at the lateral end of the mesh, creating a wider tail above the cord and a narrower one below the cord. This manoeuvre positions the cord between the two tails of the mesh and avoids the keyhole opening, which is less effective at preventing recurrence. The upper edge of the patch is sutured to the internal oblique aponeurosis using a few interrupted sutures or widely spaced continuous suture. Sharp retraction of the upper leaf of the external oblique aponeurosis from the internal oblique muscle is important because it provides the appropriate amount of laxity for the patch. When the retraction is released, a true tension-free repair is taken up when the patient strains on command during the operation (if under local anaesthetic) or resumes an upright position afterwards. Using a single non-absorbable monofilament suture, the lower edges of the two tails are fixed to the shelving margin of the inguinal ligament just lateral to the completion knot of the lower continuous suture. This creates a new deep ring of mesh (**Fig. 4.7**). Some surgeons simply suture the lower edge of the upper tail to the upper edge of the lower tail.

The excess patch is trimmed on the lateral side, leaving 3–4 cm beyond the deep ring. This is tucked underneath the external oblique aponeurosis and the external oblique aponeurosis closed with a continuous suture. Unrestricted activity is encouraged and patients are expected to return to their normal activity 2–7 days after surgery.

In the past few years, there has been an explosion in different mesh types for the open repair of inguinal hernias. The plug and patch utilises a cone-shaped mass of mesh that can be inserted, tip side inwards, into either the deep or superficial rings, depending on the type of hernia. A flat mesh is then placed over the plug akin to the Lichtenstein technique. The prolene hernia system is two flat meshes secured together by a small cyclinder of mesh. The aim is to insert one mesh into the pre-peritoneal space and the

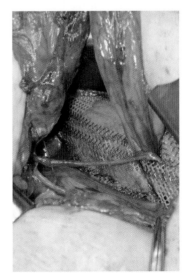

Figure 4.7 • Left inguinal hernia repair. Mesh in place. Note continuous suture attaching inferior edge of mesh to inguinal ligament and mesh fish-tailed laterally to create a new deep ring. Cord structures and ilioinguinal nerve are intact. The mesh is lying flat and 'tension' free.

other is secured akin to the Lichtenstein technique. There is also the open pre-peritonel approach with the Kugel patch, for example. All these alternatives report good results in the hands of experts, but the open flat mesh technique in its various forms, akin to the Lichtenstein technique, remains the commonest technique in Western countries to date. It is also the author's prejudice that if a mesh is to be inserted into the pre-peritoneal space, it makes sense to do this under direct vision using a laparoscope rather than using a largely blind, blunt finger dissection technique.

Laparoscopic repair

The alternative to an open operation is a laparoscopic approach. Ger is credited with the first laparoscopic approach to hernia, repairing indirect hernias with a stapling instrument developed for this purpose.[18,19] In parallel, Gazayerli described a suture repair technique through a transabdominal approach, approximating the transversus abdominis aponeurotic arch and the iliopubic tract.[20] After the repair is completed, the peritoneum is re-approximated. Since the early 1990s, laparoscopic hernia repair has evolved from simple closure of a small indirect hernia, through the placement of mesh plugs and a small mesh patch over the internal ring, to the current use of large pieces of prosthetic mesh to reinforce the lower abdominal wall.

The rationale for the use of large mesh sheets placed into the pre-peritoneal space was based on the surgical experience of the open pre-peritoneal hernia repair, especially in the treatment of recurrent hernias.[21] Although a variety of laparoscopic repairs have been described, they can be categorised in general according to the approach used to expose the defect. Three exposures are used: the intraperitoneal approach, in which the prosthesis is placed as an onlay graft over the peritoneum; the transabdominal pre-peritoneal (TAPP) repair; and the totally extraperitoneal (TEP) repair.

Intraperitoneal prosthetic repair

In the intraperitoneal repair with an onlay graft, the prosthesis is placed within the peritoneal cavity. The technique is well described by Toy and Smoot.[22] Compared to the TAPP and TEP approaches, it has the advantages of being less time-consuming to perform and requires no dissection of the pre-peritoneal space. It has the disadvantage of leaving the prosthetic material exposed within the peritoneal cavity and has a higher recurrence rate. It is the author's view that this operation is very much an operation of last resort, when other open or laparoscopic techniques have failed. It is possible that when better non-stick meshes become available, combined with glue fixation, this technique may gain in popularity.

Transabdominal pre-peritoneal prosthetic repair

TAPP repair is one of the most popular approaches used for laparoscopic herniorrhaphy, particularly in Europe. The abdomen is insufflated with carbon dioxide and the laparoscope introduced through an umbilical incision. Two accessory trocars, placed well above and slightly medial to the anterior superior iliac spines, are used to provide access for the dissecting instruments and the stapler. After both groins have been inspected, a second incision is made in the pelvic peritoneum several centimetres above the hernia defect, typically in line with the level of the anterior iliac spine, and the peritoneum then peeled away to expose the hernia defect. The peritoneum is dissected bluntly away from the abdominal wall, allowing the hernia sac to be inverted and dissected free of adherent tissue. Pre-peritoneal fat is removed to allow identification of the transversus abdominis arch, the pubic tubercle, the iliopubic tract and Cooper's ligament. A prosthetic mesh of approximately $10\,cm \times 15\,cm$ is inserted and manipulated into position so that it covers the entire myopectineal orifice. Some surgeons fix the mesh in place with staples, sutures or glue, although there is little evidence to support such practices. The peritoneum is closed over the mesh with staples or sutures. This approach has the advantage of permitting inspection of the abdomen in general, and of the opposite side in particular, enabling bilateral repairs to be performed if necessary. In addition, exposure is usually excellent. The disadvantage is that a wider dissection is required to accommodate the mesh than is used in the intraperitoneal onlay procedure. In addition, the intra-abdominal incision presents the possibility of injury to intraperitoneal structures and a second peritoneal incision in the groin increases the potential for adhesion formation and late bowel obstruction.

Totally extraperitoneal prosthetic repair

TEP repair is a laparoscopic adaptation of the open posterior pre-peritoneal approach first described by Annandale.[23] The laparoscope is introduced into the pre-peritoneal space through an infra-umbilical incision. The pre-peritoneal space is dissected towards the symphysis pubis, Cooper's ligament and the iliac vessels with a blunt instrument or space-making balloon. Carbon dioxide is insufflated into the pre-peritoneal space to maintain exposure. Care must be taken to avoid entering the peritoneum; if this occurs, loss of pressure in the pre-peritoneal space can result, making exposure more difficult. A venting Verres needle in the right iliac fossa will usually resolve this problem, or alternatively a structural balloon attached to the umbilical port will help to keep the pre-peritoneal space open. Two additional 5-mm ports are inserted, either in the right and left iliac fossa, after extending the dissection laterally or in the midline below the umbilicus. Direct hernial sacs usually reduce with ease, but an indirect hernial sac may need more work. The key landmark here is the vas. The indirect hernial sac lies above and lateral to the vas, taking the dissection away from the iliac vessels, preventing their inadvertent injury. A mesh of minimum size 10 cm×15 cm is used to cover all the inguinal and femoral myopectineal orifices, ensuring good cover laterally and superiomedially. As with TAPP repairs, there is now good evidence that suturing, tacking or stapling of mesh does not reduce the risk of hernia recurrence but is a cause of postoperative chronic pain.[24] The author does occasionally tack the mesh, confined mainly to the patient with a very large direct hernial defect or when there has been more bleeding than usual, especially patients on aspirin. In all circumstances tacks are placed medial to the inferior epigastric vessels and superior to the pubic bone only. More recently, the author has attempted laparoscopic suture closure of large direct inguinal hernias with a non-absorbable suture rather than using tacks. The TEP approach avoids the risks of entering the peritoneal cavity and subsequent intraperitoneal adhesion formation.

There is little evidence to support TEP versus TAPP and the technique used is largely down to the individual surgeon. The author's preference is the TEP approach, with the TAPP approach reserved for recurrence after a previous TEP or open intraperitoneal operations.

> ✔✔ Laparoscopic repair of inginual hernias causes less acute and chronic pain, thus earlier return to work, less infection, fewer wound complications and less numbness than the open operation. It is currently the preferred technique recommended by the National Institute for Clinical Excellence (NICE) for recurrent inguinal hernias and bilateral primary inguinal hernias, and an alternative operation for primary unilateral hernias.[25]

Complications

Complications of herniorrhaphy include recurrence, urinary retention, ischaemic orchitis and testicular atrophy, wound infection and nerve injuries (neuromas of the ilioinguinal or genitofemoral nerves). A wide variation in recurrence rates is reported in the literature, depending on both the surgical technique employed and the method and length of follow-up (questionnaire, physical examination, etc.). In general, papers comparing mesh to suture repair note lower recurrence rates in the mesh group.[26] Nevertheless, the percentage of recurrent to primary hernia repair has remained largely constant in Lothian, Scotland over the past 30 years at around 10%. Perhaps the only role for suture repair

remains in the adolescent age group, where perhaps a herniotomy alone is insufficient and the risks of mesh insertion not merited. There has been a suggestion that mesh repairs in the groin can affect fertility in males.[27] This is a very controversial area, as the occurrence of a hernia per se in the young is associated with reduced fertility. There is no convincing evidence to support the view that a mesh repair affects fertility except when there is obviously direct trauma to the vas or vessels to the testicle.

The complication that is becoming the benchmark for comparing hernia repairs is the incidence of chronic pain, rather than recurrence rate. Risk factors for chronic pain include nerve damage, preoperative pain in the hernia, young age, pain at other sites of the body, postoperative complications and psychosocial features.[28] Pain response to a standardised heat stimulus appears to be a useful tool in assessing risk of postoperative chronic pain.[29]

Suture, mesh or laparoscopic repair?

> ✔ The Shouldice technique using suture repair rather than mesh is still carried out in many centres worldwide and numerous publications have reported recurrence rates of 1–2%.[30] To date, the Lichtenstein tension-free repair has the largest number of published repairs with the lowest recurrence rates. Lichtenstein and colleagues published a multicentre series of 22 300 hernioplasties performed by this technique, with a recurrence rate of 0.77%.[31]

The 2004 NICE report commented on 37 randomised controlled trials that compared laparoscopic with open mesh repair of inguinal hernias in a total of 5560 participants.[25] The report summarised these results, stating that the laparoscopic repair as compared to an open repair was associated with less acute pain and thus a quicker return to daily activites and work, fewer wound complications such as haematoma, seroma and infection, and less risk of chronic pain. There was a similar recurrence rate and a similar risk of major vessel, bowel or bladder injury (except for a slightly higher risk for the TAPP repair). However, the laparoscopic repair took longer to perform and was a more expensive option. The cost of open surgery has to be set against the price of open surgery for the patient and society, namely more acute and chronic pain, more time off work and more wound complications. This is borne out by a cost–benefit analysis using the same data as the 2004 NICE report.[32] Unilateral hernia open flat mesh repair was the least costly option, but it provided fewer quality-adjusted life-years compared to both TAPP and TEP. Also, laparoscopic repair for bilateral hernias reduces both operating times and convalescence period, equating to greater cost-effectiveness. In addition, repair of an occult hernia on the other side may also be performed, enhancing the benefit of the laparoscopic procedure.

✅✅ Mesh repair using the Lichtenstein technique has the lowest worldwide recurrence rate for primary inguinal hernias. The laparoscopic repair is associated with less early and late pain, earlier return to normal activities and work, but is more expensive. It is, however, the preferred technique for the repair of recurrent and bilateral hernias.[25,32]

Recent publications now demonstrate that laparoscopic repairs, whether unilateral or bilateral, can be performed more quickly than open repair.[33,34] The only downside to laparoscopic hernia surgery is the need for general anaesthesia. While small numbers have been done under local or regional techniques, these have been confined to young fit patients, for whom avoidance of a general anaesthetic is not necessary. Nevertheless, in many Western countries open inguinal hernias are still predominantly repaired under general anaesthetic.

Contralateral repair

Inguinal hernia arises as a design fault, both anatomically and at the level of collagen metabolism, so there is every reason why it should be a bilateral disease. Furthermore, clinical assessment of bilateral or unilateral hernia has a false positive and negative rate of around 10%. The rate of development of a contralateral inguinal hernia following open repair is around 25% at 10 years.[26] The Edinburgh experience is that time from first repair to contralateral repair in the laparoscopic era is about half the time compared to open hernia repair. It could be argued that the larger mesh inserted laparoscopically places more strain on the contralateral side. An alternative hypothesis is that following laparoscopic repair, patients are more likely to volunteer for repair of the contralateral side as the operation is less painful. It is thus the author's practice to offer the majority of patients a bilateral laparoscopic repair, unless the laparoscopic approach is contraindicated and the patient unfit or elderly.

Recurrent inguinal hernias

The repair of recurrent inguinal hernia remains a common operation and there is now some evidence to suggest that the increasing use of mesh may be having a small effect in reducing the number of recurrent hernia repairs[26,35] (see section on prophylactic hernia repair at the end of this chapter).

As a result there is little role now for suture repair of recurrent inguinal hernias, and a re-recurrence rate of 30% for the Bassini technique has been reported.[36] The McVay procedure and transversalis repair are not commonly employed and the results are probably of historic interest only. In centres where alloplastic material is unavailable or too expensive for routine use, the Shouldice technique is probably the technique of choice.[37]

Prosthetic mesh repair of recurrent inguinal hernias

The Lichtenstein repair remains the commonest operation for recurrent inguinal hernias. Rate of re-recurrence depends to an extent on the length of follow-up, but is typically under 10%. Since its introduction, excellent results have been reported with the mesh plug method.[38] The transinguinal pre-peritoneal prosthetic repair/Rives procedure tends to be reserved for selected cases and is not indicated for the majority of recurrent inguinal hernias.[39] When an open pre-peritoneal approach is used with pre-peritoneal mesh implantation, the re-recurrence rate ranges between 0.5% and 25% after an observation period of up to 10 years, suggesting that this technique may require a degree of surgical experience for success.[40,41] Divergent results are also reported for the Stoppa technique, with re-recurrence rates varying between 1% and 12%.[42,43] The most likely explanation for this wide variation is that the size and type of recurrence probably varied between the reporting centres, and there is variation in the length and the quality of the follow-up.

Laparoscopic repair of recurrent inguinal hernias

The 2004 NICE[25] report acknowledges that after a previous open repair, laparoscopic repair is the preferred technique. The advantages of the laparoscopic approach include: elimination of one of the commonest causes of recurrence, the missed hernia; allowing the surgeon to identify those patients with complex hernias; and covering the entire myopectineal orifice, buttressing the intrinsic collagen deficit, thereby overcoming one of the causes of late recurrence. The complication rate is low, and the majority of such repairs are as easy as primary laparoscopic repair. The data from the Swedish Hernia Registry would support the benefit of a pre-peritoneal repair (open or laparoscopic) for recurrent inguinal hernia following a previous open non-peritoneal repair.[44] The type of surgery following recurrence after a previous laparoscopic repair is less well defined, and is more governed by surgeon preference and expertise. It is the author's opinion that an open mesh repair is the best option following a failed TAPP repair, and a TAPP repair for a failed TEP repair. The TAPP approach allows assessment as to why the TEP repair failed, and maintains the speedier recovery of the laparoscopic approach over open repair. However, the significant adhesions following a TAPP make a redo TAPP much more difficult, but still possible in experienced hands.

The asymptomatic hernia

Traditional teaching used to suggest that once an inguinal hernia was detected, it merited repair to prevent hernia-related complications unless the patient was not fit for such surgery. However, increasing awareness of complications following hernia repair, particularly chronic pain, has questioned this approach. Two randomised trials have reported similar results but come to different conclusions.[45,46] In essence, chronic pain on follow-up is similar between the operation group and the watchful waiting group. However, significant numbers in the watchful waiting group crossed over to the surgery arm because of increasing symptoms, but it is likely that such patients would tolerate complications of surgery better than if they were asymptomatic at the time of the surgery. Also, the risk of incarceration or strangulation is much lower than previously thought. Thus, following informed consent, surgery or watchful waiting for an asymptomatic hernia is appropriate. The younger the patient, or less fit the patient on presentation, then perhaps the earlier surgery should be offered, with suitable informed consent of the risks, benefits and alternatives to the proposed surgery.

✓✓ Repair of an asymptomatic hernia does not increase the incidence of chronic pain as compared to a wait and see policy. Either treatment option is acceptable with appropriate informed consent.[45,46] The majority of wait and see patients will cross over to surgery with time as their hernia increases in size and/or becomes more symptomatic.

Femoral hernia

Femoral hernia represents the third commonest type of primary hernia. It accounts for approximately 20% of hernias in women and 5% in men, strangulation being the initial presentation in 40%.

Anatomy

The femoral canal occupies the most medial compartment of the femoral sheath, extending from the femoral ring above to the saphenous opening below. It contains fat, lymphatic vessels and the lymph node of Cloquet. It is closed above by the septum crurale, a condensation of extraperitoneal tissue pierced by lymphatic vessels, and below by the cribriform fascia. The femoral ring is bounded anteriorly by the inguinal ligament and posteriorly by the iliopectineal (Cooper) ligament, the pubic bone and the fascia over the pectineus muscle. Medially, the boundary is the edge of the lacunar ligament, while laterally it is separated from the femoral vein by a thin septum (Fig. 4.4).

Aetiology

Femoral hernias are considered to be acquired, possibly as a result of increased abdominal pressure on the background of disturbed collagen metabolism. A postulated mechanism is the insinuation of fat into the femoral ring secondary to raised intra-abdominal pressure. This bolus of fat drags along pelvic peritoneum to develop a peritoneal sac. Once the peritoneal sac has moved the short distance down the canal and out of the femoral orifice, the sac becomes apparent. The hernia not only becomes visible and palpable, but the contents of the sac become at risk of incarceration and strangulation. The incidence of femoral herniation increases with age, and a potential mechanism for this involves the muscle bulk adjacent to the distal femoral canal. Normally, the iliopsoas and pectineus muscle bundles encroach on the canal and thus act as a barrier to the development of a femoral hernia. With the natural atrophy of muscle tissue that occurs with senescence, the actual volume of muscle within the canal decreases, allowing positive intra-abdominal pressure to push the peritoneum into the canal. This would explain the high rate of femoral hernia among elderly women as well as men. In women of all ages, the muscle mass is not as great as in men. Consequently, women are predisposed to femoral hernias with any condition that increases intra-abdominal pressure, such as pregnancy or obesity.

Management

The treatment of femoral hernia is surgical repair due to the invariable presence of incarceration and the associated risk of strangulation. Several operative approaches have been described: the low approach (Lockwood), the high approach (McEvedy) and the inguinal approach (Lothiessen). To these can now be added the laparoscopic approach.

Operative details
The low approach (Lockwood)
The low approach is based on a groin-crease incision and dissection of the femoral hernia sac below the

inguinal ligament. The anatomical layers covering the sac should be peeled away and the sac opened to inspect its contents. Once empty, the neck of the sac is pulled down, ligated as high as possible and redundant sac excised. The neck then retracts through the femoral canal and the canal is closed with a plug or cylinder of polypropylene mesh, anchored to the inguinal ligament and iliopectineal ligament with non-absorbable sutures. Suturing of the iliopectineal ligament to the inguinal ligament may result in tension due to the rigidity of these structures and may predispose to recurrence.

Transinguinal approach (Lothiessen)

Techniques of femoral repair that open the posterior inguinal wall for exposure and repair (the inguinal approaches of Lothiessen, Bassini, Shouldice, McVay–Cooper, Halsted and Andrews) should rarely be used. This technique usually involves ligation and division of the inferior epigastric vessels at the medial border of the internal inguinal ring followed by incision of the transversalis fascia to expose the extraperitoneal space and the femoral hernia sac. This is reduced and the defect closed by either suture (as in the original description) or, increasingly, mesh. However, the need to incise the natural fascial barrier in Hasselbach's triangle for exposure results in this technique being inferior to either the low or high approach, both of which leave the inguinal floor intact.

High approach (McEvedy)

The high approach was classically based on a vertical incision made over the femoral canal and continued upwards above the inguinal ligament. This has now been replaced with a transverse 'unilateral' Pfannenstiel incision, which can be extended to form a complete Pfannenstiel incision if a formal laparotomy is required. The dissection is continued through the subcutaneous tissue to the anterior rectus sheath. This can either be divided transversely or longitudinally, following which transversalis fascia is incised, the rectus muscle retracted medially and the pre-peritoneal space entered. The femoral hernia sac is identified medial to the iliac vessels and reduced by traction. If the hernia is incarcerated, the sac may be released by incising the insertion of the iliopubic tract into Cooper's ligament at the medial margin of the femoral ring. The sac is then opened, the contents dealt with appropriately and the sac ligated at its neck. The hernioplasty may then be completed by either suturing the iliopubic tract to the posterior margin of Cooper's ligament or by insertion of a prosthetic mesh, either as a sheet covering the whole of the myopectineal opening or as a mesh plug. The wound is closed in layers. This technique is particularly useful in the presence of

strangulated femoral hernias as it is easy to convert to laparotomy for bowel resection.

Laparoscopic approach

The laparoscopic approach is the same as for inguinal hernias and may employ the TAPP or TEP technique. The femoral ring is easily seen during either of these approaches and, indeed, visualisation of the whole of the myopectineal opening is frequently quoted as one of the advantages of laparoscopic herniorrhaphy. Small series of laparoscopic femoral hernia surgery have been reported with excellent results on short-term follow-up.[47,48]

Incisional hernia

Aetiology

Incisional hernias are unique in that they are the only hernia to be considered iatrogenic. The cause of wound complications after laparotomy is multifactorial, conditioned by local and systemic factors and by preoperative, perioperative and postoperative factors. Several factors including advanced age, pulmonary disease, morbid obesity, malignancy and intra-abdominal infection are associated with impaired wound healing and predispose patients to serious wound complications such as wound dehiscence, wound infection and incisional herniation. It is always easy to blame the patient for complications! But surgeon or technical factors influencing wound complications include surgical technique and suture material choices.

What is the best way to close the abdominal wall? It is amazing that today we still don't know for sure. A recent review[49] proposed mass closure (as compared to layered closure), continuous (as compared to interrupted sutures) absorbable monofilament (as compared to non-absorbable monofilament and absorbable multifilament) with a suture length to wound length ratio of 4:1. However, studies continue to challenge such doctrine. A recent randomised controlled trial (RCT)[50] comparing polypropylene to polydioxanone demonstrated no significant difference, and the 4-year incisional hernia rate was 23.7% and 30.2 %, respectively. Another recent RCT[51] demonstrated no significant difference between interrupted and continuous sutures. Controversy over the 4:1 ratio also exists. This ratio can be achieved by big bites far apart or small bites close together. A recent RCT[52] reported a 50% reduction in wound infection and a 67% reduction in incisional hernia rates in the 2–0 polydioxanone 20-mm-needle small bite arm compared to more conventional closure techniques. Using such a suture technique, suture to wound length ratios greater than 4:1 were not associated with increasing wound complications.[53] Further trials are in progress to evaluate this and other techniques in wound closure to minimise the risks of the burst abdomen (sometimes called an acute hernia or deep wound dehiscence), wound infection and incisional hernia. Indeed, incisional hernia is the commonest complication of a laparotomy. The development of an incisional hernia is inevitable if there is separation of the fascia by 12 mm at 12 weeks, so it is not difficult to see that the events that lead to an incisional hernia are determined early in the healing phase, and technical issues are likely to have a significant part to play.

✓✓ Closure of a laparotomy wound to minimise incisional hernia formation includes:[49]
1. mass closure;
2. simple running technique;
3. absorbable monofilament;
4. suture length to wound length ratio of at least 4:1.

Management

The diagnosis of an incisional hernia is usually easy except in the very obsese. However, computed tomography (CT) scanning is helpful to identify the size of the defect and the state of the adominal wall muscles (**Fig. 4.8**).

The large number of surgical procedures described in the literature to repair incisional hernias illustrates that no single technique has stood out as being effective. While 50% of incisional hernias occur within 1 year after the primary operation, 10–18% are diagnosed more than 5 years later. Any study reporting re-recurrence rates following incisional hernia repair should therefore ideally have at least 5 years of follow-up data for analysis. Unfortunately,

prospective randomised trials comparing different types of incisional hernia repair are lacking and the majority of studies are retrospective.

As a consequence of the disappointing data on mesh-free repair of incisional hernias, including the Mayo ('vest-over-pants') procedure, meshes were introduced to strengthen the abdominal wall repair. Several different techniques were developed: inlay, onlay and sublay (**Fig. 4.9**). Mesh implantation as an inlay does not achieve any strengthening of the abdominal wall and is essentially a suture repair at the muscle/fascia mesh interface. It has the highest recurrence rate of the three techniques. The results of randomised trials comparing mesh to suture repair demonstrate a clear advantage for mesh repair, even for small hernias.[54,55] However, incisional hernia should be considered an incurable disease, mesh just increasing the time from repair to recurrence.[56] Although suture repair is now rarely indicated, it might still have a role in young women who wish repair of an incisional hernia but are also contemplating further pregnancy.

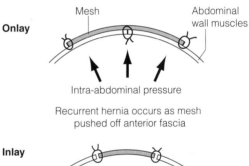

Recurrent hernia occurs as mesh pushed off anterior fascia

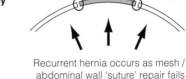

Recurrent hernia occurs as mesh / abdominal wall 'suture' repair fails

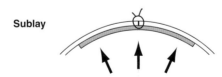

Recurrent hernia minimised as intra-abdominal pressure pins the mesh against the abdominal wall

Figure 4.9 • Cross-sectional appearance of mesh position in incisional hernia repair. Reproduced from Schumpelick V, Klinge V. Immediate follow-up results of sublay polypropylene repair in primary or recurrent incisional hernias. In: Schumpelick V, Kingsnorth AN (eds) Incisional hernia. Berlin:Springer-Verlag 1999; pp312-26. With kind permission of Springer Science+Business Media.

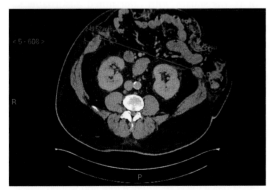

Figure 4.8 • CT scan of a large incisional hernia demonstrating loss of domain. The gap between the medial ends of the left and right recti muscles on this slice is 25 cm.

✔✔ Mesh repair of incisional hernia reduces the recurrence rate, even for small hernias.[54,55]

Mesh repair

The onlay technique remains the commonest technique in the West, largely because it is relatively easy to perform. The technique is dependent on closure of the anterior abdominal wall and adequate fixation of the mesh to the fascia and a minimum overlap of 5–8 cm is recommended. If the connection between the mesh and the fascia is lost, a buttonhole hernia develops at the edge of the mesh. Good results can be reported with attention to detail, namely wide overlap of the mesh, and obliteration of large skin flaps with fibrin glue.[57] However, for many surgeons the relatively high rate of hernia recurrence, seroma formation and mesh infection make this operation a poor option for the patient.

The sublay technique is the procedure favoured by the author. A mesh in the sublay position is not only sutured into position but is also held in place by the intra-abdominal pressure. Mesh in this position is therefore able to strengthen the abdominal wall both by mechanical sealing and by the induction of strong scar tissue. Several authors have compared the recurrence rate in a single institution where all three techniques have been used.[58,59] Both these studies clearly demonstrate the superior results achieved by the sublay technique.

Open sublay repair

The sublay operation begins by excising the old scar and performing a laparotomy. Adhesions tend to be maximal at the neck of the sac, so entering the abdominal cavity through the hernia sac is usually straightforward. It is helpful to mobilise adhesions off the underside of the anterior abdominal wall. It is not the author's routine practice to mobilise all the bowel adhesions unless there is a good history of recurrent episodes of obstruction. The sublay space is then developed, which is the space anterior to the posterior rectus sheath, although this becomes pre-peritoneal below the semi-arcuate line. Care should be taken to mobilise the inferior epigastric vessels up with the belly of the rectus muscle to minimise bleeding. It is also important to preserve as many of the intercostal nerves as possible to minimise muscle denervation (**Fig. 4.10**). The pre-peritoneal space can be developed behind the pelvis, akin to a TEP repair, especially if the hernia arises in a Pfannensteil incision. Superiorly, the sublay space can be developed behind the xiphisternum if necessary. The posterior rectus sheath is divided on either side close to the linea alba to expose the area known as the fatty triangle (**Fig. 4.11**). The posterior rectus sheath is approximated with an absorbable suture. The mesh is cut to size, aiming to have at least a 6-cm overlap

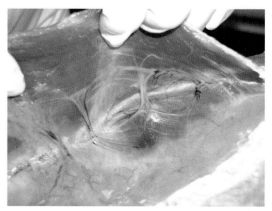

Figure 4.10 • Fresh cadaveric dissection of the retromuscular space for sublay incisional hernia. Used with permission of Dr J Conze, Aachen, Germany.

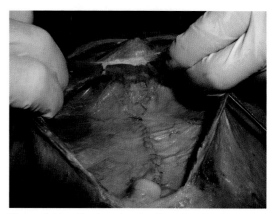

Figure 4.11 • Fresh cadaveric dissection demonstrating the fatty triangle by division of the posterior rectus sheath as it attaches to the linea alba. This allows development of the sublay space behind the xiphisternum. Used with permission of Dr J Conze, Aachen, Germany.

in all directions. This mesh is sutured to the posterior rectus sheath with interrupted absorbable sutures, avoiding any obvious nerves. These sutures are purely to hold the mesh flat until it is encased in fibrous tissue. A suction drain is often left anterior to the mesh. Any further redundant skin and hernial sac is excised and the anterior rectus sheath closed with an absorbable suture, as is the skin, minimising any subcutaneous dead space. The cross-sectional appearance is illustrated in **Fig. 4.12**. If an abdominoplasty is performed at the same time, then further drains are placed to the subcutaneous space.

✔ The open sublay technique for incisional hernia repair has a lower recurrence rate and wound complication rate compared to onlay or inlay repair techniques.[58,59] Randomised trials comparing the three mesh position techniques are lacking.

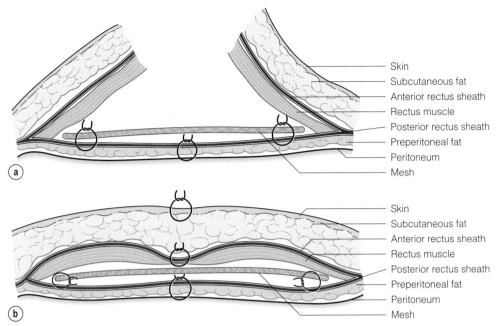

Skin
Subcutaneous fat
Anterior rectus sheath
Rectus muscle
Posterior rectus sheath
Preperitoneal fat
Peritoneum
Mesh

Skin
Subcutaneous fat
Anterior rectus sheath
Rectus muscle
Posterior rectus sheath
Preperitoneal fat
Peritoneum
Mesh

Figure 4.12 • (a) Cross-sectional appearance of peritoneum closure showing the sublay position of the mesh, which is fixed to the posterior sheath of the rectus muscle with an interrupted absorbable suture. **(b)** The anterior and posterior rectus sheath is closed continuously.

Laparoscopic repair

The laparoscopic (intraperitoneal) approach has also been applied to incisional hernias. The laparoscopic approach has the advantages of shorter hospital stay, lower analgesic requirements, fewer wound complications and an earlier return to normal activities over open surgery. However, while the complication rate is lower overall when compared to surgery, there is concern that when complications do arise with the laparoscopic approach, they are more likely to be life threatening or require further surgery to deal with compared to open surgery.[60] Furthermore, the cosmetic result for larger hernias may not be as good as there is no abdominoplasty component to the laparoscopic approach. Remember, the majority of patients wish surgery for their incisional hernia because of the cosmetic deformity rather than symptoms related to the hernia. The author reserves the laparoscopic approach for smaller incisional hernias, with a hernial neck size less than 10 cm and when cosmesis is not an issue. Two current controversies exist in the technique, related to (i) the method of fixation of the mesh and (ii) whether the hernia defect should be closed or not. The method of mesh fixation divides surgeons between those who believe transfascial sutures to be essential to prevent hernia recurrence and those who believe such sutures cause chronic pain postsurgery and their use should be avoided. The author prefers a double-crown tack technique (two rings of tacks around the hernia defect), although there is a lack of quality studies to make this an evidence-based decision. The recent introduction of absorbable tacks may reduce the risk of chronic pain and bowel adhesion to the tacks. Centring the mesh over the hernial defect is important to minimise hernia recurrence. The mesh can be centred with a central stitch,[61] although two or four corner sutures are probably more accurate.

What about closure of the defect? Bridging of the defect is recognised to be a problem at open surgery, so why bridge with laparoscopic surgery? It is clear that once adhesions to the abdominal wall are taken down, inserting a mesh and tacking it in place are usually quick and easy. Closing the defect is thus not attractive to the majority of laparoscopic surgeons, introducing tension and perhaps increasing postoperative pain. However, many groups are talking about pseudo-recurrence[62] – the redevelopment of a bulge at the hernia site several years after laparoscopic repair as the mesh slides into the hernia sac. Whether closing (either completely or partially) will reduce recurrence and pseudo-recurrence is still unknown but would seem likely.

One of the main long-term risks of the laparoscopic repair of incisional hernias is the placement of the mesh in direct contact with the intra-abdominal structures. As mentioned earlier, the use of meshes that have one side coated with a relatively non-adhesive material will help reduce (but not abolish) adhesion formation to the mesh. The other main risk is infection of the mesh, which is nearly always due to contamination from a bowel injury. Care should be taken with any adhesiolysis to minimise bowel injury with thermal sources such as diathermy and ultracision dissection kept to a minimum. The current consensus is that if the colon is injured, then it should be repaired, laparoscopically or open, according to the skills of the surgeon and no mesh inserted at this time. The patient can return in a number of months for a further attempt at repair. If the small bowel is injured with minimal contamination, then laparoscopic repair, washout and mesh insertion is acceptable. If there is significant small-bowel injury and risk of failure of the bowel repair, then no mesh should be inserted. The patient should be observed in hospital and if they remain well 4–5 days later, then it is appropriate to re-laparoscope the patient and if no continuing contamination/infection is observed, the laparoscopic mesh repair is completed. The use of antibiotic-impregnated mesh may allow a change to this policy with placement of such a mesh at the same time as bowel injury and repair.[63]

Emergency hernia surgery

Much of what has been mentioned above is applicable to hernia repair in the emergency situation. However, there are a few dilemmas that occur more frequently in the emergency setting. Patients who present as an emergency but have no bowel compromise can be treated as per elective hernia surgery. When bowel is compromised, especially when there has been significant contamination, current opinion is that synthetic mesh should not be used. However, there is little in the way of evidence apart from anecdote to support such a view and this view has been challenged.[64] The case for biological mesh in such scenarios is also lacking in evidence.[65] For those who support the laparoscopic approach, it is not unreasonable to offer this in the emergency setting and laparoscope the patient with an irreducible inguinal hernia. If the bowel can be reduced and is viable, then convert the operation to a TEP and place mesh as usual. If the bowel is compromised, then resect the bowel through a small incision and return 6 weeks later for a TEP. In the emergency incisional/ventral hernia setting, if the hernia is large, then proceed directly to open sublay mesh repair. If the hernia is smaller, then laparoscopy and intra-abdominal mesh are appropriate if there is no bowel compromise. If there is bowel ischaemia, then convert to the open sublay repair. The use of mesh in the sublay space in the emergency setting should not be associated with an increase in mesh infection as it lies external to the peritoneal cavity, but clearly each case will need to be assessed individually.

Emergency hernia surgery remains a high-risk surgical procedure, with the main risk factor for postoperative mortality being infarcted bowel.[66,67] Such operations should not be left to junior members of the surgical and anaesthetic teams. Appropriate resuscitation, followed by timely and appropriate surgery, may save lives. Occasionally, the techniques of damage limitation surgery (see Chapter 13) may be appropriate.

> ✅ Bowel infarction is the main risk factor for mortality in emergency hernia surgery.[66,67]

Port-site hernia

This is a hernia with an increasing incidence associated with the increase in laparoscopic surgery. Insertion of larger ports through the midline as opposed to more laterally appears to be a significant risk factor. This is especially true in the presence of a divarification of the recti or an unrecognised umbilical hernia. There is little evidence to support closure of the fascia except when a cut-down is performed for the first port. The use of dilating rather than cutting trocar tips may reduce the incidence of port-site hernia formation.

Antibiotic prophylaxis in hernia surgery

In general, elective hernia surgery to the groin and ventral regions does not require antibiotic prophylaxis.[68,69] However, as the risk of bowel injury is always present in incisional hernia surgery, it would be reasonable to give routine antibiotic prophylaxis for such surgery. Patients at increased risk of infection, including the immunocompromised, skin conditions with higher bacterial carriage such as psoriasis and in the emergency setting, all merit antibiotic prophylaxis.

All theatres have bacteria (called colony-forming units) in the circulating theatre air. It therefore makes sense to open the mesh just before it is required during the operation. Changing to fresh gloves before the handling of the mesh, minimising mesh contact with the skin and inserting the mesh deep to the subcutaneous tissues may all help reduce the risk of mesh contamination. The author uses a gentamicin solution (240 mg gentamicin in 250 mL normal saline) to irrigate larger meshes following insertion, although there is no evidence-based medicine to support this manoeuvre. Methicillin-resistant *Staphylococcus aureus* (MRSA) bacteria have been found on mesh several years after insertion, so prophylaxis to MRSA is appropriate if a previous repair has been complicated by MRSA infection.

> ✅✅ Antibiotic prophylaxis is unnecessary for uncomplicated elective hernia surgery to the groin and ventral regions.[68,69]

Prophylatic hernia surgery

The topic of prophylactic mesh insertion to minimise subsequent hernia formation in high-risk groups of patients remains controversial. One study reduced the incidence of incisional hernia following open gastric bypass surgery from 21% to 0% by the prophylactic insertion of a polypropylene mesh in the sublay position.[70] Another study reduced the incidence of parastomal hernia following permanent end colostomy from 50% to 5% by the prophylactic insertion of a polypropylene mesh in the sublay position at 2 years' follow-up.[71] At 5 years' the rates were 81% and 13%, respectively.[72] Both studies have small patient numbers, but no increase in morbidity was noted in the prophylactic mesh group. It is likely that prophylactic mesh to minimise subsequent hernia formation will become more mainstream practice. This may be supported by preoperative collagen type I/III ratio typing to perhaps select patients more at risk. This concept of collagen disease is important, and introduces the notion that hernia repair of any type will fail if the patient lives long enough. It is true that some surgeons' repairs last longer than others, so technical factors remain important, and mesh repairs at any time point are more likely to be intact compared to a suture repair.[56] (Re-operation rates are a surrogate for recurrence rates, although re-operation will underestimate the true recurrence rate.) However, a hernia repair at present is a patch-up job, and will probably fail eventually (if the patient lives long enough). Nevertheless, randomised trials in patients at high risk of developing incisional hernia are ongoing.

Management of an infected mesh

In general, an infected mesh has to be removed or exposed to the surface. If the mesh is lying in a pool of pus with no adherence to the patient, then the only option is removal of the mesh. If the mesh is partly embedded in tissue, then if there is adequate drainage through an open wound, many infected meshes will slowly granulate over and remain sound. However, sometimes chronic sinuses will develop and the only option is excision of these along with as much of the visible mesh as possible. Not all patients who require mesh removal will develop a hernia recurrence, although the majority probably will at some stage in the future.[73] It is the author's opinion that it is best to remove as much of the mesh foreign body as possible, control the sepsis and return at a later date for further repair. The use of biological mesh in a contaminated field is rarely indicated. The use of vacuum-assisted dressing to control the fluid exudates from the wound may aid wound care in such patients.

Key points

- Herniorrhaphy is one of the commonest operations performed.
- Techniques advanced considerably during the 1990s.
- The use of prosthetic mesh should now be considered for the repair of all hernias.
- The laparoscopic approach may be more appropriate than a traditional open approach.
- Recurrent hernias may be best managed in specialist centres or by surgeons with a specialist interest in hernia surgery who are technically competent to perform both open and laparoscopic procedures.
- A multidisciplinary approach, including plastic surgeons, may be appropriate for complex, multiply recurrent hernias.

References

1. Wagh PV, Leverich AP, Sun CN, et al. Direct inguinal herniation in men: a disease of collagen. J Surg Res 1974;17:425–33.

2. Si Z, Rhanjit B, Rosch R, et al. Impaired balance of type I and type III procollagen mRNA in cultured fibroblasts of patients with incisional hernia. Surgery 2002;131:324–31.

3. Junge K, Klinge U, Rosch R, et al. Decreased collagen typeI/III in patients with recurring hernia after implantation of alloplastic prostheses. Langenbecks Arch Surg 2004;389:17–22.

4. Junge K, Klinge U, Prescher A, et al. Elasticity of the anterior abdominal wall and impact for reparation of incisional hernias using mesh implants. Hernia 2001;5:113–8.

5. Klinge U, Klosterhalfen B. Modified classification of surgical meshes for hernia repair based on the analyses of 1,000 explanted meshes. Hernia. 2012; 16:251-8.

6. Cobb WS, Kercher KW, Heniford BT. The argument for lightweight polypropylene mesh in hernia repair. Surg Innov 2005;12:63–9.

7. Akolekar D, Kumar S, Khan LR, et al. Comparison of recurrence with lightweight composite polypropylene mesh and heavyweight mesh in laparoscopic totally extraperitoneal inguinal hernia repair: an audit of 1232 repairs. Hernia 2008;12: 39–43.

8. Holm JA, de Wall LC, Steyerberg EW, et al. Intraperitoneal polypropylene mesh hernia repair complicates subsequent abdominal surgery. World J Surg 2007;31:423–9.

9. LeBlanc KA, Booth WV. Laparoscopic repair of incisional abdominal hernias using expanded polytetrafluoroethylene: preliminary findings. Surg Laparosc Endosc 1993;3:39–41.

10. Askar OM. Aponeurotic hernias: recent observations upon paraumbilical and epigastric hernias. Surg Clin North Am 1984;64:315–29.

11. Sibley III WL, Lynn HB, Harris LE. A 25-year study of infantile umbilical hernias. Surgery 1964;55:462–70.

12. Mayo WJ. An operation for the radical cure of umbilical hernia. Ann Surg 1901;34:276–8.

13. Rowe MI, Clatworthy Jr HW. Incarcerated and strangulated hernias in children. Arch Surg 1970;101:136–43.

14. Schier F. Laparoscopic inguinal hernia repair – a prospective personal series of 542 children. J Pediatr Surg 2006;41:1081–4.

15. Kurlan MZ, Web PB, Piedad OH. Inguinal herniorrhaphy by the Mitchell Banks technique. J Pediatr Surg 1972;7:427–31.

16. Hughson W. The persistence or performed sac in relation to oblique inguinal hernia. Surg Gynecol Obstet 1925;41:610–4.

17. Lichtenstein IL, Shulman AG, Amid PK, et al. The tension-free hernioplasty. Am J Surg 1989; 157:188–93.

18. Ger R. The management of certain abdominal hernias by intra-abdominal closure of the neck. Ann R Coll Surg Engl 1982;64:342–5.

19. Ger R, Monroe K, Duvivier R, et al. Management of indirect inguinal hernias by laparoscopic closure of the neck of the sac. Am J Surg 1990; 159:370–6.

20. Gazayerli MM. Anatomical laparoscopic hernia repair of direct or indirect inguinal hernias using the transversalis fascia and iliopubic tract. Surg Laparosc Endosc 1992;2:49–52.

21. Nyhus LM, Pollak R, Bombeck CT, et al. The preperitoneal approach and prosthetic buttress repair for recurrent hernia. Ann Surg 1988; 203:733–8.

22. Toy FK, Smoot Jr RT. Laparoscopic herniorrhaphy update. Laparoendosc Surg 1992;2:197–9.

23. Annandale T. Case in which a reducible oblique and direct inguinal and femoral hernia existed on the same side and were successfully treated by operation. Edinb Med J 1876;27: 1087–9.

24. Taylor C, Layani L, Liew V, et al. Laparoscopic inguinal hernia repair without mesh fixation, early results of a large randomized clinical trial. Surg Endosc 2008;22:757–63.

25. National Institute for Clinical Excellence. Laparoscopic surgery for inguinal hernia repair. Technology Appraisal Guidance 83. London: NICE; 2004. Available at www.nice.org.uk/TA083guidance [accessed 02.08.12].
    An excellent meta-analysis of open versus laparoscopic inguinal hernia repair.

26. van Veen RN, Wijsmuller AR, Vrijland WW, et al. Long term follow up of a randomized clinical trial of non-mesh versus mesh repair of primary inguinal hernia. Br J Surg 2007;94:506–10.

27. Fitzgibbons RJ. Can we be sure polypropylene mesh causes infertility. Ann Surg 2005;241:559–61.

28. Franneby U, Sandblom G, Nordin P, et al. Risk factors for long-term pain after hernia surgery. Ann Surg 2006;244:212–9.

29. Aasvang EK, Gmaehle E, Hansen JB, et al. Predictive risk factors for persistent postherniotomy pain. Anaesthesiology 2010;112:957–69.
    Chronic pain can be predicted prior to surgery with simple bedside tests.

30. Shouldice EB. The Shouldice repair for groin hernias. Surg Clin North Am 2003;83: 1163–87.

31. Shulman AG, Amid PK, Lichtenstein IL. The safety of mesh repair for primary inguinal hernias. Am Surg 1992;58:255–9.

32. McCormack K, Wake B, Perez J, et al. Laparoscopic surgery for inguinal hernia repair: systematic review of effectiveness and economic evaluation. Health Technol Assess 2005;9:1–203.
   Cost analysis of laparoscopic compared to open surgery using the same data that were used for the 2004 NICE report (Ref. 25 above).

33. Duff M, Mofidi R, Nixon SJ. Routine laparoscopic repair of primary unilateral inguinal hernias – a viable alternative in the day surgery unit? Surgeon 2007;5:209–12.

34. Eklund A, Rudberg C, Smedberg S, et al. Short-term results of a randomized clinical trial comparing Lichtenstein open repair with totally extraperitoneal laparoscopic inguinal hernia repair. Br J Surg 2006;93:1060–8.

35. Atkinson HDE, Nicol SG, Purkayastha S, et al. Surgical management of inguinal hernia: retrospective cohort study in southeastern Scotland 1985–2001. Br Med J 2004;329:1315–6.

36. Herzog U. Das Leistenhernienrezidiv. Schweiz Rundsch Med Prax 1990;79:1166–9.

37. Wantz GE. The Canadian repair: personal observations. World J Surg 1989;13:516–21.

38. Shulman AG, Amid PK, Lichtenstein IL. The plug repair of 1402 recurrent inguinal hernias: 20-year experience. Arch Surg 1990;125:265–7.

39. Bendavid R. The rational use of mesh in hernias: a perspective. Int Surg 1992;77:229–31.

40. Fong Y, Wantz GE. Prevention of ischaemicorchitis during inguinal hernioplasty. Surg Gynecol Obstet 1992;174:399–402.

41. Schaap HM, van de Pavoordt H, Bast TJ. The preperitoneal approach in the repair of recurrent inguinal hernias. Surg Gynecol Obstet 1992;174:460–4.

42. Beets GL, Dirkoen CD, Go PM, et al. Open or laparoscopic mesh repair for recurrent inguinal hernia. A randomised controlled trial. Surg Endosc 1999;13:323–7.

43. Langer I, Herjog U, Schuppisser JP, et al. Preperitoneal prosthesis implantation in surgical management of recurrent inguinal hernia. Retrospective evaluation of our results 1989–1994. Chirurg 1996;67:394–402.

44. Sevonius D, Gunnarsson U, Nordin P, et al. Recurrent groin hernia surgery. Br J Surg 2011;98:1489–94.

45. O'Dwyer PJ, Norrie J, Alani A, et al. Observation or operation for patients with an asymptomatic inguinal hernia. A randomized clinical trial. Ann Surg 2006;244:167–73.
   The first randomised trial on surgery versus no surgery in the asymptomatic hernia.

46. Fitzgibbons RJ, Giobbie-Hurder A, Gibbs JO, et al. Watchful waiting vs repair of inguinal hernia in minimally symptomatic men. A randomized clinical trial. JAMA 2007;295:285–92.

47. Yalamarthi S, Kumar S, Stapleton E, et al. Laparoscopic totally extraperitoneal mesh repair for femoral hernia. J Laparoendosc Adv Surg Tech A 2004;14:358–61.

48. Hermandez-Richter T, Schardey HM, Rau HG, et al. The femoral hernia. An ideal approach for the transabdominal preperitoneal technique (TAPP). Surg Endosc 2000;14:736–40.

49. Ceydeli A, Rucinski J, Wise L. Finding the best abdominal closure: an evidence-based review of the literature. Curr Surg 2005;62:220–5.

50. Bloemen A, van Dooren P, Huizinga BF, et al. Randomized clinical trial comparing polypropylene or polydioxanone for midline abdominal wall closure. Br J Surg 2011;98:633–9.

51. Seiler CM, Bruckner T, Diener MK, et al. Interrupted or continuous slowly absorbable sutures for closure of primary elective midline abdominal incisionals: a multicentre randomized trial (INSECT). Ann Surg 2011;249:576–82.

52. Millbourn D, Cengiz Y, Israelsson LA. Effect of stitch length on wound complications after closure of midline incisions. A randomized controlled trial. Arch Surg 2009;144:1056–9.

53. Millbourn D, Cengiz Y, Israelsson LA. Risk factors for wound complications in midline abdominal incisions related to the size of the stitches. Hernia 2011;15:261–6.

54. Luijendijk RW, Hop WC, van den Tol MP, et al. A comparison of suture repair with mesh repair for incisional hernia. N Engl J Med 2000;343:392–8.
   The first randomised trial to demonstrate the benefit of mesh in reducing recurrence in incisional hernia repair.

55. Burger JW, Luijendijk RW, Hop WC, et al. Long term follow up of a randomized controlled trial of suture versus mesh repair of incisional hernia. Ann Surg 2004;240:578–83.

56. Flum DR, Horvath K, Koepsell T. Have outcomes of incisional hernia repair improved with time. Ann Surg 2003;237:129–35.

57. Kingsnorth AN, Shahid MK, Valliattu AJ, et al. Open onlay mesh repair for major abdominal wall hernias with selective use of component separation and fibrin sealant. World J Surg 2008;32:26–30.

58. Langer C, Liersch T, Kley C, et al. Twenty five years of experience in incisional hernia surgery. A comparative retrospective study of 432 incisional hernia repairs. Chirurg 2003;74:638–45.

59. de Vries Reilingh TS, van Geldere D, Langenhorst BLAM, et al. Repair of large midline incisional hernias with polypropylene mesh: comparison of three operative techniques. Hernia 2004;8:56–9.

60. Kaafarani HM, Hur K, Campasano M, et al. Classification and valuation of post-operative complications in a randomized trial of open versus laparoscopic ventral herniorrhaphy. Hernia 2010;14:231–5.

61. Motson RW, Engledow AH, Medhurst C, et al. Laparoscopic incisional hernia repair with a self-centring suture. Br J Surg 2006;93:1549–53.

62. Tse GH, Stutchfield BM, Duckworth AD, et al. Pseudo-recurrence following laparoscopic ventral and incisional hernia repair. Hernia 2010;14: 583–8.

63. LeBlanc KA, Elieson MJ, Corder JM. Enterotomy and mortality rates of laparoscopic incisional and ventral hernia repair: a review of the literature. JSLS 2007;11:408–14.

64. Kelly ME, Behrman SW. The safety and efficacy of prosthetic hernia repair in clean-contaminated and contaminated wounds. Am Surg 2002;68: 524–9.

65. Ventral Hernia Working Group. Incisional ventral hernias: review of the literature and recommendations regarding the grading and technique of the repair. Surgery 2010;148:544–58.

66. Nilsson H, Stylianidis G, Haapamaki M, et al. Mortality after groin hernia surgery. Ann Surg 2007;245:656–60.

67. Derici H, Unalp HR, Bozdaq AD. Factors affecting morbidity and mortality in incarcerated abdominal wall hernia. Hernia 2007;11:341–6.

68. Sanchez-Manuel FJ, Lozano-Garcia J, Seco-Gil JL. Antibiotic prophylaxis for hernia repair. Cochrane Database Syst Rev 2007; CD003769.
The latest meta-analysis on this topic.

69. SIGN. Antibiotic prophylaxis in surgery. Guideline 104. 2008. www.sign.ac.uk [accessed 02.08.12].
The SIGN website allows all guidelines produced to date to be downloaded for free. An excellent reference source on current best practice in a variety of medical and surgical conditions.

70. Strzelczyk JM, Szymanski D, Nawicki ME, et al. Randomised trial of post operation hernia prophylaxis in open bariatric surgery. Br J Surg 2006;93:1347–50.

71. Janes A, Cenqiz Y, Israelsson LA. Preventing parastomal hernia with a prophylactic mesh. Arch Surg 2004;139:1356–8.

72. Janes A, Cenqiz Y, Israelsson LA. Preventing parastomal hernia with a prosthetic mesh: a 5-year follow-up of a randomized study. World J Surg 2009;33:118–21.

73. Fawole AS, Choperala RP, Ambrose NS. Fate of the inguinal hernia following removal of infected prosthetic mesh. Hernia 2006;10:58–61.

5

Organisation of emergency general surgical services and the early assessment and investigation of the acute abdomen

Simon Paterson-Brown

Introduction

The management of emergency surgery has undergone huge changes over the last 5 years as both surgeons and hospital managers have finally recognised that it is not only a major part of 'general surgery', but also associated with a significant morbidity and mortality, accounting for a large part of hospital resources. The American College of Surgeons National Surgical Quality Improvement Project recently examined the results of emergency appendicectomy, cholecystectomy and colorectal resections in 95 hospitals between 2005 and 2008.[1] They found that the risk of severe morbidity or death was 3.7% in the 30 788 appendicectomies performed, 6.37% in the 5824 cholecystectomies and 41.56% in the 8990 colorectal resections. Interestingly, they also identified that in 7–10% of hospitals good or bad performance could be generalisable across the three procedures, suggesting that there are 'best' and 'worse' practices to be identified.

Reduced bed days and improvements in patient care are, not surprisingly, associated with earlier and better clinical decision-making, prompt and appropriate surgery, along with reductions in readmissions and later requirements for surgery. Until recently, many surgical units throughout the world continued their elective work in tandem with their on-call commitments and, as a result, getting timely surgical intervention on all but the sickest emergency patients was difficult, resulting in delayed operations, usually going on late into the night and often carried out by junior surgical trainees. However, over the last few years, due to a number of factors, this has all changed. The increased number of surgical admissions to many hospitals, associated with regional reorganisation of surgical services[2,3] and the associated increase in workload,[4] the reduced experience of surgical trainees due to the reduction in junior doctors' hours and training period,[5] and the recognition that early assessment by experienced senior surgeons with timely surgical intervention,[6] preferably by someone with an interest in that condition, have led to a recognition that a radical change in the provision of acute general surgical services was required. The Association of Surgeons of Great Britain and Ireland (ASGBI) held a consensus meeting on the future of emergency general surgery in 2006, subsequently publishing their conclusions,[7] which are summarised in Box 5.1. A subsequent survey of consultant surgeons in the UK by the ASGBI[8] reported that: only 55% considered they were able to care well for their emergency patients; the workload was increasing with junior support decreasing; only 19% had comprehensive interventional radiology service out of hours; 55% had inadequate access to an emergency theatre; current pressure within the NHS favoured elective over emergency work; many felt they could not argue the case for change at a local level; and many felt that helpful changes would include national standards of practice and of service delivery, proper theatre access, and increased separation of elective and emergency work.

1. There is evidence that there is wide variation in the quality of emergency general surgery (EGS).
2. EGS is a huge clinical service with approximately 1000 finished consultant episodes per 100 000 population per year.
3. All hospitals should have a named surgeon responsible for the clinical leadership of EGS.
4. Emergency admissions must have dedicated resources and senior surgical personnel readily available.
5. There must be a clear and identifiable separation of delivery of emergency and elective care.
6. Local circumstances will determine model of delivery.
7. Timely access to diagnostic services (particularly radiology) and emergency theatre should be provided.
8. The assessment, prioritisation and management of emergency general surgical patients should be the responsibility of accredited general surgeons.
9. An essential prerequisite for accreditation in general surgery is competence to manage unselected general surgical emergencies.
10. The largest component of EGS is GI surgery.
11. The emergency general surgeon should remain competent in trauma management.
12. Vascular surgery is undergoing significant changes and in future will probably not be involved in EGS.
13. Dedicated breast surgeons are unlikely to be involved in EGS in the future.
14. Surgeons managing EGS should be as committed to continuing medical education related to EGS in a manner equivalent to their elective surgical practice.
15. The care of emergency surgical patients should be delivered to equal standards as those accepted for elective surgical practice.

Organisation of emergency general surgical services

Separation of elective and emergency surgery

Where in the past the continuity of care for surgical patients was maintained by the 'middle grade' surgical team, current rotas are now primarily of a shift pattern where the maximum time worked per week is around 48 hours, and as a result consultants find they rarely work with the same trainees[9] and continuity of care is reduced.[10] One solution to this problem was the introduction of the 'surgeon of the day', first suggested in 1995,[11]

and then fully implemented in Edinburgh, UK, as the 'emergency team' in 1997.[12] With this system, the whole surgical team (consultant and supporting junior staff) have no elective commitments for their time on call and, although unfortunately shift working remains essential in many countries due to restricted working hours, the same trainees take part in the emergency team for extended periods of time. Their subsequent attachment to elective activity then no longer suffers from the disruption associated with on-call shifts, a state of affairs that enhances both emergency and elective training opportunities. This 'emergency team' system, with various adaptations according to local requirements,[13] has now been adopted in many units throughout the UK and increasingly worldwide. Two recent publications from the Association of Surgeons of Great Britain and Ireland include descriptions on the different ways that individual hospitals and regions in the UK have changed their service in order to improve the provision of emergency surgical services.[14,15] Box 5.2 provides recommendations published by the Royal College of Surgeons of England[16] for the separation of elective and emergency general surgery.

The emergency team undoubtedly improves the ability of the consultant general surgeon, as well as the middle grade team, to provide safe and effective emergency care, but requires other conditions to be met if this is to be both efficient and cost-effective, not only in terms of lost elective activity for the consultant but also training opportunities for the surgical trainees. These include easy access to radiological imaging, a dedicated emergency operating theatre with full (and senior) anaesthetic support available 24 hours each day,[17] enough surgical admissions to make the system worthwhile, and a distinct and dedicated admission area for emergency patients to be assessed. This is particularly useful in the assessment of patients with equivocal clinical signs, such as in early appendicitis, where the value of 'active observation' with reassessment after 2–3 hours by the same surgeon, repeated thereafter as necessary, is well established.[18]

✔✔ Emergency general surgery should be provided by a team that is free of elective commitments. All emergency general surgical patients should be admitted to a single dedicated admission area within the hospital, where they can be assessed and reviewed by the admitting surgical team. This should be supported by easy access to an emergency operating theatre and appropriate and timely radiological investigations.[7,16]

1. A physical separation of services, facilities and rotas works best, although a separate unit on the same site is preferable to a completely separate location.

2. The presence of senior surgeons for both elective and emergency work will enhance patient safety and the quality of care, and ensure that training opportunities are maximised.

3. The separation of emergency and elective surgical care can facilitate protected and concentrated training for junior surgeons providing consultants are available to supervise their work.

4. Creating an 'emergency team', linked with a 'surgeon of the week', is a good method of providing dedicated and supervised training in all aspects of emergency and elective care.

5. Separating emergency and elective services can prevent the admission of emergency patients (both medical and surgical) from disrupting planned activity and vica versa, thus minimising patient inconvenience and maximising productivity for the hospital. The success of this will largely depend on having sufficient beds and resources for each service.

6. Hospital-acquired infections can be reduced by the provision of protected elective wards and avoiding admissions from the emergency department and transfers from within/outside the hospital.

7. The improved use of IT (information technology) solutions can assist with separating workloads (for example, scheduling systems for appointments and theatres, telemedicine, picture archiving and communication systems, etc.), although it is recognised that developments in IT for the NHS are generally behind schedule.

8. High-volume specialities are particularly suited to separating two strands of work. Other specialities can also benefit by having emergencies seen by senior surgeons – this can help to reduce unnecessary admissions, deal with ward emergencies and facilitate rapid discharge.

Subspecialisation in emergency general surgery

Along with the recognition that emergency surgery deserves more attention and support has also come the recognition that specialist conditions are often better treated by surgeons with a particular interest and experience in that subspeciality. This has of course been recognised for some time in the elective performance of a number of surgical procedures, including oesophagectomy, gastrectomy, abdominal aortic aneurysm repair, lung lobectomy, cardiac surgery and colectomy,[19,20] and although mainly thought to be related to hospital and surgeon volumes,[21] specialisation of the surgical team is also an important factor.[22] However, there are now data available to support similar improvements in patient outcomes for emergency conditions, such as acute gallstone disease[23,24] and acute colorectal disorders.[25] This is not surprising considering the subspecialisation that has occurred in general surgery over the last decade,[26] with consultant surgeons now being expected to deal with surgical conditions in the emergency situation that they no longer see in their elective practice. Reports of the separation of upper and lower elective and emergency gastrointestinal (GI) services in one region of Scotland have been encouraging. Not only has there been a significant increase in the number of patients with acute gallstone problems undergoing the same admission laparoscopic cholecystectomy,[27] there have also been improvements in the management of perforated duodenal ulcers,[28] and acute diverticulitis where patients have a lower mortality and fewer stomas.[29] The challenge now is for all those surgeons involved in the development and provision of emergency surgical care to produce on-call rotas that allow, where possible, patients with specific subspeciality conditions to be treated and operated upon by surgeons with a specific interest in that area. This will undoubtedly involve reorganisation of regional emergency surgical services, bringing together a wider group of surgeons for the on-call rota, with the ability to provide both upper and lower GI cover. The political hurdles of closing some emergency services in some hospitals in order to provide these larger emergency surgical units in other hospitals must be overcome if the undoubted improvements in patient care associated with dedicated emergency surgical services delivered by surgical teams with appropriate subspeciality expertise are to be realised, while at the same time providing robust junior doctor rotas that comply with the appropriate working time directives.

Early assessment of the acute abdomen

Attempts to improve preoperative diagnosis and early management of patients with acute abdominal pain are continuously being made; this section discusses all the current available techniques and the evidence for their incorporation into emergency surgical practice. For the purposes of most studies looking at acute abdominal pain, the broad definition is taken as 'abdominal pain of less than 1 week's duration requiring admission to hospital, which has not been previously treated or investigated'. However, this must be accepted as a fairly loose definition.

For an emergency team system to work efficiently the surgical team must have rapid access to diagnostic blood tests and appropriate imaging, which should include plain and contrast radiology, both diagnostic and interventional (percutaneous drainage and biopsy), ultrasound (US) and computed tomography (CT). Furthermore, plain radiography evaluated by senior radiologists substantially enhances senior surgical assessment of patients with acute abdominal pain, resulting in reduced surgical admissions.[30] All these modalities are discussed below.

Conditions associated with abdominal pain

Many studies have looked at the spectrum of patients admitted to hospital with acute abdominal pain and the approximate percentage represented by each condition is now well understood. Figures from one study[31] appear to be fairly representative (Box 5.3). In this study the 30-day mortality in 1190 emergency admissions was 4%, with a perioperative mortality of 8%. Not surprisingly, the mortality rate was age related, with perioperative mortality in patients below 60 years being 2%, rising to 12% in those 60–69 years and reaching 20% in patients over the age of 80 years. Laparotomy for irresectable disease was the most common cause of perioperative mortality (28%), with ruptured abdominal aortic aneurysm (23%), perforated peptic ulcer (16%) and colonic resections (14%) all being associated with significant perioperative mortality.

What stands out from all the studies on acute abdominal pain published over the last few decades is the high incidence of non-specific abdominal pain (NSAP), with published figures of 40% or more.[32] NSAP usually reflects a failure of diagnosis, as many of these patients do have a cause for the pain and it has been shown that further investigations, such as laparoscopy, can reduce the overall incidence of NSAP to around 27%.[33]

Some authors have examined this diagnosis of NSAP further and describe a certain number of alternative conditions that could be related (Box 5.4),[32] including abdominal wall pain[34] and rectus nerve entrapment.[35] In some cases of NSAP, detection of abdominal wall tenderness (increased abdominal pain on tensing the abdominal wall

Box 5.3 • Conditions that may present with acute abdominal pain

Non-specific abdominal pain (NSAP) (35%)
Acute appendicitis (17%)
Intestinal obstruction (15%)
Urological causes (6%)
Gallstone disease (5%)
Colonic diverticular disease (4%)
Abdominal trauma (3%)
Abdominal malignancy (3%)
Perforated peptic ulcer (3%)
Pancreatitis (2%)

Conditions contributing 1% or less
Exacerbation of peptic ulcer
Ruptured abdominal aortic aneurysm
Gynaecological causes (these may go unnoticed as NSAP)
Inflammatory bowel disease
Medical conditions
Mesenteric ischaemia
Gastroenteritis
Miscellaneous

Reproduced from Irvin TT. Abdominal pain: a surgical audit of 1190 emergency admissions. Br J Surg 1989; 76:1121–5. © British Journal of Surgery Society Ltd. Reproduced with permission. Permission is granted by John Wiley & Sons Ltd on behalf of the BJSS Ltd.

Box 5.4 • Causes of non-specific abdominal pain[32]

Viral infections
Bacterial gastroenteritis
Worm infestation
Irritable bowel syndrome
Gynaecological conditions
Psychosomatic pain
Abdominal wall pain[34]
• Iatrogenic peripheral nerve injuries
• Hernias
• Myofascial pain syndromes
• Rib tip syndrome
• Nerve root pain
• Rectus sheath haematoma

muscles) may be a useful diagnostic test.[36] Possible causes of abdominal wall pain are also given in Box 5.4. The major problem with making a diagnosis of NSAP is in missing serious underlying disease, and the late Tim de Dombal demonstrated that 10% of patients over the age of 50 years who were admitted to hospital with acute abdominal pain were subsequently found to have intra-abdominal malignancy.[37] Half of these patients had colonic carcinoma and the major concern was that 50% of the patients who were subsequently proved to have intra-abdominal cancer were discharged from hospital with a diagnosis of NSAP.

Acute gynaecological conditions such as pelvic inflammatory disease and ovarian cyst accidents are another group of diagnoses that may often be included under the umbrella of NSAP, simply because of failure to take a good history or examination or even perform a thorough pelvic examination, whether digitally, ultrasonographically or at operation. In one study from a general surgical unit, gynaecological causes represented 13% of all diagnoses in a consecutive series of all emergency admissions (both male and female) initially presumed to be 'surgical' in origin.[38] As many of these patients present with 'query appendicitis', accurate assessment is essential if unnecessary operations are to be avoided, and even then the diagnosis may remain hidden unless the surgeon examines the pelvic organs once a normal appendix has been found. However, with the increased use of diagnostic laparoscopy, discussed later in this chapter, these conditions are now being recognised by the emergency surgeon with much greater frequency. Early recognition and appropriate treatment of pelvic inflammatory disease may help to avoid potentially serious long-term sequelae and must be encouraged.[39] Indeed, the condition of Curtis–Fitz-Hugh syndrome, when transperitoneal spread of pelvic inflammatory disease produces right upper quadrant pain due to perihepatic adhesions, is now well recognised and care must be taken to differentiate this from acute biliary conditions.[40]

Although much is made of possible 'medical' causes of acute abdominal pain in surgical textbooks, the incidence of conditions such as myocardial infarction, lobar pneumonia and some metabolic disorders is extremely small, though many still masquerade as NSAP. However, the possibility of such conditions must still be borne in mind during the clinical assessment of all patients with acute abdominal pain: one study has shown that 19 of 1168 children (1.6%) admitted to hospital with acute abdominal pain had pneumonia as the sole cause of symptoms.[41] It is therefore still extremely important to recognise these medical conditions when they do present, before exploratory surgery, as the mortality can be significantly increased.[42]

History and examination (including computer-aided diagnosis)

In the early 1970s, de Dombal et al.[43] in Leeds and Gunn[44] in Edinburgh developed a computer program based on Bayesian reasoning that produced a list of probable diagnoses for individual patients with acute abdominal pain. They demonstrated that the accuracy of clinical diagnosis could be improved by around 20%, and a subsequent multicentre study confirmed this finding.[45] Furthermore, these studies showed that there was a reduction in the unnecessary laparotomy rate and bad management errors (patients whose surgery is incorrectly delayed). When the reasons for the improvement in diagnostic accuracy associated with the use of computer-aided diagnosis (CAD) were examined, there appeared to be three main factors involved: (i) peer review and audit, which is invariably associated with improved results in most aspects of medical management;[46] (ii) an educational factor related to feedback;[47] and (iii) probably of greatest significance, the use of structured data sheets on to which the history and examination findings were documented before being entered into the computer program. One study went on to demonstrate that the diagnostic accuracy of junior doctors improved by nearly 20% when they used structured data sheets alone, without going on to use the CAD program.[48] The same study also demonstrated that medical students assessing patients with the structured data sheets and then using the CAD program reached similar levels of diagnostic accuracy to qualified doctors. Other studies have since confirmed similar improvements in clinical decision-making following the introduction of these data sheets.[49]

> ✓✓ The message from all these studies is clear: a good history and examination remain essential for both diagnostic accuracy and good clinical decision-making, and the use of a structured data sheet helps the clinician to achieve this objective.[8,9,45]

The aim of both the history and examination is to determine a diagnosis and clinical decision. There are undoubtedly specific features associated with all acute abdominal conditions that are well established; however, it remains the ability to identify the presence or absence of peritoneal inflammation that probably has the greatest influence on the final surgical decision. In other words, the presence or absence of guarding and rebound tenderness, and a history of pain on coughing, correlates well with the presence of peritonitis.[50] The differential diagnosis of acute appendicitis from NSAP is always difficult, particularly in children, and both guarding and rebound tenderness are significantly more likely to be present in acute appendicitis.[51] There was always great emphasis in the past on the importance of a rectal examination in patients with suspected acute appendicitis to elicit tenderness within the pelvis. However, when rebound tenderness is detected in the lower abdomen, as evident by pain on gentle percussion, further examination by rectal examination has been shown to provide no new information.[52] Rectal examination can therefore be avoided in such patients and reserved for those patients without rebound tenderness or where specific pelvic disease needs to be excluded. Measurement of temperature has also been shown to be relatively non-discriminatory in the early assessment of the acute abdomen.[53] Urgent urinary microscopy should be carried out on anyone with any symptoms that could relate to the urinary tract and it is a good principle to dip test the urine on admission of every patient with acute abdominal pain.

Initial blood investigations and early decision-making

After the initial assessment (history and examination) of patients with acute abdominal pain, steps should be taken towards resuscitation, pain relief and further diagnostic tests as required. There is very good evidence to support the early administration of opiate analgesia in patients with acute abdominal pain, and a recent Cochrane systematic review confirmed that patient comfort was improved without detrimentally affecting surgical decision-making.[54]

✔✔ The early administration of opiate analgesia in patients with acute abdominal pain improves patient comfort without adversely affecting clinical decision-making.[54]

Once the initial assessment has been completed, the surgeon will reach a differential diagnosis and, perhaps more importantly, a clinical decision: early operation definitely required, early operation definitely not required or need for early operation uncertain. Clearly, further investigations in the first category are unlikely to influence management, with the exception of a serum amylase level, which may reveal acute pancreatitis.[55] Further investigations in the group in which the surgeon considers early operation is not required can be organised on a more leisurely basis, and it is not surprising that it is in the group in which the surgeon is uncertain as to whether early operation is required that most difficulty exists.[56] Most of the uncertainty relates to 'query appendicitis', particularly in the young female, but also involves patients with intestinal obstruction and the elderly patient, in whom the diagnosis of mesenteric ischaemia must always be considered.[57]

✔✔ Early diagnosis in patients with mesenteric ischaemia is particularly important as survival after surgery is much better in those with venous thrombosis than those with arterial thrombosis.[58]

In the assessment of the role of subsequent investigations in the acute abdomen, it is important to identify their potential influence on clinical decision-making rather than evaluating them purely on diagnostic potential.

Although blood tests are often useful as a baseline, their influence on the diagnosis of acute abdominal pain remains unclear, with the exception of serum amylase[55] and increasingly serum lipase[59] or acute pancreatitis (see also Chapter 8). Studies examining the influence of white cell concentration[60] and C-reactive protein[61,62] in patients with 'query appendicitis' have concluded that serial white cell counts are useful (compared with a single measurement). Although isolated C-reactive protein levels may also be fairly non-discriminatory, when they are interpreted with white cell count and both are normal, acute appendicitis is unlikely.[63]

✔✔ Overall, inflammatory markers are poor discriminators of conditions such as appendicitis when looked at individually, but when combined and used with history and clinical findings of peritoneal irritation they achieve a high discriminatory power.[64] Thus, routine measurement of the white cell count and C-reactive protein in patients with acute abdominal pain can be justified, not only for a baseline with which to compare subsequent levels depending on clinical progress, but also to be interpreted along with all other clinical and biochemical findings.

Liver function tests are of course an essential investigation in the early assessment of the acute abdomen where acute biliary disease is suspected.[65]

The other area that has attracted great interest in the role of blood tests for aiding diagnosis in the acute abdomen is intestinal ischaemia, whether from strangulated obstruction or mesenteric ischaemia and infarction. Estimation of acid–base status to assess the degree of metabolic acidosis is often a late change and measurement of serum phosphate, lactate, kinase, creatine, lactate dehydrogenase, alkaline phosphatase, diamineoxidase and porcine ileal peptide have all been shown to be unreliable.[58] A recent study, however, has demonstrated the use of a combined clinico-radiological score for predicting the risk of strangulation in small-bowel obstruction.[66] This will be discussed in more detail later.

Radiological investigations

With advances in technology and improved radiological techniques, the radiologist is playing an ever more important role in the diagnosis of patients with acute abdominal pain. Furthermore, abdominal ultrasonography and plain radiography evaluated by senior radiologists substantially enhance senior surgical assessment of patients with acute abdominal pain, resulting in reduced surgical admissions.[67]

Plain radiology

The role of plain radiology in the investigation of the acute abdomen has been extensively examined. Until recently there was general consensus that the erect chest radiograph was the most appropriate investigation for the detection of free intraperitoneal gas, with use of the lateral decubitus film if either the erect chest film could not be taken (due to the patient's condition) or was equivocal. This no longer seems to be true following a report from Taiwan, where ultrasonography was shown to be superior to the erect chest radiograph, with a sensitivity of 92% in the detection of pneumoperitoneum compared with only 78% for plain radiology.[68] Undoubtedly there will be operator dependence and for now the erect chest radiograph should still be the initial test for suspected perforation (**Fig. 5.1**). Failure to detect free gas under the diaphragm in a patient with suspected intestinal obstruction can then be further investigated by US, CT or contrast radiology, as discussed below. The erect chest radiograph remains important for excluding chest conditions such as acute lobar pneumonia that can present as acute upper abdominal pain (**Fig. 5.2**).

Plain abdominal radiography is still carried out unnecessarily in a large number of patients,[69] and it could be significantly reduced if its use is limited to those patients where it might provide some diagnostic help, such as suspected intestinal obstruction, suspected perforation (**Fig. 5.3**) and exacerbation of colitis.[70]

✅✅ The use of the supine abdominal radiograph should be limited to patients with suspected intestinal obstruction, suspected perforation and exacerbation of colitis, as indicated in the guidelines produced by the Royal College of Radiologists.[71]

Similar controversy exists in the use of erect abdominal radiographs for the assessment of patients with suspected intestinal obstruction. Most surgeons still prefer both views (erect and supine) on the basis that in those patients in whom the supine radiograph is normal or equivocal the erect film may be helpful.[72]

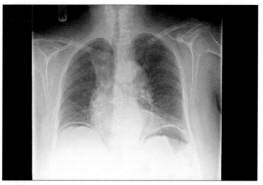

Figure 5.1 • Erect chest radiograph in a patient with a perforated duodenal ulcer. Note the free intraperitoneal air under both hemidiaphragms.

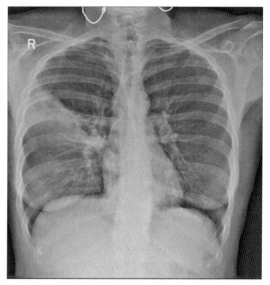

Figure 5.2 • Erect chest radiograph in a patient with acute right-sided pneumonia.

Contrast radiology

It has been recognised for many years that gastrointestinal contrast studies can be used to evaluate acute gastrointestinal conditions.[73] Its main function remains the assessment of both large- and small-bowel obstruction and possible gastrointestinal perforation. However, with the increasing availability of multi-slice CT (see below) this role is dwindling.

Perforated peptic ulcer

Although the erect chest radiograph is recognised as the most appropriate first-line investigation for a suspected perforated peptic ulcer, in approximately 50% of patients no free gas can be identified on the

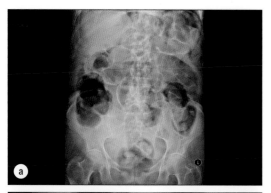

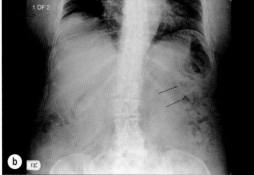

Figure 5.3 • Plain supine abdominal radiographs demonstrating free intraperitoneal air **(a)** in a patient with a perforated duodenal ulcer and retroperitoneal air **(b)** in a patient with perforated diverticular disease.

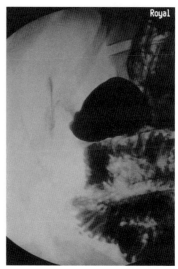

Figure 5.4 • Supine abdominal radiograph taken 20 minutes after the oral administration of 50 mL of water-soluble contrast material in a patient with a suspected perforated peptic ulcer in whom the erect chest radiograph was normal. Note the small trickle of contrast through the perforation. These findings were confirmed at laparotomy. Reproduced from Ellis BW, Paterson-Brown S (eds). Hamilton Bailey's emergency surgery, 13th edn. London: Hodder Arnold, 2000. With kind permission from Taylor Francis.

radiograph.[74] This leaves the emergency surgeon with three options: (i) to review the diagnosis, such as reconsidering acute pancreatitis; (ii) to proceed to laparotomy based on the clinical findings alone; or (iii) particularly if there are reasonable grounds for uncertainty, to arrange for either a CT with oral contrast or a water-soluble contrast study. The latter will confirm or refute the presence of an ongoing leak (**Fig. 5.4**), but will not differentiate between the patient without a perforation and one in whom the perforation has sealed. The addition of US,[68] as already discussed, and increasingly CT in this scenario may help by revealing free abdominal air and fluid in the patient whose perforation has sealed spontaneously. As has been well understood for quite some time now, many patients with perforated peptic ulcers can be managed non-operatively;[75] with this knowledge, the assessing surgeon has plenty of time to resuscitate the patient and make efforts to confirm or refute the diagnosis before rushing to emergency surgery. Patients who might be considered for non-operative treatment of their perforation should have a contrast meal to confirm spontaneous sealing of the perforation. This topic is discussed in more detail in Chapter 6.

Small-bowel obstruction

Surgery for small-bowel obstruction is performed for one of two reasons: first, there has been failure of non-operative management; second, there is clinical suspicion of impending strangulation. Although plain abdominal radiographs are useful in establishing the diagnosis of small-bowel obstruction, they cannot differentiate between strangulated and non-strangulated gut. The criteria on which strangulated intestine must be suspected are well established: peritonism, fever, tachycardia and leucocytosis.[76] However, even when the diagnosis is suspected, the changes at operation are often irreversible and resection required. Some workers have looked at serum markers such as phosphate and lactate concentrations[58] to help identify patients with possible strangulation in order to allow earlier surgery, but unfortunately they are unreliable. As in other areas of acute abdominal imaging, US also appears to be able to contribute to the diagnosis of intestinal obstruction,[77] but the problem of detecting early ischaemic changes in small-bowel obstruction remains largely unsolved. There is little doubt that water-soluble contrast studies in patients with small-bowel obstruction are useful in detecting those patients who are not likely to settle with non-operative management.[78] A randomised trial comparing water-soluble contrast follow-through versus conventional management in patients with suspected adhesive small-bowel obstruction demonstrated a significantly shorter time to surgery and therefore overall hospital stay in the group receiving the contrast study.[79] Water-soluble contrast material also allows quicker resolution of symptoms.[80] In general, failure of water-soluble contrast to reach the caecum by 4 hours strongly suggests that surgical intervention is likely to be required, and better sooner than later (**Fig. 5.5**). Water-soluble contrast follow-through is also useful in the assessment of early postoperative obstruction in order to identify those patients with an ileus from those with mechanical obstruction who need re-operation.[81]

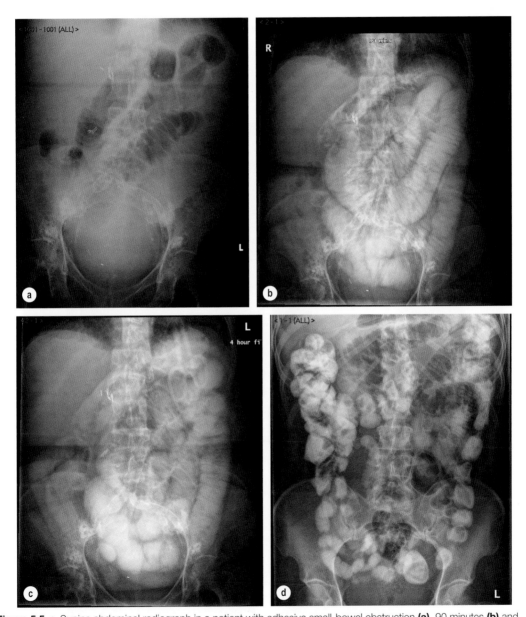

Figure 5.5 • Supine abdominal radiograph in a patient with adhesive small-bowel obstruction **(a)**, 90 minutes **(b)** and 4 hours **(c)** after oral administration of 50 mL of water-soluble contrast material. Note failure of contrast to reach the caecum and the obvious small-bowel obstruction. Laparotomy confirmed small-bowel obstruction due to adhesions. **(d)** A post-contrast 4-hour film in a patient with suspected small-bowel obstruction from the plain abdominal radiograph but on this occasion contrast has reached the colon by 4 hours and no surgery was required.

✅✅ In patients with small-bowel obstruction early administration of a water-soluble contrast material should be considered as it allows those patients who require surgery to be identified sooner and those that will settle non-operatively to do so quicker than patients managed conventionally.[79,80] A systematic review and meta-analysis of the diagnostic and therapeutic role of water-soluble contrast in adhesive small-bowel obstruction found that it was effective in predicting the need for surgery, as well as actually reducing the need for operation and shortened hospital stay.[82]

A recent clinicopathological score has been developed to predict the risk of strangulated small-bowel obstruction[66] and is discussed in more detail below under CT imaging. More detailed information on the surgical management of small-bowel obstruction is provided in Chapter 9.

Large-bowel obstruction

The management algorithm for large-bowel obstruction has now become well established following the more widespread recognition that colonic pseudo-obstruction could not be distinguished from mechanical obstruction on plain radiographs alone (**Fig. 5.6a,b**).[83] The decision that all patients with suspected large-bowel obstruction should now undergo a contrast enema (**Fig. 5.6c,d**) before laparotomy has probably been the most important factor in reducing not only the unnecessary operation rate for pseudo-obstruction, but also the associated mortality.

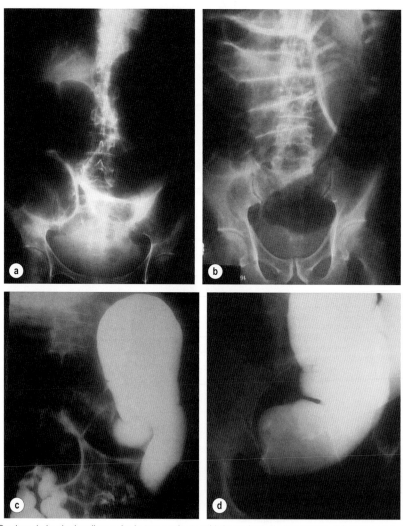

Figure 5.6 • Supine abdominal radiographs in two patients with large-bowel obstruction. **(a)** Patient A has pseudo-obstruction. **(b)** Patient B has mechanical obstruction. **(c,d)** Water-soluble contrast enema confirmed pseudo-obstruction in patient A **(c)** and an obstructing carcinoma of the sigmoid colon in patient B **(d)**.

Patients with acute colonic pseudo-obstruction present with similar history and clinical signs to the patient with a mechanical obstruction. Although factors recognised as precipitating pseudo-obstruction, such as dehydration, electrolyte abnormalities, pelvic and spinal surgery, acid–base imbalance and so on, may alert the clinician as to the possible cause, it cannot be confirmed without further investigation. As the treatment for one is non-operative and for the other is usually operative, accurate assessment is essential.

> ✔✔ All patients with a suspected large-bowel obstruction should undergo some form of contrast examination to exclude pseudo-obstruction.[83]

The surgical management of both large-bowel obstruction and the next topic, acute diverticulitis, is covered in more detail in Chapter 10.

Acute diverticulitis

The majority of patients who present with symptoms and signs of acute diverticulitis can be managed non-operatively, with the exception of those patients who have overt peritonitis from perforation. Although US in experienced hands might identify a thickened segment of colon, perhaps with an associated paracolic collection of fluid, invariably there is too much gas for adequate assessment and quite significant collections can go unnoticed. For this reason clinicians have attempted to evaluate other modalities, such as water-soluble contrast radiology and CT. The former has the ability to identify an ongoing 'leak', the latter a perforation and collection. Both of these pieces of information may be of use to the surgeon in reaching a decision to operate, even though the ultimate decision must be based on clinical rather than radiological criteria. Overall, CT has been shown in a prospectively randomised trial to be superior to contrast enemas in both the evaluation of inflammation and identification of a collection.[84]

Ultrasonography (US)

The use of US is now one of the mainstays of investigation of the acute abdomen. Accurate detection of small amounts of intraperitoneal fluid associated with conditions such as perforated peptic ulcer, acute cholecystitis, acute appendicitis, strangulated bowel and ruptured ovarian cysts can be very helpful in alerting the clinician to the possible severity of the patient's symptoms. Furthermore, reports on the accuracy of US in the detection of specific conditions such as acute cholecystitis and appendicitis are impressive. The presence of free fluid, gallstones, a thickened gallbladder wall and a positive ultrasonographic Murphy sign are all good indicators of acute cholecystitis.[85] US is the first-line investigation for acute biliary disease, with a sensitivity greater than 95% for the detection of acute cholecystitis.[86] As the most appropriate management of these patients is now laparoscopic cholecystectomy during the same admission, and if possible within 48 hours,[87] early US examination on any patient with suspected acute biliary disease should be undertaken soon after admission (see also Chapter 8).

In experienced hands US has been shown to be able to detect an acutely inflamed non-perforated appendix with a sensitivity of 81% and specificity of 100%.[88] Because the technique relies on visualising a non-compressible swollen appendix (**Fig. 5.7**), the sensitivity for perforated appendicitis is much lower (29%). When a scoring system is used for both clinical diagnosis and ultrasonographic findings, the addition of the latter increases the diagnostic accuracy for acute appendicitis.[89,90] Clearly, it would be inappropriate to scan everyone with suspected appendicitis, but where the diagnosis is uncertain, particularly in women, the case for US scanning is strong, as many alternative diagnoses can be detected.[91]

Other areas where US is specifically used to assess the acute abdomen are abdominal aortic aneurysms, renal tract disease and acute gynaecological emergencies. US may also have a role to play in the diagnosis of strangulated small-bowel obstruction, by detecting dilated non-peristaltic loops of bowel in association with free intraperitoneal fluid.[92] US can also be useful in detecting acute abdominal wall problems, such as rectus sheath haematoma (**Fig. 5.8**), and differentiating them from intra-abdominal pathology.[93] US also has a role in the early assessment of patients with blunt abdominal trauma,[94] and this is covered in detail in Chapter 13.

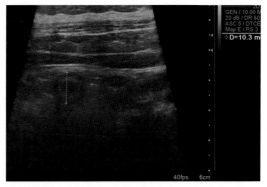

Figure 5.7 • Ultrasound examination on a patient with acute appendicitis. Note the non-compressible thick-walled hollow organ (appendix) beneath the probe.

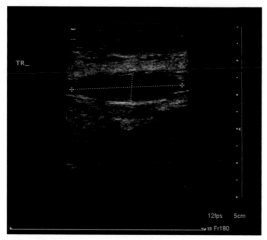

Figure 5.8 • Ultrasound of the abdominal wall demonstrating a rectus sheath haematoma.

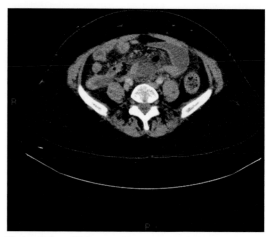

Figure 5.9 • CT image with intravenous contrast demonstrating perforated appendicitis.

Computed tomography (CT)

The place of CT in the early assessment of the acute abdomen has received wide attention over the last few years following the introduction of multislice CT and recognition of the excellent images that can be produced, especially if intravenous (i.v.) contrast is used. Its role in the investigation of the severity of acute diverticulitis has already been discussed[84] and it can also be used to identify miscellaneous intra-abdominal collections resulting from other conditions. Attempts to improve the diagnostic accuracy of acute appendicitis using CT have been impressive, with 98% accuracy in 100 consecutive patients with suspected appendicitis (**Fig. 5.9**), of whom 53 had acute appendicitis.[95] However, irrespective of the cost and availability issue, the diagnosis of acute appendicitis can usually be made without the aid of imaging studies and care must be taken to ensure that such investigations are used to complement rather than to replace the clinical assessment of patients with suspected appendicitis.[96] Because of the associated risks of i.v. contrast in some individuals as well as excessive radiation exposure, particularly in the younger patients, the role of non-contrast CT has been examined in a systematic review of seven studies.[97] This review concluded that non-contrast helical CT provides an acceptably high accuracy (sensitivity of 92.7% and specificity of 96.1%) for the diagnosis of acute appendicitis in adult patients.

A randomised study from Cambridge that examined the effect of early CT (within 24 hours of admission) compared to standard investigations on patients with undifferentiated acute abdominal pain demonstrated an improvement in diagnostic accuracy in patients undergoing early CT, but no difference in length of stay or mortality.[98] Further analysis

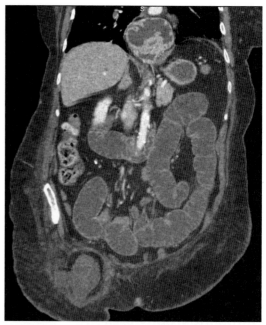

Figure 5.10 • CT image with intravenous contrast demonstrating small-bowel obstruction due to an incarcerated inguinal hernia. With thanks to Dr Dilip Patel, Consultant Radiologist, Royal Infirmary, Edinburgh.

of the same data demonstrated that another advantage of early CT was in the detection of unexpected significant primary and secondary diagnoses.[99] These findings were confirmed in another more recent randomised trial comparing plain radiology with early low-dose abdominal CT.[100] In addition to its overall role in the investigation of the acute abdomen, CT is also extremely useful specifically in the detection of gastrointestinal obstruction (**Fig. 5.10**), perforations

(**Fig. 5.11**), along with indications of the site of perforation,[101] intestinal ischaemia (**Fig. 5.12**)[102] and bleeding (**Fig. 5.13**), as well as abdominal wall problems (**Fig. 5.14**). Multislice CT with intravenous and rectal contrast can also be useful in the detection and differentiation of different types of colitis, including ulcerative, Crohn's, pseudo-membranous and *Clostridium difficile* colitis.[103] A clinicoradiological score has recently been developed to predict the risk of strangulated small-bowel obstruction using duration of pain (lasting 4 days or more), elevated C-reactive protein (>75 mg/L), leucocyte count (>10 × 10⁹/L), the presence of guarding, at least 500 mL of fluid as seen on CT and reduced enhancement of the small bowel on CT. The risk of ischaemia in 233 consecutive patients studied with small-bowel obstruction was 6% in patients with a score of 1 or less (one point for each variable) compared to a sensitivity of 67.7% and specificity of 90.8% in requiring resection for a score of 3 or more.[66] Overall, 138 of the patients in this study underwent surgery, of whom 45 required intestinal resection.

Despite the relatively high diagnostic accuracy of CT in the assessment of the acute abdomen, and particularly acute appendicitis, the main drawbacks remain cost and radiation exposure.[104] As a result the role of CT in the early assessment of patients with acute abdominal pain should still be limited to those in whom there remains uncertainty as to either diagnosis or decision to operate after initial assessment.

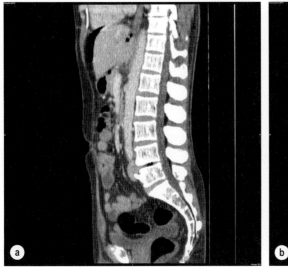
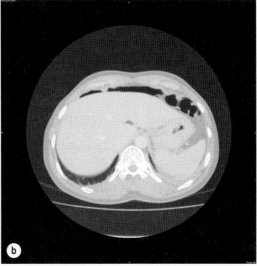

Figure 5.11 • **(a)** Sagittal view of a CT scan with intravenous contrast demonstrating free intraperitoneal gas from a perforated peptic ulcer. Note the free air anterior to the liver. **(b)** Axial view of the same patient showing free air above the liver. With thanks to Dr Dilip Patel, Consultant Radiologist, Royal Infirmary, Edinburgh.

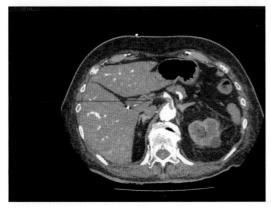
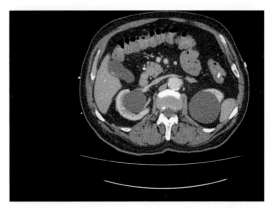

Figure 5.12 • CT angiogram demonstrating coeliac axis thrombus.

Figure 5.13 • CT angiogram demonstrating contrast in the mid descending colon from bleeding diverticular disease.

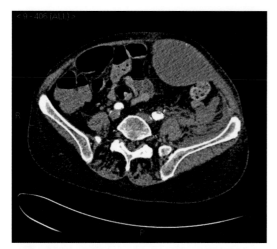

Figure 5.14 • CT image with intravenous contrast demonstrating a large rectus sheath haematoma.

Magnetic resonance imaging (MRI)

With the increased use of CT in the investigation of the acute abdomen it was only a matter of time before attention turned to the role of MRI, which is not associated with the radiation exposure of CT. MRI can undoubtedly differentiate an acutely inflamed appendix from a normal one[105] and therefore is useful in pregnant patients, where the diagnosis of acute appendicitis can be difficult.[106] However, a review of academic centres in North America reported that radiologists still preferred CT to MRI in the second and third trimester to investigate acute abdominal pain.[107]

Laparoscopy

Laparoscopy is now an integral part of the emergency surgeon's armamentarium, for both diagnosis and treatment of acute abdominal conditions. Laparoscopy significantly improves surgical decision-making when used as a diagnostic tool,[108] particularly when the need for operation is uncertain.[56] With the increasing use of laparoscopic appendicectomy (see Chapter 9), most patients with suspected appendicitis can now undergo diagnostic laparoscopy followed by laparoscopic appendicectomy if the diagnosis of acute appendicitis is confirmed (**Fig. 5.15**). Even if a policy of laparoscopic appendicectomy is not followed, all females with suspected acute appendicitis should still undergo diagnostic laparoscopy because the diagnostic error is more than twice that of males,[109] usually due to underlying gynaecological conditions (**Figs 5.16** and **5.17**). When used as a diagnostic tool in patients admitted to hospital with suspected acute non-specific

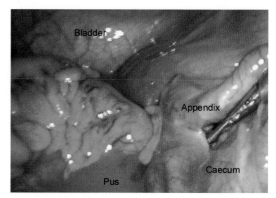

Figure 5.15 • Laparoscopy showing an acutely inflamed appendix with pelvic peritonitis.

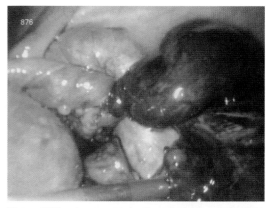

Figure 5.16 • Laparoscopic view of a torsion of the right fallopian tube with ischaemia of the distal tube and ovary.

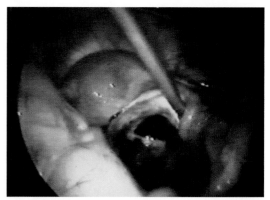

Figure 5.17 • Laparoscopic view of a haemorrhagic ovarian cyst.

abdominal pain, some of whom of course subsequently turn out to have a surgical cause, early laparoscopy versus observation has been shown to be of benefit. Two randomised studies[110,111] have demonstrated that the associated improved diagnostic accuracy in the patients undergoing laparoscopy converts to a reduced hospital stay, and in one of the studies[110] an improved quality of life (assessed 6 weeks after discharge from hospital).

The decision on what to do if a normal appendix is seen at laparoscopy is discussed in detail in Chapter 9, and there are differing arguments for and against its removal. What is essential is that the patient must be clearly told the diagnosis made at laparoscopy and the procedure performed. It has been shown that around 27% of patients undergoing laparoscopy for acute abdominal pain could either not remember what had happened or their recall was incorrect.[112] This included knowledge as to whether the appendix had been removed or not.

✅✅ It is clear that there is now overwhelming evidence in support of the use of diagnostic laparoscopy in the management of patients with acute abdominal pain in whom the need for surgery is uncertain and particularly women with suspected appendicitis.[108,110,111]

Key points

- The art of good management of patients with acute abdominal pain lies in an accurate history, careful examination and logical decision-making, taking into account results from all appropriate and available investigations.
- Regular reassessment of patients is an essential part of this process and facilities should be provided so that emergency patients are kept in an area of the hospital where regular review is facilitated.
- The ability to provide adequate emergency surgical care, with careful observation, reassessment and early access to the operating theatre, is best provided by dedicated emergency surgical teams without elective commitments.
- Swift access to investigations and an emergency theatre is an essential requisite for the appropriate management of patients with acute abdominal pain.
- Although emergency subspecialisation has great attractions for the overall care of the emergency patient with complex problems, this area of development will depend very much on local resources, requirements and workload.

References

1. Ingraham AM, Cohen ME, Bilimoria KY, et al. Comparison of 30-day outcomes after emergency general surgical procedures: potential for targeted improvement. Surgery 2010;148:217–38.

2. Senate of Surgery of Great Britain and Ireland. Reconfiguration of surgical, accident and emergency and trauma services in the UK. http://www.rcseng.ac.uk/publications/docs/reconfiguration.html; 2004.

3. Black A. Reconfiguration of surgical, accident and emergency and trauma services in the UK. Br Med J 2004;328:178–9.

4. Watkin DFL, Layer GT. A 24-hour snapshot of emergency general surgery in the UK. Ann R Coll Surg Engl 2002;84(Suppl):194–9.

5. Beecham L. New Scottish CMO criticises training reforms. Br Med J 1996;313:947.

6. Campling EA, Devlin HB, Hoile RW, et al. Report of the National Confidential Enquiry into Perioperative Deaths 1990. London: HMSO; 1992.

7. Association of Surgeons of Great Britain and Ireland. Emergency general surgery: the future. A consensus statement. www.asgbi.org.uk; June 2007 [accessed 10.11.12].
   This consensus statement provides details of the current problems in the provision of emergency general surgery and recommendations for improving practice.

8. Anderson ID. ASGBI emergency surgery survey 2010. Association of Surgeons of Great Britain and Ireland Newsletter 2010;31:12–159.

9. Hilton JR, Shiralkar SP, Samsudin A, et al. Disruption of the on-call surgical team. Ann R Coll Surg Engl 2002;84(Suppl.):50–3.

10. Ledwidge SFC, Bryden E, Halestrap P, et al. Continuity of care of emergency surgical admissions:impact on SPR training. Surgeon 2008;6:136–8.

11. Kelly MJ. Off-duty for consultants in the week? It can be done! Ann R Coll Surg Engl 1995;77(Suppl.):257–9.

12. Addison PDR, Getgood A, Paterson-Brown S. Separating elective and emergency surgical care (the emergency team). Scott Med J 2001;46:48–50.

13. Tincknell L, Burton S, Cooke C, et al. The emergency surgical team – the way forward in emergency care? Ann R Coll Surg Engl 2009;91:18–22.

14. Emergency surgery. J Assoc Surg Great Britain and Ireland 2012;36:2–19.

15. Anderson ID, Markham NI, Cripps N, et al. Issues in professional practice: emergency general surgery. London: Association of Surgeons of Great Britain and Ireland; May 2012. http://www.asgbi.org.uk/en/publications/issues_in_professional_practice.cfm [accessed 10.11.12].

16. The Royal College of Surgeons of England. Separating emergency and elective surgical care: recommendations for practice. http://www.rcseng.ac.uk/publications/docs/separating_emergency_and_elective.html; 2007. Strong support and recommendations for the separation of emergency and elective surgical care.

17. Calder FR, Jadhav V, Hale JE. The effect of a dedicated emergency theatre facility on emergency operating patterns. J R Coll Surg Edinb 1998;43:17–9.

18. Thomson HJ, Jones PF. Active observation in acute abdominal pain. Am J Surg 1986;152:522–5.

19. Halm EA, Lee C, Chassin MR. Is volume related to outcome in health care? A systematic review and methodologic critique of the literature. Ann Intern Med 2002;137:511–20.

20. Hannan EL, Radzyner M, Rubin D, et al. The influence of hospital and surgeon volume on in-hospital mortality for colectomy, gastrectomy and lung lobectomy in patients with cancer. Surgery 2002;131:6–15.

21. Paterson-Brown S. Surgical volume and clinical outcome. Br J Surg 2007;94:523–4.

22. Smith JAE, King PM, Lane RHS, et al. Evidence of the effect of 'specialisation' on the management of surgical outcome and survival from colorectal cancer in Wessex. Br J Surg 2003;90:583–92.

23. Mercer SJ, Knight JS, Toh SKC, et al. Implementation of a specialist-led service for the management of gallstone disease. Br J Surg 2004;91:504–8.

24. Young AL, Cockbain AJ, White AW, et al. Index admission laparoscopic cholecystectomy for patients with acute biliary symptoms: results from a specialist centre. HPB (Oxford) 2010;12:270–6.

25. Darby CR, Berry AR, Mortensen N. Management variability in surgery for colorectal emergencies. Br J Surg 1992;79:206–10.

26. Dawson EJ, Paterson-Brown S. Emergency general surgery and the implications for specialisation. Surgeon 2004;2:165–70.

27. Simpson DJ, Wood AM, Paterson HM, et al. Improved management of acute gallstone disease after regional surgical subspecialisation. World J Surg 2008;32:2690–4.

28. Robson AJ, Richards JMJ, Nixon SJ, et al. The effect of surgical subspecialisation on outcomes in peptic ulcer disease complicated by perforation and bleeding. World J Surg 2008;32:1456–61.

29. Boyce SA, Bartolo DCC, Paterson HM, The Edinburgh Coloproctology Unit. Subspecialist emergency management of diverticulitis is associated with reduced mortality and fewer stomas. Colorectal Dis 2012; Sept 11. Epub ahead of print.

30. Cochrane RA, Edwards AT, Crosby DL, et al. Senior surgeons and radiologists should assess emergency patients on presentation: a prospective randomised controlled trial. J R Coll Surg Edinb 1998;43:324–7.

31. Irvin TT. Abdominal pain: a surgical audit of 1190 emergency admissions. Br J Surg 1989;76:1121–5.

32. Gray DWR, Collin J. Non-specific abdominal pain as a cause of acute admission to hospital. Br J Surg 1987;74:239–42.

33. Paterson-Brown S. The acute abdomen: the role of laparoscopy. In: Williamson RCN, Thompson JN, editors. Baillière's clinical gastroenterology: gastrointestinal emergencies, Part 1. London: Baillière Tindall; 1991. p. 691–703.

34. Gallegos NC, Hobsley M. Abdominal wall pain: an alternative diagnosis. Br J Surg 1990;77:1167–70.

35. Hall PN, Lee APB. Rectus nerve entrapment causing abdominal pain. Br J Surg 1988;75:917.

36. Gray DWR, Seabrook G, Dixon JM, et al. Is abdominal wall tenderness a useful sign in the diagnosis of non-specific abdominal pain? Ann R Coll Surg Engl 1988;70:233–4.

37. de Dombal FT, Matharu SS, Staniland JR, et al. Presentation of cancer to hospital as 'acute abdominal pain'. Br J Surg 1980;67:413–6.

38. Paterson-Brown S, Eckersley JRT, Dudley HAF. The gynaecological profile of acute general surgery. J R Coll Surg Edinb 1988;33:13–5.

39. Pearce JM. Pelvic inflammatory disease. Br Med J 1990;300:1090–1.

40. Shanahan D, Lord PH, Grogono J, et al. Clinical acute cholecystitis and the Curtis–Fitz-Hugh syndrome. Ann R Coll Surg Engl 1988;70:45–7.

41. Ravichandran D, Burge DM. Pneumonia presenting with acute abdominal pain in children. Br J Surg 1996;83:1706–8.

42. Blidaru P, Blidaru A, Popa G. False acute abdomen in emergency surgery. Br J Surg 1996;83(Suppl. 2):61–2.

43. de Dombal FT, Leaper DJ, Staniland JR, et al. Computer-aided diagnosis of acute abdominal pain. Br Med J 1972;2:9–13.

44. Gunn AA. The diagnosis of acute abdominal pain with computer analysis. J R Coll Surg Edinb 1976;21:170–2.

45. Adams ID, Chan M, Clifford PC, et al. Computer aided diagnosis of acute abdominal pain: a multicentre study. Br Med J 1986;293:800–4.

A large study involving eight centres, 250 doctors and 16 737 patients demonstrated an improvement in diagnostic accuracy, reduction in the incidence of perforated appendicitis and bad management errors associated with the use of the computer.

46. Batstone GF. Educational aspects of medical audit. Br Med J 1990;301:326–8.

47. Marteau TM, Wynne G, Kaye W, et al. Resuscitation: experience without feedback increases confidence but not skill. Br Med J 1990;300:849–50.

48. Lawrence PC, Clifford PC, Taylor IF. Acute abdominal pain: computer aided diagnosis by non-medically qualified staff. Ann R Coll Surg Engl 1987;69:233–4.

This paper demonstrates that medical students assessing patients with acute abdominal pain using a structured pro-forma and then CAD have the same diagnostic accuracy as medical staff who use the pro-forma but not CAD.

49. Paterson-Brown S, Vipond MN, Simms K, et al. Clinical decision-making and laparoscopy versus computer prediction in the management of the acute abdomen. Br J Surg 1989;76:1011–3.

The addition of structured patient pro-formas without CAD significantly improved clinical decision-making and laparoscopy.

50. Bennett DH, Tambeur LJMT, Campbell WB. Use of coughing test to diagnose peritonitis. Br Med J 1994;308:1336–7.

51. Williams NMA, Johnstone JM, Everson NW. The diagnostic value of symptoms and signs in childhood abdominal pain. J R Coll Surg Edinb 1998;43:390–2.

52. Dixon JM, Elton RA, Rainey JB, et al. Rectal examination in patients with pain in the right lower quadrant of the abdomen. Br Med J 1991;302:386–8.

53. Howie CR, Gunn AA. Temperature: a poor diagnostic indicator in abdominal pain. J R Coll Surg Edinb 1984;29:249–51.

54. Manterola C, Astudillo P, Losada H, et al. Analgesia in patients with acute abdominal pain. Cochrane Database Syst Rev 2011;(1):CD005660; PMID 21249672 [update of Cochrane Database Syst Rev 2007; (3):CD005660].

This Cochrane systematic review analysed 51 papers and concluded that the use of opioid analgesics in patients with acute abdominal pain is helpful in terms of patient comfort and does not adversely affect decision-making.

55. Clavien PA, Burgan S, Moossa AR. Serum enzymes and other laboratory tests in acute pancreatitis. Br J Surg 1989;76:1234–43.

56. Paterson-Brown S, Eckersley JRT, Sim AJW, et al. Laparoscopy as an adjunct to decision-making in the acute abdomen. Br J Surg 1986;73:1022–4.

57. Bradbury AW, Brittenden J, McBride K, et al. Mesenteric ischaemia: a multi-disciplinary approach. Br J Surg 1995;82:1446–59.

58. Schoots IG, Koffeman DA, Levi M, et al. Systematic review of survival after acute mesenteric ischaemia according to disease aetiology. Br J Surg 2004;91:17–27.

Data from 45 observational studies including 3692 patients were reviewed. Prognosis after acute mesenteric venous thrombosis is better than for arterial ischaemia, and that for arterial embolism is better than that for arterial thrombosis.

59. Dervenis C, Johnson CD, Bassi C, et al. Diagnosis, objective assessment of severity, and management of acute pancreatitis. Santorini Consensus Conference. Int J Pancreatol 1999;25:195–210.

60. Thompson MM, Underwood MJ, Dookeran KA, et al. Role of sequential leucocyte counts and C-reactive protein measurements in acute appendicitis. Br J Surg 1992;79:822–4.

61. Davies AH, Bernau F, Salisbury A, et al. C-reactive protein in right iliac fossa pain. J R Coll Surg Edinb 1991;36:242–4.

62. Gronroos JM, Gronroos P. Leucocyte and C-reactive protein in the diagnosis of acute appendicitis. Br J Surg 1999;86:501–4.

63. Sengupta A, Bax G, Paterson-Brown S. White cell count and C-reactive protein measurement in patients with possible appendicitis. Ann R Coll Surg Engl 2009;91(2):113–5.

64. Andersson REB. Meta-analysis of the clinical and laboratory diagnosis of appendicitis. Br J Surg 2004;91:28–37.

Systematic Medline search of 28 diagnostic variables in 24 studies.

65. Peng WK, Sheikh Z, Paterson-Brown S, et al. Role of liver function tests in predicting common bile duct stones in acute calculous cholecystitis. Br J Surg 2005;92:1241–7.

66. Schwenter F, Poletti PA, Platon A, et al. Clinicoradiological score for predicting the risk of strangulated small bowel obstruction. Br J Surg 2010;97:1119–25.

67. Cochrane RA, Edwards AT, Crosby DL, et al. Senior surgeons and radiologists should assess emergency patients on presentation: a prospective randomised controlled trial. J R Coll Surg Edinb 1998;43:324–7.

68. Chen S-C, Yen Z-S, Wang H-P, et al. Ultrasonography is superior to plain radiology in the diagnosis of pneumoperitoneum. Br J Surg 2002;89:351–4.

69. Anyanwu AC, Moalypour SM. Are abdominal radiographs still overutilised in the assessment of acute abdominal pain? A district general hospital audit. J R Coll Surg Edinb Irel 1998;43:267–70.

70. Bell DJ, Woo EK. Are abdominal radiographs still overutilised in the assessment of acute abdominal pain? (letter). Surgeon 2006;4:60–1.

71. Royal College of Radiologists working party. Making the best use of a department of clinical radiology: guidelines for doctors. 5th ed. London; 2003.

72. Traill ZC, Nolan DJ. Imaging of intestinal obstruction. Br J Hosp Med 1996;55:267–71.

73. Ott DJ, Gelfand DW. Gastrointestinal contrast agents: indications, uses and risks. JAMA 1983;249:2380–4.

74. Wellwood JM, Wilson AN, Hopkinson BR. Gastrografin as an aid to the diagnosis of perforated peptic ulcer. Br J Surg 1971;58:245–9.

75. Crofts TJ, Park KGM, Steele RJC, et al. A randomized trial of non-operative treatment for perforated peptic ulcer. N Engl J Med 1989;320:970–3.

76. Stewardson RH, Bombeck CT, Nyhus LM. Critical operative management of small bowel obstruction. Ann Surg 1978;187:189–93.

77. Ogata M, Mateer JR, Condon RE. Prospective evaluation of abdominal sonography for the diagnosis of bowel obstruction. Ann Surg 1996;223:237–41.

78. Brochwocz MJ, Paterson-Brown S, Murchison JT. Small bowel obstruction: the water-soluble follow-through revisited. Clin Radiol 2003;58:393–7.

79. Lee JF-Y, Meng WC-S, Leung K-L, et al. Water soluble contrast follow-through in the management of adhesive small bowel obstruction: a prospective randomized trial. Ann Coll Surg HK 2004;8:120–6.
A randomised prospective trial of 150 patients with suspected adhesive small-bowel obstruction demonstrated that the group given water-soluble contrast studies received surgery significantly sooner (42 vs. 65 h) and had a significantly shorter hospital stay (5 vs. 7 days) than the group treated conventionally. The incidence of surgical intervention in both groups was the same.

80. Burge J, Roadley G, Donald J, et al. Randomised controlled trial of gastrografin in adhesive small bowel obstruction. Aust N Z J Surg 2005;75:672–4.
A randomised trial of 40 patients with suspected adhesive small-bowel obstruction treated conventionally or given gastrografin. Four patients in each group required surgery. Time to resolution of symptoms was significantly quicker in the group given gastrografin.

81. Sajja SBS, Schein M. Early postoperative small bowel obstruction. Br J Surg 2004;91:683–91.

82. Branco BC, Barmparas G, Schnuriger B, et al. Systematic review and meta-analysis of the diagnostic and therapeutic role of water soluble contrast agent in adhesive small boiwel obstruction. Br J Surg 2010;97:47–8.
Fourteeen prospective studies were analysed and confirmed that water-soluble contrast radiography predicted the need for surgery, reduced the need for surgery and shortened hospital stay in patients with adhesive small-bowel obstruction.

83. Dudley HAF, Paterson-Brown S. Pseudo-obstruction. Br Med J 1986;292:1157–8.
Leading article that provides the history of pseudo-obstruction and the relevant papers in relation to diagnosis and treatment.

84. Ambrosetti P, Becker C, Terrier F. Colonic diverticulitis: impact of imaging on surgical management. A prospective study of 542 patients. Eur Radiol 2002;12:1145–9.

85. Laing FC, Federie MP, Jeffrey RB, et al. Ultrasonic evaluation of patients with acute right upper quadrant pain. Radiology 1981;140:449–55.

86. Samuels BL, Freitas JE, Bree RL, et al. A comparison of radionuclide hepatobiliary imaging and real-time ultrasound for the detection of acute cholecystitis. Radiology 1983;47:207–10.

87. Peng WK, Sheikh Z, Nixon SJ, et al. Role of laparoscopic cholecystectomy in the early management of acute gall bladder disease. Br J Surg 2005;92:586–91.

88. Puylaert IBCM, Rutgers PF, Lalisang RI, et al. A prospective study of ultrasonography in the diagnosis of appendicitis. N Engl J Med 1987;317:666–9.

89. Gallego MG, Fadrique B, Nieto MA, et al. Evaluation of ultrasonography and clinical diagnostic scoring in suspected appendicitis. Br J Surg 1998;85:37–40.

90. Douglas CD, Macpherson NE, Davidson PM, et al. Randomised controlled trial of ultrasonography in diagnosis of acute appendicitis, incorporating the Alvarado score. Br Med J 2000;321:919–22.

91. McGrath FP, Keeling F. The role of early sonography in the management of the acute abdomen. Clin Radiol 1991;44:172–4.

92. Ogata M, Mateer JR, Condon RE. Prospective evaluation of abdominal sonography for the diagnosis of bowel obstruction. Ann Surg 1996;223:237–41.

93. Klingler PJ, Wetscher G, Glaser K, et al. The use of ultrasound to differentiate rectus sheath hematoma from other acute abdominal disorders. Surg Endosc 1999;13:1129–34.

94. Stengel D, Bauwens K, Sehouli J, et al. Systematic review and meta-analysis of emergency ultrasonography for blunt abdominal trauma. Br J Surg 2001;88:901–12.

95. Rao PM, Rhea JT, Novelline RA, et al. Effect of computed tomography of the appendix on treatment of patients and use of hospital resources. N Engl J Med 1998;338:141–6.

96. Unlu C, de Castro MMN, Tuynman JB, et al. Evaluating routine diagnostic imaging in acute appendicitis. Int J Surg 2009;7:451–597.

97. Molstrom C, Johar S. Is contrast needed for CT in the diagnosis of appendicitis? A systematic review of the literature. AccessMedicine from McGraw-Hill; 2011. www.AccessMedicine.com; [accessed 10.11.12].

98. Sala E, Watson CJE, Beadsmoore C, et al. A randomized, controlled trial of routine early abdominal computed tomography in patients presenting with non-specific acute abdominal pain. Clin Radiol 2007;62(10):961–9.

99. Sala E, Beadsmoore C, Gibbons D, et al. Unexpected changes in clinical diagnosis: early abdomino-pelvic computed tomography compared with clinical evaluation. Abdom Imaging 2009;34(6):783–7.

100. Nguyen LK, Wong DD, Fatovich DM, et al. Low-dose computed tomography versus plain abdominal radiography in the investigation of an acute abdomen. Aust N Z J Surg 2012;82(1–2):36–41.

101. Imatu M, Awai K, Nakayama Y, et al. Multidetector CT findings suggesting a perforation site in the gastrointestinal tract: analysis in surgically confirmed 155 patients. Radiat Med 2007;25(3):113–8.

102. Chou CK, Mak CW, Tzeng WS, et al. CT of small bowel ischemia. Abdom Imaging 2004;29(1):18–22.

103. Thoeni RF, Cello JP. CT imaging of colitis. Radiology 2006;240(3):623–38.

104. Old JL, Dusing RW, Yap W, et al. Imaging for suspected appendicitis. Am Fam Physician 2005;71(1):71–8.

105. Nitta N, Takahashi M, Furukawa A, et al. MR imaging of the normal appendix and acute appendicitis. J Magn Reson Imaging 2005;21(2):156–65.

106. Pedrosa I, Levine D, Eyvazzadeh AD, et al. MR imaging evaluation of acute appendicitis in pregnancy. Radiology 2006;238(3):891–9.

107. Jaffe TA, Miller CM, Merkle EM. Practice patterns in imaging of the pregnant patient with abdominal pain: a survey of academic centers. AJR Am J Roentgenol 2007;189(5):1128–34.

108. Paterson-Brown S. Emergency laparoscopic surgery. Br J Surg 1993;80:279–83.
Review article showing the overwhelming evidence in support of diagnostic laparoscopy in the assessment of patients with acute abdominal pain, particularly when the diagnosis and decision to operate is in doubt.

109. Paterson-Brown S, Thompson JN, Eckersley JRT, et al. Which patient with suspected appendicitis should undergo laparoscopy? Br Med J 1988;296:1363–4.

110. Decadt B, Sussman L, Lewis MPN, et al. Randomised clinical trial of early laparoscopy in the management of acute non-specific abdominal pain. Br J Surg 1999;86:1383–6.
A randomised trial that demonstrated the improvements in diagnostic accuracy and subsequent quality of life in the group undergoing laparoscopy.

111. Morino M, Pellegrino L, Castagna E, et al. Acute non-specific abdominal pain: a randomized, controlled trial comparing early laparoscopy versus clinical observation. Ann Surg 2006;244:881–8.

112. Murphy SM, Donnelly M, Fitzgerald T, et al. Patients' recall of clinical information following laparoscopy for acute abdominal pain. Br J Surg 2004;91:485–8.

6

Perforations of the upper gastrointestinal tract

Enders K.W. Ng

Introduction

Foregut perforations are challenging surgical emergencies and the keys to success in managing these potentially life-threatening situations are timely diagnosis and appropriate intervention. This chapter summarises the latest evidence and clinical experience concerning the investigation and therapeutic options for perforation in different parts of the upper gastrointestinal tract. Owing to the potential implications for prognosis and management planning, perforations are conventionally classified according to the anatomical position and causative mechanism.

Peptic ulcer perforation

The estimated lifetime risk of perforation in peptic ulcer disease ranges from 2% to 10%.[1-3] Typical presentation includes a sudden onset of epigastric pain, which rapidly generalises to other parts of the abdomen. Some patients may report a history of dyspepsia or peptic ulcer, but such findings are absent in about one-third of the patients.[4] 'Board-like rigidity' is the most commonly mentioned physical sign, referring to the diffuse peritonitis revealed on abdominal examination. However, in the elderly and the critically ill who develop ulcer perforation during hospitalisation, the presentation can often be atypical and subtle. Diagnosis under such circumstances requires a high index of suspicion. Though subdiaphragmatic free gas on a plain erect chest X-ray (**Fig. 6.1**) is diagnostic, it is seen in no more than 70% of patients.[5]

A lateral decubitus X-ray, water-soluble contrast meal, ultrasound scan and computed tomography (CT) of the abdomen are thus invaluable additional investigations when the diagnosis is in doubt (see also Chapter 5). However, it is noteworthy that the role of CT may be limited if the onset of symptoms is less than 6 hours.[6] Pneumogastrogram was once advocated for being able to increase the diagnostic yield from 66% on plain erect X-ray to 91%.[7] However, such a practice is now abandoned because forceful intragastric air insufflation is likely to reopen some of the spontaneously sealed-off perforations. For patients with profound peritoneal signs and a serum amylase level not diagnostic of acute pancreatitis, a laparoscopy or laparotomy after resuscitation is indeed the most time-saving and efficient investigation. It has the advantage of being able to execute immediate therapeutic intervention, either laparoscopically or via an open laparotomy, once the pathology is verified.

Prognosis

Perforation accounts for the majority of deaths related to peptic ulcer disease.[8,9] Spillage of gastroduodenal contents through the perforation initiates a chemical peritonitis, which will rapidly be superimposed by bacterial infection if left untreated. This leads in turn to the systemic inflammatory response syndrome and multi-organ dysfunction associated with the bacterial translocation across the peritoneal surface. Despite surgical intervention, mortality rates remain around 5–15%.[9-11] The prognostic indicators for ulcer perforation have been widely studied,

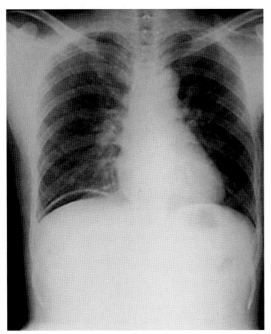

Figure 6.1 • Erect chest radiograph showing right subphrenic free gas shadow associated with a perforated peptic ulcer.

yet most published series consist of relatively small numbers of patients with marked heterogeneity in both demographics and treatment methods.

> ✅ Before the era of laparoscopic surgery, significantly higher rates of mortality were reported by Boey et al. in patients with an ulcer perforation who were admitted with major medical illness, preoperative shock and long-standing perforation (more than 24 hours). Those with no, one, two and all three risk factors at presentation were noted to have mortality rates of 0%, 10%, 45.5% and 100%, respectively.[12] This study underscores the importance of stratifying patients with ulcer perforation according to their risk of mortality, which is of relevance to the prognosis and choice of surgical intervention.

Similar findings have been reported by other multivariate analyses. Some also identified that age >65 years and perforation during hospital stay are additional predictive factors of death.[13,14] In 2001, Lee et al. compared the APACHE II score with the Boey parameters in a cohort of over 400 patients.[15] An APACHE II score >5 was found to have predictive value for increasing postoperative complications and death, whereas the Boey score only predicted mortality but not morbidity. Interestingly, in the same study, a higher Boey

score was found to be associated with an increased chance of conversion when laparoscopic repair was attempted. Albeit a precise and useful tool for research purposes, the APACHE II system is cumbersome to employ in daily practice, not to mention that the calculated score may vary with different time points of assessment.

> ✅ It is widely accepted that patient comorbidity, age >65 years, the presence of preoperative shock and long-standing perforation are associated with an increase in mortality and morbidity following perforated peptic ulcer.

A Danish group has recently published a revised prediction model, the Peptic Ulcer Perforation (PULP) score, based on a multicentre study including more than 2600 patients with perforated gastric or duodenal ulcers treated surgically over a 6-year period.[16] It comprises eight variables including (1) age over 65 years, (2) active malignancy or human immunodeficiency virus (HIV) infection, (3) cirrhosis, (4) steroid use, (5) presentation more than 24 hours after symptom onset, (6) preoperative shock, (7) serum creatinine higher than 130 μM/L and (8) the four levels of ASA score (2–5). In the study, PULP score was reported to predict postoperative 30-day mortality with an area under curve (AUC) of 0.83, which was significantly better than the conventional Boey score (AUC = 0.70) and ASA score alone (AUC = 0.78).

Treatment

Some 50% of perforated peptic ulcers have spontaneously sealed at the time of admission to hospital.[17] Such an observation has led to the sporadic advocacy of non-operative management, especially for older patients with poor premorbid status.[18] However, the non-operative approach has not been widely accepted, with the exception of a few centres. Donovan et al. were among the first to advocate use of diatrizoate meglumine (Hypaque) water-soluble contrast meal for confirmation of spontaneous sealing of the perforation.[19] In the absence of duodenal scarring and contrast extravasation, patients with subphrenic free gas were managed non-operatively with nasogastric suction and intravenous antibiotics. By implementing this preset policy, these authors were able to report an overall mortality rate of only 4.6% in a series of 249 patients.[20]

> ✅✅ The non-operative approach to the treatment of perforated peptic ulcers has been studied in a randomised trial consisting of 83 patients, of whom 40 were assigned to non-operative management

while the rest underwent immediate laparotomy.[21] After 12 hours, 28% of the patients in the non-operative group failed to improve and required surgery. Though mortality rates were comparable between the two approaches, the incidence of intra-abdominal collections and sepsis was much higher in the non-operative group. Most strikingly, patients over 70 years of age were found to be less responsive to the non-operative approach when compared to the younger patients. In concluding the study, the authors did not recommend routine use of non-operative management for peptic ulcer perforation. However, they recognised that the results suggested that patients (a) did not need to be rushed to the operating theatre and time could be more usefully spent in better preoperative resuscitation, and (b) in selected patients the non-operative approach has a role to play.

Though the majority of surgeons now advocate immediate surgical intervention for perforated peptic ulcers, there remains debate as to what constitutes the most appropriate operation. The omental repair technique first described by Graham in 1937 involves patching the perforation with a piece of detached omentum.[22] It is no longer a common practice nowadays and has been largely replaced by the pedicle omentopexy which is usually secured in place by two to three tie-over sutures (**Fig. 6.2a, b**). For a time such a simple omentopexy repair was associated with a high subsequent ulcer relapse rate.[23–25] This resulted in the popularity of adding a definitive acid-reducing procedure, such as distal gastrectomy or vagotomy, to lower ulcer recurrence.[26–29] In a prospective follow-up study, 107 selected patients with perforated pyloroduodenal ulcers undergoing omental patch closure and parietal cell vagotomy were evaluated up to 21 years later. The operative

mortality was only 0.9% and the recurrent ulcer rate by life table analysis was 7.4%, with a re-operative rate of only 1.9%.[30] As a result, emergency vagotomy was once a standard of care recommended for peptic ulcer perforation.

The addition of a truncal or highly selective vagotomy may cause little early morbidity or mortality apart from prolonging the time of anaesthesia. However, resectional surgery in the form of emergency antrectomy or distal gastrectomy has been shown to increase mortality in patients with perforated peptic ulcers, and therefore should be avoided wherever possible.[31]

All these 'definitive' surgical approaches, however, have changed over the last two decades following better understanding about the pathogenesis of peptic ulcer disease; most surgeons now prefer a much less aggressive 'damage control' tactic when treating ulcer perforations.[32,33] The availability of *Helicobacter pylori* eradication regimens and potent proton-pump inhibitors provides excellent means to alleviate patients' ulcer diathesis without the need for a definitive acid-reducing procedure. A simple omental patch repair and thorough peritoneal toileting are the only key manoeuvres needing to be done during the emergency operation. The only exception is probably those suffering from giant duodenal perforations (>2 cm), which may not be amenable to a simple patch repair (see below).[34]

Role of *Helicobacter pylori* and non-steroidal anti-inflammatory drugs (NSAIDs)

While the relationship between *Helicobacter pylori* infection and uncomplicated peptic ulcers is indisputable, the role of the bacteria in ulcer

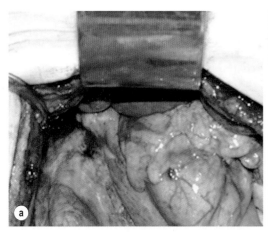
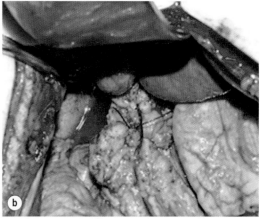

Figure 6.2 • (a) A small perforation at the juxtapyloric area. **(b)** Pedicle omental patch repair on the perforation site secured with absorbable sutures.

perforation was once enigmatic. Reported infection rates in earlier series varied markedly from 0% to 100%.[35-37] The difference in the number, timing and types of diagnostic test used to diagnose *H. pylori* infection in these studies may have accounted for the widely different findings. Furthermore, the frequency of NSAID intake can be an important confounding factor. In one consecutive series of 73 patients with perforated duodenal ulcers, intraoperative antral biopsies for rapid urease test and histopathology were taken. These revealed an *H. pylori* infection rate of 70%,[38] the figure rising to 80% if NSAID users were excluded. Some studies also reported a high proportion of NSAID use among patients with perforated gastric ulcers, especially in those without *H. pylori* infection, suggesting that these drugs may represent a factor of relevance to *H. pylori*-negative ulcer perforation.[39,40]

The more affirmative evidence confirming a causal relationship between *H. pylori* infection and non-NSAID peptic ulcer perforation comes from long-term follow-up studies. A study of 163 consecutive patients with perforated peptic ulcer managed by simple closure confirmed the strong association between persistent *H. pylori* infection and ulcer.[41] Of the 163 patients, 47.2% were found to have *H. pylori* infection during endoscopy at a mean follow-up of 6 years. Male gender and *H. pylori* were the only two independent predictive factors of ulcer relapse in the study.

In a randomised study, 99 patients with perforated duodenal ulcers and confirmed *H. pylori* infection received either 1 week of anti-*Helicobacter* therapy or 4 weeks of omeprazole.[42] Endoscopic surveillance after 1 year showed that ulcer recurrence rate decreased significantly from 38% in the control group to 4.8% in the eradication group. A recent meta-analysis has further consolidated the efficacy of *H. pylori* eradication in the prevention of ulcer relapse after simple repair of duodenal ulcer perforation.[43] The pooled incidence of 1-year ulcer relapse from three prospectively randomised trials was only 5.2% in patients treated with *H. pylori* eradication, which was significantly lower than that of the control group (35.2%).

✔✔ These two studies[42,43] confirm that medical eradication of *H. pylori* results in resolution of ulcer diathesis without the need for long-term antacid therapy or definitive surgery in patients who have undergone simple omental patch closure for perforated duodenal ulcers. The majority of patients with perforated peptic (pyloroduodenal) ulcers should be managed by simple omental patch closure, thorough peritoneal lavage, and subsequent treatment with proton inhibitors and eradication of *H. pylori* as necessary.

The role of cyclo-oxygenase-2 (COX-2)-specific inhibitors

Selective COX-2 inhibitors have been approved for symptomatic treatment of arthritis for nearly two decades. In contrast to conventional NSAIDs, COX-2 inhibitors provide anti-inflammatory effects without suppressing synthesis of prostaglandins essential for maintenance of mucosal integrity.[44] In the Celecoxib Long-term Arthritis Safety Study (CLASS), a double-blind randomised controlled trial, selective COX-2 inhibitor was confirmed to be associated with a significantly lower annualised incidence of peptic ulcer complications when compared to non-selective NSAIDs (0.44% vs 1.27%, $P = 0.04$).[45] However, such a protective effect was negated if the patient used aspirin concomitantly.[45,46] In another population-based study, a 44% increase in the annual number of prescriptions for NSAIDs (both selective and non-selective) had been recorded since the introduction of COX-2 inhibitors, but the annual hospitalisation rates for perforated peptic ulcer decreased from 17 per 100 000 person-years to 12 per 100 000 person-years during the study period.[47]

The impact of COX-2 inhibitor and traditional NSAIDs on perforation-related death was recently determined in a population cohort study.[48] While the observed 30-day mortality of the entire cohort of 2061 patients with ulcer perforation was 25%, that among NSAID and COX-2 inhibitor users was much higher, amounting to 35%. The increase in mortality associated with use of COX-2 inhibitors was similar to that of traditional NSAIDs, with an adjusted mortality rate ratio (compared to non-users of NSAIDs) of 2.0 and 1.7, respectively. COX-2 inhibitors, although being able to reduce the overall incidence of perforated ulcers, do not confer any advantage in clinical outcomes if perforation occurs. Such an observation may be related to the poor underlying comorbid condition of the patients who require extended use of NSAIDs or COX-2 inhibitor therapy.

As a result of knowing that the mortality risk is high once perforation occurs in the long-term NSAID users, protective measures against development of peptic ulcer in this group of patients have been extensively investigated. In an economic evaluation study using the Markov model and data extracted from a systematic review, the prescription of a proton-pump inhibitor (PPI) was shown to be cost-effective for people with osteoarthritis no matter whether they are taking a traditional NSAID or COX-2 selective inhibitor.[49] Importantly, the cost-effectiveness of adding a PPI remained valid even in patients at low risk of gastrointestinal adverse events.

Chapter 6

Laparoscopic versus open repair

As the ulcer diathesis is readily corrected by *H. pylori* eradication and cessation of NSAID usage, most patients with ulcer perforation can now be treated with a simple patch repair together with a thorough peritoneal washing. These operations used to mandate a midline laparotomy, but developments in minimally invasive surgery have revolutionised the surgical approach. The first laparoscopic closure of peptic ulcer perforation was reported in 1992.[50] Since then several series have been published.[51–53] However, interpretation of these data is difficult due to marked heterogeneity in the study designs, patients' demographics and the laparoscopic techniques used. With the exception of the two truly randomised trials from Hong Kong, all the others are either single-centre series or retrospective non-randomised comparative studies.[54,55] Most of them reported significantly better, albeit marginal, outcomes in the laparoscopic group, which could be due to selection bias when choosing the surgical approach for individual patients.

In a systematic review of 15 publications, the laparoscopic closure was found to be associated with significantly less analgesic use, shorter hospital stay, less wound infection and lower mortality rate compared to open surgery.[56] However, shorter operating time and less suture-site leakage were clear advantages of the open technique. Interestingly, in a more updated review comprising data extracted from 56 studies, apart from confirming the above-mentioned findings, the issue of conversion to open surgery was addressed.[57] The overall conversion rate was 12.4%, with the main reason being the size of perforation and inadequate localisation of the perforated pathology. The authors also identified that patients with a Boey score of 3, age over 70 years and symptoms persisting longer than 24 h were associated with a higher morbidity and mortality, and recommended these factors to be relative contraindications for laparoscopic intervention.

> ✔✔ Laparoscopic repair of perforated peptic ulcers results in significantly less analgesic use, shorter hospital stay, less wound infection and lower mortality rate compared to open surgery at the expense of a longer operating time and higher incidence of suture-site leakage.[56] Elderly patients and those with a Boey score of 3 and symptoms for >24 hours should undergo open surgery.[57]

Giant duodenal ulcer perforation

Giant duodenal perforation (>2 cm in diameter) remains a challenge to most surgeons because failure of omental patch repair is not uncommon (2–10%), which can lead in turn to increased morbidity rates and a resultant higher mortality (10–35%).[58,59] Converting the perforation into a controlled fistula by suturing the perforated site around an indwelling Foley catheter or T-tube was once advocated as a salvage measure. However, leakage remains a major concern with this technique and it should be reserved for patients with overtly unstable physiology to which the operative time is limited. For patients who are haemodynamically stable, a distal gastrectomy incorporating resection of the perforation-bearing duodenum is considered to be a viable option by some surgeons. However, due to pre-existing scarring and recent tissue loss, the duodenal stump thus created can be difficult to manage. Various procedures have been described, keeping in mind the friability of tissues. Nissen's double-layer closure technique,[60] catheter duodenostomy (**Fig. 6.3**),[61] lateral duodenostomy through the third part of the duodenum,[62] and making a duodenojejunostomy with a Roux-en-Y segment of jejunum[63] have all been mentioned. Nevertheless, it is noteworthy that the best way to avoid a difficult duodenal closure is to avoid an unnecessary gastrectomy, even in the presence of giant duodenal perforation. The alternatives to gastrectomy in these situations include converting the large perforation into a Finney pyloroplasty, use of omental plugging technique[64] or fashioning a controlled tube duodenostomy after primary closure of the perforation.[65] It cannot be overemphasised that most of the technical advocates are based on level III evidence only because of the rare nature of giant perforations. However, if there is no option but to proceed with a distal gastrectomy, a Roux-en-Y reconstruction is preferable as this will permit enteral nutrition in the postoperative period while the (inevitable, but hopefully controlled) duodenal fistula is allowed to close.

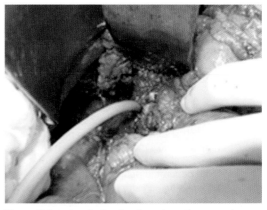

Figure 6.3 • A catheter duodenostomy for managing a difficult duodenal stump.

Perforated gastric ulcers

Reports pertaining to gastric ulcer perforation only are scarce.[66] On a statistical basis, gastric perforation tends to cluster among the elderly and is more likely to be associated with use of NSAIDs, but other possible causes include carcinoma, lymphoma and gastrointestinal stromal tumours. Perforation in the older age group carries a less favourable prognosis, partly related to their impaired physiological response to the septic insult, and more so to the delay in presentation, which is not uncommon. While simple omental patch remains the best option (after biopsying the lesion – see below), most surgeons prefer an ulcer excision if this can easily be carried out and without compromise to the stomach lumen. Formal gastric resection is not indicated unless either of these options is not possible, and this is rare.

Because a small minority of gastric perforations are malignant, and the possibility of gastric lymphoma needs to be remembered, it is essential to biopsy the ulcer edge, if it is not being excised.[67] Definitive surgery, if then required, can be carried out at a later date once the pathology has been reviewed, full staging investigations carried out, and after a full and frank discussion with the patient regarding prognosis and alternative treatment options. This is particularly true for gastric lymphoma, which can now be managed almost entirely by chemotherapy, radiotherapy or a combination of the two.

Though surgery for a perforated gastric cancer was once considered to be invariably palliative in nature, recent evidence suggests that long-term survival is still achievable in selected patients (stage I and II). A systematic review based on nine published articles encompassing 127 patients surgically treated for gastric cancer perforation reveals that the diagnosis of malignancy was known in 14–57% during the preoperative and intraoperative phases.[68] While mortality rates for emergency gastrectomy ranged from 0 to 50%, a two-stage approach was adopted in five of the nine series, and patients able to receive an R0 gastrectomy during the second-stage operation demonstrated significantly better long-term survival (median 75 months, 50% 5-year) compared with patients who had only simple closure. It highlights the importance of not taking a too pessimistic stance if the biopsy of a repaired gastric ulcer turns out to be carcinoma.

✔ Simple omental patch closure with biopsies of the ulcer edge or ulcer excision is the best option for perforated gastric ulcers. The former works surprisingly well, even for large lesions and is to be preferred where possible over resection. Gastric

resection, often at night, in difficult circumstances on a sick patient and increasingly by surgeons who may not be experienced in upper gastrointestinal surgery should only be undertaken as a last resort, when all other methods of closure are considered doomed to failure.

Oesophageal perforation

Classification

Perforation of the oesophagus can be broadly classified into iatrogenic and spontaneous. Iatrogenic perforations represent the most common cause of oesophageal perforation, with most occurring during diagnostic or therapeutic endoscopy, while some are related to para-oesophageal operations, such as fundoplication, cardiomyotomy, bariatric procedures, etc. The reported incidence of perforation for rigid oesophagoscopy is 0.11% and for fibre-optic endoscopy varies from 0.018% to 0.03%.[69,70] Therapeutic endoscopy is associated with a much higher frequency of perforation (1–10%).[71,72] Spontaneous rupture of the oesophagus (Boerhaave's syndrome) accounts for approximately 15% of perforations and classically occurs after forceful retching or vomiting, often related to an episode of binge eating and/or drinking.[73] The perforation is typically located just proximal to the oesophagogastric junction and more commonly opens into the left pleural space. Other less common causes of oesophageal perforation include foreign body penetration, traumatic endotracheal intubation, nasogastric catheterisation and the swallowing of corrosives.

Diagnosis

The overall mortality following oesophageal perforation was estimated to be 18% in a recent review covering 726 published patients.[74] Paramount in the management of this highly lethal emergency is expedient diagnosis and judicious clinical management. However, the presentation can be non-specific and may easily be confused with other disorders such as spontaneous pneumothorax/pneumomediastinum, myocardial infarction, acute pancreatitis and pneumonia. The essential attribute is to maintain a high index of suspicion, especially if a normal laparotomy has been performed. Pain is the most common symptom, which may occur anywhere from the neck to the abdominal region, depending on the location, the cause and the time elapsed between onset and presentation. Less often, dysphagia, odynophagia, dyspnoea, cyanosis and fever are other possible complaints. A preceding history of forceful vomiting,

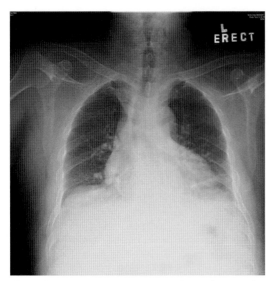

Figure 6.4 • Plain radiograph of a patient with surgical emphysema in the neck due to a mid oesophageal perforation following endoscopic ultrasound examination and transmural biopsy.

oesophageal instrumentation, para-oesophageal surgery and chest trauma should always be taken into consideration. Physical examination and plain radiograph may reveal surgical emphysema over the neck and upper chest wall (**Fig. 6.4**). Hydrothorax or pneumothorax may also be found on erect chest X-ray (**Fig. 6.5**). Hamman's sign (a crunching sound heard on chest auscultation) is found less commonly than suggested in textbooks.

The role of ancillary investigations for oesophageal perforation depends largely on the condition of the patient. If a patient is relatively stable and requires no endotracheal intubation, a water-soluble contrast swallow is a relatively easy way to confirm the diagnosis, determine the location, and assess the severity of the perforation (**Fig. 6.6**). However, for patients with profound sepsis mandating intubation and ventilatory support, a contrast-enhanced CT scan of the suspected region will be required to help establish the diagnosis (**Fig. 6.7**). A careful flexible oesophagoscopy is a very useful technique when the diagnosis is in doubt after these other investigations and often before surgery, as it confirms the exact site and length of perforation.

The management of oesophageal perforation starts with aggressive resuscitation and close monitoring of the physiological parameters. Further contamination of the mediastinum is minimised by making the patient 'nil by mouth'. Although insertion of a nasogastric tube reduces the potential for ongoing leakage from refluxed gastric contents, in the presence

of a perforation that might be managed non-operatively (see below), this will need to be inserted either under direct vision (endoscopically) or using X-ray guidance. Vigorous intravenous fluid replacement and broad-spectrum antibiotics are prescribed for control of systemic infection, and antifungal

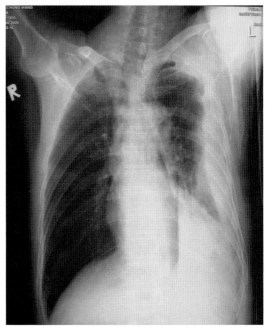

Figure 6.5 • Left hydropneumothorax revealed on decubitus chest radiograph in a patient with Boerhaave's syndrome.

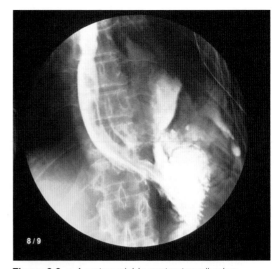

Figure 6.6 • A water-soluble contrast swallowing showing massive leak at the lower oesophagus in Boerhaave's syndrome.

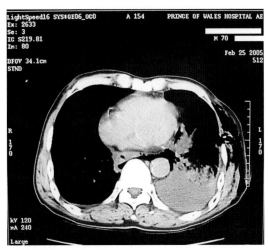

Figure 6.7 • Pneumomediastinum and left pleural effusion revealed by CT scan in a patient with lower oesophageal perforation.

therapy should also be considered. Chest drainage should be established if there is hydrothorax or hydropneumothorax and most patients require intensive care support. Subsequent management should be individualised according to the patient's clinical condition, the presence of comorbidities, the underlying oesophageal pathology, the location of perforation, and sometimes the time lapse between perforation and diagnosis. Nowadays, a multidisciplinary team approach involving medical, endoscopic and surgical management is increasingly adopted in the care of such patients.

Non-operative management

Candidates for conservative treatment, as defined by Cameron and colleagues in 1979, include those with a small perforation that does not breach the mediastinal pleura, together with mild symptoms and no evidence of systemic sepsis.[75,76] Preferably, the perforation is accompanied by a re-entry of extravasated contrast medium into the oesophageal lumen. Any sympathetic pleural effusion has to be drained, with the effluent regularly inspected to exclude fistulation. Nutritional support, either by the parenteral route or increasingly by the operative insertion of a feeding jejunostomy tube, is commenced early.

Previous experience suggests that patients who respond to non-operative management are those with small cervical tears following oesophagoscopy or traumatic endotracheal intubation, well-circumscribed intramural dissection after pneumatic dilatation for achalasia and small anastomotic leaks following oesophageal surgery.[77,78] Non-operative

treatment of spontaneous rupture (Boerhaave's syndrome) and iatrogenic perforation of the thoracic oesophagus with pleural contamination used to have a high failure rate in previously reported series and such patients were often managed by early surgical intervention. However, all this has changed over the last decade with the introduction of aggressive conservative strategy and the increasing interest in endoscopic stenting technology.

Vogel et al. were the first to advocate an 'aggressive conservative' approach in a series of 47 patients with oesophageal perforation (10 proximal and 37 thoracic).[79] Of these 47 patients, 34 were managed non-operatively with repetitive radiographs, aggressive image-guided chest drainage and operative intervention when indicated (only needed in 30% of the patients). The authors reported no mortality and an admirably high oesophageal healing rate in the series, even among patients with Boerhaave's syndrome. In another cohort study by a tertiary referral centre of 81 consecutive patients with acute oesophageal perforation managed over a 20-year period, there was a marked temporal increase in the frequency of utilising CT scan for diagnosis and treatment monitoring of the patients. The percentage of patients being treated non-operatively also increased significantly from 0% in the first 5-year cohort to 75% in the last one.[80] Parallel to these results was a marked reduction in complication rate and mean hospital stay. There was no difference in final mortality rates between patients treated with a non-operative approach and those who underwent immediate surgery.

One hindrance in promulgating wider use of the non-operative approach for oesophageal perforation lies in the difficulty of selecting appropriate candidates for this treatment while those who will benefit from early surgery are not delayed unnecessarily. The criteria set by Cameron et al. were far from evidence based, and the subsequent modification by Altorjay et al. also restricted non-operative management to patients with almost microperforation only.[81] Recently, an oesophageal perforation severity scoring system has been suggested by the Pittsburgh group.[82] Based on 10 clinical variables (old age, tachycardia, leucocytosis, pleural effusion, fever, non-contained leak, respiratory compromise, delay in diagnosis, cancer and hypotension), a maximum score of 18 can be derived at the time of admission. The prevalence of complications, mortality and the length of hospital stay were found to be significantly varied among groups with different scores (less than 2, 3–5 and more than 5). Notably the data suggested that patients with low clinical scores had worse outcomes if treated operatively when compared to those managed by the non-operative approach. These authors concluded that patients with a low clinical score, especially those with minimal mediastinal contamination and no respiratory distress, should be tried with aggressive non-operative treatment and surgical repair reserved for those with signs of deterioration.

Endoscopic stenting

An important adjunct now available in dealing with these 'minor' perforations is endoluminal stenting.[83,84] The recent development of a retrievable type of silicone-coated stent has shown some promising results (**Fig. 6.8**). In a prospective series of 18 patients with iatrogenic perforation of the oesophagus, 17 were treated with the Polyflex (Boston Scientific, Natick, MA, USA) stent in addition to chest drainage.[85] Except for one patient with a persistent leak who required operative repair, the remaining 16 had successful resolution of their perforations as confirmed by oesophagram. Most of the patients were able to resume oral intake in 72 hours, and the mean time before the stent was removed was 52 days. Alternatively, elderly and frail patients who suffer perforation following attempted dilatation of a malignant stricture can be managed by insertion of a covered permanent stent.

✅ The effectiveness of self-expandable covered stents in non-operative treatment of oesophageal rupture has been confirmed by a recent systematic review based on 25 selected studies encompassing 267 patients.[86] Due to a lack of randomised controlled trials, this study is already the best current evidence supporting the use of endoscopic stenting in treating oesophageal perforation that is not associated with profound sepsis.

The technical success rate of stenting was 99% and clinical success was achieved in 85% of patients. Though 34% of the patients had a stent-related complication (mainly stent migration), surgical intervention was required in only 13%, in whom the rupture site failed to heal completely after 6–8 weeks of stenting. These stents should be removed as soon as possible to prevent longer-term problems.

Surgical intervention

Early surgical intervention should be seriously considered if patients have profound sepsis upon admission, if adequate chest drainage cannot be achieved, or when clinical deterioration is observed

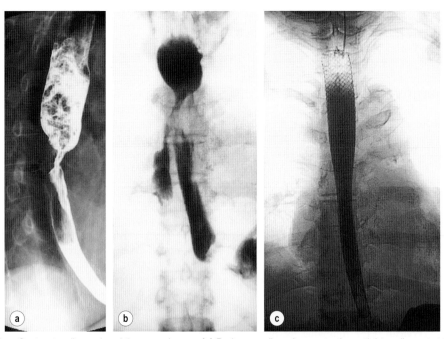

Figure 6.8 • Contrast radiography of the oesophagus. **(a)** Barium swallow demonstrating a tight malignant stricture. **(b)** Water-soluble contrast swallow after dilatation demonstrating a perforation. **(c)** Water-soluble contrast study in the same patient following insertion of an expandable metal stent, demonstrating no further leak.

after a period of aggressive non-operative management. In addition to thorough drainage of the mediastinum and the pleural space, three surgical manoeuvres for control of leakage may be applied:

1. Isolation and diversion (cervical oesophagostomy) followed by delayed staged reconstruction.
2. Primary repair of the perforation, with or without reinforcement and insertion of a T-tube, and external drainage.
3. Immediate oesophagectomy.

Oesophageal exclusion and diversion

The technique of oesophageal exclusion and diversion was described several decades ago. It involves division and closure of the oesophagus proximal and distal to the site of injury, with creation of an end-cervical oesophagostomy. Subsequently it has evolved to a side cervical oesophagostomy for proximal diversion of saliva and a staple transection of the oesophagogastric junction to prevent reflux of gastroduodenal contents back into the oesophageal lumen. Nevertheless, such an incomplete diversion often ends up with continuous soiling in the mediastinum, leading to persistent thoracic sepsis. With time, it proves to be a suboptimal treatment and is now reserved mainly for patients who are too unstable to undergo definitive repair or resection.

Primary repair

Primary repair is an appropriate option for perforations occurring less than 24 hours after the injury, because surrounding tissues are neither excessively inflamed nor ischaemic. As the laceration on the mucosal side can be much longer/wider than is appreciated from the adventitial surface, a cautious longitudinal extension of the muscular defect is often required for better assessment of the extent of the mucosal injury. Following careful debridement of the necrotic tissues along the perimeter of the perforation, the edges are then closed with interrupted absorbable sutures (**Fig. 6.9**). It may be possible, in very early perforations with very healthy tissue, to close the defect wound in two layers: first the mucosa/submucosal layer, followed by the muscular layer. However, in the majority of circumstances a single all-layer suture is adequate. Enrolment of reinforcing autogenous vascular pedicle flap remains controversial.[87,88] Most advocates of reinforcement flaps suggest an onlay patch rather than a wrap, to minimise the possibility of stricture at the repair site. A major concern with the wrap technique is the induction of an obstructive component distal to the repair site, rendering it more prone to leakage.

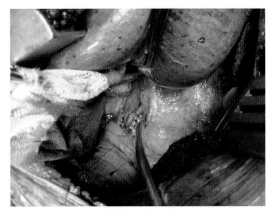

Figure 6.9 • Primary repair with interrupted absorbable stitches for a lower oesophageal rupture.

Though technically feasible, primary repair is associated with a high failure rate and many surgeons now advocate insertion of a T-tube into the perforation, which is closed around it (after debridement), producing a controlled fistula. This can be removed at a later date, often many weeks/months later, once the patient has recovered and the surrounding leakage (managed by appropriately placed chest drains) has subsided.

Immediate resection

Several series have pointed out that primary repair resulted in greater morbidity and even mortality than immediate oesophageal resection.[89–91] However, this may well relate to the underlying cause of perforation and whether the cause remains.

> ✔ In a series of 41 patients, of whom 25 patients underwent surgical repair of oesophageal perforation, about one-third had continued swallowing difficulty that mandated regular oesophageal dilation after an average of 3.7 years.[92] A high incidence of functional or structural deficiency was observed after primary repair of oesophageal perforation, which indeed affected the quality of life of the patients.

Oesophagectomy is therefore a reasonable option (if the surgeon is experienced in this procedure) in patients with underlying disease (including carcinoma, if the lesion was considered operable before the perforation occurred) and if the diagnosis has been made early and the patient is in a good condition. Occasionally it may also be required in patients presenting late, in whom simple closure over a T-tube is not possible. This scenario is, however, very uncommon. (The reader is referred to the *Oesophagogastric Surgery* volume in this Companion to Specialist Surgical Practice series for more detailed information.)

> ✓ Primary repair with or without T-tube drainage is the best option for the management of oesophageal perforations depending on time from occurrence to diagnosis. Patients with an underlying condition related to the perforation, in whom the diagnosis has been made early (<24 hours) and who are in a good condition, can be considered for resection if the appropriate surgical expertise is available.

Corrosive perforation

Corrosive injury to the upper gastrointestinal tract is an entity very different from other mechanical types of oesophageal perforation. It is a notoriously difficult situation associated with dreadful rates of morbidity and mortality. While more than 80% of accidental corrosive ingestion occurs in children, injuries in adults are usually intentional, and thus more severe in extent.[93] The mortality rate ranges from 10% to 78% in cases of attempted suicide.[94,95] The severity of damage depends on the type, concentration, volume and duration of contact of the agent with the mucosal surface. Making a distinction between acid and alkali as to the extent and severity of oesophagogastric damage has been elusive. It is well known that acid induces a coagulating burn injury, which tends to be self-limiting with the coagulum formation. In contrast, alkali causes a liquefactive necrosis to the tissue, leading to dissolution of protein and collagen, saponification of fats, and thrombosis of blood vessels. All these incur a deeper damage and even transmural perforation.

The acute management of corrosive ingestion entails a quick and efficient assessment of the patient's vital signs. Laryngeal oedema can be life threatening and establishing a patent airway is of paramount importance. Either an early endotracheal intubation or tracheostomy may be required in difficult cases before further resuscitation and management. It is generally agreed that early gentle endoscopic examination is of value for both prognostic consideration and decision-making.[96,97] Surgical intervention, such as thoracotomy, drainage, mediastinal debridement, proximal diversion of saliva with a cervical oesophagostomy and exclusion from gastric reflux, are better performed early if signs of full-thickness perforation are evident on radiological or endoscopic investigations. Reconstruction should be deferred until sepsis has subsided. More

often than not, reconstruction is done by fashioning a jejunal or colonic interposition loop through an extra-anatomical plane (e.g. the substernal or presternal routes).

Perforation after endotherapy for mucosal/submucosal tumours

Since its introduction in the 1980s, endoscopic mucosal resection (EMR) has been increasingly practised for upper gastrointestinal lesions identified at early stages.[98–100] With the snaring technique, en bloc resection used to be a challenging task as the average size of lesion removed is limited (<15 mm in diameter).[101] The recent development of new endoscopic accessories, such as the insulated-tip knife and hook knife, has opened a new horizon for such purposes.[102,103] The novel endoluminal procedure, endoscopic submucosal dissection (ESD), has virtually no limitation on the size of resection, provided that the lesion is superficial with a low chance of nodal spread.[104] However, ESD is a technically demanding procedure with a significantly higher risk of perforation compared with conventional EMR.[105,106] As most ESD-induced perforations can be recognised intraoperatively, attempts to close the defect by various techniques have been reported.[107] Fujishiro et al. described a 100% success rate of closing ESD perforations using endoscopic clips.[108] The average duration of hospital stay was only 12 days and none of the 27 patients in the series required surgical salvage. More importantly, as reported in an intermediate-term follow-up study by Ikehara et al., perforation during ESD for early oesophageal and gastric cancers has not been associated with increased risk of dissemination of the malignancy.[109]

Duodenal and jejunal perforations during endoscopic retrograde cholangiopancreatography (ERCP)

Visceral perforations due to ERCP are not uncommon, with an incidence reported to range between 0.5% and 2.1%.[110,111] The injury carries a death rate over 15%. Risk factors include older age of patients, suspected sphincter of Oddi dysfunction, a dilated duct, performance of sphincterotomy and longer duration of the procedure.[112] ERCP-related perforation can be further subclassified according to the causative mechanism and location because management strategy may vary accordingly. Stapfer et al. first described a typing system in 2000 to guide the treatment for the situation (type I: duodenal wall injury; type II: peri-Vaterian injury related to sphincterotomy; type III: distal bile duct injury probably related to guidewire or basket injury; and type IV: retroperitoneal air alone).[113] While perforation of the oesophagus and stomach due to insertion of the side-view duodenoscope can be managed as discussed in the previous sections, type I injury with lateral or medial duodenal wall tear is often related to difficult positioning of the endoscope in the attempt to obtain access to the papilla. Vulnerability further increases if there is anatomical deformity such as a stricture or tumour compression. This kind of perforation tends to be intraperitoneal, which is unlikely to be self-contained, and early surgical repair with debridement of devitalised tissue is recommended. Small perforations less than 1 cm in diameter can be closed primarily with transverse sutures in one or two layers. For perforations of a larger size, or when the diagnosis has been delayed, jejunal serosal patch, duodenal diversion or conversion to a Billroth II gastrectomy are alternative options, but to some extent the choice depends mainly on the patient's clinical condition and intraoperative findings.

Another prominent risk factor for 'scope' perforation is a history of previous Billroth II gastrectomy, because retrograde insertion of the endoscope along the afferent loop may overstretch and rupture the jejunum around the relatively fixed duodenojejunal flexure. The reported incidence under such circumstances can be as high as 10% even in expert centres and early surgical repair is usually necessary.[114,115]

In contrast, perforations resulting from endoscopic sphincterotomy (type II) or guidewire/basket (type III) are mostly retroperitoneal with a small size of leakage and therefore more amenable to non-operative therapy. Although some perforations can be identified at the time of the ERCP, many are not suspected until after the procedure. Clearly, early suspicion is raised by the presence of abdominal pain post-procedure, but the observation of a paraduodenal or perinephric gas shadow on plain abdominal radiographs is suggestive of retroperitoneal perforation. In such cases, and even if the plain X-rays are unremarkable, a CT scan of the abdomen with oral and intravenous contrast should be organised to confirm the diagnosis and extent of the perforation. Small perforations with minimal extravasation of contrast can be successfully managed by non-operative means, including nasogastric drainage, antibiotics and parenteral nutrition. Some surgeons also advocate biliary decompression by either an internal plastic stent or external nasobiliary drain. Radiologically guided percutaneous drainage is indicated if a sizeable collection is shown by the initial imaging. However, surgical intervention should be offered to patients with extensive extravasation of contrast or clinical deterioration despite initial non-operative treatment. This can be a formidable undertaking and is associated with significant morbidity and mortality. Thankfully they are relatively rare, but when they occur each patient will need to be managed according to first principles: debridement of ischaemic and damaged tissue, primary repair of the defect if possible, diversion of biliary contents (by means of a T-tube) and consideration given to duodenal exclusion (closure of pylorus and gastrojejunostomy). In such circumstances a feeding jejunostomy should also be inserted for long-term nutritional support.

✓ It has been shown in various series that one of the key prerequisites for successful non-operative management of ERCP perforations is the early recognition and diagnosis of the situation.[116,117]

Key points

- Perforations of the upper gastrointestinal tract are either spontaneous or iatrogenic.
- Early surgery is generally required for the majority of perforations as delay in diagnosis and treatment is associated with increased morbidity and mortality.
- For perforated duodenal ulcers omental patch repair followed by postoperative therapy with proton-pump inhibitors and eradication of *Helicobacter pylori*, if present, is the treatment of choice.
- For perforated gastric ulcers, either ulcer excision (if feasible) or omental patch repair and biopsy of the ulcer is all that is required. Gastric resection should not be carried out without histology unless closure cannot be achieved using these other techniques.

- Management of oesophageal perforations depends largely on whether the pleura has been breached. It can be a challenging condition and surgical strategies will depend on the expertise available. These include non-operative management, stent insertion (both permanent and removable), repair (with or without T-tube drainage) and occasionally oesophageal resection.
- Early endoscopy is a very useful technique to assess many oesophageal emergencies including corrosive injury.
- ERCP perforations vary from simple to extensive and management depends on early diagnosis and accurate assessment as to the degree of extravasation.

References

1. Coggon D, Lambert P, Langman MJ. 20 years of hospital admissions for peptic ulcer in England and Wales. Lancet 1981;1:1302–4.

2. Vaira D, Menegatti M, Miglioli M. What is the role of *Helicobacter pylori* in complicated ulcer disease? Gastroenterology 1997;113(Suppl.):S78–84.

3. Behrman SW. Management of complicated peptic ulcer disease. Arch Surg 2005;140:201–8.

4. Bornman PC, Theodorou NA, Jeffery PC, et al. Simple closure of perforated duodenal ulcer: a prospective evaluation of a conservative management policy. Br J Surg 1990;77:73–5.

5. Chen CH, Yang CC, Yeh YH. Role of upright chest radiography and ultrasonography in demonstrating free air of perforated peptic ulcers. Hepatogastroenterology 2001;48:1082–4.

6. Grassi R, Romano S, Pinto A, et al. Gastro-duodenal perforations: conventional plain film, US and CT findings in 166 consecutive patients. Eur J Radiol 2004;50:30–6.

7. Lee CW, Yip AW, Lam KH. Pneumogastrogram in the diagnosis of perforated peptic ulcer. Aust N Z J Surg 1993;63:459–61.

8. Svanes C. Trends in perforated peptic ulcer: incidence, etiology, treatment and prognosis. World J Surg 2000;24:277–83.

9. Robson AJ, Richards JM, Ohly N, et al. The effect of surgical subspecialization on outcomes in peptic ulcer disease complicated by perforation and bleeding. World J Surg 2008;32:1456–61.

10. Kujath P, Schwandner O, Bruch HP. Morbidity and mortality of perforated peptic gastroduodenal ulcer following emergency surgery. Langenbecks Arch Surg 2002;387:298–302.

11. Egberts JH, Summa B, Schulz U, et al. Impact of preoperative physiological risk profile on postoperative morbidity and mortality after emergency operation of complicated peptic ulcer disease. World J Surg 2007;31:1449–57.

12. Boey J, Choi SK, Poon A, et al. Risk stratification in perforated duodenal ulcers. A prospective validation of predictive factors. Ann Surg 1987;205:22–6.

13. Kocer B, Surmeli S, Solak C, et al. Factors affecting mortality and morbidity in patients with peptic ulcer perforation. J Gastroenterol Hepatol 2007; 22:565–70.

14. Sillakivi T, Lang A, Tein A, et al. Evaluation of risk factors for mortality in surgically treated perforated peptic ulcer. Hepatogastroenterology 2000;47:1765–8.

15. Lee FY, Leung KL, Lai BS, et al. Predicting mortality and morbidity of patients operated on for perforated peptic ulcers. Arch Surg 2001;136:90–4.

16. Møller MH, Engebjerg MC, Adamsen S, et al. The Peptic Ulcer Perforation (PULP) score: a predictor of mortality following peptic ulcer perforation. A cohort study. Acta Anaesthesiol Scand 2012;56(5):655–62.

17. Donovan AJ, Berne TV, Donovan JA. Perforated duodenal ulcer: an alternative therapeutic plan. Arch Surg 1998;133:1166–71.

18. Dascalescu C, Andriescu L, Bulat C, et al. Taylor's method: a therapeutic alternative for perforated gastroduodenal ulcer. Hepatogastroenterology 2006; 53:543–6.

19. Donovan AJ, Vinson TL, Maulsby GO, et al. Selective treatment of duodenal ulcer with perforation. Ann Surg 1979;189:627–36.

20. Berne TV, Donovan AJ. Nonoperative treatment of perforated duodenal ulcer. Arch Surg 1989;124:830–2.

21. Crofts TJ, Park KG, Steele RJ, et al. A randomized trial of nonoperative treatment for perforated peptic ulcer. N Engl J Med 1989;320:970–3.
   This randomised trial disproved the recommendation of non-operative treatment for older patients. The higher incidence of intra-abdominal sepsis and prolonged hospital stay are additional discouraging factors for conservative management in patients with peptic ulcer perforation.

22. Graham RR. Technical surgical procedures for gastric and duodenal ulcer. Surg Gynecol Obstet 1938;66:269–87.

23. Drury JK, McKay AJ, Hutchison JS, et al. Natural history of perforated duodenal ulcers treated by suture closure. Lancet 1978;2:749–50.

24. Griffin GE, Organ CH. The natural history of the perforated duodenal ulcer treated by suture placation. Ann Surg 1976;183:382–5.

25. Bornman PC, Theodorou NA, Jeffery PC, et al. Simple closure of perforated duodenal ulcer: a prospective evaluation of a conservative management policy. Br J Surg 1990;77:73–5.

26. Tanphiphat C, Tanprayoon T, Na Thalang A. Surgical treatment of perforated duodenal ulcer: a prospective trial between simple closure and definitive surgery. Br J Surg 1985;72:370–2.

27. Christiansen J, Andersen OB, Bonnesen T, et al. Perforated duodenal ulcer managed by simple closure versus closure and proximal gastric vagotomy. Br J Surg 1987;74:286–7.

28. Boey J, Lee NW, Koo J, et al. Immediate definitive surgery for perforated duodenal ulcers: a prospective controlled trial. Ann Surg 1982;196:338–44.

29. Ceneviva R, de Castro e Silva Júnior O, Castelfranchi PL, et al. Simple suture with or without proximal gastric vagotomy for perforated duodenal ulcer. Br J Surg 1986;73:427–30.

30. Jordan Jr. PH, Thornby J. Perforated pyloroduodenal ulcers. Long-term results with omental patch closure and parietal cell vagotomy. Ann Surg 1995;221:479–86.

31. Noguiera C, Silva AS, Santos JN, et al. Perforated peptic ulcer: main factors of morbidity and mortality. World J Surg 2003;27:782–7.

32. Gilliam AD, Speake WJ, Lobo DN, et al. Current practice of emergency vagotomy and *Helicobacter pylori* eradication for complicated peptic ulcer in the United Kingdom. Br J Surg 2003;90:88–90.

33. Datsis AC, Rogdakis A, Kekelos S, et al. Simple closure of chronic duodenal ulcer perforation in the era of *Helicobacter pylori*: an old procedure, today's solution. Hepatogastroenterology 2003;50(53):1396–8.

34. Gupta S, Kaushik R, Sharma R, et al. The management of large perforations of duodenal ulcers. BMC Surg 2005;5:15.

35. Reinbach DH, Cruickshank G, McColl KE. Acute perforated duodenal ulcer is not associated with *Helicobacter pylori* infection. Gut 1993;34:1344–7.

36. Sebastian M, Chandran VP, Elashaal YI, et al. *Helicobacter pylori* infection in perforated peptic ulcer disease. Br J Surg 1995;82:360–2.

37. Mihmanli M, Isgor A, Kabukcuoglu F, et al. The effect of *H. pylori* in perforation of duodenal ulcer. Hepatogastroenterology 1998;45:1610–2.

38. Ng EK, Chung SC, Sung JJ, et al. High prevalence of *Helicobacter pylori* infection in duodenal ulcer perforations not caused by non-steroidal anti-inflammatory drugs. Br J Surg 1996;83:1779–81.

39. Gisbert JP, Legido J, García-Sanz I, et al. *Helicobacter pylori* and perforated peptic ulcer prevalence of the infection and role of non-steroidal anti-inflammatory drugs. Dig Liver Dis 2004;36:116–20.

40. Bobrzyński A, Konturek PC, Konturek SJ, et al. *Helicobacter pylori* and nonsteroidal anti-inflammatory drugs in perforations and bleeding of peptic ulcers. Med Sci Monit 2005;11:CR132–5.

41. Chu KM, Kwok KF, Law SY, et al. *Helicobacter pylori* status and endoscopy follow-up of patients having a history of perforated duodenal ulcer. Gastrointest Endosc 1999;50:58–62.

42. Ng EK, Lam YH, Sung JJ, et al. Eradication of *Helicobacter pylori* prevents recurrence of ulcer after simple closure of duodenal ulcer perforation: randomized controlled trial. Ann Surg 2000;231:153–8.
    This is the first randomised trial showing significant reduction in ulcer recurrence after eradication of *Helicobacter pylori* in patients undergoing simple omental repair of perforated duodenal ulcer.

43. Tomtitchong P, Siribumrungwong B, Vilaichone RK, et al. Systematic review and meta-analysis: *Helicobacter pylori* eradication therapy after simple closure of perforated duodenal ulcer. Helicobacter 2012;17(2):148–52.
    The pooled incidence of 1-year ulcer relapse from three prospective randomised trials was only 5.2% in patients treated with *H. pylori* eradication, which was significantly lower than that of the control group (35.2%).

44. Goldstein JL, Silverstein FE, Agrawal NM, et al. Reduced risk of upper gastrointestinal ulcer complications with celecoxib, a novel COX-2 inhibitor. Am J Gastroenterol 2000;95:1681–90.

45. Silverstein FE, Faich G, Goldstein JL, et al. Gastrointestinal toxicity with celecoxib vs nonsteroidal anti-inflammatory drugs for osteoarthritis and rheumatoid arthritis: the CLASS study: a randomized controlled trial. Celecoxib Long-term Arthritis Safety Study. JAMA 2000;284:1247–55.

46. García Rodríguez LA, Barreales Tolosa L. Risk of upper gastrointestinal complications among users of traditional NSAIDs and COXIBs in the general population. Gastroenterology 2007;132(2):498–506.

47. Christensen S, Riis A, Nørgaard M, et al. Introduction of newer selective cyclo-oxygenase-2 inhibitors and rates of hospitalization with bleeding and perforated peptic ulcer. Aliment Pharmacol Ther 2007;25(8):907–12.

48. Thomsen RW, Riis A, Munk EM, et al. 30-day mortality after peptic ulcer perforation among users of newer selective COX-2 inhibitors and traditional NSAIDs: a population-based study. Am J Gastroenterol 2006;101(12):2704–10.

49. Latimer N, Lord J, Grant RL, et al. National Institute for Health and Clinical Excellence Osteoarthritis Guideline Development Group. Cost effectiveness of COX 2 selective inhibitors and traditional NSAIDs alone or in combination with a proton pump inhibitor for people with osteoarthritis. Br Med J 2009;339:b2538.

50. Nathanson LK, Easter DW, Cuschieri A. Laparoscopic repair/peritoneal toilet of perforated duodenal ulcer. Surg Endosc 1990;4:232–3.

51. Druart ML, Van Hee R, Etienne J, et al. Laparoscopic repair of perforated duodenal ulcer. A prospective multicenter clinical trial. Surg Endosc 1997;11:1017–20.

52. Katkhouda N, Mavor E, Mason RJ, et al. Laparoscopic repair of perforated duodenal ulcers: outcome and efficacy in 30 consecutive patients. Arch Surg 1999;134:845–8.

53. Lau WY, Leung KL, Zhu XL, et al. Laparoscopic repair of perforated peptic ulcer. Br J Surg 1995; 82:814–6.

54. Lau WY, Leung KL, Kwong KH, et al. A randomized study comparing laparoscopic versus open repair of perforated peptic ulcer using suture or sutureless technique. Ann Surg 1996;224:131–8.

55. Siu WT, Leong HT, Law BK, et al. Laparoscopic repair for perforated peptic ulcer: a randomized controlled trial. Ann Surg 2002;235:313–9.

56. Lunevicius R, Morkevicius M. Systematic review comparing laparoscopic and open repair for perforated peptic ulcer. Br J Surg 2005;92:1195–207.
    A systematic review of 15 publications. The laparoscopic closure was associated with significantly less analgesic use, shorter hospital stay, less wound infection and lower mortality rate compared to open surgery at a cost of a longer operating time and higher suture-site leakage.

57. Bertleff MJ, Lange JF. Laparoscopic correction of perforated peptic ulcer: first choice? A review of literature. Surg Endosc 2010;24(6):1231–9.
    A review comprising 56 studies showing an overall conversion rate of 12.4%. Patients with a Boey score of 3, age over 70 years and symptoms persisting longer than 24 hours are relative contraindications to the laparoscopic approach.

58. Booth RAD, Williams JA. Mortality of duodenal ulcer treated by simple suture. Br J Surg 1971;58:42–4.

59. Baker RJ. Perforated duodenal ulcer. In: Baker RJ, Fischer JE, editors. Mastery of surgery, 4th ed, vol. 1. Philadelphia, PA: Lippincott; 2001.

60. Burch JM, Cox CL, Feliciano DV, et al. Management of the difficult duodenal stump. Am J Surg 1991; 162:522–6.

61. Isik B, Yilmaz S, Kirimlioglu V, et al. A life-saving but inadequately discussed procedure: tube duodenostomy. Known and unknown aspects. World J Surg 2007;31(8):1616–24.

62. Ng EK, Chung SC, Li AK. Controlled duodenostomy for difficult duodenal stump. Aust N Z J Surg 1995;65(5):345–6.

63. Chung RS, DenBesten L. Duodenojejunostomy in gastric operations for postbulbar duodenal ulcer. Arch Surg 1976;111(9):955–7.

64. Jani K, Saxena AK, Vaghasia R. Omental plugging for large-sized duodenal peptic perforations: a prospective randomized study of 100 patients. South Med J 2006;99(5):467–71.

65. Lal P, Vindal A, Hadke NS. Controlled tube duodenostomy in the management of giant duodenal ulcer perforation: a new technique for a surgically challenging condition. Am J Surg 2009;198(3):319–23.

66. Wysocki A, Biesiada Z, Beben P, et al. Perforated gastric ulcer. Dig Surg 2000;17:132–7.

67. Madiba TE, Nair R, Mulaudzi TV, et al. Perforated gastric ulcer – reappraisal of surgical options. S Afr J Surg 2005;43:58–60.

68. Mahar AL, Brar SS, Coburn NG, et al. Surgical management of gastric perforation in the setting of gastric cancer. Gastric Cancer 2011;Oct 8. Epub ahead of print.

69. Wesdorp IC, Bartelsman JF, Huibregtse K, et al. Treatment of instrumental oesophageal perforation. Gut 1984;25:398–404.

70. Jones WG, Ginsberg RJ. Esophageal perforation: a continuing challenge. Ann Thorac Surg 1992;53:534–43.

71. Adamek HE, Jakobs R, Dorlars D, et al. Management of esophageal perforations after therapeutic upper gastrointestinal endoscopy. Scand J Gastroenterol 1997;32:411–4.

72. Fry LC, Mönkemüller K, Neumann H, et al. Incidence, clinical management and outcomes of esophageal perforations after endoscopic dilatation. Z Gastroenterol 2007;45:1180–4.

73. Sepesi B, Raymond DP, Peters JH. Esophageal perforation: surgical, endoscopic and medical management strategies. Curr Opin Gastroenterol 2010;26:379–83.

74. Brinster CJ, Singhai S, Lee L, et al. Evolving options in the management of esophageal perforation. Ann Thorac Surg 2004;77:1475–83.

75. Cameron JL, Kieffer RF, Hendrix TR, et al. Selective nonoperative management of contained intrathoracic esophageal disruptions. Ann Thorac Surg 1979;27:404–8.

76. Shaffer Jr. HA, Valenzuela G, Mittal RK. Esophageal perforation. A reassessment of the criteria for choosing medical or surgical therapy. Arch Intern Med 1992;152:757–61.

77. Molina EG, Stollman N, Grauer L, et al. Conservative management of esophageal nontransmural tears after pneumatic dilation for achalasia. Am J Gastroenterol 1996;91:15–8.

78. Michel L, Grillo HC, Malt RA. Operative and nonoperative management of esophageal perforations. Ann Surg 1981;194:57–63.

79. Vogel SB, Rout WR, Martin TD, et al. Esophageal perforation in adults: aggressive, conservative treatment lowers morbidity and mortality. Ann Surg 2005;241(6):1016–21.

80. Kuppusamy MK, Hubka M, Felisky CD, et al. Evolving management strategies in esophageal perforation: surgeons using nonoperative techniques to improve outcomes. J Am Coll Surg 2011;213(1):164–71.

81. Altorjay A, Kiss J, Vörös A, et al. Nonoperative management of esophageal perforations. Is it justified? Ann Surg 1997;225(4):415–21.

82. Abbas G, Schuchert MJ, Pettiford BL, et al. Contemporaneous management of esophageal perforation. Surgery 2009;146(4):749–55.

83. Hünerbein M, Stroszczynski C, Moesta KT, et al. Treatment of thoracic anastomotic leaks after esophagectomy with self-expanding plastic stents. Ann Surg 2004;240:801–7.

84. Siersema PD, Homs MY, Haringsma J, et al. Use of large-diameter metallic stents to seal traumatic nonmalignant perforations of the esophagus. Gastrointest Endosc 2003;58:356–61.

85. Freeman RK, Van Woerkom JM, Ascioti AJ. Esophageal stent placement for the treatment of iatrogenic intrathoracic esophageal perforation. Ann Thorac Surg 2007;83:2003–7.

86. van Boeckel PG, Sijbring A, Vleggaar FP, et al. Systematic review: temporary stent placement for benign rupture or anastomotic leak of the oesophagus. Aliment Pharmacol Ther 2011;33(12):1292–301.

87. Wright CD, Mathisen DJ, Wain JC, et al. Reinforced primary repair of thoracic esophageal perforation. Ann Thoracic Surg 1995;60:245–8.

88. Gouge T, Depan H, Spencer F. Experience with the Grillo pleural wrap procedure in 18 patients with perforation of the thoracic esophagus. Ann Surg 1989;209:612–7.

89. Orringer MB. Esophagectomy for esophageal disruption. Ann Thorac Surg 1990;49:35–42.

90. Altorjay A, Kiss J, Voros A. The role of esophagectomy in the management of esophageal perforations. Ann Thorac Surg 1998;65:1433–6.

91. Salo JA, Isolauri JO, Heikkila LJ, et al. Management of delayed esophageal perforation with mediastinal sepsis; esophagectomy or primary repair? J Thorac Cardiovasc Surg 1993;106:1088–91.

92. Iannettoni MD, Vlessis AA, Whyte RI, et al. Functional outcome after surgical treatment of esophageal perforation. Ann Thorac Surg 1997;64:1606–9.

93. Gumaste VV, Dave PB. Ingestion of corrosive substances by adults. Am J Gastroenterol 1992;87:1–5.

94. Ertekin C, Alimoglu O, Akyildiz H, et al. The results of caustic ingestions. Hepatogastroenterology 2004;51:1397–400.

95. Sugawa C, Lucas CE. Caustic injury of the upper gastrointestinal tract in adults: a clinical and endoscopic study. Surgery 1989;106:802–6.

96. Poley JW, Steyerberg EW, Kuipers EJ, et al. Ingestion of acid and alkaline agents: outcome and prognostic value of early upper endoscopy. Gastrointest Endosc 2004;60:372–7.

97. Rigo GP, Camellini L, Azzolini F, et al. What is the utility of selected clinical and endoscopic parameters in predicting the risk of death after caustic ingestion? Endoscopy 2002;34:304–10.

98. Hirao M, Masuda K, Asanuma T, et al. Endoscopic resection of early gastric cancer and other tumors with local injection of hypertonic saline–epinephrine. Gastrointest Endosc 1988;34:264–9.

99. Inoue H, Takeshita K, Hori H, et al. Endoscopic mucosal resection with a cap-fitted panendoscope for esophagus, stomach, and colon mucosal lesions. Gastrointest Endosc 1993;39:58–62.

100. Akiyama M, Ota M, Nakajima H, et al. Endoscopic mucosal resection of gastric neoplasms using a ligating device. Gastrointest Endosc 1997;45:182–6.

101. Korenaga D, Haraguchi M, Tsujitani S, et al. Clinicopathological features of mucosal carcinoma of the stomach with lymph node metastasis in eleven patients. Br J Surg 1986;73:431–3.

102. Ohkuwa M, Hosokawa K, Boku N, et al. New endoscopic treatment for intramucosal gastric tumors using an insulated-tip diathermic knife. Endoscopy 2001;33:221–6.

103. Chiu PW, Chan KF, Lee YT, et al. Endoscopic submucosal dissection used for treating early neoplasia of the foregut using a combination of knives. Surg Endosc 2008;22:777–83.

104. Gotoda T. Endoscopic resection of early gastric cancer. Gastric Cancer 2007;10:1–11.

105. Oda I, Saito D, Tada M, et al. A multicenter retrospective study of endoscopic resection for early gastric cancer. Gastric Cancer 2006;9:262–70.

106. Oka S, Tanaka S, Kaneko I, et al. Advantage of endoscopic submucosal dissection compared with EMR for early gastric cancer. Gastrointest Endosc 2006;64:877–83.

107. Minami S, Gotoda T, Ono H, et al. Complete endoscopic closure of gastric perforation induced by endoscopic resection of early gastric cancer using endoclips can prevent surgery. Gastrointest Endosc 2006;63:596–601.

108. Fujishiro M, Yahagi N, Kakushima N, et al. Successful nonsurgical management of perforation complicating endoscopic submucosal dissection of gastrointestinal epithelial neoplasms. Endoscopy 2006;38:1001–6.

109. Ikehara H, Gotoda T, Ono H, et al. Gastric perforation during endoscopic resection for gastric carcinoma and the risk of peritoneal dissemination. Br J Surg 2007;94:992–5.

110. Freeman ML, Nelson DB, Sherman S, et al. Complications of endoscopic sphincterotomy. N Engl J Med 1996;909–18.

111. Cotton PB, Lehman G, Vennes J, et al. Endoscopic sphincterotomy complications and their management: an attempt at consensus. Gastrointest Endosc 1991;383–93.

112. Enns R, Eloubeidi MA, Mergener K, et al. ERCP-related perforations: risk factors and management. Endoscopy 2002;34:293–8.

113. Stapfer M, Selby RR, Stain SC, et al. Management of duodenal perforation after endoscopic retrograde cholangiopancreatography and sphincterotomy. Ann Surg 2000;232(2):191–8.

114. Faylona JM, Qadir A, Chan AC, et al. Small-bowel perforations related to endoscopic retrograde cholangiopancreatography (ERCP) in patients with Billroth II gastrectomy. Endoscopy 1999;31:546–9.

115. Bagci S, Tuzun A, Ates Y, et al. Efficacy and safety of endoscopic retrograde cholangiopancreatography in patients with Billroth II anastomosis. Hepatogastroenterology 2005;52:356–9.

116. Assalia A, Suissa A, Ilivitzki A, et al. Validity of clinical criteria in the management of endoscopic retrograde cholangiopancreatography related duodenal perforations. Arch Surg 2007;142:1059–64.

117. Martin DF, Tweedle DE. Retroperitoneal perforation during ERCP and endoscopic sphincterotomy: causes, clinical features and management. Endoscopy 1990;22:174–5.

7

Acute non-variceal upper gastrointestinal bleeding

Colin J. McKay
James Lau

Introduction

A major audit of upper gastrointestinal (UGI) bleeding in the UK carried out over 15 years ago reported an incidence of 103 cases per 100 000 adults per year.[1] A much higher incidence was reported in an audit from the West of Scotland, which found 172 cases per 100 000.[2] The difference was thought to be due to regional variation in deprivation and possible *Helicobacter pylori* prevalence. Whatever the actual incidence at regional level, UGI bleeding remains a significant health problem and in Scotland alone accounts for approximately 7000 hospital admissions each year. Overall mortality from an episode of UGI bleeding was 14% in the UK study[1] and 8% in the study from the West of Scotland,[2] and both demonstrated a marked increase in mortality if bleeding occurred following hospitalisation with another complaint (33% and 44% in the respective studies). A more recent audit[3] covering patients admitted to UK hospitals during a 2-month period in 2007 demonstrated a marked reduction in the proportion of patients undergoing surgery, as well as an increase in the proportion of patients admitted with variceal bleeding. Overall mortality had fallen slightly at 10%, compared with 14% in the earlier UK audit, and the mortality of 26% for inpatients was also lower than in the pevious study. However, mortality in patients admitted with peptic ulcer bleeding had fallen from 8.8% to 5.8% and the overall reduction in mortality from 14 to 10% occurred despite the increase in incidence of variceal bleeding. Mortality is now rare in the absence of comorbidity. The typical patient with severe peptic

ulcer bleeding is now elderly, often suffering medical comorbidity and taking antiplatelet therapy. Such patients are at greater risk of death despite skilled intervention and are less able to withstand surgery should this be necessary. Although the need for surgical intervention is now much reduced with the widespread availability of skilled endoscopic haemostasis, mortality following surgery remains high. In the recent UK audit, postoperative mortality was 30% and, while this is likely to reflect the fact that surgery has become a last resort in patients who are often elderly and suffering from other conditions, there are inevitable concerns about the availability of appropriate expertise in the management of what has become an uncommon surgical emergency. As a result alternatives to surgical intervention are increasingly being employed and will be discussed in this chapter.

Aetiology

In the Rockall study[1] only 4% of patients had UGI bleeding due to varices, with the majority (35%) being attributed to peptic ulcer disease. Of some concern was the 25% of patients in this study where no cause for bleeding was identified at all, particularly as this group had a mortality of 20%. Very similar figures were reported in the Scottish study.[2] Of those patients with a diagnosis, approximately 25% were due to duodenal ulcer and 25% to peptic ulceration in the stomach, oesophagus or a combination of sites. The remainder were due to a number of other conditions, including oesophagitis, gastritis

Table 7.1 • Endoscopic diagnoses to patients who presented with acute upper gastrointestinal bleeding in the 2007 UK Audit.

Endoscopic diagnoses	Total number of patients (5004) % (n)
Peptic ulcer	36 (1826)
Varices	11 (544)
Malignancy	3.7 (187)
Oesophagitis	24 (1177)
Gastritis/ erosions	22 (1091)
Erosive duodenitis	13 (640)
Mallory-Weiss Tear	4.3 (213)
Others including vascular ectasia	2.6 (133)
No abnormality seen	17 (865)

Modified from Hearnshaw S et al. Gut 2011; 60: 1327-1335

and duodenitis, with 10% of cases explained by malignancy or Mallory–Weiss syndrome (Table 7.1). In the most recent UK audit, the proportion of patients with variceal bleeding had increased to 11%, whereas the overall proportion with peptic ulcer remained unchanged.

Initial assessment and triage

Patients with acute UGI bleeding present with haematemesis, melaena or a combination of the two. Haematemesis may be defined as the vomiting of blood from the upper gastrointestinal tract and is indicative of significant bleeding from a site in the oesophagus, stomach or duodenum. Melaena is the passage of black, tarry stools and usually indicates a bleeding site in the upper gastrointestinal tract, although bleeding from the small bowel or even the right colon may present in a similar way, depending on speed of passage. Coffee-ground vomiting (the vomiting of black, particulate material that tests positive for blood) is not indicative of active bleeding. Presentation with haematemesis is associated with an increased risk of mortality compared with melaena or coffee-ground vomiting.[4] Patients with upper gastrointestinal blood loss may occasionally present with frank rectal bleeding (haematochezia), but this is indicative of major blood loss and, not surprisingly, is associated with an increased need for transfusion, surgery and mortality.[5] A good example of this would be a patient who has previously undergone aortic aneurysm surgery who subsequently develops an aortoduodenal fistula.

Scoring systems

Many patients with UGI haemorrhage have trivial bleeding, require no intervention and can safely be discharged early. Others, however, have catastrophic bleeding and many lie between these two extremes. On initial assessment, differentiation between patients can sometimes be difficult. Two separate studies have assessed the initial, pretreatment risk factors in an attempt to enable triage of patients to appropriate early endoscopy, observation or even non-admission. In the English audit discussed above, Rockall and colleagues identified risk factors for mortality.[5] Patients with an initial score of zero (i.e. age <60, no tachycardia, no hypotension and no comorbidity) had very low mortality, although in a subsequent study 18% of patients with an initial Rockall score of zero required further intervention. Assessment of the re-bleeding risk therefore requires the full Rockall score, which necessitates endoscopic assessment. This is discussed below.

In contrast, a scoring system was developed in the West of Scotland, the aim being to allow early assessment of the need for intervention rather than risk of death.[6] The Glasgow Blatchford Score (GBS) performed significantly better than the Rockall score at predicting the need for intervention and has now been validated in prospective studies from the UK[7] and Hong Kong.[6] In particular, the GBS is the better scoring system for predicting low-risk patients who can be safely discharged. The proportion of patients with UGI haemorrhage who fulfil these low-risk criteria (i.e. a GBS of 0) is, however, low (4.6% in the Hong Kong study). The proportion of patients who require endoscopic therapy increases with higher scores. There remains a small but significant proportion of patients with low to moderately high scores who require endoscopic therapy and it is difficult to define a cut-off score beyond which urgent endoscopy becomes mandatory.

Full assessment of mortality risk demands endoscopic determination of the cause of bleeding and assessment of the appearance of any ulcer present. These findings are incorporated into the full Rockall score. This composite Rockall system has been validated in prospective studies,[8–10] but is more accurate in predicting mortality than the risk of re-bleeding[8,9] (Table 7.2).

✔ A GBS of 0 on presentation identifies a low risk group of patients who may be safely discharged without the need for urgent UGI endoscopy.

A full Rockall score should be calculated for all patients with UGI bleeding following initial endoscopic assessment.

Table 7.2 • Rockall score for predicting risk of re-bleeding or death In non-variceal UGI haemorrhage

Component	0	1	2	3
Age (years)	<60	60–79	≥80	
Shock	Pulse < 100 SBP ≥ 100 mmHg	Pulse ≥ 100 SBP ≥ 100 mmHg	SBP < 100 mmHg	
Comorbidity			IHD, cardiac failure, other major comorbidity	Renal failure, liver failure, disseminated malignancy
Diagnosis	Mallory–Weiss, no lesion, no SRH	All other diagnoses		
Stigmata of recent haemorrhage	No stigmata or dark spot		Blood in UGI tract, adherent clot, visible or spurting vessel	

IHD, ischaemic heart disease; SBP, systolic blood pressure; SRH, stigmata of recent haemorrhage.
Reproduced from Rockall TA, Logan RFA, Devlin HB et al. Variation in outcome after acute upper gastrointestinal haemorrhage. Lancet 1995; 346(8971):346–50. With permission from Elsevier.

Initial management

While it may be appropriate to consider discharge for young patients with no haemodynamic compromise and a GBS of zero, particularly where there has been no witnessed frank haematemesis, most patients with a history of UGI bleeding will be admitted for observation and endoscopy. This will entail insertion of a large-bore cannula, administration of prewarmed crystalloid or colloid as required and immediate blood samples taken for crossmatch, biochemistry, full blood count, coagulation screen and arterial blood gases. There is some evidence that admission to a dedicated UGI bleeding unit is associated with a reduction in mortality.[11] Such a unit requires a 24-hour on-call service for immediate endoscopy if required and early (within 24h) consultant-led endoscopy for all patients. Indications for urgent (out-of-hours) endoscopy vary, but the main factor determining the degree of urgency is the necessity for endostasis. Therefore, patients with evidence of continuing haemorrhage, declared either by continuing haematemesis or haemodynamic instability despite initial fluid resuscitation, require emergency endoscopy with a view to endostasis. Repeated 'coffee-ground' vomiting or melaena in a haemodynamically stable patient are of less urgent concern. Most stable patients will undergo UGI endoscopy within 24h (usually on the morning after admission). In such patients the purpose of endoscopy is twofold: firstly, patients with minor bleeds undergo full diagnostic assessment and if considered at low risk of re-bleeding can be discharged home; secondly, to identify the group of patients who have significant lesions and who require endoscopic therapy to reduce the risk of re-bleeding. This will be discussed in the next section.

Massive haemorrhage

In those patients who have evidence of haemodynamic compromise, initial resuscitation should follow the appropriate guidelines.[11] A Cochrane review of 55 trials found no evidence of any benefit of administering colloid rather than crystalloid solutions during resuscitation in critically ill patients.[12] As colloid solutions are more expensive, initial resuscitation with appropriate crystalloids is recommended.

Use of blood and blood products

Red cell replacement is likely to be required when 30% or more of the blood volume is lost. This can be difficult to assess, particularly in young patients, and clinical assessment of blood loss, coupled with the response to initial volume replacement, must guide the decision on the necessity of transfusion. Haemoglobin levels are a poor indicator of the degree of acute blood loss. It should very rarely be necessary to administer unmatched blood to such patients, but group-specific blood may be required in life-threatening haemorrhage. In the majority of patients there is usually sufficient time to allow full compatibility testing before transfusion. In patients with evidence of continuing haemorrhage, however, arrangements for emergency endoscopic intervention must be made in parallel with resuscitation.

Administration of platelets should aim to maintain a platelet count of more than 50×10^9/L, but in practice a platelet transfusion should be triggered by a count of less than 75×10^9/L in a patient with ongoing haemorrhage, and may be anticipated in a patient who has required more than two blood volumes of fluid/blood replacement. Platelet therapy may be required in the presence of a normal platelet count where a patient has been receiving antiplatelet therapy.

Coagulation factors are likely to be required when more than one blood volume has been lost. These are most commonly given in the form of fresh frozen plasma (FFP). The use of platelets, FFP and other agents such as recombinant factor VIIa should be guided by local protocols and early involvement of a haematologist.

Early pharmacological treatment

Upper gastrointestinal endoscopy is the mainstay of investigation and management of UGI bleeding, but there may also be a role for early treatment with acid suppression therapy. In vitro studies have shown that, at pH < 6, platelet aggregation and plasma coagulation are markedly reduced,[13] a situation exacerbated by the presence of pepsin. It is therefore reasonable to expect acid suppression therapy to promote clot formation and stabilisation. Six randomised trials comparing pre-endoscopy proton-pump inhibitor (PPI) therapy with histamine-2 receptor antagonist or placebo were analysed in a Cochrane review.[14] No significant impact of PPI therapy was demonstrated on mortality, surgery or re-bleeding rates. There was, however, a reduction in the proportion of patients with stigmata of recent haemorrhage at the time of endoscopy, and a reduction in the requirement for endoscopic therapy at the index endoscopy. While these findings may suggest that pre-endoscopy PPI therapy is warranted, there was no evidence of a reduction in any of the clinically significant parameters. In a large, single-centre, randomised study,[15] pre-endoscopy intravenous omeprazole infusion was associated with a reduction in the incidence of active bleeding and significant reduction in the necessity for endoscopic intervention. However, no difference was observed for re-bleeding, surgery or mortality rates, which were observed in 3%, 2% and 2% of patients, respectively. An accompanying cost-effective analysis concluded that the strategy of pre-emptive use of PPI infusion was cost-saving, probably because of reduced endoscopic therapy and hospitalisation.[16] It therefore seems reasonable to propose pre-endoscopic PPI therapy in patients admitted with UGI bleeding, but this should not delay or act as a substitute for early endoscopic intervention. There is no evidence to support the use of other agents such as somatostatin, octreotide or vasopressin in the pre-endoscopy setting, except where variceal bleeding is suspected.

✔✔ Pre-endoscopy treatment with PPIs is recommended as it reduces the number of actively bleeding ulcers and increases the number of clean-based ulcers seen at the time of endoscopy.[14]
Early use of PPI reduces the need for endoscopic intervention and hospitalisation.

Endoscopy

Upper gastrointestinal endoscopy is required for any patient with significant UGI bleeding. Patients with haemodynamic instability or evidence of continuing haemorrhage require emergency endoscopy, whereas the majority of patients will undergo endoscopy within 24 hours of admission. In a study from Hong Kong,[17] 70 patients aged less than 60 years with a clean ulcer base and stable vital signs were safely discharged on the same day as endoscopy with appropriate anti-ulcer medication. A systematic review of the literature supports a policy of early endoscopy, as this allows the safe discharge of patients with low-risk haemorrhage and improves outcome for patients with high-risk lesions.[18]

✔✔ Early endoscopy is recommended for all patients with UGI haemorrhage.[18]

Endoscopic technique

Endoscopy for UGI bleeding requires the support of a dedicated endoscopic unit with trained nursing staff, availability of additional endoscopes and equipment, ready access to anaesthetic staff and operating theatre, and, increasingly, access to interventional radiology services. These procedures are not ideal for the unsupervised trainee and should be performed or supervised by experienced consultant staff.

For the majority of stable patients, procedures can be safely carried out using standard diagnostic endoscopes. In the unstable patient or where continuing haemorrhage is suspected, the twin-channel or large (3.7-mm) single-channel endoscope is preferable and allows better aspiration of gastric contents as well as more flexibility with regard to the use of heater probes and other instruments. In unstable or obtunded patients, anaesthetic support is mandatory as an endotracheal tube should be passed before endoscopy to guard against aspiration. In rare cases, the use of a pharyngeal over-tube and gastric lavage tube is necessary to remove blood and clot from the stomach before adequate visualisation of the bleeding site can be achieved. Water is poured down the lavage tube via a funnel, which is then placed in a bucket at floor level, allowing siphoning of gastric contents. This, however, can be a time-consuming, unpleasant and messy experience, and in the presence of continuing bleeding should not be allowed to delay endostasis. The use of a tilting trolley allows repositioning of the patient, which can facilitate visualisation of the proximal stomach when obscured by blood and clot. Initially, placing the patient in an upright position may suffice, and if necessary rolling the patient into a right lateral and upright position may be needed for complete visualisation of the gastric fundus. In general, lavage is more successful in achieving visualisation than endoscopic aspiration, as endoscope working channels rapidly block with clot. Lavage can be achieved using repeated flushes of saline down the endoscope working channel or with the use of the powered endoscopic lavage catheters such as that provided with the heater probe. With experience, it should rarely be necessary to proceed to surgery or angiography because of inability to visualise the bleeding site due to blood and clot in the stomach or duodenum.

Bleeding gastric ulcers are most likely within the antrum or at the incisura (77%), or less commonly higher on the lesser curve (15%), with ulcers at other sites within the stomach being uncommon. Ulcers at the incisura and proximal lesser curvature can be readily overlooked unless the endoscope is retroflexed within the stomach. The most common site for a bleeding duodenal ulcer is the posterior wall, sometimes with involvement of the inferior and superior walls of the first part of duodenum. Superficial anterior duodenal wall ulcers can ooze, but usually these ulcers perforate. Ulcers elsewhere in the duodenum are seen in less than 10% of patients.[19] The presence of active bleeding at the time of endoscopy and the size of the ulcer, rather than its anatomical site, are the main endoscopic determinants of the risk of therapeutic failure.

Management of bleeding due to causes other than peptic ulceration

Gastritis/duodenitis

Bleeding due to gastritis or duodenitis may be associated with non-steroidal anti-inflammatory drug (NSAID) therapy or ingestion of alcohol. It may also be due to *Helicobacter pylori* and can be severe enough to cause superficial erosions. Such bleeding, however, is almost always self-limiting in the absence of bleeding disorders and therapeutic intervention is not required at the time of endoscopy. Treatment with appropriate acid suppression therapy and early discharge is usually appropriate in the absence of other comorbid illness.

Mallory–Weiss syndrome

Mallory–Weiss syndrome was first described in 1929 and refers to haematemesis following repeated or violent vomiting or retching. It is caused by a linear tear of the mucosa close to the oesophagogastric junction. It accounts for approximately 5% of patients with UGI haemorrhage and most will settle without the need for therapeutic

intervention. However, if bleeding is seen at the time of endoscopy, several approaches have been described. The simplest and most readily available technique is the injection of 1:10 000 adrenaline, as for bleeding peptic ulcers, which is sufficient in the great majority of patients.[20] Mechanical methods of endostasis such as endoscopic band ligation or clip application have not been shown to be superior to adrenaline injection alone but are appropriate alternatives, particularly when major bleeding or shock has occurred or where adrenaline injection fails to achieve endostasis.[20,21]

Oesophagitis

Gastro-oesophageal reflux disease is responsible for approximately 10% of cases of UGI haemorrhage and is rarely severe. Treatment is with oral PPI therapy.

Neoplastic disease

Major bleeding is occasionally associated with oesophageal, gastric or duodenal tumours. Gastrointestinal stromal tumours (GISTs) may present with bleeding, which can be severe in very occasional cases. Malignancies of the UGI tract commonly cause occult, chronic bleeding but major bleeding can occur and may be difficult to control endoscopically. Management will be dependent on the specific circumstances and may include endoscopic techniques such as argon plasma coagulation, angiographic embolisation or, as a last resort, surgical resection. Where possible, however, if a malignancy is suspected, non-operative methods of achieving haemostasis should be employed, allowing full staging investigations to be organised to guide appropriate management.

Dieulafoy's lesion

This rare cause of UGI bleeding is due to spontaneous rupture of a submucosal artery, usually in the stomach and often within 6 cm of the cardia. The characteristic endoscopic appearance is of a protruding vessel with no evidence of surrounding ulceration. They are commonly missed due to their small size and relatively inaccessible position. Endoscopic clip application or band ligation offers durable and definitive treatment when the lesion is identified. In a small randomised trial,[22] haemoclip application was associated with a lower rate of re-bleeding than adrenaline injection, although both achieved similar rates of initial haemostasis.

Endoscopic management of bleeding peptic ulcers

Endoscopy has a central role in the management of non-variceal UGI bleeding. It enables an early diagnosis and allows for risk stratification. Endoscopic signs or stigmata of bleeding are of prognostic value and, in patients with actively bleeding ulcers or stigmata associated with a high risk of recurrent bleeding, endoscopic therapy stops ongoing bleeding and reduces re-bleeding.[23] When compared to placebo in pooled analyses, endoscopic therapy has been shown not only to reduce recurrent bleeding, but also the need for surgery and mortality.[24,25]

Endoscopic stigmata of bleeding

Forrest et al.[26] categorised endoscopic findings of bleeding peptic ulcers into those with active bleeding, stigmata of bleeding and a clean base. A modified nomenclature has been in common use in the endoscopy literature. Laine and Peterson[27] summarised published endoscopic series of ulcer appearances in which endoscopic therapy was not used and provided crude figures in both the prevalence and rate of recurrent bleeding associated with these stigmata of bleeding. In ulcers that are actively bleeding (**Fig. 7.1**) or exhibit a non-bleeding visible vessel (NBVV; **Fig. 7.2**), endoscopic treatment should be offered. There has, however, been observer variation in the interpretation of endoscopic signs[28] and the National Institutes of Health Consensus Conference[29] defined an NBVV as 'protuberant discoloration' (Fig. 7.2). The endoscopist should search the ulcer base diligently in patients judged to have bled significantly or when there is circumstantial

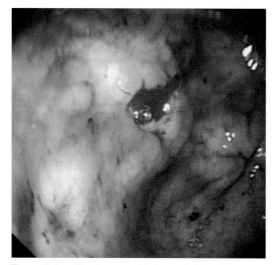

Figure 7.1 • Bleeding vessel in base of ulcer.

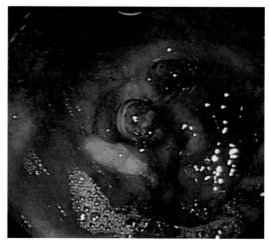

Figure 7.2 • Visible vessel.

evidence of ongoing or recent bleeding, e.g. presence of fresh blood or coffee-ground materials in the gastroduodenal tract. There has been until recently a controversy whether to wash away adherent clot overlying an ulcer (**Fig. 7.3**). Endoscopists vary in their vigour in clot irrigation before declaring a clot adherent. There have been several randomised studies and a pooled analysis has demonstrated that recurrent bleeding is reduced following clot elevation and treatment to the underlying vessel when compared to medical therapy alone.[30] Techniques for clot elevation include target irrigation using a heat probe and cheese-wiring using a snare with or without pre-injection with diluted adrenaline. One should, however, be cautious in elevation of clots overlying large deep bulbar and lesser curve ulcers as some of these may have eroded into larger arteries. A recourse to angiographic embolisation without clot elevation and possible provocation of bleeding may be a better option in sucvh cases. Ulcers with flat pigmentation and clean base (**Fig. 7.4**) are associated with minimal risk of recurrent bleeding. Stable patients with such ulcers can be discharged home early on medical treatment (Table 7.3).

✓✓ Endoscopic therapy should be applied where there is active bleeding or a non-bleeding visible vessel in the ulcer base.[23] Adherent clot should be removed and endoscopic therapy applied to the underlying vessel.[30]

Endoscopic treatment

Modalities of endoscopic treatment can be broadly categorised into: injection, thermocoagulation, haemoclipping and, recently, the use of haemostatic nano-powder.

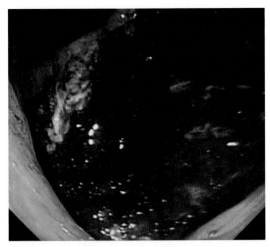

Figure 7.3 • Adherent clot.

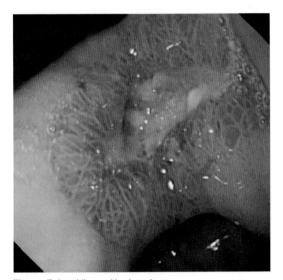

Figure 7.4 • Ulcer with clean base.

Injection

Injection therapy has been widely used because of its simplicity. Injection therapy works principally by volume tamponade. Aliquots (0.5–1 mL) are injected near the bleeding point at four quadrants using a 21- or 23-gauge injection needle. Adrenaline 1:10 000 has an added local vasoconstrictive effect. There is no role for the use of sclerosants as there have been fatal case reports of gastric necrosis following its injection and the added injection of a sclerosant such as polidocanol or sodium tetradecylsulphate after pre-injection of diluted adrenaline does not confer any advantage over injection of diluted adrenaline alone. Injection of fibrin or thrombin has been shown to be effective in some studies but repeated injections are required. These products are costly.[31,32]

Thermal methods

In a canine mesenteric artery model, contact thermocoagulation is superior to injection therapy and non-contact coagulation such as laser photocoagulation in securing haemostasis. Contact thermocoagulation using a 3.2-mm probe consistently seals arteries up to 2 mm in diameter in ex vivo models. Johnston and colleagues emphasised the need for firm mechanical tamponade before sealing of the artery with thermal energy, introducing the term 'coaptive thermocoagulation'. Mechanical compression alone stops bleeding, reduces heat-sink effect and dissipation of thermal energy. The footprint after treatment provides a clear end-point to therapy. Non-contact thermocoagulation in the form of laser photocoagulation is no longer used as a laser unit is bulky and difficult to be transported. At least in animal experiments, non-contact coagulation in the form of laser photocoagulation is not as effective as contact thermocoagulation. There has also been interest in the use of argon plasma thermocoagulation, with two randomised trials comparing this to injection sclerotherapy or heat-probe treatment, respectively.[33] Neither demonstrated any significant difference in treatment outcome.

Table 7.3 • Prevalence and outcomes of ulcers based on endoscopic appearance

Endoscopic signs	Prevalence (%)	Further bleeding (%)	Surgery (%)	Death (%)
Clean base	42	5	0.5	2
Flat spot	20	10	6	3
Adherent clot	17	22	10	7
Non-bleeding visible vessel	17	43	34	11
Active bleeding	18	55	35	11

Data from Laine L, Peterson WL. Bleeding peptic ulcer. N Engl J Med 1994; 331 (11):717–27.

Mechanical methods

Haemoclips are commonly used. Their application may be difficult in awkwardly placed ulcers such as those on the lesser curvature of the stomach and the posterior bulbar duodenum. In a meta-analysis of 15 studies with 390 patients[34] that compared haemoclipping versus injection and thermocoagulation, successful application of haemoclips (81.5%) was superior to injection alone (75.4%) but comparable to thermocoagulation (81.2%) in producing definitive haemostasis. In this pooled analysis, haemoclipping also led to a reduced need for surgery when compared to injection alone.

Hemospray®

Recently the endoscopic use of a haemostatic nanopowder was reported in a small series of 20 patients with actively bleeding peptic ulcers.[35] The powder was approved in the United States for external use in traumatic injuries. During endoscopy, the tip of a catheter is placed 1–2 cm from the ulcer. With the push of a button, the powder is then sprayed onto the bleeding ulcer with a pressurised canister with carbon dioxide. It was successful in the control of bleeding in 19 of 20 patients. Comparative studies are required to determine the efficacy of this haemostatic powder. The simplicity of its application certainly appeals to endoscopists.

Single versus combined methods

Soehendra introduced the concept of combination treatment that involved pre-injection with adrenaline allowing a clear view of the vessel, which then allowed targeted therapy using a second modality to induce thrombosis. In a meta-analysis of 16 studies and 1673 patients,[36] adding a second modality after adrenaline injection further reduces bleeding from 18.4% to 10.6% (odds ratio (OR) 0.53, 95% CI 0.4–0.69), emergency surgery from 11.3% to 7.6% (OR 0.64, 95% CI 0.46–0.90) and mortality from 5.1% to 2.6% (OR 0.51, 95% CI 0.31–0.84). In an independent meta-analysis of 22 studies (2472 patients),[37] dual therapy was shown to be superior to injection alone. However, treatment outcomes following combination treatments were not better than either mechanical or thermal therapy alone. Based on the above pooled analyses, adrenaline alone should no longer be considered an adequate treatment for bleeding peptic ulcers. The current evidence suggests that after initial adrenaline injection to stop bleeding, the vessel should either be clipped or thermocoagulated. In ulcers with a clear view to the vessel, direct clipping or thermocoagulation should yield similar results.

✔✔ Endoscopic therapy for bleeding peptic ulcers should use dual therapy or mechanical therapy rather than adrenaline injection alone in order to reduce the risk of re-bleeding.[36,37]

Limit of endoscopic therapy

As mentioned previously, the size of the bleeding artery is a critical determinant in the success of endoscopic treatment. In an ex vivo model, a vessel size of 2 mm could be consistently sealed by a 3.2-mm contact thermal device. In clinical studies that examined factors that might predict failure of endoscopic treatment, ulcer size greater than 2 cm, ulcers on the lesser curvature and ulcers on the superior or posterior wall of bulbar duodenum were consistently identified as major risk factors for recurrent bleeding.[23] These ulcers erode into large artery complexes such as the left gastric and the gastroduodenal artery, which are usually sizeable. Consideration should therefore be given to prophylactic measures against recurrent bleeding in these ulcers judged endoscopically to be at significant risk of re-bleeding.

Second-look endoscopy

Many endoscopists re-scope their patients the next morning and re-treat ulcers with remaining stigmata of bleeding. In a pooled analysis on the role of second-look endoscopy,[38] the authors found a modest 6.2% reduction in the absolute risk of re-bleeding (number needed to treat (NNT) to reduce one episode of recurrent bleeding). The NNT for reduction of surgery and surgery was 58 and 97, respectively. A subsequent meta-analysis and a third meta-analysis carried out for an international consensus conference confirmed that routine second-look endoscopy did reduce the incidence of re-bleeding. The findings were strongest in studies including a high proportion of high-risk ulcers. However, in many of these trials, adrenaline injection alone was used. The role of second-look endoscopy following dual therapy or mechanical therapy remains unclear. In addition, adjuvant treatment with PPI therapy following endoscopic haemostasis can be expected to reduce the benefit of second-look endoscopy even further. With aggressive first endoscopic treatment, the risk of complications, especially perforation, with second treatment is substantial. There may, however, be a role for second-look endoscopy in selected high-risk patients, although this would require further studies and the most recent international consensus guidelines did not recommend this approach on the basis of the available evidence.[23]

✔✔ Second-look endoscopy is not indicated as a routine if primary optimum endoscopic haemostasis has been performed.[23]

Pharmacological management of bleeding peptic ulcers

Acid suppression

It has been shown in an in vitro study that platelet aggregation is dependent on plasma pH. It is thought that a pH of 6 is critical for clot stability and an intragastric pH above 4 inactivates stomach pepsin, preventing the digestion of clots.[13] To raise intragastric pH consistently above 6, a high-dose PPI given intravenously is required. The antisecretory effect of histamine receptor antagonists, due to tolerance, is less reliable than PPIs. In a study from the Hong Kong group,[39] a 3-day course of high-dose omeprazole infusion given after endoscopic therapy to bleeding ulcers reduced the rate of recurrent bleeding from 22.5% to 6.7% at day 30. The majority of recurrent bleeding occurred within the first 3 days of endoscopic treatment. This trial demonstrated the importance of early endoscopic triage, selecting only the high-risk ulcers for aggressive endoscopic treatment followed by profound acid suppression. In a Cochrane systematic review of 24 controlled trials and 4373 patients,[40] PPI treatment was shown to reduce re-bleeding (pooled rate of 10.6% vs. 17.3%, OR 0.49, 95% CI 0.37–0.65) as well as surgery (pooled rate of 6.1% vs. 9.3%, OR 0.61, 95% CI 0.48–0.78) when compared with placebo or histamine-2 receptor antagonist. There was no evidence of an effect on all-cause mortality, although when the analysis was confined to patients with high-risk stigmata (active bleeding or visible vessels) there was an associated reduction in mortality with PPI therapy. A multicentre study randomised 767 patients from 91 hospitals in 16 countries to intravenous esomeprazole or placebo following successful endoscopic haemostasis.[41] Esomeprazole was associated with significant reductions in re-bleeding and endoscopic re-intervention rates and non-significant reductions in mortality and the need for surgery.

✔✔ High-dose intravenous PPI therapy (80 mg omeprazole followed by 8 mg/h for 72 h) is recommended for patients with active bleeding or visible vessels at the time of endoscopy.[40]

Surgical management of bleeding peptic ulcers

The first UK audit revealed a mortality of 24% in those patients (251 of 2071, 12%) who required surgery for bleeding peptic ulcers.[1] However, in 78% of these patients, no previous attempt at endoscopic haemostasis had been made. In the most recent UK audit,[3] surgery was required in only 1.9% of patients but mortality remained high in this group (30%). The high mortality is probably related to an aged population, with the mean age at 68, and the high incidence of comorbidity. In some patients with severe comorbid illnesses and bleeding peptic ulcer, gastrointestinal haemorrhage is an agonal event. Bleeding ulcers that fail endostasis are typically 'difficult' ulcers – larger chronic ulcers that erode into major arterial complexes. The decline in elective ulcer surgery also means the atrophy of surgical techniques in dealing with these ulcers. Ideally, a specialist team with an experienced upper gastrointestinal surgeon should be involved in managing these patients.

Although emergency ulcer surgery has diminished significantly, it has an important gatekeeping role in the management algorithm. The clear indication for surgery is loosely defined as 'failure of endoscopic treatment'. In a patient with massive bleeding that cannot be controlled by endoscopy, immediate surgery should obviously follow. Similarly, in a patient with bleeding controlled at endoscopy, most clinicians would adopt a non-operative approach. However, the difficulty lies in deciding the exact role of surgery in ulcers judged to have a high risk of recurrent bleeding (e.g. >2 cm and at difficult locations), in whom endoscopic haemostasis has been initially successful. Increasingly, angiographic embolisation is replacing emergency surgery in these circumstances.

Choice of surgical procedure for bleeding peptic ulcers

The choice of surgical procedure for bleeding peptic ulcers, when required, has not been adequately examined in the era following routine eradication of *Helicobacter pylori* and high-dose PPI therapy. Many surgeons maintain that under-running of ulcers alone combined with acid suppression using high-dose PPI therapy is safer than definitive surgery by either gastric resection or vagotomy. Two randomised studies looking at the different surgical procedures used to control bleeding peptic ulcers have been reported,[42,43] but both predate the PPI and routine *H. pylori* eradication era and therefore their results must be interpreted with considerable caution. One of these was a multicentre study comparing minimal surgery (under-running the vessel or ulcer excision alone plus intravenous histamine receptor antagonist) versus definitive ulcer surgery (vagotomy and pyloroplasty or partial gastrectomy) in patients with gastric and duodenal ulcers.[42] The trial was terminated, however, because of the high rate of fatal re-bleeding in the minimal surgery group (6 of 62 vs. 0 of 67, P = 0.02).

The other trial was carried out by the French Association of Surgical Research and included only bleeding duodenal ulcers.[43] The patients in this trial were randomly assigned to either under-running plus vagotomy and drainage (58 patients) or partial gastrectomy (60 patients). Recurrent bleeding occurred in 10 of 58 patients (17%) after under-running and vagotomy. In the group assigned to partial gastrectomy, only two patients (3%) re-bled and both recovered without the need for further surgery. The rate of duodenal stump leak in the gastrectomy group was 8 in 60 (13%). When the results were analysed on an intention-to-treat basis, and those with duodenal leaks after re-operations for re-bleeding in the under-running and vagotomy group were included, duodenal leak rate was similar in both groups (7/58 vs. 8/60). The mortality in both groups was similar (22% after vagotomy and 23% after gastrectomy). In the era of PPI therapy, the role of vagotomy has disappeared. A proper ligation of the gastroduodenal artery complex including the right gastroepiploic and the transverse pancreatic branches is the key to avoid recurrent bleeding.

In a survey of UK surgeons reported in 2003, more than 80% of respondents rarely or never perform vagotomy for bleeding peptic ulcer.[44] Despite the absence of recent randomised evidence, surgeons have clearly adopted a more conservative approach based on the efficiency of PPI treatment and *H. pylori* eradication in the healing of peptic ulceration. With improvements in endoscopic therapy and the increasing age and comorbidity of patients, the risks of definitive ulcer surgery may outweigh any potential benefit from reduction in re-bleeding. For duodenal ulcer haemorrhage, longitudinal duodenotomy is carried out and control of bleeding achieved by digital pressure or by grasping the posterior duodenal wall in tissue forceps. If possible, preservation of the pylorus is preferred, but extension of the duodenotomy to include the pylorus may be required if access is difficult. Control of bleeding may be aided by mobilisation of the duodenum (Kocher's manoeuvre), allowing pressure to be applied posteriorly. In the majority of patients, simple under-running of the bleeding vessel can be achieved using 0 or 1/0 absorbable sutures above and below the bleeding point, ensuring deep enough tissue penetration to completely occlude the vessel. Due to the variation in anatomy of the gastroduodenal artery (**Fig. 7.5**), four or five sutures should be placed to ensure enduring haemostasis. The duodenotomy can then be closed longitudinally or converted into a formal pyloroplasty if the pylorus has been divided.

In cases of a massive duodenal ulcer, it may be necessary to exclude the ulcer, perform a distal gastrectomy and close the distal duodenum. This can be a challenging procedure in an elderly, unstable patient, particularly where duodenal thickening and scarring prevent safe stump closure. In this situation it may be better to anticipate a controlled duodenal

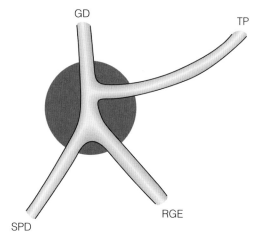

Figure 7.5 • The anatomy of the gastroduodenal (GD) artery complex with confluence of several branches into the artery itself. RGE, right gastroepiploic artery; SPD, superior pancreatico-duodenal artery; TP, transverse pancreatic. Reproduced from Berne CJ, Rosoff L. Peptic ulcer perforation of the gastroduodenal artery complex: clinical features and operative control. Ann Surg 1969; 169:141–4. With permission from Lippincott, Williams & Wilkins.

fistula by closing the duodenal stump around a Foley catheter rather than attempting more complex closures, such as with the Billroth I reconstruction.

In the case of surgery for a bleeding gastric ulcer, the common scenario is for the ulcer to be located high on the lesser curve of stomach. Anterior gastrotomy, identification of the bleeding site and simple under-running of the ulcer (with biopsy of the ulcer edge) is the procedure of choice, and is also suitable for rare cases of Mallory–Weiss tear or a Dieulafoy lesion that does not respond to endoscopic management. In the rare case of a distal gastric ulcer that does not respond to endoscopic therapy, there may occasionally be a case for ulcer excision or even distal gastrectomy, but it is difficult to justify such a course of action in the hands of a non-specialist surgeon, and simple under-running should be the aim in the majority of patients.

✔ The choice of operation in patients with bleeding peptic ulcers who have failed endoscopic treatment should involve, where possible, simple under-running of the bleeding ulcer, without either vagotomy or gastric resection. Biopsies should be taken from the edge of a gastric ulcer.

Management of recurrent bleeding

The decision on management of patients who re-bleed after initial endoscopic control can be difficult. In a randomised study that compared endoscopic re-treatment to surgery in such patients,[45] endoscopic re-treatment secured bleeding again in 75% of patients. With intention-to-treat analysis, complications following endoscopic re-treatment were significantly less when compared to those who received surgery. The gastrectomy rate in the surgery group was 50%. In a subgroup analysis, those re-bleeding with hypotensive shock from ulcers greater than 2 cm were less likely to respond to a repeat endoscopic treatment. It is therefore suggested that a selective approach can be used in re-bleeding patients. Patients with smaller ulcers and subtle signs of re-bleeding should be re-endoscoped and therapy repeated, often with successful outcome. If not successful, surgery should obviously follow. It remains probable that patients with large chronic ulcers and in shock are better treated by expeditious surgery without recourse to endoscopic re-treatment. Some of these patients may benefit from early 'elective/pre-emptive' surgery or (increasingly) angiographic embolisation.

> ✅ Management of re-bleeding following successful endostasis will depend on the specific circumstances. Further endoscopic haemostasis may be appropriate for many patients,[46] but high-risk ulcers, particularly those where good endostasis was difficult to achieve at the first procedure, may be better considered for surgery or even transarterial angiographic embolisation.

The role of selective mesenteric embolisation

Transarterial angiographic embolisation (TAE) is an alternative rescue procedure for bleeding duodenal ulcers and the technique has been in use for over two decades. In the 1980s, there were reports of visceral infarcts[46,47] following TAE, and its use was restricted to a small group of patients with refractory bleeding considered unfit for surgical intervention. With advances in embolisation techniques and specifically the use of superselective coiling (**Fig. 7.6**), the success rate in the control of bleeding has been reported to be between 64% and 91%, and mortality between 5% and 25%. There have since been two retrospective comparative studies comparing angio-embolisation with surgery,[48,49] involving a total of 179 patients of whom 72 had TAE and 107 underwent surgery. In the Hong Kong series,[48] re-bleeding was higher after TAE compared with surgery but complications were higher in the surgical group and overall mortality was similar at 25% for TAE and 30% for surgery. The Swedish study[49] had a lower mortality in both groups (3% and 14% for TAE and surgery, respectively), perhaps reflecting different selection criteria, but again there were no significant differences between the TAE and surgical groups. In the latter comparative study, the lack of outcome difference and the more advanced age in the TAE group suggest that TAE may be at least as good an option as surgery in the management of refractory ulcer bleeding. TAE is certainly now the procedure of choice in the small group of patients who re-bleed after surgery, but a randomised controlled study comparing surgery and TAE in this group of patients would be of great interest. Similarly, the role of semi-elective TAE following successful endostasis in patients considered at high risk of re-bleeding or death has not been studied, but is another area where further research may be interesting.

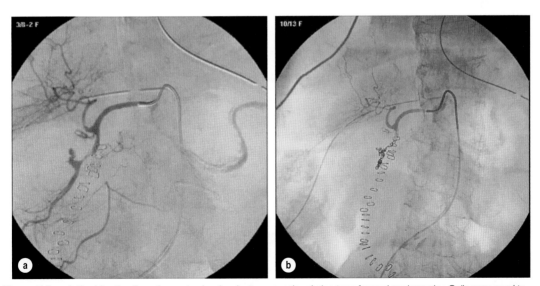

Figure 7.6 • Active bleeding from the gastroduodenal artery complex during transfemoral angiography. Coils were used to embolise the artery leading to cessation of bleeding.

✅ Transarterial embolisation should be considered in patients who re-bleed following surgery for bleeding peptic ulcers and as an alternative to surgery when endoscopic haemostasis has failed, provided appropriate facilities and expertise are available. This may be particularly useful in elderly patients with medical comorbidity. TAE should also be considered as a possible pre-emptive treatment option in high-risk surgical patients who are at high risk of re-bleeding after endostasis.

Helicobacter pylori eradication

A Cochrane review[50] concluded that *H. pylori* eradication was associated with a significant reduction in the risk of re-bleeding compared with no *H. pylori* eradication, from 20% to 2.9%. If antisecretory therapy was continued, the risk was 5.6%, still significantly higher than achieved with *H. pylori* eradication. The overall risk of re-bleeding following *H. pylori* eradication was less than 1% per year. It is therefore of concern that in a UK review of consultant behaviour, fewer than 60% routinely tested patients for *H. pylori* following treatment for complicated peptic ulcers.[44]

✅✅ Following treatment for bleeding duodenal ulcer, patients should be tested for *H. pylori* and receive eradication therapy where appropriate. Patients should have further testing to ensure successful eradication.[50]

Use of NSAIDs

In patients who continue to require NSAIDs, co-therapy with PPI reduces recurrence in peptic ulcers and bleeding. In these patients, H. pylori should first be tested and treated if confirmed. A randomized controlled trial compared the use of a traditional NSAID plus a PPI to COX-2 inhibitors and found that the rate of further ulcer complications is between 4-6% in 6 months.[51] A subsequent randomized trial combined the use of COX-2 inhibitor to PPI and compared them to the use of a COX-2 inhibitor alone.[52] At 1 year, the use of COX-2 inhibitor alone was associated with a rate of 8.9% in recurrent bleeding. The risk of recurrent bleeding was completely abolished in those who the combined treatment. COX-2 inhibitor plus PPI appears to offer the best protection to these high risk patients.

Summary

The challenge posed by peptic ulcer bleeding has altered with the increasing age of the population at risk and the increasing availability of skilled therapeutic endoscopy. Failure of endoscopic haemostasis is increasingly uncommon but the surgical challenge presented by the elderly patient with refractory bleeding from a large ulcer is considerable. Successful management of UGI bleeding will involve the close cooperation of a multidisciplinary team, which will increasingly include interventional radiologists, aided by local protocols based on evidence-based best practice (**Fig. 7.7**).

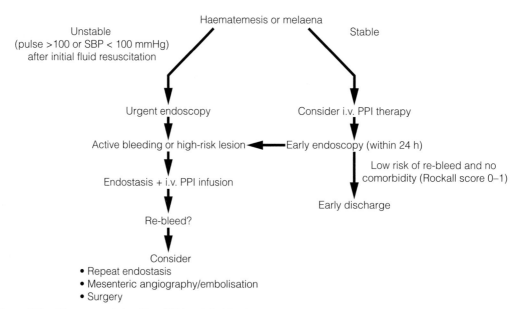

Figure 7.7 • Management algorithm. SBP, systolic blood pressure.

Key points

- A full Rockall score should be calculated for all patients with UGI bleeding following initial endoscopic assessment.
- Pre-endoscopy treatment with PPIs is recommended as it reduces the risk of active bleeding at the time of endoscopy and may reduce the need for endoscopic intervention.
- Early endoscopy should be performed on all patients with UGI bleeding/haemorrhage.
- Endoscopic therapy should be applied where there is active bleeding or a non-bleeding visible vessel in the ulcer base. Adherent clot should be removed and endoscopic therapy applied to the underlying vessel.
- Endoscopic therapy for bleeding peptic ulcers should involve use of dual therapy or mechanical therapy rather than adrenaline injection alone in order to reduce the risk of re-bleeding.
- High-dose intravenous PPI therapy (80 mg omeprazole followed by 8 mg/h for 72 h) is recommended for patients with active bleeding or visible vessels at the time of endoscopy.
- The choice of operation in patients with bleeding peptic ulcers who have failed endoscopic treatment should involve, where possible, simple under-running of the bleeding ulcer, without either vagotomy or gastric resection.
- Management of re-bleeding following successful endoscopic haemostasis will depend on the specific circumstances. Further endoscopic haemostasis may be appropriate for many patients but those with high-risk ulcers, particularly where good endostasis was difficult to achieve at the first procedure, may be better considered for surgery or transarterial angiographic embolisation.
- Following treatment for bleeding duodenal ulcer, patients should be tested for *H. pylori* and receive eradication therapy where appropriate. Patients should have further testing to ensure successful eradication.

References

1. Rockall TA, Logan RF, Devlin HB, et al. Incidence of and mortality from acute upper gastrointestinal haemorrhage in the United Kingdom. Steering Committee and members of the National Audit of Acute Upper Gastrointestinal Haemorrhage. Br Med J 1995;311(6999):222–6.

2. Blatchford O, Davidson LA, Murray WR, et al. Acute upper gastrointestinal haemorrhage in west of Scotland: case ascertainment study. Br Med J 1997;315(7107):510–4.

3. Hearnshaw SA, Logan RF, Lowe D, et al. Acute upper gastrointestinal bleeding in the UK: patient characteristics, diagnoses and outcomes in the 2007 UK audit. Gut 2011;60(10):1327–35.

4. Wilcox CM, Alexander LN, Cotsonis G. A prospective characterization of upper gastrointestinal hemorrhage presenting with hematochezia. Am J Gastroenterol 1997;92(2):231–5.

5. Rockall TA, Logan RF, Devlin HB, et al. Variation in outcome after acute upper gastrointestinal haemorrhage. The National Audit of Acute Upper Gastrointestinal Haemorrhage. Lancet 1995;346(8971):346–50.

6. Pang SH, Ching JY, Lau JY, et al. Comparing the Blatchford and pre-endoscopic Rockall score in predicting the need for endoscopic therapy in patients with upper GI hemorrhage. Gastrointest Endosc 2010;71(7):1134–40.

7. Stanley AJ, Dalton HR, Blatchford O, et al. Multicentre comparison of the Glasgow Blatchford and Rockall Scores in the prediction of clinical endpoints after upper gastrointestinal haemorrhage. Aliment Pharmacol Ther 2011;34(4):470–5.

8. Vreeburg EM, Terwee CB, Snel P, et al. Validation of the Rockall risk scoring system in upper gastrointestinal bleeding. Gut 1999;44(3):331–5.

9. Sanders DS, Carter MJ, Goodchap RJ, et al. Prospective validation of the Rockall risk scoring system for upper GI hemorrhage in subgroups of patients with varices and peptic ulcers. Am J Gastroenterol 2002;97(3):630–5.

10. Sanders DS, Perry MJ, Jones SG, et al. Effectiveness of an upper-gastrointestinal haemorrhage unit: a prospective analysis of 900 consecutive cases using the Rockall score as a method of risk standardisation. Eur J Gastroenterol Hepatol 2004;16(5):487–94.

11. Stainsby D, MacLennan S, Thomas D, et al. Guidelines on the management of massive blood loss. Br J Haematol 2006;135(5):634–41.

12. Perel P, Roberts I. Colloids versus crystalloids for fluid resuscitation in critically ill patients. Cochrane Database Syst Rev 2007;(4)CD000567.

13. Green Jr FW, Kaplan MM, Curtis LE, et al. Effect of acid and pepsin on blood coagulation and platelet aggregation. A possible contributor prolonged gastroduodenal mucosal hemorrhage. Gastroenterology 1978;74(1):38–43.

14. Sreedharan A, Martin J, Leontiadis GI, et al. Proton pump inhibitor treatment initiated prior to endoscopic diagnosis in upper gastrointestinal bleeding. Cochrane Database Syst Rev 2010;(7) CD005415.
   This systematic review of randomised trials found no effect of pre-endoscopy PPI therapy on mortality but there was a significant reduction in active bleeding and the need for intervention at the time of endoscopy.

15. Lau JY, Leung WK, Wu JC, et al. Omeprazole before endoscopy in patients with gastrointestinal bleeding. N Engl J Med 2007;356(16):1631–40.

16. Tsoi KK, Lau JY, Sung JJ. Cost-effectiveness analysis of high-dose omeprazole infusion before endoscopy for patients with upper-GI bleeding. Gastrointest Endosc 2008;67(7):1056–63.

17. Lai KC, Hui WM, Wong BC, et al. A retrospective and prospective study on the safety of discharging selected patients with duodenal ulcer bleeding on the same day as endoscopy. Gastrointest Endosc 1997;45(1):26–30.

18. Spiegel BM, Vakil NB, Ofman JJ. Endoscopy for acute nonvariceal upper gastrointestinal tract hemorrhage: is sooner better? A systematic review. Arch Intern Med 2001;161(11):1393–404.
   This systematic review of 23 studies concluded that early endoscopy improved outcome in patients with UGI bleeding in all risk categories.

19. Wong SK, Yu LM, Lau JY, et al. Prediction of therapeutic failure after adrenaline injection plus heater probe treatment in patients with bleeding peptic ulcer. Gut 2002;50(3):322–5.

20. Park CH, Min SW, Sohn YH, et al. A prospective, randomized trial of endoscopic band ligation vs. epinephrine injection for actively bleeding Mallory–Weiss syndrome. Gastrointest Endosc 2004;60(1):22–7.

21. Huang SP, Wang HP, Lee YC, et al. Endoscopic hemoclip placement and epinephrine injection for Mallory–Weiss syndrome with active bleeding. Gastrointest Endosc 2002;55(7):842–6.

22. Park CH, Sohn YH, Lee WS, et al. The usefulness of endoscopic hemoclipping for bleeding Dieulafoy lesions. Endoscopy 2003;35(5):388–92.

23. Barkun AN, Bardou M, Kuipers EJ, et al. International consensus recommendations on the management of patients with nonvariceal upper gastrointestinal bleeding. Ann Intern Med 2010;152(2):101–13.
   These are the most recently published comprehensive guidelines on the management of UGI bleeding based on studies published to date and include data from published and new meta-analyses as well as expert opinion.

24. Cook DJ, Guyatt GH, Salena BJ, et al. Endoscopic therapy for acute nonvariceal upper gastrointestinal hemorrhage: a meta-analysis. Gastroenterology 1992;102(1):139–48.

25. Sacks HS, Chalmers TC, Blum AL, et al. Endoscopic hemostasis. An effective therapy for bleeding peptic ulcers. JAMA 1990;264(4):494–9.

26. Forrest JA, Finlayson ND, Shearman DJ. Endoscopy in gastrointestinal bleeding. Lancet 1974;2(7877):394–7.

27. Laine L, Peterson WL. Bleeding peptic ulcer. N Engl J Med 1994;331(11):717–27.

28. Laine L, Freeman M, Cohen H. Lack of uniformity in evaluation of endoscopic prognostic features of bleeding ulcers. Gastrointest Endosc 1994;40(4):411–7.

29. Consensus Conference. Therapeutic endoscopy and bleeding ulcers. JAMA 1989;262(10):1369–72.

30. Kahi CJ, Jensen DM, Sung JJ, et al. Endoscopic therapy versus medical therapy for bleeding peptic ulcer with adherent clot: a meta-analysis. Gastroenterology 2005;129(3):855–62.
   A pooled analysis of several randomised studies demonstrated that recurrent bleeding is reduced following clot elevation and treatment to the underlying vessel when compared to medical therapy alone.

31. Kubba AK, Murphy W, Palmer KR. Endoscopic injection for bleeding peptic ulcer: a comparison of adrenaline alone with adrenaline plus human thrombin. Gastroenterology 1996;111(3):623–8.

32. Rutgeerts P, Rauws E, Wara P, et al. Randomised trial of single and repeated fibrin glue compared with injection of polidocanol in treatment of bleeding peptic ulcer. Lancet 1997;350(9079):692–6.

33. Havanond C, Havanond P. Argon plasma coagulation therapy for acute non-variceal upper gastrointestinal bleeding. Cochrane Database Syst Rev 2005;(2)CD003791.

34. Sung JJ, Tsoi KK, Lai LH, et al. Endoscopic clipping versus injection and thermo-coagulation in the treatment of non-variceal upper gastrointestinal bleeding: a meta-analysis. Gut 2007;56(10):1364–73.

35. Sung JJ, Luo D, Wu JC, et al. Early clinical experience of the safety and effectiveness of Hemospray in achieving hemostasis in patients with acute peptic ulcer bleeding. Endoscopy 2011;43(4):291–5.

36. Calvet X, Vergara M, Brullet E, et al. Addition of a second endoscopic treatment following epinephrine injection improves outcome in high-risk bleeding ulcers. Gastroenterology 2004;126(2):441–50.

37. Marmo R, Rotondano G, Piscopo R, et al. Dual therapy versus monotherapy in the endoscopic treatment of high-risk bleeding ulcers: a meta-analysis of controlled trials. Am J Gastroenterol 2007;102(2):279–89; quiz 469.
   These two meta-analyses provide compelling evidence that addition of a second endoscopic therapy is better than adrenaline alone.

38. Marmo R, Rotondano G, Bianco MA, et al. Outcome of endoscopic treatment for peptic ulcer bleeding: Is a second look necessary? A meta-analysis. Gastrointest Endosc 2003;57(1):62–7.

39. Lau JY, Sung JJ, Lee KK, et al. Effect of intravenous omeprazole on recurrent bleeding after endoscopic treatment of bleeding peptic ulcers. N Engl J Med 2000;343(5):310–6.

40. Leontiadis GI, Sharma VK, Howden CW. Proton pump inhibitor treatment for acute peptic ulcer bleeding. Cochrane Database Syst Rev 2006;(1): CD002094.
    This Cochrane review of randomised trials found that high-dose PPI therapy reduced re-bleeding, surgery and mortality rates following endotherapy for high-risk ulcers.

41. Sung JJ, Barkun A, Kuipers EJ, et al. Intravenous esomeprazole for prevention of recurrent peptic ulcer bleeding: a randomized trial. Ann Intern Med 2009;150(7):455–64.

42. Poxon VA, Keighley MR, Dykes PW, et al. Comparison of minimal and conventional surgery in patients with bleeding peptic ulcer: a multicentre trial. Br J Surg 1991;78(11):1344–5.

43. Millat B, Hay JM, Valleur P, et al. Emergency surgical treatment for bleeding duodenal ulcer: oversewing plus vagotomy versus gastric resection, a controlled randomized trial. French Associations for Surgical Research. World J Surg 1993;17(5):568–74.

44. Gilliam AD, Speake WJ, Lobo DN, et al. Current practice of emergency vagotomy and *Helicobacter pylori* eradication for complicated peptic ulcer in the United Kingdom. Br J Surg 2003;90(1):88–90.

45. Lau JY, Sung JJ, Lam YH, et al. Endoscopic retreatment compared with surgery in patients with recurrent bleeding after initial endoscopic control of bleeding ulcers. N Engl J Med 1999;340(10):751–6.

46. Shapiro N, Brandt L, Sprayregan S, et al. Duodenal infarction after therapeutic Gelfoam embolization of a bleeding duodenal ulcer. Gastroenterology 1981;80(1):176–80.

47. Trojanowski JQ, Harrist TJ, Athanasoulis CA, et al. Hepatic and splenic infarctions: complications of therapeutic transcatheter embolization. Am J Surg 1980;139(2):272–7.

48. Wong TC, Wong KT, Chiu PW, et al. A comparison of angiographic embolization with surgery after failed endoscopic hemostasis to bleeding peptic ulcers. Gastrointest Endosc 2011;73(5):900–8.

49. Eriksson LG, Ljungdahl M, Sundbom M, et al. Transcatheter arterial embolization versus surgery in the treatment of upper gastrointestinal bleeding after therapeutic endoscopy failure. J Vasc Interv Radiol 2008;19(10):1413–8.

50. Gisbert JP, Khorrami S, Carballo F, et al. Meta-analysis: *Helicobacter pylori* eradication therapy vs. antisecretory non-eradication therapy for the prevention of recurrent bleeding from peptic ulcer. Aliment Pharmacol Ther 2004;19(6):617–29.
    This Cochrane review included seven studies and a reduction in re-bleeding rates following *H. pylori* eradication compared with antisecretory therapy and no eradication.

51. Chan FK, Hung LC, Suen BY, Wu JC, Lee KC, Leung VK, et al. Celecoxib versus diclofenac and omeprazole in reducing the risk of recurrent ulcer bleeding in patients with arthritis. N Engl J Med 2002;347(2)104–10.

52. Chan FK, Wong VW, Suen BY, Wu JC, Ching JY, Hung LC, et al. Combination of a cyclo-oxygenase-2 inhibitor and a proton-pump inhibitor for prevention of recurrent ulcer bleeding in patients at very high risk: a double-blind, randomised trial. Lancet 2007;369(1)621–6.

Pancreaticobiliary emergencies

Mark Duxbury

Introduction

The clinical benefits of subspecialisation in pancreaticobiliary surgery are now widely accepted and are supported by a considerable body of evidence.[1] However, the nature of surgical service provision often demands that pancreaticobiliary emergencies be treated by surgeons with principal specialist interests lying outside upper gastrointestinal surgery. The aim of this chapter is to provide an overview of current evidence relating to the treatment of the more commonly encountered pancreaticobiliary emergencies, including the management of acute cholecystitis, acute cholangitis, acute pancreatitis, and pancreaticobiliary disease in pregnancy, for the emergency general surgeon.

Biliary colic and acute cholecystitis

The majority of acute gallbladder disorders are due to gallstones and have a range of clinical presentations.

Pathogenesis

In the emergency setting, biliary colic or acute cholecystitis are the most common presentations of symptomatic cholelithiasis and it is often difficult at the initial assessment to distinguish between the two conditions as they form part of a continuum. Biliary colic is thought to occur following the impaction of a gallstone within the cystic duct or gallbladder infundibulum, leading to gallbladder obstruction. In a functioning gallbladder, obstruction results in marked gallbladder contraction with the perception of pain. Following disimpaction of the stone, the pain subsides. Disimpacted gallstones may either fall back into the gallbladder or pass into the common bile duct (CBD).

Persistent gallbladder obstruction leads to acute mural inflammation, although there is often a poor correlation between the clinical presentation and the histopathological features of acute and chronic inflammation in the gallbladder wall. Initially, in acute cholecystitis, the inflammatory process within the gallbladder is sterile; however, bacterial colonisation of the obstructed bile and inflamed tissue occurs and may result in an empyema of the gallbladder. Further, if the inflammatory process is particularly severe, gallbladder ischaemia and necrosis can occur, with the risk of gallbladder perforation and subsequent biliary peritonitis.

Clinical presentation

Biliary colic presents with severe upper abdominal pain in the epigastric and right upper quadrant regions, commonly with radiation to the back or shoulders. Although termed 'colic', the pain is usually constant when present, but remits after a period of minutes to hours. Pain may be provoked by eating, and the patients frequently describe an association with ingestion of fatty foods. A history of previous similar episodes may be obtained. Palpation of the abdomen may reveal epigastric/right upper quadrant tenderness but no evidence of peritoneal irritation. Blood investigations are usually normal.

In acute cholecystitis the pain is localised to the right upper quadrant, and also may radiate to the back or right shoulder tip. Because of peritoneal irritation the pain is exacerbated by movement and breathing. Commonly, the patient is nauseated and may have vomited. Systemic signs of inflammation including tachycardia and pyrexia may be present and abdominal examination will typically reveal right upper quadrant tenderness with signs of localised peritonitis. Classically, Murphy's sign (acute tenderness during palpation below the tip of the right ninth rib elicited on inspiration) can be observed in patients with acute cholecystitis. A tender gallbladder may occasionally be palpable in the right upper quadrant, particularly in the presence of an empyema. Haematological investigations typically demonstrate a leucocytosis and liver function tests (LFTs) may be mildly deranged. An obstructive picture to the LFTs may be a consequence of choledocholithiasis, but may also be a consequence of impacted gallstones in Hartmann's pouch pressing on or eroding into the common hepatic duct (Mirizzi syndrome) or contiguous inflammation affecting the biliary tree or adjacent hepatic parenchyma.

Initial radiological imaging

Transabdominal ultrasound is the initial investigation of choice in both biliary colic and acute cholecystitis and has a sensitivity of greater than 95% for detecting gallstones (see also Chapter 5). In addition, ultrasound (US) can demonstrate signs of acute inflammation such as gallbladder wall thickening, pericholecystic fluid and a positive sonographic Murphy's sign (**Fig. 8.1**). US may also demonstrate gas in the gallbladder wall in patients with emphysematous cholecystitis. Newer techniques of colour velocity imaging and power Doppler ultrasound can provide additional information, and may therefore be helpful in distinguishing patients with true acute cholecystitis from those with upper abdominal pain and incidental cholelithiasis. In addition, transabdominal ultrasound can detect the presence of biliary tree dilatation, which may indicate choledocholithiasis, although the sensitivity for choledocholithiasis may be significantly impaired by obesity or gas within overlying bowel. In patients where US is equivocal either computed tomography (CT) or magnetic resonance imaging (MRI) can be helpful (Fig. 8.1).

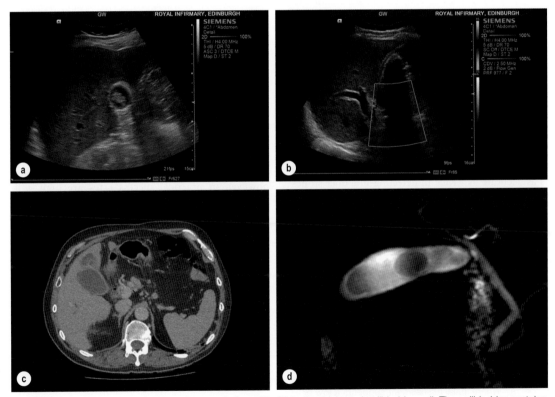

Figure 8.1 • (a) Ultrasound features of acute cholecystitis. Note the thickened gallbladder wall. The gallbladder contains stone and debris. This patient was also tender on pressing the transducer on to the gallbladder (sonographic Murphy's sign). **(b)** Addition of colour Doppler to help identify associated anatomy. **(c)** Axial CT image demonstrates cholecystitis with gallbladder wall thickening and adjacent parenchymal inflammatory changes in the liver. **(d)** Coronal MRCP reconstruction with a single calculus in the gallbladder and normal biliary tree.

Radionucleotide scintigraphy has historically been reported to have greater accuracy in diagnosing acute cholecystitis than standard US techniques. However, these techniques are time-consuming, involve the use of radiopharmaceuticals, and their use is now generally restricted to individuals who are clinically suspected of having abnormal gallbladder function in the presence of a normal ultrasound scan (gallbladder dyskinesia).

Management of patients with acute gallbladder disease and suspected bile duct stones

Concomitant choledocholithiasis may be indicated by obstructive LFTs or US evidence of biliary dilatation and/or evidence of ductal calculi. In the acute setting several additional factors may complicate the decision-making process. Most importantly, if there are signs of generalised peritonitis, operative intervention cannot be deferred and investigation for CBD calculi becomes of secondary importance. In this situation, any ductal stones can be looked for at operation. It is also important to bear in mind the clinical overlap between acute cholangitis and acute cholecystitis, and patients with cholangitis due to CBD calculi may have upper abdominal tenderness and guarding. An appropriate index of suspicion together with findings on US should result in such individuals being appropriately treated for their ductal calculi.

In the majority of patients with acute biliary colic or cholecystitis who have deranged LFTs there will be an opportunity to assess the CBD preoperatively. The management options include endoscopic retrograde cholangiopancreatography (ERCP) or magnetic resonance cholangiopancreatography (MRCP). MRCP has the advantage that it is non-invasive and is as accurate as ERCP in detecting bile duct stones (**Fig. 8.2**),[2] as well as providing valuable additional information about more complex presentations, e.g. Mirizzi syndrome (**Fig. 8.3**). Nowadays, ERCP is reserved for therapeutic intervention, e.g. sphincterotomy and stone removal or stenting, rather than for diagnosis (**Fig. 8.4**).

✓ Guidelines on the management of CBD stones published by the British Society of Gastroenterology recommend that where initial assessment, based on clinical features, liver function tests and ultrasound findings, suggests a high probability of CBD calculi, then it is reasonable to proceed directly to ERCP if this is considered the treatment of choice.[3] Where initial assessment suggests a low or uncertain index of suspicion for CBD calculi, then it is recommended that patients undergo MRCP or endoscopic ultrasound (EUS), with ERCP reserved for those with abnormal or equivocal results.

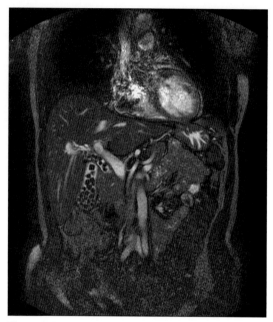

Figure 8.2 • MRCP demonstrating gallbladder stones and extensive choledocholithiasis extending into the intrahepatic biliary tree. The patient underwent laparoscopic cholecystectomy and bile duct exploration.

An alternative management strategy is to undertake intraoperative cholangiography during acute cholecystectomy (**Fig. 8.5**). If a ductal stone is demonstrated on intraoperative cholangiography, the options are to undertake laparoscopic CBD exploration, convert to an open procedure with exploration of the CBD or to perform a postoperative ERCP or, in some cases, intraoperative ERCP. The potential risk with adoption of a postoperative ERCP strategy is failure to cannulate at endoscopy; however, in practice, success rates are high with experienced endoscopists and few patients require further surgery.

✓✓ Systematic reviews of studies reporting the outcome of laparoscopic CBD exploration report morbidity rates of between 2% and 17% and mortality rates of 1–5%.[4] This is comparable to ERCP, with a Cochrane review of randomised controlled trials concluding that there was no clear difference in primary success rates, morbidity or mortality between the two approaches.[5] However, it is important to note that the majority of these studies involved elective as well as emergency patients.

Although laparoscopic CBD exploration is a logical extension to laparoscopic cholecystectomy and is now becoming much more widely practised, the associated inflammation around Calot's triangle

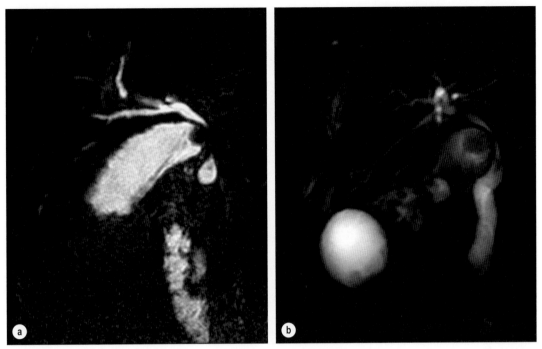

Figure 8.3 • Coronal MRCP reconstruction demonstrates Mirizzi syndrome.

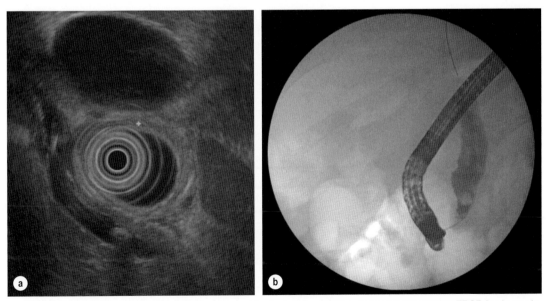

Figure 8.4 • **(a)** EUS demonstrates a distal common bile duct stone. **(b)** The stone was removed at ERCP (endoscopic retrograde cholangiopancreatography). With thanks to Dr Ian Penman, Consultant Gastroenterologist, Royal Infirmary of Edinburgh, UK.

and the CBD in patients with acute cholecystitis may make laparoscopic exploration difficult and/or hazardous. A suggested algorithm for the management of patients with suspected biliary colic/acute cholecystitis and suspected CBD stones is described in **Fig. 8.6**.

Treatment

Biliary colic

The initial treatment for biliary colic consists of adequate analgesia and antiemetics. Although opiate analgesia is widely prescribed, non-steroidal

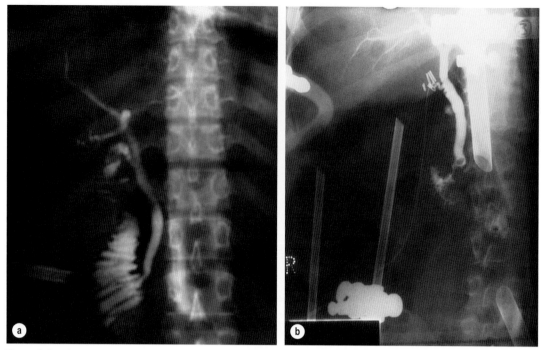

Figure 8.5 • Intraoperative cholangiograms obtained during laparoscopic cholecystectomy demonstrating a non-obstructing calculus in the cystic duct **(a)** and distal common bile duct **(b)**.

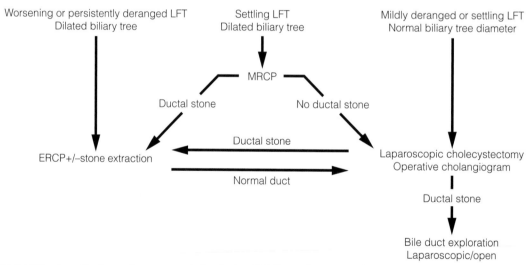

Figure 8.6 • Investigation and management of patients with biliary colic or acute cholecystitis and suspected bile duct stones. ERCP, endoscopic retrograde cholangiopancreatography; LFT, liver function tests; MRCP, magnetic resonance cholangiopancreatography.

anti-inflammatory drugs (NSAIDs) are also effective in relieving pain. Moreover, studies have suggested that NSAIDs can reduce the number of patients progressing from biliary colic to acute cholecystitis. Early laparoscopic cholecystectomy should be offered.

Acute cholecystitis

Initial therapy in acute cholecystitis includes intravenous fluid resuscitation, analgesia, a nil-by-mouth regimen and administration of intravenous antibiotics. Although the initial inflammation is sterile, secondary infection with aerobic

Gram-negative organisms, enterococci and anaerobes occurs. *Clostridium perfringens* infection of the necrotic gallbladder may be a particular complication in the diabetic patient. Few data exist to support the optimum antibiotic regimen and local microbiology recommendations should be followed, although a second- or third-generation cephalosporin combined with metronidazole is frequently prescribed.

Urgent surgical intervention is indicated in those patients with generalised peritonitis arising from a gallbladder perforation or in those with emphysematous cholecystitis (**Fig. 8.7**). Outwith these circumstances, the therapeutic options are to remove the gallbladder, either during the index admission or, electively, at a later admission. Early operation has the advantage of prompt definitive therapy but surgical intervention may be technically more difficult. The rationale for deferred surgery is to allow for resolution of inflammation, but the patient remains at risk of exacerbations during the 'waiting' period, leading to readmission and increased healthcare-associated costs. In addition, as many surgeons can attest, subsequent 'delayed' surgery may still be technically very demanding. Several randomised trials over the last 15 years comparing early versus late laparoscopic cholecystectomy for acute cholecystitis have now confirmed that early laparoscopic cholecystectomy is both safe and has significant benefits for patients. Conversion rate, hospital stay and complications are all significantly lower in the early surgery group.[6–8] A meta-analysis of five randomised clinical trials comparing early versus delayed laparoscopic cholecystectomy for acute cholecystitis has demonstrated that there is no difference in conversion rate or incidence of bile duct injury and the total hospital stay is shorter.[9]

The benefits of early laparoscopic cholecystectomy over early open cholecystectomy have also been assessed.[10] A total of 63 patients with acute cholecystitis were randomised to either early laparoscopic cholecystectomy (*n*=32) or early open cholecystectomy (*n*=31). Conversion to the open procedure was required in five patients randomised to laparoscopic cholecystectomy. Although there were no deaths or bile duct injuries in either group, the postoperative complication rate was significantly higher in the open group (*P*=0.0048): seven patients (23%) had major and six (19%) had minor complications after open cholecystectomy, whereas only one (3%) minor complication occurred after the laparoscopic procedure. Both the postoperative hospital stay (median 4 days vs. 6 days; *P*=0.0063) and duration of sick leave (mean 13.9 days vs. 30.1 days; *P* <0.0001) were significantly shorter in the laparoscopic group.

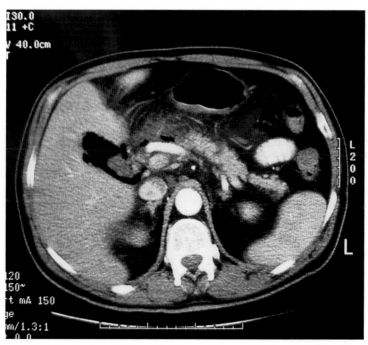

Figure 8.7 • CT image of emphysematous cholecystitis demonstrating gas in the gallbladder wall with extension into the hepatoduodenal ligament.

☑☑ Early laparoscopic cholecystectomy should be attempted in all patients with acute cholecystitis who are fit for surgery, recognising that there will be some in whom the acute inflammation prevents adequate visualisation of the anatomy and conversion will be required.[6–10]

It therefore follows that patients admitted to hospital as an emergency with acute biliary colic should also be offered early laparosocpic cholecystectomy.

Antibiotic cover for urgent cholecystectomy

☑☑ Antibiotic therapy following successful early cholecystectomy for acute non-gangrenous cholecystitis does not need to be continued beyond 12 hours.[11]

Non-surgical options for decompressing the gallbladder in acute cholecystitis

Although early laparoscopic cholecystectomy is optimal management for acute cholecystitis, surgery may not be feasible in some patients because of comorbid conditions. In these patients US-guided percutaneous cholecystostomy is a useful alternative (**Fig. 8.8**). If the diagnosis is in doubt, such as might be the case in the critically ill patient on the intensive care unit, percutaneous cholecystostomy can also be diagnostic,[12] with successful drainage of the gallbladder possible in up to 90% of patients.[13] Although cannulation of the gallbladder may be achieved through a transperitoneal approach, a transhepatic approach is to be preferred because of the lower risk of biliary peritonitis and the earlier maturation of the cholecystostomy tract. Following insertion of the drainage tube into the gallbladder,

free drainage is established. On occasions, simple aspiration of the gallbladder may be effective; however, a recent randomised trial concluded that placement of a percutaneous cholecystostomy drain was associated with a superior clinical response rate.[14] With effective intervention, clinical improvement usually occurs within 24–48 hours; therefore, in those in whom rapid improvement does not occur, a complication, either of the original acute cholecystitis (gallbladder necrosis and/or perforation) or of the cholecystostomy tube placement (bile leak, visceral perforation, bleeding, etc.), should be suspected and surgical intervention should be reconsidered. The cholecystostomy tube should be maintained until a mature fistula tract is achieved, which usually forms within 3 weeks. Contrast radiology in the form of a 'tubogram' may be undertaken in order to confirm drain position, cystic and common bile duct patency, as well as the presence and site of any calculi.

A randomised clinical trial assessing the role of percutaneous cholecystostomy in patients with acute cholecystitis who are high-risk surgical candidates included 123 patients with acute cholecystitis and an Acute Physiological and Chronic Health Evaluation (APACHE) II score of 12 or greater.[15] Patients were randomised to either percutaneous cholecystostomy (PC; *n*=60) or to conservative therapy (C; *n*=63). Percutaneous cholecystostomy was associated with a number of major complications in the initial stages of the trial, although this appeared to be due to the use of non-locking drains inserted under CT guidance. A change in technique to US transhepatic placement of locking drains helped to lower procedure-related complications. Nevertheless, in this trial rates of clinical resolution (PC 86% vs. C 87%) and mortality (PC 17.5% vs. C 13%) were similar between the two groups.

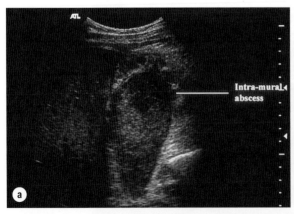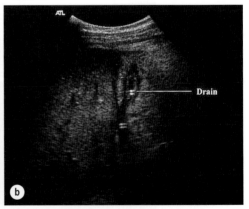

Figure 8.8 • Ultrasound of a patient with acute cholecystitis. **(a)** Before treatment; note the microabscesses within the thickened gallbladder wall. **(b)** After successful percutaneous transhepatic drainage. With thanks to Dr Paul Allan, Consultant Radiologist, Royal Infirmary of Edinburgh, UK.

✓✓ Percutaneous cholecystostomy should only be used in those patients not fit for surgery whose symptoms do not improve rapidly on standard non-operative therapy.[15]

The results of the current multicentre randomised controlled (CHOCOLATE) trial, comparing percutaneous cholecystostomy with laparoscopic cholecystectomy, are awaited.[16]

In patients who have not been offered early cholecystectomy for their acute cholecystitis, including those who have undergone cholecystostomy, following disease resolution, definitive therapy directed towards the gallbladder needs to be considered. Recurrent symptoms will occur in approximately one-third of patients who have previously had acute calculous cholecystitis and have not undergone definitive treatment.[17] Therefore, interval cholecystectomy following optimisation of any comorbid disease should be considered. In those patients in whom surgical intervention is absolutely contraindicated, the cholecystostomy tube may be left in situ for a more prolonged period. Cholelithiasis may then be treated by percutaneous extraction of the gallstones or, less commonly, by direct dissolution with a solvent such as methyl-*tert*-butyl ether. However, recurrence of gallstones following these therapies is common, with studies suggesting that 10–20% of all patients treated by these methods develop further symptoms.[18–20] As a result of these limitations, such approaches are not widely employed.

Management of acute gallstone disease in pregnancy

Non-obstetric acute abdominal pain is relatively common in pregnancy, causes being similar to those in non-pregnant patients, and transabdominal US and MRI are the primary imaging modalities. Laparoscopic cholecystectomy is generally a safe therapeutic option in pregnancy.[21] Although traditionally invasive approaches during the first trimester have been avoided, more recent data indicate that minimally invasive surgery can be conducted with relative safety in the first trimester.[22,23] Biliary imaging may be performed with intraoperative ultrasound, or with limited exposure fluoroscopy and foetal shielding. Management decisions must be based on the efficacy or otherwise of non-operative measures, fully informed consent and with foetal–maternal benefits being considered on an individual basis.

Gallbladder torsion

Torsion of the gallbladder is rare, may be partial or complete and can result in gallbladder necrosis. It can present with clinical and radiological features of acute cholecystitis without gallstones. Treatment is by cholecystectomy.

Acute acalculous cholecystitis

Acute inflammation of the gallbladder can occur in the absence of gallstones and is termed acute acalculous cholecystitis (AAC). Although AAC may present as a complication of a number of clinical conditions, it occurs most frequently in the critically ill or postoperative patient. Despite the fact that AAC is an uncommon entity, it does appears to be increasing in frequency.[24] Observational studies have suggested that AAC occurs in 0.004–0.05% of patients undergoing surgery.[25,26] Although much less common than gallstone-induced acute cholecystitis, the mortality rate of AAC is significantly higher, in part reflecting the patient population affected.[24]

The pathogenetic mechanisms in AAC are not clear. Most recent evidence suggests that AAC is a consequence of microvascular ischaemia resulting in gallbladder inflammation. Studies have demonstrated that the gallbladder arterial and capillary network is reduced and irregular in AAC compared with that in acute cholecystitis.[27] Furthermore, in animal models, the induction of a vasculitic process through the activation of factor XII causes AAC. As indirect evidence, AAC can occur as a consequence of systemic lupus erythematosus, polyarteritis nodosa and antiphospholipid syndrome. In critical illness states, gallbladder microvascular ischaemia probably occurs as a manifestation of the systemic inflammatory response syndrome.

The diagnosis of AAC is often difficult. Because it occurs principally in critically ill patients and in those who have recently had abdominal surgery, the symptoms and signs may be masked by coexisting problems. The critically ill patient may be sedated and/or ventilated, limiting the availability of historical information, and abdominal signs may be masked by sedation or drug-induced paralysis in the critical care setting. In the postoperative patient, abdominal signs may be limited by wound pain, and other more operation-specific complications may be considered as a cause for changes in the clinical condition.

Unfortunately, diagnostic imaging may also be unhelpful. Although US signs of AAC have been described (dilated gallbladder, gallbladder wall thickening, pericholecystic fluid and gallbladder sludge), these are not diagnostic. In a prospective series of 21 critically ill patients, all study subjects had gallbladder abnormalities on at least one occasion during serial US examinations; however, only four patients required intervention for AAC.[28] Similarly, although CT may demonstrate gallbladder abnormalities, these signs may again be non-diagnostic. Cholescintigraphy may be the most accurate method of identifying AAC. In a retrospective study of 27 patients with AAC, cholescintigraphy detected AAC in 9 of 10 patients (90%), whereas CT detected AAC in 8 of 12 (67%) and US detected AAC in 2 of 7 (29%).[29] However, these results must be viewed cautiously as every patient did not undergo all investigations. Moreover, other series have suggested a high incidence of false-positive cholescintigraphy scans in critically ill patients.[30] Because of the inaccuracy of imaging studies, the definitive diagnosis of AAC may only be made at laparotomy or diagnostic laparoscopy.[31] AAC must therefore be considered in all critically ill or postoperative patients with right upper quadrant pain, deranged LFTs or unexplained sepsis. With the difficulty of diagnosis in mind, one prospective study assessed the benefit of percutaneous cholecystostomy in 82 critically ill patients with unexplained sepsis.[32] In 48 patients (59%) there was rapid improvement in the clinical condition within 48 hours but ultrasound did not predict which patients would respond to cholecystostomy.

The optimal therapeutic strategy in AAC is not clear. In all patients, broad-spectrum antibiotic therapy should be instituted as 65% of bile cultures will be positive, with *Escherichia coli* the most common organism. Therapeutic interventions include cholecystostomy with or without interval cholecystectomy, or early cholecystectomy. Several series have demonstrated that percutaneous cholecystostomy is not only an effective immediate intervention but may also constitute definitive treatment as the likelihood of recurrent episodes is small.[33,34] However, early cholecystectomy has been advocated because necrosis of the gallbladder may occur in up to 63% of cases,[29,35] with perforation occurring in approximately 15%. It would therefore appear reasonable to manage AAC in critically ill patients with initial percutaneous cholecystostomy, but in the absence of rapid clinical improvement a complication should be presumed and cholecystectomy carried out. In those patients managed successfully by percutaneous cholecystostomy there does not appear to be an absolute requirement for interval cholecystectomy.

✔ A high index of suspicion is required for the diagnosis of AAC in critically ill patients.[32] Percutaneous cholecystostomy under either US or CT guidance is the primary treatment unless there are signs of overt peritonitis when cholecystectomy is indicated. Failure to improve after cholecystostomy is also an indication for cholecystectomy.

Acute cholangitis

Acute cholangitis may be defined as an acute pyogenic infection within the biliary tree. Because of the possibility of rapid disease progression, acute cholangitis is a potentially life-threatening condition that requires urgent therapeutic intervention.

Pathogenesis

Acute cholangitis arises as a consequence of biliary stasis with subsequent bacterial infection. Although a number of pathological processes may lead to biliary stasis, the most common underlying causes of acute cholangitis are bile duct calculi, malignant bile duct obstruction and biliary stent occlusion. Biliary obstruction need not be complete as acute cholangitis can arise in a partially obstructed biliary system. Under normal conditions bile is sterile; however, in 58% of individuals with asymptomatic ductal calculi, bile cultures will be positive, indicating bacterial colonisation.[36] In those progressing to acute cholangitis, cholangiovenous reflux of bacteria and bacterial products occurs because of increasing hydrostatic pressure within the biliary tree. This cholangiovenous reflux results in bacteraemia and the induction of a systemic inflammatory response, and it is this response, leading to organ dysfunction, that is responsible for the morbidity and mortality in acute cholangitis. Decompression of the biliary tree removes the inflammatory insult.

Aerobic Gram-negative bacilli (*E. coli*, *Klebsiella*, *Pseudomonas* species), enterococcus and anaerobes are the most common organisms cultured from the bile of patients with acute cholangitis.[36] In up to 50% of patients, anaerobic organisms may be associated with aerobic organisms. In the elderly, polymicrobial infection is more common than monomicrobial infection, and again concomitant anaerobic infection occurs in the majority. In approximately 35% of patients, blood cultures will be positive for the same organisms that are found in the bile.[37] The route of bacterial biliary colonisation is not clear; however, the types of bacteria involved suggest that they are derived from the intestinal tract.

Presentation

The presentation of acute cholangitis can be variable, ranging from mild symptoms and signs to overwhelming septic shock. Classically, patients with acute cholangitis present with the symptoms and signs that constitute Charcot's triad: upper abdominal pain, jaundice and pyrexia. However, the complete triad may be present in as few as 22% of patients.[38] In the elderly patient, the presentation may be subtle, with signs of an acute confusional state being common and deranged LFTs being the only pointer to the diagnosis. Similarly, acute cholangitis must be included in the differential diagnosis for any patient presenting with rigors. It is not uncommon for patients who have previously had endoscopic biliary stents to present with a rigor as the major feature of an obstructed and infected stent. At the other end of the spectrum, acute cholangitis can present with signs of septic shock and evidence of multiple organ dysfunction. Because the progression to septic shock can be rapid in patients with biliary obstruction, the diagnosis of acute cholangitis must be considered in any patient presenting with jaundice and signs of sepsis.

Investigation

Cholestatic LFTs are found in the majority of patients with acute cholangitis, demonstrating elevated bilirubin, alkaline phosphatase and γ-glutamyl transferase. However, serum bilirubin may be normal in acute cholangitis arising in a partly obstructed biliary tree because the remaining unobstructed liver is able to compensate. A neutrophilia is typical and serum amylase may also be raised. Deranged coagulation tests can occur, either as a consequence of prolonged biliary obstruction resulting in vitamin K deficiency, or due to disseminated intravascular coagulation. Blood cultures must be obtained as soon as possible.

The initial radiological investigation of choice is transabdominal US. This may demonstrate signs of bile duct obstruction, although false-negative scans can occur. Ultrasound may also determine the underlying pathology. CT can identify biliary dilatation in 78% of patients with acute cholangitis as well as the level of obstruction in 65% and the cause of the obstruction in 61%;[39] however, the initial information obtained is no greater than with US.

Although the determination of the exact site and nature of the bile duct obstruction may require direct visualisation with either ERCP or percutaneous transhepatic cholangiography (PTC), the true value of these procedures is their potential for therapeutic intervention. For this reason, although MRCP has recently been reported to be accurate in identifying biliary obstruction and the underlying obstructing lesion, it does not have an early role in managing patients with acute cholangitis.

Management

Initial resuscitation aims to achieve adequate oxygen delivery, administration of an appropriate volume of intravenous fluid and appropriate analgesia. Efficacy of therapy is assessed by close monitoring of vital signs and, because of the potential for rapid decompensation, management of the patient in a high-dependency unit is usually required (see also Chapter 16).

Aerobic Gram-negative bacilli are the most common organisms in acute cholangitis and therefore empirical therapy with antibiotics covering these bacteria should be commenced. In addition, because anaerobic bacteria, although rarely cultured from blood, are frequently found in bile cultures in association with aerobic bacteria, antibiotic regimens should also have anaerobic activity. Piperacillin is an extended-spectrum penicillin with activity against aerobic Gram-negative bacilli, enterococcus and anaerobes. The addition of the β-lactamase inhibitor tazobactam increases the spectrum of activity.

> ✓✓ In a randomised clinical trial involving 96 patients with acute cholangitis, piperacillin had similar efficacy to combination therapy with ampicillin and tobramycin, achieving clinical cure or significant improvement in 70% of patients.[40] Another randomised trial assessing single antibiotic therapy[37] demonstrated that intravenous ciprofloxacin alone improved the clinical condition in 85% of cases and had similar efficacy to a combination of ceftazidime, ampicillin and metronidazole.

Although appropriate antibiotic therapy is important, relief of biliary obstruction is crucial to successful disease resolution. Emergency operative intervention is associated with significant risk, with a reported mortality of 20% and a 50% complication rate for patients with severe acute cholangitis.[41] As a result, the mainstay of treatment now is endoscopic bile duct drainage, with improved results compared with surgical intervention.[42]

> ✓✓ The benefits of endoscopic therapy over surgery in patients with acute cholangitis were confirmed several years ago in a randomised controlled trial, with significantly fewer complications and lower mortality in those undergoing endoscopic drainage.[42,43]

The method used to achieve non-surgical biliary drainage would appear to be less important than simply achieving adequate drainage. Within the confines of a randomised trial, one study[44] demonstrated that biliary decompression in acute cholangitis with a biliary stent inserted without a sphincterotomy was as efficacious as insertion of a nasobiliary drain. In patients in whom ERCP is unsuccessful, drainage by PTC should be undertaken in the acute situation, even in patients who do not have a dilated intrahepatic biliary tree.[45] Once external drainage has been achieved in the first instance, the placement of a biliary stent can be organised as a staged procedure.

In the case of gallstone-related acute cholangitis, following resolution of the episode of acute cholangitis, adequate clearance of the bile duct should be confirmed by direct cholangiography, ERCP, high-quality MRCP or operative cholangiography. Cholecystectomy should be undertaken if there are no contraindications in order to reduce the risk of further gallstone-related problems.[46,47]

Acute pancreatitis

Acute pancreatitis is defined as an acute inflammatory process of the pancreas, with variable involvement of other regional or remote organ systems.[48] It is a common acute illness, with epidemiological data from the Health Service Statistics Division in Scotland reporting an annual incidence of 318 cases per million (365 cases per million in men, 275 cases per million for women).[49] Analysis of patterns of incidence in this particular population (which has remained relatively constant over the past decade) suggests an increase in the incidence of acute pancreatitis, particularly in those over 40 years of age. Similar increases in the incidence of acute pancreatitis have also been observed in Germany, Finland and Denmark. The factors giving rise to the observed increased incidences are not clear; however, at least in Finland, the increase in the incidence of acute pancreatitis is strongly correlated with an increase in alcohol consumption.

In practical terms the management of acute pancreatitis can be divided into two broad phases. The first phase includes the establishment of diagnosis, severity stratification, initial resuscitation and the choice of appropriate disease-specific initial therapy. The second phase relates to those with severe disease who will usually require further intervention for intra-abdominal complications or support for ongoing multiple organ failure. Guidelines[50–52] suggest that patients with complications arising from severe acute pancreatitis are most appropriately managed in a unit with specialist expertise and therefore this chapter only focuses on the initial phase of management.

Within this chapter the terminology used to describe patients with acute pancreatitis is in keeping with definitions agreed by the 1992 Atlanta consensus conference (Box 8.1).[48] The Atlanta classification attempted to introduce uniformity in the description of clinical severity and the various complications of the disease; however, with increasing

---

Box 8.1 • Terminology relating to acute pancreatitis as defined by the Atlanta consensus conference

Mild acute pancreatitis
Minimal organ dysfunction and an uneventful recovery

Severe acute pancreatitis
Associated with organ failure and/or local complications such as necrosis, abscess or pseudocyst

Acute fluid collections
Occur early in the course of acute pancreatitis, are situated in or near the pancreas, and always lack a wall of granulation or fibrous tissue

Pancreatic necrosis
Diffuse or focal areas of non-viable pancreatic parenchyma, typically associated with peripancreatic fat necrosis

Acute pseudocysts
Collection of pancreatic juice surrounded by a wall of fibrous or granulation tissue

Pancreatic abscess
Circumscribed intra-abdominal collection of pus arising in close proximity to the pancreas, but containing little or no pancreatic necrosis, which arises as a consequence of acute pancreatitis

---

understanding of the pathophysiology of pancreatitis, improved imaging techniques and newer therapeutic strategies, steps are being taken to revise the classification of acute pancreatitis. Alternative classification techniques have already been proposed[53] but still suffer from significant limitations as prognostic or predictive tools. A revision of the Atlanta criteria and management guidelines is anticipated.

Aetiology

Acute pancreatitis may be caused by a wide variety of aetiological agents (Box 8.2), although the majority of cases are due to either gallstones or alcohol excess. Recent epidemiological studies have demonstrated that alcohol excess is an increasingly frequent cause of acute pancreatitis. The prevalence of idiopathic acute pancreatitis varies between reported series and is probably a function of the degree of investigation undertaken to identify a cause. Recent UK guidelines state that no more than 20% of patients should be labelled as having idiopathic acute pancreatitis.[51]

Pathogenesis

The mechanisms through which each aetiological agent causes pancreatic acinar cell injury are not clear. However, after the initial pancreatic insult, it

Common

Gallstones

Alcohol

Uncommon

Trauma

Endoscopic retrograde cholangiopancreatography

Sphincterotomy

Biliary manometry

Pancreatic duct obstruction

Ampulla of Vater neoplasia

Drugs

Azathioprine

Metabolic

Hypercalcaemia

Hyperlipidaemia

Infection

Mumps

Coxsackie B

HIV

Vascular

Vasculitis

Cardiopulmonary bypass

Hereditary pancreatitis

is believed that regardless of the aetiological agent the pathogenetic mechanisms of disease progression in acute pancreatitis are similar. Following pancreatic acinar cell injury, local pancreatic inflammation occurs. Although the inflammatory process may remain confined to the pancreas and peripancreatic tissues, a systemic inflammatory response may be triggered. This systemic inflammatory response is characterised by the systemic activation of leucocytes and endothelial cells and the secretion of proinflammatory cytokines, and is responsible for the development of the organ dysfunction that characterises severe acute pancreatitis. It is not clear why some patients develop severe acute pancreatitis whilst others with similar aetiological agents develop mild acute pancreatitis; however, there is evidence to implicate both excessive proinflammatory mediators and decreased anti-inflammatory mechanisms.

Clinical presentation

Presenting symptoms may range from mild discomfort to overwhelming abdominal pain. Typically, patients present with increasing epigastric/central abdominal pain radiating through to the back. This pain may be eased by sitting forward. Nausea is a

predominant early symptom, with associated vomiting or retching. Before presenting with gallstone-induced acute pancreatitis, patients may have had symptoms consistent with biliary colic. Likewise, in alcohol-induced acute pancreatitis, patients will often have a long history of alcohol ingestion and/or recent binge drinking.

Signs of cardiovascular and respiratory dysfunction may be present. Examination may reveal abdominal signs ranging from localised epigastric tenderness to generalised peritonitis. More specific signs of severe acute pancreatitis include periumbilical bruising (Cullen's sign) and flank bruising (Grey Turner's sign; **Fig. 8.9**).

Diagnosis (see also Chapter 5)

Traditionally, the diagnosis of acute pancreatitis has depended on the detection of a serum amylase concentration more than three times the upper limit of normal. However, hyperamylasaemia may occur in several other conditions (Box 8.3), and a serum amylase concentration above the 'diagnostic' threshold does not definitely indicate acute pancreatitis. Conversely, acute pancreatitis may exist with serum amylase concentrations below this threshold.

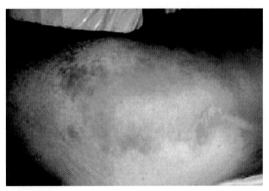

Figure 8.9 • Grey Turner's sign in severe acute pancreatitis. Reproduced from Powell JJ, Parks RW. Diagnosis and early management of acute pancreatitis. Hosp Med 2003; 64:150–5. With permission from the BJHM.

Acute pancreatitis

Pancreatic pseudocyst

Mesenteric infarction

Perforated viscus

Acute cholecystitis

Diabetic ketoacidosis

In those patients with a prolonged history prior to admission to hospital, serum amylase concentrations may have normalised. Amylase measurement therefore needs to be timely. Serum amylase levels do not provide prognostic information, nor can they be followed in order to monitor the early disease process. However, very high levels of serum amylase on admission are often suggestive of a gallstone aetiology.

Because of the limitations of the serum amylase test, other markers have been used to diagnose acute pancreatitis. Serum lipase is perhaps the most common and is more sensitive and specific than serum amylase. Moreover, because of its longer half-life, serum lipase is more accurate if there has been a delay in obtaining the initial sample.[50] However, as with serum amylase, serum lipase concentrations do not correlate with disease severity. In contrast, newer markers such as urinary trypsinogen activation peptide and serum carboxypeptide B activation peptide provide both diagnostic and prognostic information, although these are not assayed routinely in most units.

Although the vast majority of cases of acute pancreatitis can be diagnosed either clinically or biochemically, contrast-enhanced CT may be required in equivocal cases (**Fig. 8.10**).

Finally, in a few patients, laparotomy may be required to confirm the diagnosis of acute pancreatitis while refuting other potential diagnoses such as acute mesenteric ischaemia or a perforated peptic ulcer. The decision to undertake diagnostic laparotomy should not be made lightly as there is evidence that early operation has an adverse effect on outcome in acute pancreatitis.[54] In contrast, patients with acute intestinal ischaemia may present with abdominal pain and hyperamylasaemia and diagnostic delay may be critical. If the pancreas appears normal on CT, and in the absence of a firm diagnosis, laparoscopy or laparotomy should be considered if there are ongoing signs of peritonitis. Clearly, access to CT on a 24-hour basis is a prerequisite for this strategy.

Establishment of aetiology

Following diagnosis, usually confirmed biochemically, transabdominal US should be undertaken in all patients with acute pancreatitis within 24 hours to determine the presence or absence of gallstones. For those patients in whom alcohol is thought to be the causative agent, an accurate alcohol history must be taken, with corroborative information being obtained from other sources as necessary. In patients where alcohol is effectively excluded as a causative agent and no other biochemical cause is identified, it is reasonable to repeat transabdominal US. Endoscopic ultrasound should be considered for patients without an identified aetiology as this may demonstrate biliary microlithiasis (**Fig. 8.11**), in which case cholecystectomy should be considered.

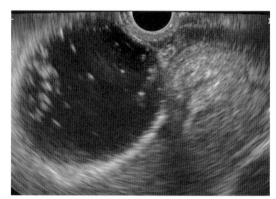

Figure 8.11 • Endoscopic ultrasound detection of gallbladder microlithiasis in a patient with recurrent pancreatitis. Transabdominal ultrasound was normal. Following laparoscopic cholecystectomy there have been no further episodes of pancreatitis. Courtesy of Dr Ian Penman, Edinburgh

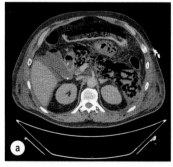
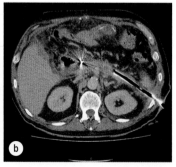
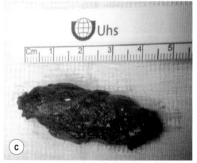

Figure 8.10 • **(a)** Contrast-enhanced CT image of severe acute pancreatitis demonstrating extensive necrosis with gas. **(b)** A radiologically guided drain has been placed. **(c)** Minimally invasive necrosectomy was performed to remove solid debris.

Management

General guidelines

> ✓✓ Guidelines for the initial management of acute pancreatitis have been published by the 1997 Santorini consensus conference,[50] the British Society of Gastroenterology,[51] the American College of Gastroenterology,[52] the Japanese Society of Abdominal Emergency Medicine[55,56] and the International Association of Pancreatology.[57] Their recommendations are broadly similar and are described below.

Initial resuscitation

As in other acute abdominal emergencies, initial therapy is aimed at adequate resuscitation (see also Chapter 16). Provision of oxygen to maintain arterial oxygen saturation, intravenous fluid therapy and adequate analgesia constitute the mainstays of therapy. In addition, the correction of metabolic abnormalities such as hyperglycaemia or hypocalcaemia may require administration of intravenous insulin or calcium. Patients with acute pancreatitis should be started on some form of thromboprophylaxis (see also Chapter 14). Antacid therapy with H_2 antagonists, proton-pump inhibitors or other gastroprotective agents may be commenced as prophylaxis against upper gastrointestinal haemorrhage in those patients with severe disease.

Severity stratification

Following resuscitation, patients should be categorised into either prognostically mild or severe disease, allowing decisions to be taken regarding the degree of monitoring, supportive care and intervention appropriate for each patient. Subjective clinical assessment of prognosis is inaccurate and a validated prognostic scoring system should be used. A number of systems currently exist and can be divided as follows:

- Multiple factor scoring systems – Glasgow,[58–60] Ranson[61] and APACHE II.[62]
- Biochemical scoring systems – C-reactive protein (CRP)[63] and the Hong Kong system based on glucose and urea.[64]
- Immunological scoring – interleukin (IL)-6.[65]
- Radiological scoring – Balthazar[66] and Helsinki.[67]

It should be noted that the Ranson score is based on a North American population with alcohol as the predominant aetiological agent, whereas the Glasgow score is designed for use in a typical British population of gallstone-predominant disease.

Furthermore, practical confusion can result from the fact that there are at least three versions of the 'Glasgow' score: the original publication in 1978[58] and subsequent modifications in 1981[59] and 1984.[60] An APACHE II score of 9 or more has been validated for predicting prognostic severity in acute pancreatitis,[68] although a number of clinical trials have used lower cut-off points in order to predict severe disease, resulting in lower positive predictive values. Although an APACHE II score can be generated soon after admission, unlike the Ranson and Glasgow systems, it has the disadvantage of requiring collation of a sizeable number of variables. Comparative studies of the commonly used scoring systems have reported that no single system is superior to the others.[69] Accuracy to predict prognosis is typically 75–80%; however, a recent modification of the APACHE II system, which includes a clinical assessment of obesity (APACHE-O score), has been suggested to further improve predictive accuracy[70] and accuracy rates as high as 95% have been reported using computerised artificial neural networks.[71]

Finally, it should be noted that the currently used prognostic systems are a one-off or static assessment and serial or dynamic assessment may provide a more accurate determination of outcome. Indeed, it would appear that it is not the presence of organ dysfunction at presentation that is important in determining outcome, rather it is the response to initial resuscitation. Several authors have demonstrated that clinical outcome is worst in patients with persistent organ dysfunction, as manifested by worsening or static organ dysfunction scores following initial resuscitation, compared with patients whose organ dysfunction scores improve.[72–74]

Imaging in acute pancreatitis

As already mentioned, US should be performed in order to confirm or exclude the presence of gallstones. Following this, all patients with prognostically 'severe' acute pancreatitis should undergo contrast-enhanced CT between the third and tenth days of admission to determine the presence of pancreatic necrosis.[51]

Specific therapies for acute pancreatitis

The majority of patients recover from an episode of acute pancreatitis without complication and require little intervention. However, despite intense biomedical research activity there remains a dearth of effective specific therapies for severe acute pancreatitis. The importance of vigorous volume resuscitation and careful monitoring and treatment for metabolic, respiratory, renal and cardiac complications cannot be overemphasised. However, in addition to this supportive care, the therapeutic options are limited. Several randomised controlled trials have assessed the role of early ERCP and prophylactic antibiotics; however, controversy still persists regarding the relative values of both these therapeutic options. These treatments, together with other potential therapeutic options, are reviewed below.

Early ERCP

Early ERCP with endoscopic sphincterotomy (ES) in gallstone-induced acute pancreatitis aims to remove impacted ductal gallstones, thereby eliminating the initiating stimulus and hopefully reducing pancreatic inflammation. Three randomised trials assessing early ERCP have been published. They have produced some conflicting results and so it is worth discussing the results in some detail.

Neoptolemos et al.[75] randomised 121 patients with gallstone-induced acute pancreatitis, 53 of whom had prognostically severe disease, to either early ERCP ($n=59$) or conventional therapy ($n=62$). Although there was no difference in mortality between the two groups (1 for ERCP vs. 5 for conventional therapy; $P=0.23$), there was a significant reduction in total complications (17% ERCP vs. 34% conventional; $P=0.03$) and duration of hospital stay (median 9.5, range 6–36 days ERCP vs. 17.0, range 4–74 days conventional; $P=0.035$) in those patients with prognostically severe disease. Similarly, Fan et al.[76] randomised 195 patients with acute pancreatitis, of whom 127 had gallstone-induced disease and 81 had prognostically severe disease, to either early ERCP ($n=97$) or conventional therapy ($n=98$). Again, there was no significant difference in mortality rates between the two groups (5 for ERCP vs. 9 for conventional therapy; $P=0.276$). However, there was a significant reduction in the incidence of biliary sepsis following ERCP in those with prognostically severe acute pancreatitis (0% ERCP vs. 20% conventional; $P=0.008$). Moreover, in those patients with gallstones a significant reduction in overall morbidity was observed (16% ERCP vs. 33% conventional; $P=0.003$).

In contrast, a multicentre trial undertaken by Folsch et al.[77] randomised 238 patients with gallstone-induced acute pancreatitis but without evidence of biliary obstruction to undergo either early ERCP ($n=126$) or conventional management ($n=112$). In total only 46 patients had prognostically severe disease. In contrast to the previous studies, the mortality rate was higher in the groups undergoing ERCP (10 for ERCP vs. 4 for conventional therapy; odds ratio (OR) 4.57, 95% confidence interval (CI) 0.67–62.7; $P=0.16$). Furthermore, ERCP was associated with an increased rate of respiratory failure (15 for ERCP vs. 5 for conventional, OR 5.16, 95% CI 1.63–22.9; $P=0.03$). Because of the trend towards increased mortality and the significantly increased rate of respiratory failure in those undergoing ERCP, the trial supervisory committee terminated the study early.

The Dutch Acute Pancreatitis Study Group reported an observational multicentre study in eight university medical centres and seven major teaching hospitals involving 153 patients with predicted severe acute biliary pancreatitis without cholangitis who were enrolled in a randomised multicentre probiotic trial and who were prospectively followed. Conservative treatment or ERCP within 72 hours after symptom onset were compared, management being based on the discretion of the treating physician. Patients without and with cholestasis (bilirubin: >40 μmol/L and/or common bile duct dilatation) were analysed separately. In the 51% of patients with cholestasis, ERCP was associated with fewer complications than conservative treatment (25% vs. 54%, $P=0.020$; multivariate adjusted OR 0.35, 95% CI 0.13–0.99, $P=0.049$). Mortality was non-significantly lower after ERCP (6% vs. 15%, $P=0.213$, multivariate adjusted OR 0.44; 95% CI 0.08–2.28, $P=0.330$). In patients without cholestasis, ERCP was not associated with reduced complications (45% vs. 41%, $P=0.814$; multivariate adjusted OR 1.36, 95% CI 0.49–3.76, $P=0.554$) or mortality (14% vs. 17%, $P=0.754$; multivariate adjusted OR 0.78, 95% CI 0.19–3.12, $P=0.734$).[78]

✔✔ Rationalisation of the results of the fully reported trials suggests that early ERCP/ES is of benefit in patients with prognostically severe gallstone-induced acute pancreatitis with evidence of cholangitis or biochemical evidence of obstructive liver function tests (serum bilirubin >90 μmol/L).[75–79]

Antibiotic therapy

The administration of prophylactic antibiotics in acute pancreatitis is based on the hypothesis that the prevention of infected pancreatic necrosis would improve outcome. Numerous studies have been undertaken to investigate this hypothesis and differing results have led to much debate. Early clinical studies did not show any benefit, possibly due to inclusion of patients with a low risk of infection or because antibiotics with poor pancreatic penetration were used. In the light of these conflicting reports and more recent meta-analyses the details of these studies are worth considering further.

In a multicentre trial published in 1993,[80] 74 patients with CT-proven pancreatic necrosis were randomised to receive either imipenem or no initial antibiotic therapy. Pancreatic infection was significantly reduced in the antibiotic-treated group (30% vs. 12%; $P<0.001$). Furthermore, rates of non-pancreatic infection were also significantly reduced; however, antibiotic therapy had no effect on the development of multiple organ failure, the need for operative intervention or on the mortality rate.

A Finnish study[81] randomised 60 patients with CT-proven pancreatic necrosis to receive either prophylactic intravenous cefuroxime or antibiotics only when there were clinical indications of infection. Although there was no difference in the rates of pancreatic infections between the two groups (30% cefuroxime vs. 40% control), prophylactic cefuroxime significantly reduced the mean number of infectious complications per patient (1.0 vs. 1.8; $P<0.01$), mainly through a marked fall in the number of urinary tract infections. There was also a significant reduction in mortality in patients treated with cefuroxime (23.3% vs. 3.3%; $P=0.028$), although this was not associated with any difference in local pancreatic infection.

Another study[82] randomised 23 patients with alcohol-induced severe acute pancreatitis to either standard medical therapy or standard medical therapy plus intravenous ceftazidime, amikacin and metronidazole. Antibiotic therapy resulted in a significant reduction in the number of patients with proven infections (0 vs. 7; $P<0.03$), but there was no significant reduction in mortality rates. Schwarz et al.[83] reported a randomised controlled trial of 26 patients with CT-proven pancreatic necrosis in which the combination of ofloxacin and metronidazole lessened the physiological disturbance found in severe acute pancreatitis, but did not prevent or delay the development of infected pancreatic necrosis.

Subsequently two further studies were published that compared different antibiotic regimens in patients with necrotising pancreatitis. The first of these,[84] a multicentre, randomised controlled trial involving 60 patients with pancreatic necrosis, observed that intravenous imipenem was more effective than perfloxacin at reducing rates of both infected pancreatic necrosis (34% vs. 10%; $P=0.034$) and extrapancreatic infection (44% vs. 20%; $P=0.059$), but had no effect on the mortality rate. The second of these studies again examined the effect of imipenem[85] in a randomised trial comparing the prophylactic use of imipenem with the therapeutic use of imipenem in patients with severe acute pancreatitis and CT-proven pancreatic necrosis. Patients enrolled in the prophylactic arm received imipenem from the time of admission, whereas patients in the therapeutic arm only commenced imipenem following the development of signs suggesting the development of infected pancreatic necrosis (pyrexia, leucocytosis, raised CRP, in the absence of another source of infection). There was no significant difference in the number of patients requiring necrosectomy or in the mortality rate between the two groups.

The largest randomised placebo-controlled, double-blind trial on the use of prophylactic antibiotics was published in 2004.[86] This multicentre study randomised 114 patients to receive either ciprofloxacin in combination with metronidazole or placebo. Only patients with a predicted severe attack were included, defined either by an elevated serum C-reactive protein above 150 mg/L or by pancreatic necrosis on CT scan. No beneficial effects with regard to reduction of pancreatic infection, systemic complications or hospital mortality were demonstrated; however, a shift to open antibiotic treatment was more frequent in patients receiving placebo, suggesting a subgroup of patients may warrant antibiotic treatment.

Using a different strategy aimed at eliminating the reservoir from which bacteria arise to colonise pancreatic necrosis, Luiten et al.[87] evaluated the role of selective gut decontamination. In a multicentre trial, 102 patients with prognostically severe acute pancreatitis were randomised to either conventional therapy or conventional therapy supplemented with selective gut decontamination using oral and rectal colistin, amphotericin and norfloxacin. In addition, patients in the selective gut decontamination group received intravenous cefotaxime until aerobic Gram-negative bacteria were eliminated from the oral cavity and rectum. Selective gut decontamination reduced rates of pancreatic infection compared with the control group (38% vs. 18%; $P=0.03$). Although there was a reduction in mortality from 35% in the control group to 22% in the selective decontamination group, it did not reach significance ($P=0.19$). However, when allowing for differences in disease severity, multivariate analysis suggested a significant survival benefit following gut decontamination ($P=0.048$). Although the results of this trial appear promising, selective gut decontamination is not regarded as a standard for the prevention of pancreatic infection because of the difficulties of drug administration in the intensive care setting.

The inconsistencies among these trials may result from the relatively small number of patients per study and the limited statistical power to detect such differences. There is also considerable heterogeneity in patient selection and the antibiotics used. Other differences include variety in the non-antibiotic treatments, such as fluid resuscitation, enteral nutrition and timing of surgical intervention. Although many published guidelines recommend the use of antibiotics in patients with severe acute pancreatitis, none of the published randomised trials is in itself of sufficient power to mandate antibiotic prophylaxis.

In an attempt to strengthen the evidence regarding the use of antibiotic prophylaxis in acute pancreatitis, several meta-analyses have been performed. In 1998, Golub et al.[88] undertook a meta-analysis of all trials that had been published up to that point and reported that in patients with severe disease, the risk of death fell from 18.2% in patients not receiving antibiotic prophylaxis to 5.3% in those receiving prophylaxis (log odds ratio −0.32 to −2.44; $P=0.008$). Similarly, Sharma and Howden[89] undertook a meta-analysis of three of the trials utilising broad-spectrum antibiotics in patients with severe disease. They suggested that antibiotic prophylaxis resulted in a 12.3% (95% CI 2.7–22%) absolute risk reduction in mortality rate, with eight (95% CI 5–37) patients needing treatment to prevent one death.

More recent meta-analyses, however, do not support the use of prophylactic antibiotics in patients with severe acute pancreatitis. In 2006, Mazaki et al.[90] analysed six trials and concluded that prophylactic antibiotics were not associated with a statistically significant reduction in infected necrosis (relative risk 0.77, CI 0.54–1.12; $P=0.173$), non-pancreatic infections (relative risk 0.71, CI 0.32–1.58), surgical intervention (relative risk 0.78, CI 0.55–1.11) or mortality (relative risk 0.78, CI 0.44–1.39), but were associated with a significant reduction in hospital stay. In 2007, de Vries et al.[91] undertook a meta-analysis on six trials and reported that prophylactic antibiotics had no significant effect on infection of pancreatic necrosis (absolute risk reduction 0.055, CI −0.084 to 0.194) or mortality (absolute risk reduction 0.058, CI −0.017 to 0.134).

Furthermore, there is concern that the use of potent antibiotics may increase the rate of fungal-associated infected pancreatic necrosis and in turn adversely affect outcome. The use of antibiotic therapy has been shown to alter the organisms involved in the development of infected pancreatic necrosis,[92] and it has been suggested that higher rates of fungal infection have been reported in recent studies.[93] There is currently debate as to whether fungal-associated infected pancreatic necrosis is associated with increased mortality; however, a recent randomised trial of antifungal therapy in patients with severe acute pancreatitis showed a definite reduction in the incidence of fungal infection in the treatment group.[94]

✔✔ In the light of all these conflicting studies, it is clear that further trials are needed to clarify the role of antibiotic and antifungal prophylaxis in acute pancreatitis. At present, a pragmatic approach is that routine administration of prophylactic antibiotics to all patients with predicted severe acute pancreatitis is not indicated, but should be considered in those patients with evidence of pancreatic necrosis who appear septic (with leucocytosis, fever and/or organ failure). If blood and other cultures are subsequently found to be negative and no source of infection is identified, antibiotics should be discontinued. If positive microbiological cultures are obtained, appropriate antibiotics should be continued based on microbiological sensitivities.[88–91]

Early enteral nutrition

In those patients with severe acute pancreatitis the systemic inflammatory response may be maintained by intestinal dysfunction, leading to bacterial translocation from the intestinal lumen. Intestinal dysfunction may in part be a consequence of the nil-by-mouth regimen, leading to a loss of luminal nutrition in the intestine. The provision of enteral nutrition aims to ameliorate intestinal dysfunction, thereby reducing the systemic inflammatory response and improving outcome.

This hypothesis was assessed in a randomised study of 32 patients with acute pancreatitis who received either early enteral nutrition through an endoscopically placed feeding tube, or parenteral nutrition following central or peripheral venous cannulation.[95] Enteral nutrition appeared to be well tolerated, with no patients developing a significant complication from the study intervention. Importantly, enteral nutrition was able to supply a similar caloric intake to parenteral nutrition. However, the patients in the study had relatively mild disease and thus no significant differences in clinical outcome were observed, although enteral nutrition was associated with a significant reduction in the cost of patient care.

A similar study that randomised 34 patients with acute pancreatitis to receive, in addition to standard therapy, either early enteral nutrition or parenteral nutrition demonstrated that the introduction of early enteral nutrition was associated with a significant reduction in CRP and APACHE II scores.[96] Furthermore, in those receiving parenteral nutrition, serum anti-endotoxin IgM antibody levels increased, whereas they remained unchanged in those receiving enteral nutrition.

In contrast to the previous two studies, all patients in the randomised controlled trial reported by Kalfarentzos et al.[97] had prognostically severe disease. In total, 38 patients were randomised to receive either enteral nutrition or parenteral nutrition. Enteral nutrition was delivered distal to the ligament of Treitz through a radiologically placed feeding tube. Even in this population of patients with severe disease, enteral nutrition was well tolerated, with the protein and caloric intake equalling that administered to the patients receiving parenteral nutrition. This ability to provide adequate nutrition via the enteral route appeared to translate into a clinical benefit. In those patients receiving enteral nutrition there were significantly fewer complications and a significant reduction in the number of infectious episodes. Further, the cost of nutritional support in the enteral feeding group was one-third of that in the parenteral nutrition group.

A slightly different study randomised 27 patients with prognostically severe acute pancreatitis to either enteral nutrition or standard care, where parenteral nutrition was not instituted from the outset.[98] Although no major complications arose from the provision of enteral nutrition, it was not possible to meet full nutritional requirements. In contrast to previous studies, enteral nutrition did not appear to affect markers of the inflammatory response (IL-6, tumour necrosis factor receptors and CRP). Moreover, the institution of enteral nutrition was associated with a significant deterioration in gut barrier function.

A large study from China[99] randomised 96 patients with severe pancreatitis to parenteral nutrition versus nasojejunal feeding. Measures of inflammation including CRP and IL-6 decreased earlier with enteral nutrition, as did APACHE II scores. Furthermore, mucosal permeability was improved, as inferred by urine endotoxin levels.

In an attempt to determine the efficacy of both enteral nutrition and antibiotic prophylaxis, Olah et al.[100] undertook a two-phase study. In the first phase, patients within 72 hours of the onset of prognostically severe acute pancreatitis were 'randomised' to either parenteral nutrition or enteral nutrition delivered by a nasojejunal feeding tube. In this phase of the study there was no significant difference in the rates of septic complications between the two treatment groups. The second phase of the study was a prospective cohort study, with all patients being given enteral nutrition and imipenem with prophylactic intent, with subsequent comparison of outcome measures obtained in phase 2 with those obtained in phase 1. Following their analysis, the authors of this study stated that the combination of enteral nutrition and antibiotic prophylaxis significantly reduced the rate of septic complications and the requirement for surgical intervention when compared with parenteral nutrition. However, the results of the study have to be interpreted with caution. The initial phase of the study was not truly 'randomised', with patients being allocated to treatment groups according to date of birth, whereas the second phase involved comparison of historical cohorts. Both of these flaws may have resulted in bias.

Another small study randomised 17 patients with prognostically severe acute pancreatitis (APACHE II score=6) to either enteral nutrition through a nasojejunal tube ($n=8$) or parenteral nutrition ($n=9$).[101] Not surprisingly, given the small numbers enrolled in the trial, there was no significant difference in morbidity between the two treatment groups, although the use of enteral nutrition was associated with an earlier institution of normal diet and resumption of normal bowel opening.

The interpretation of the results of all the published trials assessing the role of enteral nutrition and the subsequent translation of these into evidence-based clinical practice is difficult. Firstly, all the trials have insufficient power to determine the effects of enteral nutrition on the most relevant outcome measures of morbidity and mortality. The conclusions of two meta-analyses, one of which reported on six studies[102] and the other on two of the six studies,[103] were contradictory. In one, enteral nutrition was favoured;[103] in the other, the interpretation was that there were insufficient data upon which to make firm judgments.[102] Secondly, all the randomised trials to date have delivered enteral nutrition through a nasojejunal feeding tube requiring either radiological or endoscopic placement. However, a prospective observational study has reported that successful nasogastric feeding can be achieved in patients with severe acute pancreatitis.[104] Early nasogastric and nasojejunal feeding appear equivalent in patients with objectively graded severe acute pancreatitis.[105] Thirdly, other than the trial conducted by Powell et al.,[98] enteral nutrition was compared with early parenteral nutrition. In general, it is not standard practice to commence parenteral nutrition in patients immediately following admission with acute pancreatitis. Furthermore, it is possible that the observed 'benefits' from the institution of enteral nutrition, as compared with parenteral nutrition, are in fact due to the induction of deleterious effects by parenteral nutrition. It has been demonstrated that a nil-by-mouth regimen and the institution of parenteral nutrition in normal volunteers is associated with an increased inflammatory response following a stimulus,[106] and malnourished patients have an impairment of intestinal function and increased markers of the acute-phase response. Furthermore, the use of parenteral nutrition in acute pancreatitis is associated with a significant increase in line sepsis when compared with standard management.[107]

The Dutch PYTHON multicentre trial[108] plans to recruit 208 patients with predicted severe acute pancreatitis and randomise to a very early (<24 h) start of enteral nutrition versus introducing oral diet and enteral nutrition if necessary at around 72 hours after admission. The 3-year trial is designed to determine whether very early feeding reduces the combined end-point of mortality or infections.

✓✓ Although there is no definitive evidence demonstrating that early enteral nutrition improves outcome in severe acute pancreatitis, all published studies demonstrate that enteral nutrition is feasible, safe and does not exacerbate the disease process. Further trials are required to determine the impact of early enteral nutrition in predicted severe acute pancreatitis on infectious complications and disease outcome.[102,103]

Other potential treatment strategies

Probiotic therapy

The use of probiotic therapy in acute pancreatitis is based on the hypothesis that colonisation of the proximal gastrointestinal tract by pathogenic bacteria is a precursor to the development of infected pancreatic necrosis. Probiotic therapy therefore aims to establish colonisation of the gastrointestinal tract by non-pathogenic bacteria, thereby reducing the risk of infective complications. This hypothesis was tested by randomising 45 patients with acute pancreatitis, 32 of whom had severe disease, to receive either live *Lactobacillus plantarum* ($n=22$) or killed *Lactobacillus plantarum* ($n=23$) delivered via a nasojejunal feeding tube, along with oat fibre as a bacterial substrate.[109] All patients received a standard enteral nutrition formula in addition to the live or killed *L. plantarum*. Within this trial, probiotic therapy appeared to reduce the risk of developing either infected pancreatic necrosis or abscess. One patient who received live *L. plantarum* developed pancreatic infection compared with seven patients in the control group ($P=0.023$).

The controversial PROPATRIA trial, a multicentre randomised, double-blind, placebo-controlled trial, recruited 298 patients with predicted severe acute pancreatitis (Acute Physiology and Chronic Health Evaluation (APACHE II) score ≥8, Imrie score ≥3 or CRP >150 mg/L) within 72 hours of onset of symptoms to receive a multispecies probiotic preparation ($n=153$) or placebo ($n=145$), via the enteral route twice daily for 28 days. An unexpected more than doubling in mortality in the treatment arm was reported.[110] This trial provoked extensive discussion regarding its design, execution, analysis and safety monitoring.

✓✓ As a result of the current evidence available, the use of probiotics in patients with severe acute pancreatitis cannot be recommended.[109,110]

Anticytokine therapy

With increased understanding of the pathogenetic mechanisms in acute pancreatitis, it is hoped that novel therapies will be developed that can perturb these mechanisms and improve outcome. Indeed, a large number of agents that either antagonise the proinflammatory response or augment the anti-inflammatory response have been demonstrated to ameliorate disease severity in animal models of acute pancreatitis. However, it should be noted that in these studies the agent is usually administered before or immediately after the induction of acute pancreatitis, a scenario that does not translate to the clinical situation. One such agent to undergo clinical trials was lexipafant, a high-affinity platelet-activating factor receptor antagonist, which acts as a general down-regulator of the proinflammatory cytokine response. On the basis of encouraging results from initial trials, a large multicentre trial recruiting 1500 patients was undertaken. Although the trial results have not been formally reported, it is widely known that there was no improvement in mortality following the use of lexipafant, and that the manufacturers are now no longer pursuing this drug as a treatment for severe acute pancreatitis.

It is expected that further drugs that perturb the pathogenetic mechanisms of acute pancreatitis will be developed and will undergo clinical trials.

Prognosis

Current UK guidelines provide targets for mortality rates in acute pancreatitis.[51] These guidelines state that overall mortality should be less than 10% of patients admitted with acute pancreatitis, with a mortality rate less than 30% in those with prognostically severe disease. Certainly, epidemiological data published in 1999 suggested that there had been a significant reduction in mortality rates between 1984 and 1995.[49]

Treatment of gallstones in acute gallstone pancreatitis

In 1988, before laparoscopic surgery, Kelly and Wagner[111] randomised 165 patients with gallstone-induced acute pancreatitis to either early ($n=83$) or late ($n=82$) biliary surgery, with early surgery being undertaken within 48 hours of admission. In those with mild acute pancreatitis ($n=125$) there was no significant difference in outcome between the two groups (morbidity: early 6.7% vs. late 3.3%, $P>0.10$; mortality: early 3.1% vs. late 0%, $P>0.10$). However, in those with severe acute pancreatitis ($n=40$) early biliary surgery resulted in a significant increase in morbidity and mortality (morbidity: early 82.6% vs. late 17.6%, $P<0.001$; mortality: early 47.8% vs. late 11%, $P<0.025$). A recent prospective study[112] randomised 50 patients with mild gallstone pancreatitis to laparoscopic cholecystectomy performed within 48 hours of admission, regardless of the resolution of abdominal pain or serum biochemistry, or performed once pain had resolved and biochemistry was normalising. The primary end-point, hospital length of stay, was significantly shorter in the early surgery group, with no apparent impact on the technical difficulty of the procedure or perioperative complication rate. However, careful patient selection for such early surgery remains important as other considerations may influence decision-making, such as further investigation and/or treatment of abnormal LFTs, persistent fever and so on, which may complicate assessment of the patient after laparoscopic cholecystectomy. As a result most surgeons still prefer to wait a few days until the acute attack has resolved before proceeding (still during the same hospital admission) with removal of the gallbladder.

✔✔ British Society of Gastroenterology guidelines recommend that patients with gallstone-induced mild acute pancreatitis should undergo cholecystectomy (laparoscopic) during the same hospital admission unless a clear plan for definitive treatment within the following 2 weeks has been made.[51] In patients with severe comorbid disease contraindicating cholecystectomy, definitive treatment may be provided by ERCP and ES. In those with gallstone-induced severe disease, cholecystectomy should be delayed until disease resolution or undertaken as an additional procedure during surgery for a complication of the acute pancreatitis.

Managing the acute sequelae of acute pancreatitis

Infected necrosis

Many patients with pancreatic necrosis require minimal if any local intervention.[113] In those patients requiring intervention, an individualised approach is required. The interventional approaches to infected necrosis can be viewed as lying along a spectrum of 'invasiveness'. The optimal therapeutic approach will depend on the patient's condition and the morphology and extent of the pancreatic or peripancreatic necrosis. Many patients with infected necrosis can be managed with radiologically guided percutaneous drainage alone. Minimally invasive necrosectomy techniques, e.g. minimally invasive retroperitoneal pancreatic necrosectomy (MIRP) and videoscopic-assisted retroperitoneal

debridement (VARD), as well as radiologically guided limited incision open necrosectomy, have gained popularity and may result in lesser physiological insult than more traditional open necrosectomy. These patients should be managed within a specialist pancreatic unit where appropriate repertoire of interventional techniques is available.

Haemorrhage

Advances in imaging and endovascular intervention capabilities have increased the options available for patients that develop acute bleeding in association with pancreatic necrosis, often the result of pseudoaneurysm or true aneurysm formation. CT angiography is generally the preferred initial modality to localise the site of haemorrhage. Once the bleeding vessel is localised, directed transarterial embolisation can be attempted and, in many cases, obviates the need for a technically challenging laparotomy in an unwell patient with a 'hostile abdomen'.

Iatrogenic pancreaticobiliary emergencies

ERCP-related complications

The most common complications of ERCP and ES are pancreatitis, cholangitis, haemorrhage and duodenal perforation. Pancreatitis is managed in the same way as pancreatitis of any other aetiology. Cholangitis will commonly respond to antibiotic treatment, provided biliary drainage has been achieved at ERCP, either by effective stent placement or by clearing the biliary tree. Haemostasis can frequently be achieved endoscopically using local adrenaline injection into the papilla. However, should endoscopic haemostasis be ineffective, an operative approach may be required, particularly in a haemodynamically unstable patient. Generally, haemostasis can be achieved at laparotomy via a duodenotomy. Localisation of the ampulla, placement of the duodenotomy and initial tamponade can be facilitated by insertion of a Fogarty catheter via the cystic duct, through the ampulla. Definitive haemostasis can then achieved by direct suture similar to that carried out during a surgical 'sphincteroplasty'. Care should be taken to avoid suturing the pancreatic duct and the use of a small cannula or probe can be helpful here.

Perforation may be apparent at the time of ERCP, but should be suspected in patients who develop severe pain or systemic physiological compromise following ERCP. CT is the preferred modality for diagnosis of perforation as the perforation is frequently retroperitoneal (**Fig. 8.12**). Small perforations may seal spontaneously and can, in some

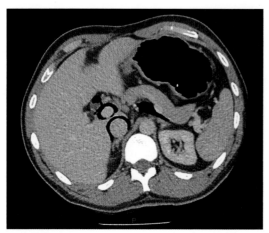

Figure 8.12 • CT image demonstrates retroperitoneal gas in a patient with iatrogenic perforation at ERCP.

cases, be managed non-operatively by placing the patient nil by mouth, then initiating nasogastric tube drainage and systemic antibiotic treatment. The patient's nutritional status also requires careful attention. Should sepsis develop, a collection should be suspected and actively sought. Percutaneous drainage of the retroperitoneum may be required, although operative debridement should not be delayed if the patient's condition is not improved by percutaneous drainage, or if this approach is ineffective in controlling the collection. Again, referral to a specialist unit may be advisable as these complications can be difficult to treat and have a significant mortality.

Post-pancreatectomy haemorrhage

This potentially life-threatening complication is fortunately relatively uncommon but may present to the non-pancreatic surgeon. A 'herald bleed' may precede major haemorrhage and in most cases following pancreaticoduodenectomy, the bleeding arises from the gastroduodenal artery stump. In patients sufficiently stable for transfer to radiology, CT angiography and endovascular treatment with embolisation may be sufficient to control haemorrhage. In patients requiring emergency laparotomy, mortality rates are significant.

Key points

- Laparoscopic cholecystectomy is the gold standard intervention for the management of biliary colic and acute cholecystitis. Laparoscopic cholecystectomy during the index admission is both feasible and safe in patients with acute cholecystitis.
- Percutaneous cholecystostomy may be undertaken in those patients with acute cholecystitis who do not respond to conservative management and who have significant comorbidity contraindicating emergency surgical intervention. Percutaneous cholecystostomy may be the definitive therapy in patients with acute acalculous cholecystitis.
- Intravenous antibiotics and endoscopic drainage of the biliary tree form the basis of management for patients with acute cholangitis. Definitive management of acute cholangitis secondary to choledocholithiasis includes cholecystectomy in order to reduce the risk of further gallstone-related complications.
- Acute pancreatitis is an increasingly common life-threatening illness. Initial management of severe acute pancreatitis involves appropriate resuscitation and organ support.
- Routine administration of prophylactic antibiotics to all patients with predicted severe acute pancreatitis is not indicated, but should be considered in those patients with evidence of pancreatic necrosis who appear septic.
- Early ERCP and ES should be undertaken in patients with gallstone-induced severe acute pancreatitis and evidence of either acute cholangitis or significant biliary obstruction (serum bilirubin >90 μmol/L).
- Surgery has little role in the initial management of severe acute pancreatitis.
- Cholecystectomy should be undertaken in all patients with gallstone-induced acute pancreatitis during the index admission or within the next 2 weeks unless they have ongoing problems from severe disease or are unfit for surgery. In those unfit for surgery ERCP and ES should be considered as definitive treatment.
- Complicated severe acute pancreatitis should be managed in a specialist unit.

References

1. Birkmeyer JD, et al. Hospital volume and surgical mortality in the United States. N Engl J Med 2002;346:1128–37.

2. Varghese JC, Farrell MA, Courtney G, et al. A prospective comparison of magnetic resonance cholangiopancreatography with endoscopic retrograde cholangiopancreatography in the evaluation of patients with suspected biliary tract disease. Clin Radiol 1999;54:513–20.

3. Williams E, Green J. Guidelines on the management of common bile duct stones (CBDS). Gut 2008;57:1004–21.

4. Tranter SE, Thompson MH. Comparison of endoscopic sphincterotomy and laparoscopic exploration of the common bile duct. Br J Surg 2002;89:1495–504.
   Systematic review illustrating that laparoscopic exploration of the common bile duct may be a better way of removing stones than endoscopic sphincterotomy with laparoscopic cholecystectomy.

5. Martin DJ, Vernon DR, Toouli J. Surgical versus endoscopic treatment of bile duct stones. Cochrane Database Syst Rev. 2006: CD003327.
   No clear difference was found in primary success rates, morbidity or mortality between the two approaches in the above two studies.

6. Lo CM, Liu CL, Fan ST, et al. Prospective randomized study of early versus delayed laparoscopic cholecystectomy for acute cholecystitis. Ann Surg 1998;227:461–7.
   A randomised study of 99 patients to either early (within 72 hours) or delayed laparoscopic cholecystectomy. Early surgery was associated with a lower conversion rate (early 11% vs. delayed 23%; $P=0.174$), lower complication rate (early 13% vs. delayed 29%; $P=0.07$), shorter total hospital stay (early 6 days vs. delayed 11 days; $P<0.001$) and shorter recuperation period (early 12 days vs. delayed 19 days; $P<0.001$).

7. Lai PB, Kwong KH, Leung KL, et al. Randomized trial of early versus delayed laparoscopic cholecystectomy for acute cholecystitis. Br J Surg 1998;85:764–7.
   A randomised study of 104 patients to either early ($n=53$) or delayed ($n=51$) laparoscopic cholecystectomy. Surgery would appear to have been more difficult in the early group as manifested by significantly longer operating times (123 vs. 107 min; $P=0.04$); however, this did not translate into a higher conversion rate (early 21% vs. delayed 24%; $P=0.74$). Morbidity rates were similar between the two groups, with no bile duct injuries reported. Early surgery was associated with a significant reduction in overall hospital stay (7.6 vs. 11.6 days; $P<0.001$).

8. Johansson M, Thune A, Blomqvist A, et al. Management of acute cholecystitis in the laparoscopic era: results of a prospective, randomized clinical trial. J Gastrointest Surg 2003;7:642–5.
   A study of 145 patients randomised to early laparoscopic cholecystectomy within the first 7 days (early; $n=71$) or to interval cholecystectomy at 6–8 weeks (late; $n=74$). In the late group, 26% failed conservative therapy and required urgent laparoscopic cholecystectomy. On an intention-to-treat basis, analysis demonstrated no significant difference in conversion rates (early 31% vs. delayed 29%; $P=0.78$) or complications, although one major bile duct injury occurred in the delayed group. There was a reduction in overall hospital stay (early 5, range 3–63 days, vs. delayed 8, range 4–50 days; $P<0.05$).

9. Gurusamy K, Samraj K, Gluud C, et al. Meta-analysis of randomised controlled trials on the safety and effectiveness of early versus delayed laparoscopic cholecystectomy for acute cholecystitis. Br J Surg 2010;97:141–50.
   This meta-analysis of five randomised controlled trials demonstrated no difference in conversion rate or incidence of bile duct injury and a shorter total hospital stay in the early surgery group.

10. Kiviluoto T, Siren J, Luukkonen P, et al. Randomised trial of laparoscopic versus open cholecystectomy for acute and gangrenous cholecystitis. Lancet 1998;351:321–5.
    There was a significantly lower complication rate in the laparoscopic group, with shorter hospital stay and quicker return to work.

11. Lau WY, Yuen WK, Chu KW, et al. Systemic antibiotic regimens for acute cholecystitis treated by early cholecystectomy. Aust N Z J Surg 1990;60:539–43.
    In a randomised trial of 203 patients, the continuation of cefamandole for 12 hours after surgery had equal efficacy with a prolonged dosage schedule of 7 days but was associated with fewer adverse drug reactions.

12. Lo LD, Vogelzang RL, Braun MA, et al. Percutaneous cholecystostomy for the diagnosis and treatment of acute calculous and acalculous cholecystitis. J Vasc Interv Radiol 1995;6:629–34.

13. McGahan JP, Lindfors KK. Percutaneous cholecystostomy: an alternative to surgical cholecystostomy for acute cholecystitis? Radiology 1989;173:481–5.

14. Ito K, Fujita N, Noda Y, et al. Percutaneous cholecystostomy versus gallbladder aspiration for acute cholecystitis: a prospective randomized controlled trial. AJR Am J Roentgenol 2004;183:193–6.

15. Hatzidakis AA, Prassopoulos P, Petinarakis I, et al. Acute cholecystitis in high-risk patients: percutaneous cholecystostomy vs conservative treatment. Eur Radiol 2002;12:1778–84.
    A randomised trial of 123 patients with acute cholecystitis. Rates of clinical resolution and mortality were similar between the percutaneous cholecystostomy and conservative therapy groups.

16. Kortram K, van Ramshorst B, Bollen TL, et al. Acute cholecystitis in high risk surgical patients: percutaneous cholecystostomy versus laparoscopic cholecystectomy (CHOCOLATE Trial): study protocol for a randomized controlled trial. Trials 2012;13:7.

17. Vetrhus M, Soreide O, Nesvik I, et al. Acute cho-lecystitis: delayed surgery or observation. A randomized clinical trial. Scand J Gastroenterol 2003;38:985–90.

18. McDermott VG, Arger P, Cope C. Gallstone recurrence and gallbladder function following percutaneous cholecystolithotomy. J Vasc Interv Radiol 1994;5:473–8.

19. Courtois CS, Picus DD, Hicks ME, et al. Percutaneous gallstone removal: long-term follow-up. J Vasc Interv Radiol 1996;7:229–34.

20. Hellstern A, Leuschner U, Benjaminov A, et al. Dissolution of gallbladder stones with methyl tert-butyl ether and stone recurrence: a European survey. Dig Dis Sci 1998;43:911–20.

21. Hernandez Estrada AI, Aguirre Osete X, Pedraza Gonzalez LA. Laparoscopic cholecystectomy in pregnancy. Five years experience at the Spanish Hospital of Mexico and literature review. Ginecol Obstet Mex 2011;79:200–5.

22. Dhupar R, Smaldone GM, Hamad GG. Is there a benefit to delaying cholecystectomy for symptomatic gallbladder disease during pregnancy? Surg Endosc 2010;24:108–12.

23. Chiappetta Porras LT, Nápoli ED, Canullán CM, et al. Minimally invasive management of acute biliary tract disease during pregnancy. HPB Surg 2009;2009:829020.

24. Glenn F, Becker CG. Acute acalculous cholecystitis. An increasing entity. Ann Surg 1982;195:131–6.

25. Inoue T, Mishima Y. Postoperative acute cholecystitis: a collective review of 494 cases in Japan. Jpn J Surg 1988;18:35–42.

26. Devine RM, Farnell MB, Mucha Jr P. Acute cholecystitis as a complication in surgical patients. Arch Surg 1984;119:1389–93.

27. Hakala T, Nuutinen PJ, Ruokonen ET, et al. Microangiopathy in acute acalculous cholecystitis. Br J Surg 1997;84:1249–52.

28. Helbich TH, Mallek R, Madl C, et al. Sonomorphology of the gallbladder in critically ill patients. Value of a scoring system and follow-up examinations. Acta Radiol 1997;38:129–34.

29. Kalliafas S, Ziegler DW, Flancbaum L, et al. Acute acalculous cholecystitis: incidence, risk factors, diagnosis, and outcome. Am Surg 1998;64:471–5.

30. Kalff V, Froelich JW, Lloyd R, et al. Predictive value of an abnormal hepatobiliary scan in patients with severe intercurrent illness. Radiology 1983;146:191–4.

31. Almeida J, Sleeman D, Sosa JL, et al. Acalculous cholecystitis: the use of diagnostic laparoscopy. J Laparoendosc Surg 1995;5:227–31.

32. Boland GW, Lee MJ, Leung J, et al. Percutaneous cholecystostomy in critically ill patients: early response and final outcome in 82 patients. AJR Am J Roentgenol 1994;163:339–42.

33. Shirai Y, Tsukada K, Kawaguchi H, et al. Percutaneous transhepatic cholecystostomy for acute acalculous cholecystitis. Br J Surg 1993;80:1440–2.

34. Sugiyama M, Tokuhara M, Atomi Y. Is percutaneous cholecystostomy the optimal treatment for acute cholecystitis in the very elderly? World J Surg 1998;22:459–63.

35. Shapiro MJ, Luchtefeld WB, Kurzweil S, et al. Acute acalculous cholecystitis in the critically ill. Am Surg 1994;60:335–9.

36. Csendes A, Burdiles P, Maluenda F, et al. Simultaneous bacteriologic assessment of bile from gallbladder and common bile duct in control subjects and patients with gallstones and common duct stones. Arch Surg 1996;131:389–94.

37. Sung JJ, Lyon DJ, Suen R, et al. Intravenous ciprofloxacin as treatment for patients with acute suppurative cholangitis: a randomized, controlled clinical trial. J Antimicrob Chemother 1995;35:855–64.
A randomised trial assessing single antibiotic therapy demonstrated that intravenous ciprofloxacin alone improved the clinical condition in 85% of patients and had similar efficacy to a combination of ceftazidime, ampicillin and metronidazole.

38. Csendes A, Diaz JC, Burdiles P, et al. Risk factors and classification of acute suppurative cholangitis. Br J Surg 1992;79:655–8.

39. Balthazar EJ, Birnbaum BA, Naidich M. Acute cholangitis: CT evaluation. J Comput Assist Tomogr 1993;17:283–9.

40. Thompson Jr JE, Pitt HA, Doty JE, et al. Broad spectrum penicillin as an adequate therapy for acute cholangitis. Surg Gynecol Obstet 1990;171:275–82.
A randomised clinical trial involving 96 patients with acute cholangitis in which piperacillin had similar efficacy to combination therapy with ampicillin and tobramycin, achieving clinical cure or significant improvement in 70% of patients.

41. Lai EC, Tam PC, Paterson IA, et al. Emergency surgery for severe acute cholangitis. The high-risk patients. Ann Surg 1990;211:55–9.
Retrospective study of 86 patients. All patients had ductal exploration under general anaesthesia. Study identifies markers of 'high risk': comorbidity, pH <7.4, total bilirubin >90 μmol/L, platelet count <150×10⁹/L and serum albumin <30 g/L. For high-risk patients, non-operative intervention may be preferable.

42. Lai EC, Mok FP, Tan ES, et al. Endoscopic biliary drainage for severe acute cholangitis. N Engl J Med 1992;326:1582–6.
A randomised controlled trial comparing endoscopic biliary drainage with surgical decompression in 82 patients with severe acute cholangitis as manifested by signs of shock or progression of the disease despite appropriate antibiotics. In those undergoing endoscopic therapy there were fewer complications (34% vs. 66%; P>0.05) but more importantly a significant reduction in mortality (10% vs. 32%; P<0.03).

43. Tokyo guidelines for the management of acute cholangitis and cholecystitis. Proceedings of a consensus meeting, April 2006, Tokyo, Japan. J Hepatobiliary Pancreat Surg 2007;14:1–121.

44. Lee DW, Chan AC, Lam YH, et al. Biliary decompression by nasobiliary catheter or biliary stent in acute suppurative cholangitis: a prospective randomized trial. Gastrointest Endosc 2002;56:361–5.

45. Pessa ME, Hawkins IF, Vogel SB. The treatment of acute cholangitis. Percutaneous transhepatic biliary drainage before definitive therapy. Ann Surg 1987;205:389–92.

46. Boerma D, Rauws EA, Keulemans YC, et al. Wait-and-see policy or laparoscopic cholecystectomy after endoscopic sphincterotomy for bile-duct stones: a randomised trial. Lancet 2002;360:761–5.

47. Targarona EM, Ayuso RM, Bordas JM, et al. Randomised trial of endoscopic sphincterotomy with gallbladder left in situ versus open surgery for common bileduct calculi in high-risk patients. Lancet 1996;347:926–9.

48. Bradley 3rd. EL. A clinically based classification system for acute pancreatitis. Summary of the International Symposium on Acute Pancreatitis, Atlanta, GA, September 11 through 13, 1992. Arch Surg 1993;128:586–90.

49. McKay CJ, Evans S, Sinclair M, et al. High early mortality rate from acute pancreatitis in Scotland, 1984–1995. Br J Surg 1999;86:1302–5.

50. Dervenis C, Johnson CD, Bassi C, et al. Diagnosis, objective assessment of severity, and management of acute pancreatitis. Santorini consensus conference. Int J Pancreatol 1999;25:195–210.
An important consensus statement.

51. UK Working Party on Acute Pancreatitis. UK guidelines for the management of acute pancreatitis. Gut 2005;54(Suppl. 3):iii1–9.
Current UK guidelines, likely to be revised soon.

52. Banks PA, Freeman ML. Practice guidelines in acute pancreatitis. Am J Gastroenterol 2006;101:2379–400.
Useful summary of management guidelines.

53. Petrov MS, Windsor JA. Classification of the severity of acute pancreatitis: how many categories make sense? Am J Gastroenterol 2010;105:74–6.

54. Mier J, Leon EL, Castillo A, et al. Early versus late necrosectomy in severe necrotizing pancreatitis. Am J Surg 1997;173:71–5.
Single institution randomised study (n=41) demonstrating that early intensive conservative treatment with late necrosectomy for selected cases is the preferred approach for severe necrotising pancreatitis.

55. Mayumi T, Takada T, Kawarada Y, et al. Management strategy for acute pancreatitis in the JPN Guidelines. J Hepatobiliary Pancreat Surg 2006;13:61–7.

56. Mayumi T, Ura H, Arata S, et al. Evidence-based clinical practice guidelines for acute pancreatitis: proposals. J Hepatobiliary Pancreat Surg 2002;9:413–22.
Summary of evidence-based guidelines, albeit in 2002.

57. Uhl W, Warshaw A, Imrie C, et al. IAP guidelines for the surgical management of acute pancreatitis. Pancreatology 2002;2:565–73.
Summary of evidence to 2002.

58. Imrie CW, Benjamin IS, Ferguson JC, et al. A single-centre double-blind trial of Trasylol therapy in primary acute pancreatitis. Br J Surg 1978;65:337–41.

59. Osborne DH, Imrie CW, Carter DC. Biliary surgery in the same admission for gallstone-associated acute pancreatitis. Br J Surg 1981;68:758–61.

60. Blamey SL, Imrie CW, O'Neill J, et al. Prognostic factors in acute pancreatitis. Gut 1984;25:1340–6.

61. Ranson JH, Rifkind KM, Roses DF, et al. Prognostic signs and the role of operative management in acute pancreatitis. Surg Gynecol Obstet 1974;139:69–81.

62. Knaus WA, Draper EA, Wagner DP, et al. APACHE II: a severity of disease classification system. Crit Care Med 1985;13:818–29.

63. de Beaux AC, Goldie AS, Ross JA, et al. Serum concentrations of inflammatory mediators related to organ failure in patients with acute pancreatitis. Br J Surg 1996;83:349–53.

64. Fan ST, Lai EC, Mok FP, et al. Prediction of the severity of acute pancreatitis. Am J Surg 1993;166:262–9.

65. Pezzilli R, Billi P, Miniero R, et al. Serum interleukin-6, interleukin-8, and beta 2-microglobulin in early assessment of severity of acute pancreatitis. Comparison with serum C-reactive protein. Dig Dis Sci 1995;40:2341–8.

66. Balthazar EJ, Robinson DL, Megibow AJ, et al. Acute pancreatitis: value of CT in establishing prognosis. Radiology 1990;174:331–6.

67. Schroder T, Kivisaari L, Somer K, et al. Significance of extrapancreatic findings in computed tomography (CT) of acute pancreatitis. Eur J Radiol 1985;5:273–5.

68. Larvin M, McMahon MJ. APACHE-II score for assessment and monitoring of acute pancreatitis. Lancet 1989;2:201–5.

69. Wilson C, Heath DI, Imrie CW. Prediction of outcome in acute pancreatitis: a comparative study of APACHE II, clinical assessment and multiple factor scoring systems. Br J Surg 1990;77:1260–4.

70. Triester SL, Kowdley KV. Prognostic factors in acute pancreatitis. J Clin Gastroenterol 2002;34:167–76.

71. Mofidi R, Duff MD, Madhavan KK, et al. Identification of severe acute pancreatitis using an artificial neural network. Surgery 2007;141:59–66.

72. Buter A, Imrie CW, Carter CR, et al. Dynamic nature of early organ dysfunction determines outcome in acute pancreatitis. Br J Surg 2002;89:298–302.

73. Johnson CD, Abu-Hilal M. Persistent organ failure during the first week as a marker of fatal outcome in acute pancreatitis. Gut 2004;53:1340–4.

74. Mofidi R, Duff MD, Wigmore SJ, et al. Association between early systemic inflammatory response, severity of multiorgan dysfunction and death in acute pancreatitis. Br J Surg 2006;93:738–44.

75. Neoptolemos JP, Carr-Locke DL, London NJ, et al. Controlled trial of urgent endoscopic retrograde cholangiopancreatography and endoscopic sphincterotomy versus conservative treatment for acute pancreatitis due to gallstones. Lancet 1988;2:979–83.
Early ERCP with sphincterotomy resulted in fewer complications and shorter hospital stay.

76. Fan ST, Lai EC, Mok FP, et al. Early treatment of acute biliary pancreatitis by endoscopic papillotomy. N Engl J Med 1993;328:228–32.
Hospital mortality rate was slightly lower in the group undergoing emergency ERCP with or without endoscopic papillotomy. Subsequent comments on this paper are also worth reading.

77. Folsch UR, Nitsche R, Ludtke R, et al. Early ERCP and papillotomy compared with conservative treatment for acute biliary pancreatitis. The German Study Group on Acute Biliary Pancreatitis. N Engl J Med 1997;336:237–42.
Prospective multicentre study: 126 patients were randomly assigned to early ERCP with sphincterotomy, when appropriate, and 112 patients were assigned to conservative management. In patients with acute biliary pancreatis, without obstructive jaundice, early ERCP and sphincterotomy were not found to be beneficial.

78. van Santvoort HC, Besselink MG, de Vries AC, et al. Early endoscopic retrograde cholangiopancreatography in predicted severe acute biliary pancreatitis: a prospective multicenter study. Ann Surg 2009;250:68–75.

79. Nitsche R, Folsch UR. Endoscopic sphincterotomy for acute pancreatitis: arguments against. Ital J Gastroenterol Hepatol 1998;30:562–5.

80. Pederzoli P, Bassi C, Vesentini S, et al. A randomized multicenter clinical trial of antibiotic prophylaxis of septic complications in acute necrotizing pancreatitis with imipenem. Surg Gynecol Obstet 1993;176:480–3.

81. Sainio V, Kemppainen E, Puolakkainen P, et al. Early antibiotic treatment in acute necrotising pancreatitis. Lancet 1995;346:663–7.

82. Delcenserie R, Yzet T, Ducroix JP. Prophylactic antibiotics in treatment of severe acute alcoholic pancreatitis. Pancreas 1996;13:198–201.

83. Schwarz M, Isenmann R, Meyer H, et al. Antibiotic use in necrotizing pancreatitis. Results of a controlled study. Dtsch Med Wochenschr 1997;122:356–61.

84. Bassi C, Falconi M, Talamini G, et al. Controlled clinical trial of pefloxacin versus imipenem in severe acute pancreatitis. Gastroenterology 1998;115:1513–7.

85. Nordback I, Sand J, Saaristo R, et al. Early treatment with antibiotics reduces the need for surgery in acute necrotizing pancreatitis – a single-center randomized study. J Gastrointest Surg 2001;5:113–20.

86. Isenmann R, Runzi M, Kron M, et al. Prophylactic antibiotic treatment in patients with predicted severe acute pancreatitis: a placebo-controlled, double-blind trial. Gastroenterology 2004;126:997–1004.

87. Luiten EJ, Hop WC, Lange JF, et al. Controlled clinical trial of selective decontamination for the treatment of severe acute pancreatitis. Ann Surg 1995;222:57–65.

88. Golub R, Siddiqi F, Pohl D. Role of antibiotics in acute pancreatitis: a meta-analysis. J Gastrointest Surg 1998;2:496–503.

89. Sharma VK, Howden CW. Prophylactic antibiotic administration reduces sepsis and mortality in acute necrotizing pancreatitis: a meta-analysis. Pancreas 2001;22:28–31.

90. Mazaki T, Ishii Y, Takayama T. Meta-analysis of prophylactic antibiotic use in acute necrotizing pancreatitis. Br J Surg 2006;93:674–84.
Three examples of articles presenting arguments for and against the use of antibiotics in severe acute pancreatitis.

91. de Vries AC, Besselink MG, Buskens E, et al. Randomized controlled trials of antibiotic prophylaxis in severe acute pancreatitis: relationship between methodological quality and outcome. Pancreatology 2007;7:531–8.
A useful assessment of methodological quality of studies in the field concludes that adequate evidence for the routine use of antibiotic prophylaxis in severe acute pancreatitis is lacking.

92. Howard TJ, Temple MB. Prophylactic antibiotics alter the bacteriology of infected necrosis in severe acute pancreatitis. J Am Coll Surg 2002;195:759–67.

93. Beger HG, Rau B, Isenmann R, et al. Antibiotic prophylaxis in severe acute pancreatitis. Pancreatology 2005;5:10–9.

94. He YM, Lv XS, Ai ZL, et al. Prevention and therapy of fungal infection in severe acute pancreatitis: a prospective clinical study. World J Gastroenterol 2003;9:2619–21.

95. McClave SA, Greene LM, Snider HL, et al. Comparison of the safety of early enteral vs parenteral nutrition in mild acute pancreatitis. JPEN J Parenter Enteral Nutr 1997;21:14–20.

96. Windsor AC, Kanwar S, Li AG, et al. Compared with parenteral nutrition, enteral feeding attenuates the acute phase response and improves disease severity in acute pancreatitis. Gut 1998;42:431–5.

97. Kalfarentzos F, Kehagias J, Mead N, et al. Enteral nutrition is superior to parenteral nutrition in severe acute pancreatitis: results of a randomized prospective trial. Br J Surg 1997;84:1665–9.

98. Powell JJ, Murchison JT, Fearon KC, et al. Randomized controlled trial of the effect of early enteral nutrition on markers of the inflammatory response in predicted severe acute pancreatitis. Br J Surg 2000;87:1375–81.

99. Zhao G, Wang CY, Wang F, et al. Clinical study on nutrition support in patients with severe acute pancreatitis. World J Gastroenterol 2003;9:2105–8.

100. Olah A, Pardavi G, Belagyi T, et al. Early nasojejunal feeding in acute pancreatitis is associated with a lower complication rate. Nutrition 2002;18:259–62.

101. Gupta R, Patel K, Calder PC, et al. A randomised clinical trial to assess the effect of total enteral and total parenteral nutritional support on metabolic, inflammatory and oxidative markers in patients with predicted severe acute pancreatitis (APACHE II > or =6). Pancreatology 2003;3:406–13.

102. Al-Omran M, Groof A, Wilke D. Enteral versus parenteral nutrition for acute pancreatitis. Cochrane Database Syst Rev. 2003; CD002837.
A meta-analysis of six studies concluded that there were insufficient data on which to make any firm judgment.

103. Marik PE, Zaloga GP. Meta-analysis of parenteral nutrition versus enteral nutrition in patients with acute pancreatitis. Br Med J 2004;328:1407.
A meta-analysis of two of the six studies reported in Ref. 102 demonstrated an advantage for the enteral route.

104. Eatock FC, Brombacher GD, Steven A, et al. Nasogastric feeding in severe acute pancreatitis may be practical and safe. Int J Pancreatol 2000;28:23–9.

105. Eatock FC, Chong P, Menezes N, et al. A randomized study of early nasogastric versus nasojejunal feeding in severe acute pancreatitis. Am J Gastroenterol 2005;100:432–9.

106. Fong YM, Marano MA, Barber A, et al. Total parenteral nutrition and bowel rest modify the metabolic response to endotoxin in humans. Ann Surg 1989;210:449–56.

107. Sax HC, Warner BW, Talamini MA, et al. Early total parenteral nutrition in acute pancreatitis: lack of beneficial effects. Am J Surg 1987;153:117–24.

108. Bakker OJ, van Santvoort HC, van Brunschot S, et al. Pancreatitis, very early compared with normal start of enteral feeding (PYTHON trial): design and rationale of a randomised controlled multicenter trial. Trials 2011;12:73.

109. Olah A, Belagyi T, Issekutz A, et al. Randomized clinical trial of specific lactobacillus and fibre supplement to early enteral nutrition in patients with acute pancreatitis. Br J Surg 2002;89:1103–7.
A randomised trial of 45 patients, of which 32 had severe pancreatitis. Probiotic therapy appeared to reduce the risk of developing either infected pancreatic necrosis or abscess. One patient who received live *Lactobacillus plantarum* developed pancreatic infection compared with seven patients in the control group (*P*=0.023).

110. Besselink MG, van Santvoort HC, Buskens E, et al. Probiotic prophylaxis in predicted severe acute pancreatitis: a randomised, double-blind, placebo-controlled trial. Lancet 2008;371:651–9.
A controversial trial of 298 patients that reported a more than doubling of mortality in the probiotic group.

111. Kelly TR, Wagner DS. Gallstone pancreatitis: a prospective randomized trial of the timing of surgery. Surgery 1988;104:600–5.

112. Aboulian A, Chan T, Yaghoubian A, et al. Early cholecystectomy safely decreases hospital stay in patients with mild gallstone pancreatitis: a randomized prospective study. Ann Surg 2010;251:615–9.

113. van Santvoort HC, Bakker OJ, Bollen TL, et al. A conservative and minimally invasive approach to necrotizing pancreatitis improves outcome. Gastroenterology 2011;141:1254–63.

9

Acute conditions of the small bowel and appendix

Peter Lamb

Introduction

Acute disease of the small bowel, from which appendicitis is considered separately, contributes substantially to the workload of the general surgeon and often patients will present as emergencies. There are many causes of acute small-bowel disease and disease in any intra-abdominal organ or the peritoneum may involve the small bowel secondarily. The pattern of acute small-bowel disease varies with the age of the patient: some conditions are more common in young people, others in an older population. The incidence of acute surgical small-bowel pathology is difficult to estimate but is probably second to appendicitis as the site of disease requiring urgent surgical intervention. Acute small-bowel disease manifests itself in one of three main ways: (i) obstruction, (ii) peritonitis and (iii) haemorrhage. These categories are not mutually exclusive and more than one type of process may exist in each clinical episode. Treatment of small-bowel disease may be operative or conservative, and the timing of surgical intervention requires as much consideration as the causes and specific treatment of small-bowel disease.

Small-bowel obstruction

Although there are many causes of small-bowel obstruction (Box 9.1), the commonest cause in the developed world is adhesions secondary to previous surgery (approximately 60% of episodes), followed by malignancy. By comparison, in the developing world the most common cause is hernia. A large retrospective study using Scottish National Health Service data estimated that 5.7% of all hospital admissions following abdominal and pelvic surgery over a 10-year period were directly related to adhesions.[1] In order to avoid unnecessary surgery and to ensure the correct surgical approach is employed, an attempt should be made to diagnose the cause of the obstruction preoperatively where possible, or at least to eliminate conditions that might require special treatment. In practice, however, the cause of the obstruction is often diagnosed at operation. A retrospective study of 102 patients undergoing surgery for adhesive small-bowel obstruction carried out between 1987 and 1992, and followed up for 14 years, reported that a total of 273 further episodes of obstruction occurred, requiring 237 hospital admissions.[2] Nearly half of these further episodes resulted in more surgery.

Mechanism

The small bowel responds to obstruction by the onset of vigorous peristalsis. This produces colicky pain, usually in the central abdomen, as the small bowel is of midgut embryological origin. As the obstruction develops, the proximal intestine dilates and fills with fluid, producing systemic hypovolaemia. Further fluid is lost through vomiting, which occurs early if the obstruction is proximal. As the process continues the risk of complications increases and if the blood supply is compromised, infarction and perforation will occur. If the blood supply remains intact and the

Within the lumen

Gallstone

Food bolus

Bezoars

Parasites (e.g. *Ascaris*)

Enterolith

Foreign body

Within the wall

Tumour

Primary

    Small-bowel tumour

        Carcinoma

        Lymphoma

        Sarcoma

    Carcinoma of caecum

Secondary

Inflammation

Crohn's disease

Radiation enteritis

Postoperative stricture

Potassium chloride stricture

Vascultides (e.g. scleroderma)

Outside the wall

Adhesions

Congenital

    Bands

Acquired

    Postoperative

    Inflammatory

    Neoplastic

    Chemical (e.g. starch, talc)

    Pharmacological (e.g. practolol)

Hernia

Primary

    Congenital (e.g. diaphragmatic)

    Acquired (e.g. inguinal, femoral, etc.)

Secondary

    Incisional hernia

    Internal postoperative hernia (e.g. lateral space, mesenteric defect)

bowel is readily decompressed by vomiting and subsequent nasogastric drainage, peristalsis will eventually stop, leaving grossly dilated, non-functioning bowel. In the former scenario the pain, initially colicky, will become continuous, whereas in the latter even the colicky pain may cease as peristalsis stops.

Presentation

The typical clinical presentation of small-bowel obstruction is central abdominal colicky pain, vomiting (often bile stained), abdominal distension and a reduction or absence of flatus. Vomiting may be less of a feature and a greater degree of abdominal distension observed if the blockage is in the distal ileum – in which case the vomiting often becomes 'faeculant' as the stagnant small-bowel contents become degraded by bacterial colonisation. Bowel sounds increase and may be audible to the patient. Localised peritonitic pain and tenderness may develop and this suggests incipient strangulation. In some patients there may be an obvious causative feature such as an irreducible hernia. The presence of surgical scars is important, as is any history of previous intra-abdominal pathology.

Although small-bowel obstruction can occur without the development of abdominal pain, the absence of this symptom should be viewed with caution. This is particularly the case in postoperative patients, where small-bowel obstruction and intestinal ileus can be difficult to differentiate. The history and examination of the patient should be sufficiently detailed to allow a diagnosis of small-bowel obstruction and to determine possible causes. Complicated small-bowel obstruction, with ischaemia or perforation, should be readily detectable by marked abdominal tenderness. It is essential to assess the patient's general state, particularly the degree of dehydration and its effect on the patient, so that adequate resuscitation is undertaken prior to any planned surgical treatment.

Initial management

The aim of management is to adequately resuscitate patients, confirm the diagnosis and to identify possible bowel strangulation before gangrene and perforation occurs, so that early surgery can be arranged. There is less urgency in the recognition of non-strangulating obstruction, and a period of decompression and intravenous fluid resuscitation may allow resolution to occur without surgery. However, failure of the obstruction to resolve after 48–72 hours is usually an indication for surgical intervention.

The first step in management is fluid resuscitation and patients often require several litres of normal saline with potassium supplementation or Hartmann's solution in the first few hours after admission. Patients with a long history are likely to be severely dehydrated, with an alkalosis and associated hypokalaemia, the former due to loss of hydrogen ions in the vomit and the latter from renal compensation. Urinary catheterisation is essential to monitor response to resuscitation and measurement of central venous pressure can be helpful in the elderly, particularly those patients with coexisting morbidity. Adequate fluid replacement should be given before any surgical intervention is planned and can be given rapidly if required, even in the elderly, provided appropriate monitoring is used (see also Chapter 16).

Decompression of the stomach with a nasogastric tube will reduce vomiting in most patients, help to decompress the bowel and reduce the risk of airway contamination from aspiration. Fluid lost from the nasogastric tube should be replaced with additional intravenous crystalloids (normal saline or Hartmann's solution) and potassium supplements. Analgesia should be given early and in adequate doses, with opiates the most commonly used. This will not mask signs of peritonitis and there is no justification for withholding adequate analgesia while waiting for further clinical assessment[3] (see also Chapter 5). However, the analgesia requirement should be reviewed regularly, especially in the early stages of management, as a persistent requirement for increasing amounts of opiate analgesia is a strong sign that underlying strangulation is a possibility and surgery indicated. Again, as in all emergency patients, antithromboembolic prophylaxis should be commenced early and continued until resolution (see Chapter 14).

Investigation

The investigations undertaken in patients with small-bowel obstruction are aimed at:

1. assessing the general state of the patient;
2. confirming the diagnosis of small-bowel obstruction;
3. identifying which patients should undergo early surgery (those with a high risk of strangulation) and those in whom a non-operative approach is appropriate.

Radiological investigations are discussed in detail in Chapter 5. Contrast-enhanced computed tomography (CT; **Fig. 9.1**) is increasingly used in the early assessment of patients with small-bowel obstruction, both to identify the underlying cause (particularly malignancy) and to identify features of possible strangulation. CT features of intraperitoneal free fluid, mesenteric oedema and lack of the 'small-bowel faeces sign', in combination with a history of vomiting, have been reported to be highly predictive of requiring operative intervention.[4] There is also evidence to support the role of oral contrast studies, with the passage of contrast to the colon at 4 hours being a good predictor that obstruction will resolve

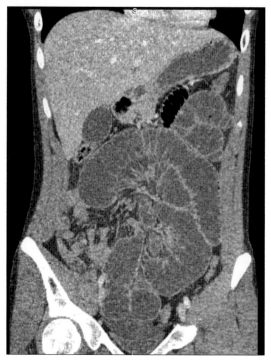

Figure 9.1 • Multislice CT scan with intravenous contrast demonstrating small-bowel obstruction. With thanks to Dr Dilip Patel, Consultant Radiologist, Royal Infirmary, Edinburgh.

with non-operative treatment.[5] The current view is that, although these tests may aid management, identifying patients with possible strangulation remains difficult, and the surgeon must base much of the decision-making on clinical assessment.

Non-operative management

Intravenous fluids and nasogastric aspiration are the two components of the 'drip and suck' regimen, which is the first-line treatment for most patients with obstruction, particularly when the underlying cause is thought to be adhesions, as spontaneous resolution will occur in the majority. As mentioned earlier, this treatment plan should be abandoned at the first suggestion of underlying strangulation. Although non-operative management can be continued for several days in the absence of any suggestion of strangulation, surgical exploration is generally indicated if the obstruction fails to resolve after 48–72 hours. In some patients with known extensive adhesions from multiple previous explorations, it might be worth waiting longer and if so attention should be paid to nutritional support, sometimes necessitating insertion of a central line for parenteral feeding (see Chapter 17).

✔️✔️ In the absence of clinical or CT signs (free fluid, mesenteric oedema, small-bowel faeces sign, devascularised bowel) of strangulation, or patients with partial obstruction, initial non-operative management is appropriate. These patients are good candidates for a trial of water-soluble contrast medium with both diagnostic and therapeutic purposes. The appearance of water-soluble contrast in the colon on X-ray within 24 hours from administration predicts resolution. In the absence of signs of strangulation or peritonitis non-operative treatment can be prolonged up to 72 hours (Bologna Guidelines for Diagnosis and Management of Adhesive Small Bowel Obstruction – 2010).[6]

Surgical management

The particular circumstances of any given patient determine the need for surgical intervention, but some of the commonest features in decision-making are listed in Box 9.2.

Operative principles

Once a decision to operate has been made, patients should be fully resuscitated, treatment of comorbidity optimised and the stomach emptied with a nasogastric tube. The wide range of possible surgical procedures should be explained to the patient. Prophylactic antibiotics and antithromboembolic prophylaxis (if not already started) should be administered.

Generally, a midline incision is the most flexible when the diagnosis is unknown. If the patient has a previous midline incision, this should be excised

Box 9.2 • Small-bowel obstruction: indications for surgery

Absolute indication (surgery as soon as patient resuscitated)
Generalised peritonitis
Visceral perforation
Irreducible hernia
Localised peritonitis

Relative indication (surgery within 24 hours)
Palpable mass lesion
'Virgin' abdomen
Failure to improve (continuing pain, high nasogastric aspirates)

Trial of initial conservative treatment (with further investigations)
Incomplete obstruction
Previous surgery
Advanced malignancy
Diagnostic doubt (possible ileus)

and extended cranially or caudally so that the peritoneal cavity can be entered through a 'virgin' area. Loops of small bowel may be densely adherent to the back of the old scar and attempts to enter the peritoneal cavity through this area can result in an inadvertent enterotomy. This is clearly best avoided, particularly if the bowel wall is grossly distended, friable and diseased.

Having entered the abdominal cavity, the first step is to identify the point at which the dilated bowel proximal to the obstruction changes to collapsed distal bowel. It is important to demonstrate that such a change is present as this confirms the diagnosis of mechanical obstruction and identifies the obstructing point. The presence of uniformly dilated small bowel, or no definite point of change in diameter of the bowel, suggests that the clinical diagnosis of mechanical obstruction may be incorrect. Dilated bowel can be decompressed, usually by milking the contents proximally and aspirating via a large-bore nasogastric tube. If the small-bowel contents will not easily pass to the stomach or the bowel is so friable that retrograde decompression might produce a tear, then a suction catheter may be inserted through a small enterotomy. Where possible this should be carried out through non-diseased bowel. Decompression is particularly useful in distal obstruction when a large number of dilated loops can be difficult to handle and make subsequent abdominal closure difficult. The fluid within the bowel makes it heavy and if it is removed from the abdominal cavity, it should be handled with care so that the mesentery is not damaged. The large surface area of dilated loops results in considerable insensible fluid loss and if it is anticipated that the viscera will lie outside the abdominal cavity for a significant length of time, it should be placed in a waterproof 'bowel' bag or wrapped in moist swabs.

Having identified the point of obstruction, the cause is dealt with. If it is due to adhesions, they should be divided as completely as possible. Although it is not necessary or helpful to divide every last adhesion within the abdomen (as these will inevitably re-form), enough should be divided to confirm that there remains no possible site of obstruction between the duodenojejunal (DJ) flexure and the caecum. It is essential to recognise the patient in whom the clinical diagnosis of mechanical small-bowel obstruction is incorrect, as the presence of adhesions does not in itself confirm the diagnosis.

The small bowel should be resected if it is clearly ischaemic or there is disease or narrowing in the bowel at the point of obstruction, and an anastomosis may be carried out if both ends of the bowel are healthy. If the viability of a segment of bowel is unclear then it should be wrapped in warm moist swabs for several minutes and re-examined.

Where viability remains in doubt it should be resected. Even after removing the obstruction, exteriorisation of the bowel may be indicated if there is generalised disease of the bowel and when an anastomotic dehiscence might be more likely. An ileostomy may be indicated in patients with Crohn's disease as part of their long-term management, and the possibility of such a step should be recognised, considered and discussed with the patient before undertaking the laparotomy. When the viability of large sections of bowel is unclear or the patient is unstable a reasonable option is to resect clearly ischaemic bowel and return the stapled ends to within the abdomen. A planned re-look laparotomy is then performed at 24–36 hours, when either an anastomosis or exteriorisation of bowel ends can be performed, depending on the patient's condition.

There has been considerable research aimed at reducing the development of further adhesions after surgery. There is some evidence that the intraperitoneal administration of icodextrin 4% solution (ADEPT®) at the end of surgery reduces intraabdominal adhesion formation and the risk of reobstruction. In a randomised trial the small-bowel obstruction recurrence rate was 2% (2/91) in the icodextrin groups versus 11% (10/90) in the control group after a mean follow-up period of 41.4 months ($P<0.05$). However, no difference was found in the need for laparotomy.[7]

Abdominal closure should be carried out using a mass closure technique. There are some patients with gross obstruction or repeated procedures in whom, even after relief of obstruction, the oedematous bowel makes closure impossible. In these patients the use of a vacuum-assisted closure dressing or prosthetic mesh to allow temporary closure, with subsequent removal and formal closure a few days later, should be considered. If at subsequent surgery it is still not possible to approximate the fascial edges, alternative techniques can be used: the mesh can be left in situ and the wound edges mobilised and closed over the top; a component separation technique can be used to allow fascial closure; or vacuum-assisted closure dressings can be continued and the abdomen managed as a laparostomy. Further discussions on abdominal sepsis and dehiscence are covered in Chapter 18.

Special conditions

Radiation enteritis
Patients can present with an acute abdomen during radiotherapy due to radiation enteritis or with acute-on-chronic attacks many years later. Patients in the former scenario can present considerable diagnostic difficulties as they are often neutropenic or suffering other side-effects of their treatment. The possibility of a primary pathology, such as acute appendicitis, arising during the course of radiotherapy must also be borne in mind but, where possible, surgical exploration is best avoided.

A more common acute presentation is with adhesions due to previous radiotherapy and these patients normally have obstructive symptoms. Again, a non-operative management policy is the best course as laparotomy is fraught with difficulty. The adhesions are often dense and, if the small bowel is inadvertently injured, there is a significant risk that it might not heal whether it is repaired or anastomosed.

Malignant obstruction
Primary tumours of the small bowel are rare but can be the cause of acute small-bowel obstruction: surgical management at laparotomy will depend on the exact nature of the disease.

A more common problem is the patient with advanced intra-abdominal malignancy, with or without a past history of surgical treatment for malignancy, who presents with bowel obstruction. If the obstruction fails to settle or rapidly recurs, there is usually time to carry out appropriate investigations to determine the extent of the disease prior to surgery. CT is important in identifying a single area of obstruction, which might be amenable to surgery, as compared to extensive intra-abdominal disease without a single point of obstruction.

Ascites can be a confusing factor in such a patient and aspiration for cytology to confirm widespread malignancy can be helpful. Clearly in the presence of advanced and disseminated malignancy laparotomy should be avoided at all costs. However, if the obstructive symptoms are difficult to manage non-operatively and the patient is otherwise in reasonable condition, a laparotomy may be useful in the short term. When surgery is necessary, the exact procedure will depend on the operative findings. The choice usually lies between resection and bypass.

It is also important to recognise that not all patients have obstruction due to their malignant process. One study of patients who presented with obstruction following previous treatment of intra-abdominal malignancy reported that in around one-third of such patients the obstruction was due to a cause other than secondary malignancy.[8] In a study from Japan of 85 patients who had previously undergone surgery for gastric cancer and who were subsequently re-admitted to hospital with intestinal obstruction, the cause was benign adhesions in 20%.[9]

The results of bypass entero-enterostomy for malignant adhesions are generally poor, with short periods of patient survival. For this reason there is growing expertise among palliative care physicians in the medical management of intestinal obstruction.[10] The principles involve the use of fluid diet, steroids and octreotide. The results of such management are variable but it does offer the opportunity to spare a patient the morbidity of laparotomy in the terminal phase of their disease.

Abdominal wall hernia

Any hernia can present with intestinal obstruction **(Figs 9.2** and **9.3)** and if presentation is delayed, gangrene may have occurred and a bowel resection may be necessary. A Richter hernia involves part of the circumference of the bowel wall and the lumen is not obstructed. Infarction of the trapped bowel wall segment can still occur and there will be exquisite localised tenderness over a potential hernia site; the indication for surgical intervention is usually clinically apparent.

Any patient with acute symptoms of a hernia that is irreducible should have urgent surgery, with repair carried out in the usual way. In the presence of obstruction necessitating bowel resection, it is probably best to avoid the use of a prosthetic mesh if possible. When there has been gross contamination of the surrounding area, the risk of complications is increased and a full treatment course of antibiotics should be given. In most cases, a direct approach

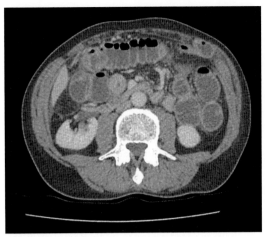

Figure 9.3 • Multislice CT image with intravenous contrast demonstrating small-bowel obstruction secondary to a left-sided Spigelian hernia.

to the hernia is appropriate. For a strangulated femoral hernia a 'high' McEvedy approach usually provides optimum access for both hernia repair and bowel resection if required. The incarcerated tissue may reduce under anaesthesia and it is unlikely, should this occur, that there will have been strangulation. However, the bowel loops must be inspected from within the hernia sac to ensure that a gangrenous loop of bowel or a strictured segment has not dropped back into the abdominal cavity (see also Chapter 4).

A final consideration is the patient who has an asymptomatic hernia who develops acute intestinal obstruction and who then demonstrates signs of an apparently irreducible swelling in the site of the hernia. The intestinal obstruction raises intra-abdominal pressure and this will, in turn, produce the irreducible hernia. The unwary may find the hernia difficult to reduce and, in their efforts to do so, can elicit tenderness. It is worth obtaining a plain abdominal radiograph in all patients with an irreducible hernia and apparent bowel obstruction. The absence of dilated small-bowel loops, or the presence of a dilated colon, should suggest the possibility that the apparently 'incarcerated' hernia is a secondary effect of some other intra-abdominal pathology. If in doubt, a CT scan may help reach the correct diagnosis preoperatively and allow planning of surgery. In such cases consideration will need to be given for a formal laparotomy rather than a local approach over the hernia.

Enterolith obstruction

Enterolith obstruction is rare: the commonest types are gallstone ileus and bezoars.

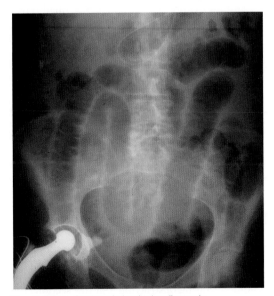

Figure 9.2 • Supine abdominal radiograph demonstrating small-bowel obstruction in a patient with an irreducible femoral hernia.

Gallstone ileus typically occurs in the elderly female and is due to the development of a cholecystoduodenal fistula after an episode of acute cholecystitis with ongoing chronic inflammation. The gallstone may be visible on a plain abdominal radiograph and gas can often be seen within the biliary tree. At surgery the stone should be removed via a proximal enterotomy and the intestine proximal to the obstruction carefully palpated to exclude the presence of a second stone. In these circumstances the gallbladder should be left alone, as cholecystectomy can be difficult and is usually unnecessary.

Bezoars may arise in psychiatric patients, the normal population after over-indulging in particular types of food (e.g. oranges and peanuts), and those who have ingested a foreign body. Rarely, they can occur with material that is collected within a jejunal diverticulum.

Intussusception

In children, acute presentation is usually to the paediatric department and the main differential diagnosis is gastrointestinal (GI) infection. This is discussed in more detail in Chapter 12. Intussusception in adults is usually caused by tumours of the bowel, often metastatic deposits, which should be treated on their merits once detected at laparotomy.

Connective tissue disorders

There are several systemic connective tissue disorders that can affect the GI tract and result in a loss of peristaltic power. These patients generally present with chronic symptoms and the presence of the underlying disorder is established. Occasionally, symptoms suggesting acute GI obstruction are present and the differentiation between full mechanical obstruction and ileus can be difficult. Expectant management of these patients should be pursued whenever possible. The obstructed episode may progress to perforation of the bowel and if peritonitis is present, the perforated bowel should be resected and consideration given to bringing the proximal bowel out as an ileostomy, depending on the site and state of disease. In addition, postoperative ileus is common and the differentiation of a further episode of mechanical obstruction or continuing ileus presents a diagnostic challenge.

Intestinal obstruction in the early postoperative period

GI ileus can occur after any abdominal operation. The surgeon may also be asked to see patients who have undergone gynaecological, orthopaedic or

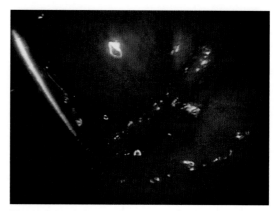

Figure 9.4 • Laparoscopic view of a band adhesion. With thanks to Luigi Sussman, Auckland, New Zealand.

cardiac procedures who have apparent bowel obstruction. Each case must be judged on its merits but the differentiation between true mechanical obstruction and paralytic ileus can be difficult. In patients who genuinely have a mechanical obstruction, appropriate surgical intervention is frequently delayed as a result of this diagnostic dilemma. In these patients, the use of water-soluble contrast small-bowel studies and contrast-enhanced CT is often helpful and should be considered early.[11]

Laparoscopy

Following the development of laparoscopic surgery, there have been reports regarding the use of laparoscopic surgery in the treatment of small-bowel obstruction.[12,13] Open surgery is the preferred method for surgical treatment of strangulating small-bowel obstruction as well as after failed non-operative management. However, in selected patients and with appropriate surgical skills, a laparoscopic approach can be attempted using an open access technique. Laparoscopic adhesiolysis may be suitable during a first episode of small-bowel obstruction, particularly when there has been limited previous surgery and/or a single band is anticipated, such as might occur in a patient who has previously had an appendicectomy but no other major abdominal surgery (**Fig. 9.4**). A low threshold for open conversion should be maintained.[6,12]

Peritonitis

Small-bowel pathology may present as an acute abdomen, with either localised or generalised peritonitis. This may represent the end-stage of any condition causing obstruction, but this section considers conditions that present with primarily inflammatory signs.

Crohn's disease

Crohn's disease is a chronic relapsing inflammatory disease that can affect any part of the GI tract. A common presentation is inflammation of the terminal ileum and this occasionally presents as an acute abdomen. The small bowel alone is affected in approximately 30% of patients and the small bowel and colon together in 50%. The incidence of Crohn's disease is highest in the USA, the UK and Scandinavia and is rare in Asia and Africa, suggesting that dietary factors may be important. Similar to appendicitis, the disease can appear at any age but is most frequent in young adults and there may be a familial tendency. It is thought that the disease is most likely due to an immunological disorder, although the exact mechanism remains unclear although the final pathway is probably a microvasculitis in the bowel wall. Where possible, the management of patients with Crohn's disease should be undertaken by a surgeon with a special interest in this condition and the reader is referred to the much more detailed account of this disease in the *Colorectal Surgery* volume of the *Companion to Specialist Surgical Practice* series.[14] Only first principles for managing an acute episode are discussed in this chapter.

Presentation

An acute clinical episode typically presents with abdominal pain, diarrhoea and fever, and can occur in a patient who has previously been entirely well. An acute presentation is more likely in young adults, hence the differential diagnosis of Crohn's disease in patients with suspected appendicitis.

Two other clinical presentations occur, although they are less likely to be acute. First, resolving Crohn's disease will produce fibrosis in the ileum that can cause obstructive symptoms. These tend to be subacute or chronic and an acute presentation with small-bowel obstruction is rare. Second, entero-enteric or enterocutaneous fistula occurs in Crohn's disease because of the transmural inflammation that is a characteristic histological finding.

Investigation

A patient who presents with right iliac fossa pain, with symptoms that are more insidious than typical appendicitis, should give rise to clinical suspicion. Inflammatory markers may be markedly elevated (white cell count, platelet count, alkaline phosphatase, erythrocyte sedimentation rate), but these are not specific to Crohn's disease. An ultrasound scan may show thickening of the bowel wall or a mass, and contrast-enhanced CT will provide more detailed information.

Surgery for acute Crohn's disease presenting de novo

If a patient with known Crohn's disease presents with an acute flare-up, or during first presentation the diagnosis of Crohn's disease is established before surgery, the patient should be referred to a surgeon with a special interest in this condition.[15] However, the diagnosis may only be suspected at the time of operation, and the surgeon must proceed according to first principles. In the presence of a localised inflammatory mass or stricture, resection and primary anastomosis may be appropriate. If surgery has been carried out for suspected appendicitis and a normal appendix with ileocaecal Crohn's disease is discovered, the appendix should be removed with careful repair of the caecum, so that the possible diagnosis of acute appendicitis is ruled out of any future attacks of pain. No further action needs to be taken at this time for the Crohn's disease and appropriate investigation and treatment can be initiated in the postoperative period. Fortunately, extensive small-bowel Crohn's disease is an uncommon finding at laparotomy, but in this situation the bare minimum should be carried out. If a stricture is found it should be resected, to treat the problem and to confirm the diagnosis. If multiple strictures are found multiple stricturoplasties can be carried out, with full-thickness biopsies taken for histology. The differential diagnosis of lymphoma should also be considered.

Mesenteric ischaemia

Mesenteric ischaemia can be due to embolism or thrombosis, arterial or venous, and may be acute or chronic. Chronic mesenteric ischaemia is also termed 'mesenteric claudication' and is usually caused by a stenosis in the proximal part of the superior mesenteric artery. Patients develop cramp-like abdominal pains after eating, caused by the increased oxygen requirements to the small intestine, which cannot be met by increased blood flow because of the stenosis. The disease is usually associated with atherosclerosis and the investigation of choice is mesenteric angiography. This condition is discussed in more detail in the *Vascular and Endovascular Surgery* volume of the *Companion to Specialist Surgical Practice* series and is not discussed further here. These patients should be transferred to a specialist vascular surgeon.

Acute mesenteric ischaemia can affect any part of the GI tract, but is most common in the small bowel and colon. Acute ischaemia to the small bowel will usually produce infarction, whereas ischaemia to the large bowel presents with bloody diarrhoea and abdominal pain, which will usually settle over the course of a few days and is often termed 'ischaemic colitis'. Delayed strictures may occur.

Acute small-bowel ischaemia is caused by either thrombosis or embolus. Thrombosis may occur in the superior mesenteric artery or its branches, usually associated with underlying atherosclerosis. Embolus is often associated with atrial fibrillation, when an atrial thrombus dislodges and impacts itself in the superior mesenteric artery distribution. Venous thrombosis in the distribution of the superior mesenteric vein is a less common cause of acute small-bowel ischaemia but may be related to increased blood coagulability, portal vein thrombosis, dehydration, infection, compression and vasoconstricting drugs.

Early detection of acute mesenteric ischaemia is difficult (see Chapter 5) and failure to detect this condition early continues to be one of the major causes of morbidity and mortality. The diagnosis is more common in the elderly patient who gives a history of vague but worsening abdominal pain. There may be a background history of atherosclerosis, but not invariably so. Initial examination findings can be unremarkable, lulling the clinician into a false sense of security.

The investigations for possible mesenteric ischaemia are discussed in detail in Chapter 5. CT with intravenous contrast performed as a diagnostic test for the 'acute abdomen' may suggest the diagnosis, but CT angiography (**Fig. 9.5**) is more useful if the

diagnosis is suspected. Patients in whom a diagnosis is suspected should be resuscitated and prepared for laparoscopy or laparotomy. Once the diagnosis has been confirmed, a decision must be made as to whether the ischaemic bowel is salvageable by vascular reconstruction. If the underlying cause is thrombosis, then resection should be performed; however, if an embolus is present, then in selected patients exploration of the superior mesenteric artery with removal of the embolus may save an extended small-bowel resection.[16] This procedure is difficult and may require associated vascular reconstruction. Advice should be sought from a specialist vascular surgeon.

If surgical resection is carried out, primary anastomosis may be performed, providing the blood supply to both proximal and distal margins is adequate. If embolectomy and reconstruction have been performed, or there is doubt about the margins, then anastomosis should be deferred. In this situation the distal and proximal ends of bowel should be stapled off and returned to the abdomen, with re-exploration planned within 48 hours. At re-operation an anastomosis may be performed or the ends brought out as stomas if anastomosis is contraindicated. Attention must be given in the postoperative period to the general condition of the patient in order that any possible secondary ischaemic event can be detected early.

Unfortunately, for the majority of patients with mesenteric ischaemia the small intestine is beyond salvage at the time of laparotomy and requires resection. If the whole of the superior mesenteric artery has been affected, the majority of the small bowel and part of the proximal colon will often be involved and no resection should be performed. These patients should receive intravenous opiates and be kept well sedated, as death will occur shortly afterwards.

> ✓✓ Overall prognosis is better following acute mesenteric venous infarction as compared to acute mesenteric arterial ischaemia, and survival better following arterial embolism as compared to arterial thrombosis.[17]

Meckel's diverticulum

Meckel's diverticulum is a remnant of the omphalomesenteric or vitelline duct. It arises from the antimesenteric border of the distal ileum approximately 60 cm from the iliocaecal valve. It may contain ectopic tissue, usually gastric, and is estimated to be present in approximately 2% of the population. Meckel's diverticulum may remain asymptomatic throughout life, particularly if it has

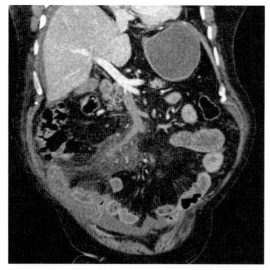

Figure 9.5 • Multislice CT image with intravenous contrast demonstrating ischaemic bowel due to superior mesenteric vein thrombosis. With thanks to Dr Dilip Patel, Consultant Radiologist, Royal Infirmary, Edinburgh.

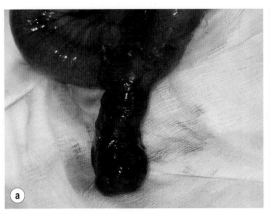
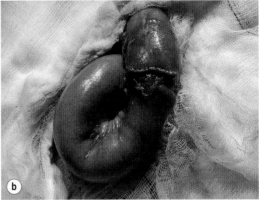

Figure 9.6 • **(a)** Acutely inflamed Meckel's diverticulum identified at laparotomy. **(b)** Operative view after resection of the Meckel diverticulum shown in (a).

a broad base and does not contain ectopic gastric mucosa. Occasionally, a band may exist between Meckel's diverticulum and the umbilicus, which can cause small-bowel obstruction. This should be treated as for a congenital band adhesion, although resection of the diverticulum should accompany division of the band. Occasionally, the diverticulum may intussuscept, also causing obstruction. Again, this will require reduction and excision. The other two common complications of Meckel's diverticulum are inflammation, when the patient presents with signs and symptoms similar to acute appendicitis, and haemorrhage. Acute inflammation is rarely suspected before surgery and the patient is usually diagnosed on the operating table (**Fig. 9.6a**) once a normal appendix has been found through a right iliac fossa incision or at laparoscopy. In the presence of inflammation, a Meckel's diverticulum should be excised and the small bowel repaired (**Fig. 9.6b**). Occult GI bleeding may occur from a Meckel's diverticulum that contains ectopic gastric mucosa and the diagnosis is usually established by CT angiogram. The treatment is again surgical resection.

Haemorrhage

Disease of the small intestine is an occasional cause of acute GI haemorrhage.[18] There are no specific clinical features that distinguish the small bowel as the source rather than the colon, except that the blood loss may be less 'fresh' and more like melaena. As discussed in Chapter 7, it is important to exclude bleeding from a gastroduodenal source at an early stage by upper GI endoscopy. The most commonly encountered causes are vascular malformation, jejunal diverticulae, peptic ulceration in a

Meckel's diverticulum, and small-bowel tumour. These are all treated by resection.

It is important to try to identify the site of bleeding before surgery, as one of the major problems at operation is that a vascular abnormality may produce no external signs. The mobility and variable anatomical layout of the small bowel mean that it can even be difficult to identify a bleeding point that has been demonstrated by imaging. CT angiography is recommended (**Fig. 9.7a**),[18] and if a bleeding point is found, formal angiography may allow a catheter to be passed into the mesenteric branches as close as possible to the bleeding point and left in position to aid surgical localisation (**Fig. 9.7b**). In selected patients, the vessel may be embolised and then at surgery the ischaemic segment can be resected. If this has not been possible, intraoperative enteroscopy may be helpful. Occasionally, the only option is to place segmental soft bowel clamps throughout the small intestine, resecting the segment that fills up with blood after a period of waiting. Blind resection is often unrewarding and the risks of rebleeding are high. If no bleeding point can be identified, the surgeon can either close the abdomen and await events, hoping that further bleeding does not occur (and this can often be the case), or divide the small bowel around its midpoint, bringing out two stomas. Subsequent bleeding can then be identified to one or other side and enteroscopy used to localise it further.

Acute appendicitis

Acute appendicitis is the most common intra-abdominal surgical emergency that requires operation, with an incidence of 7–12% in the population of USA and Europe. Although frequently described

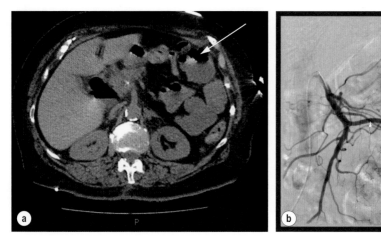

Figure 9.7 • **(a)** CT angiogram with intravenous contrast demonstrating a bleeding point in the jejunum. **(b)** Mesenteric angiogram demonstrating embolisation of the bleeding point shown in (a). With thanks to Dr Jim Gordon-Smith, Consultant Radiologist, Royal Infirmary, Edinburgh.

as a childhood illness, the peak incidence is towards 30 years of age. It is slightly more common in males (1.3–1.6:1) but the operation of appendicectomy is more common in women because of other mimicking conditions. The reader is referred to Chapter 5 for description of some of the general features and investigation of patients with acute abdominal pain, many of which relate directly to acute appendicitis.

Pathology

The aetiology of acute appendicitis is bacterial infection secondary to blockage of the lumen by faecoliths, parasitic worms, tumours of caecum or the appendix, or enlargement of lymphoid aggregates within the appendix wall. In many cases, the cause of the obstruction remains unknown. There is little seasonal variation but there may be a familial tendency. The incidence has been falling since the 1930s, presumably because of improved living standards and general hygiene. Changes in dietary habits, such as an increase in dietary fibre, may also be a factor as appendicitis is less common in countries with a high roughage diet (e.g. central Africa).

The pathology of acute appendicitis is classically described as suppurative, gangrenous or perforated. Typically, there is full-thickness inflammation of the appendix wall. As the disease progresses, adjacent tissues, particularly the omentum, may also become inflamed. Haemorrhagic ulceration and necrosis in the wall indicate gangrenous appendicitis, and subsequent perforation may be associated with a localised periappendiceal mass/abscess or generalised peritonitis.

Clinical features

The presentation of acute appendicitis varies widely but the classical history is of central abdominal pain over 12–24 hours migrating to the right iliac fossa. Nausea and vomiting frequently occur and although diarrhoea is less common, when present it can be confused with gastroenteritis. On examination, the patient usually exhibits a low-grade pyrexia and localised peritonism in the right lower quadrant.

Appendicitis can occur at any age; although the main peak is in young adults, there is a second peak around the seventh decade. The condition is most difficult to diagnose at the extremes of age: in the very young because of the lack of history and frequent late presentation, and in the elderly because of a wide list of differential diagnoses and often less impressive physical signs.

A further factor that may produce atypical signs is the variation in the position of the appendix. A retrocaecal appendix can give rise to tenderness in the right loin and/or right upper quadrant, whereas a pelvic appendix may be associated with very little abdominal discomfort but marked tenderness on rectal examination and a history of diarrhoea. Rectal examination tends to be of little value in the diagnosis of acute appendicitis unless the organ lies in the pelvis. If the diagnosis has been established from abdominal examination, rectal examination contributes very little additional information.[19]

Acute appendicitis is one of a dwindling number of conditions in which a decision to operate may be based solely on clinical findings. In this context, the description of classic history and/or the presence of localised peritonism are highly predictive of acute appendicitis. The risk of morbidity and mortality is significantly increased if the appendix perforates; thus, to err on the side of overdiagnosing acute appendicitis remains accepted best surgical practice. As discussed in Chapter 5, if in doubt, laparoscopy offers an alternative to what may turn out to be an unnecessary laparotomy.

Investigations

The majority of these investigations are discussed at length in Chapter 5.

Urinalysis is essential, particularly in women. Although pus cells and microscopic haematuria can occur in appendicitis, their absence may be useful in excluding significant urinary tract disease. The presence of organisms on microscopy may confirm the diagnosis of urinary tract infection. Pyelonephritis or pyonephrosis may be difficult to differentiate clinically from an acutely inflamed retrocaecal appendix. In such cases urgent investigation of the urinary tract is indicated to exclude these diagnoses prior to appendicectomy. Ultrasound is often used to identify gynaecological causes of pain and may visualise an inflamed appendix (**Fig. 9.8**), but cannot reliably be used to exclude appendicitis.

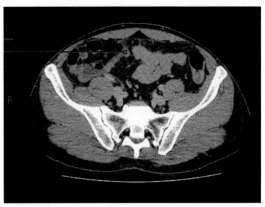

Figure 9.9 • Multislice CT image with intravenous contrast demonstrating an acutely inflamed appendix.

There has been an increasing trend towards using CT (**Fig. 9.9**) in the assessment of patients with acute lower abdominal pain, since the potential role of CT in acute appendicitis was first reported.[20] A recent meta-analysis concluded that CT has reduced negative appendicectomy rates, and even proposed the routine use of CT in adult patients with suspected appendicitis.[21] At present, due to the radiation involved, it is reasonable to proceed directly to laparoscopy for young, fit patients with a high clinical suspicion of appendicitis. As discussed in Chapter 5, ultrasonography can also be helpful. However, there should be a low threshold for CT imaging when there is diagnostic doubt, particularly in older patients, and for those in whom the risks of laparoscopy are increased, due to comorbidities, previous abdominal surgery or morbid obesity.

Differential diagnosis

Just as appendicitis should be considered in any patient with abdominal pain, many other abdominal emergencies must be considered in the differential diagnosis of acute appendicitis. Some of the more common conditions that present in a similar fashion include gastroenteritis, mesenteric lymphadenitis, gynaecological diseases, right-sided urinary tract disease and disease of the distal small bowel. Gynaecological disorders are probably the most important group because the removal of a normal appendix is highest in young women. Acute salpingitis, Mittelschmerz pain and complications of ovarian cyst may all be difficult to differentiate. Torsion of an ovarian cyst usually presents with a notable acute onset of pain and may sometimes

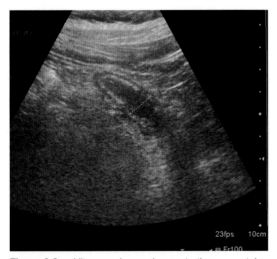

Figure 9.8 • Ultrasound scan demonstrating an acutely inflamed appendix.

be distinguished on clinical grounds. It is important to recognise ruptured ectopic pregnancy, and females of childbearing age should routinely have a pregnancy test (although it must be remembered that appendicitis is not uncommon in the first trimester of pregnancy).

The continuing development of imaging techniques and laparoscopic surgery has prompted the view that the previous proportion of normal appendices removed in the 'open surgery' era (typically up to 20% of patients operated on) was unacceptably high. Although it is clearly advantageous to spare patients unnecessary surgery, the morbidity and mortality of failing to diagnose appendicitis until perforation has occurred is greater than that associated with the removal of a normal appendix. If the diagnostic tools discussed in Chapter 5 are not readily available, the best policy remains early surgery when there is clinical suspicion of acute appendicitis.

Management

A positive diagnosis of acute appendicitis requires urgent surgery as any further delay will result in a higher proportion of perforation.[22,23] Where the diagnosis is in doubt, in patients who are systemically well and/or have mild signs, early exploration in the middle of the night is not indicated and these patients can be safely observed with regular review or investigations as described in Chapter 5. The incidence of perforation in this subgroup of patients is no higher than if they are taken to theatre for early exploration.[24,25] Intravenous antibiotics may be given once a decision has been made to operate or to actively treat acute appendicitis non-operatively.

Surgical treatment

Conventional appendicectomy

A classical appendicectomy incision is made over the point of maximum tenderness and this usually lies on a line between the anterior superior iliac spine and umbilicus in the right iliac fossa (McBurney's point). The skin incision should be horizontal and placed in a skin crease if possible to achieve a satisfactory cosmetic result. The abdominal wall muscles may be separated in the traditional 'muscle splitting' fashion or the abdominal cavity may be entered at the lateral margin of the rectus muscle, with retraction of the muscle fibres medially.

Once the abdominal cavity has been entered, the appendix should be located by gentle palpation and it may be most easily mobilised from the inflammatory adhesions by finger dissection. If it is obviously inflamed, it should be removed, lavage performed and no further laparotomy carried out. If the appendix is macroscopically normal, examination should be undertaken of the terminal ileum (for at least 60 cm to exclude an inflamed Meckel's diverticulum) and small-bowel mesentery and pelvis, both by palpation and direct visualisation. Any free peritoneal fluid should be examined and cultured. The presence of bile staining indicates bowel perforation at some point, such as perforated peptic ulcer, and faecal fluid indicates colonic perforation. In both cases a full laparotomy is indicated. In the former situation, it is best to close the right iliac fossa incision in preference to an upper midline, but in the latter condition some surgeons advocate extending the right iliac fossa incision across to the left as a muscle-cutting lower abdominal transverse incision. If in doubt, a midline incision is best.

It used to be traditional teaching to bury the appendix stump but there is now general recognition that simple ligation of the stump is adequate.[26] If the appendix has perforated at the base, formal repair of the caecal pole is advised. Leaving an excessively long stump should be avoided as this can become ischaemic and produce symptoms postoperatively. Peritoneal lavage should always be carried out but surgical drains are unnecessary unless there is an established abscess cavity.

All patients should receive prophylactic broad-spectrum antibiotics against the risk of wound infection, which is the commonest complication of appendicectomy.[27,28] A single dose is as effective as three doses for wound prophylaxis. For perforated appendicitis, a 5-day treatment course of antibiotics is used by many surgeons, although there are limited data to support this view. When patients can tolerate diet, completing the course of antibiotics orally has been shown to reduce hospital stay without additional complication.[29] Although the risk of deep vein thrombosis is relatively low in young patients, prophylaxis is best administered as a routine as not all patients will make a swift recovery and early postoperative mobilisation may be delayed.

> ✔✔ Prophylactic antibiotics should be administered in all patients undergoing appendicectomy for acute appendicitis in order to reduce the risk of wound infection.[27,28]

Laparoscopic appendicectomy

The advantages of laparoscopic appendicectomy over the open approach have been extensively studied over the last 15 years, although individual studies have produced conflicting results.[30–35]

✓✓ A recent Cochrane database systematic review of 67 studies has confirmed the benefit of the laparoscopic approach in relation to less pain, faster recovery and a lower incidence of wound infections. However, it suggests that there is an increase in intra-abdominal abscesses (odds ratio 1.87) in patients undergoing a laparoscopic procedure. A laparoscopic approach was generally recommended for patients with suspected appendicitis, especially young female, obese and working patients.[36]

The increase in abscesses may of course reflect problems with surgical technique or poor patient selection. There is no reason why the laparoscopic approach should have a higher complication rate, if performed correctly, and indeed it brings with it the possibility of performing a better lavage than at open surgery. The increased abscesses reported may relate to inadequate removal of the lavage fluid (see below).

As skill in laparoscopic techniques has become more widespread, laparoscopic appendicectomy has become increasingly common.[37] It seems reasonable to proceed with laparoscopic appendicectomy for any patient in whom an acutely inflamed appendix is discovered during diagnostic laparoscopy, providing the surgeon has the relevant skills. Large and obese patients probably benefit more from the laparoscopic approach due to the larger wound required at open surgery.

Technique

The basic principles of laparoscopic appendicectomy mirror those of conventional open surgery. The appendix mesentery is usually divided first and may be cauterised with electrocoagulation at the level of the appendix, tied in continuity with ligatures or controlled by application of haemostatic clips. The appendix itself is usually ligated with a preformed loop ligature. An alternative, effective and rapid technique is to apply an endoscopic stapling device to the mesoappendix. The appendix can then be removed after further application of the stapler or by using a pre-tied ligature. Unfortunately, such stapling devices are expensive.

The inflamed appendix should usually be removed in a retrieval bag as it is important to remove the appendix through the abdominal wall without contaminating the soft tissues. A friable or perforated appendix should be handled gently and care taken to remove all debris, including any loose faecolith. A thorough lavage is essential in contaminated cases to prevent postoperative abscess formation. In the authors' institution it is standard practice in such cases to leave a drain in the pelvis to remove any residual lavage fluid in the immediate postoperative period (this may often be removed after 12–24 hours). In patients with generalised contamination from a perforated appendix, it must be remembered that the advantages of the laparoscopic approach are small, as even if the operation can be completed laparoscopically these patients rarely recover quickly due to the systemic nature of their disease. If conversion to open surgery is required then the laparoscope can be used to transilluminate the abdominal wall, allowing accurate placement of a conventional surgical incision, which it may be possible to keep to a smaller size than would otherwise have been used.

There have been various descriptions of operative technique for laparoscopic appendicectomy and different positions for port placement. If ports are placed low in the abdominal wall, the cosmetic result may be improved. One approach is to place working ports at the umbilicus and in the suprapubic region, with the camera port in the left iliac fossa.

One of the reported complications of laparoscopic appendicectomy is leaving too long a stump and risking recurrent symptoms.[38] Care must therefore be taken to ensure that the entire appendix has been fully mobilised to avoid this complication.

The normal appendix at open surgery

In practice, if a standard incision has been made for a planned open appendicectomy, a normal appendix should probably be removed in every patient, including those with Crohn's disease that affects the caecum, in order to prevent future diagnostic dilemma. The removal of a normal appendix may still be associated with morbidity; the wound infection rate is the same as for removal of a non-perforated inflamed appendix. The main long-term complication is small-bowel obstruction. This has been examined in a historical cohort study of 245–400 patients in Sweden with population-based matched controls.[39] This study calculated the cumulative risk of surgically treated small-bowel obstruction following open appendicectomy to be 1.3% after 30 years compared with 0.21% for non-operated controls. Higher risk was associated with those patients undergoing appendicectomy for other conditions, a perforated appendix and a normal appendix.

The normal appendix at laparoscopy

The complication rate associated with open removal of a normal appendix is 17–21%, depending on whether other conditions have been identified.[40,41] The long-term sequelae of laparoscopic removal of a normal appendix remain relatively unknown, but the rate is hopefully less. Removal of a normal appendix at diagnostic laparoscopy is not mandatory and should not usually be undertaken if a definite alternative diagnosis for the patient's symptoms, such as pelvic inflammatory disease, is established.

There is more debate about what should be done if a normal appendix is seen and no other condition can be identified to account for the patient's symptoms. In this scenario, there are two arguments in favour of removing the appendix. (i) There is a small incidence of appendicitis on histological examination of a macroscopically normal appendix.[42,43] One study evaluating the ability of laparoscopy to discriminate between a normal and an inflamed appendix demonstrated a sensitivity of 92% and a specificity of 85% if an appendix with isolated mucosal inflammation was considered to be inflamed.[44] (ii) Removal of the appendix prevents diagnostic dilemma in a patient who continues to suffer from abdominal symptoms and signs following laparoscopy. The counter argument is that the clinical significance of isolated mucosal inflammation in an otherwise normal appendix remains highly debatable, and that all operative interventions or procedures are associated with some form of risk.

Surgeons will have their own opinions on this matter and decisions may vary between patients and the clinical presentation. The final course of action has to be left to the operating surgeon and the patient should be counselled about the options preoperatively. In a patient who has required repeated admissions to hospital with recurring right iliac fossa pain, it would make sense to remove the appendix, even if normal, to at least exclude appendicitis from the differential diagnosis on any possible future admissions.

Non-surgical treatment

It has been suspected for many years that not only can acute appendicitis settle spontaneously, returning with recurrent symptoms at a later date, but that it can be successfully treated in some patients with antibiotics, providing there are no signs of overt peritonitis. The former is supported by a study which reported that 71 of 1084 patients (6.5%) who underwent appendicectomy for acute appendicitis admitted to similar symptoms 3 weeks to 12 years previously.[45] The latter is supported by a number of randomised trials comparing antibiotic treatment versus appendicectomy in patients with suspected appendicitis.[46–49] The difficulty with such a strategy is highlighted by one recent trial, carried out in 243 patients, which found that despite CT assessment 18% of patients were identified at surgery to have unexpected complicated appendicitis.[49] Furthermore, 12% of those

treated with antibiotics required appendicectomy within 30 days and a further 26% developed recurrent appendicitis requiring surgery within 1 year. A recent Cochrane review of five low to moderate quality randomised trials (901 patients) found that 73% of patients treated with antibiotics were cured (including recurrence within 1 year) within 2 weeks without major complications, compared to 97% of patients who directly underwent appendicectomy.[50]

It therefore follows that when a diagnosis of acute appendicitis is suspected appendicectomy should be carried out, and that surgery remains the gold standard treatment for acute appendicitis. Antibiotic treatment might be used as an alternative treatment in the absence of overt peritonitis in specific patients where there are factors that favour a non-operative approach. However, this decision must be made in the knowledge that regular review is essential, surgery is indicated if resolution does not take place within 12–24 hours or the patient deteriorates, and that there is a significant risk of recurrent symptoms during the next 12 months.

Treatment of atypical presentation of acute appendicitis

Appendix mass

The natural history of acute appendicitis left untreated is that it will either resolve, become gangrenous and perforate, or become walled off by a mass of omentum and small bowel. The latter situation prevents inflammation spreading to the abdominal cavity yet resolution of the condition is delayed. Such a patient usually presents with a longer history (1 week or more) of right lower quadrant abdominal pain, appears systemically well and has a tender palpable mass in the right iliac fossa. This condition is best managed non-operatively as the risk of perforation has passed and removal of the appendix at this late stage can be difficult and is associated with a significant complication rate. A recent meta-analysis reported that the non-operative treatment of complicated appendicitis (appendix mass or abscess) is associated with a decrease in complications compared to acute appendicectomy, with a similar duration of hospital stay.[51] The differential diagnosis includes Crohn's disease in younger patients and carcinoma of the caecum in older patients. Confirmation is obtained from ultrasound or CT and it is not uncommon for these investigations to reveal an underlying abscess.[52] However, if the patient remains systemically well, non-operative treatment can still be pursued with percutaneous drainage of any fluid collections if required (see below). Following resolution of the symptoms and mass, further investigations, which might include CT and colonoscopy, must be used to exclude these other conditions.

In the past, routine interval appendicectomy (6 weeks to 3 months) was considered essential to prevent recurrent symptoms in the young and to exclude carcinoma in the elderly. However, providing carcinoma can be excluded by other means, routine interval appendicectomy is no longer recommended. In the majority of patients the appendix has been destroyed and in one study only 9% of patients treated non-operatively for an appendix mass subsequently developed recurrent symptoms, and all did so within 5 months.[52]

> ✔✔ A systematic review has confirmed that non-operative management of an appendix mass will be successful in the majority of patients and recurrence of symptoms is low. As a result the routine use of interval appendicectomy is no longer justified.[53]

Appendix abscess

In some patients the appendix becomes walled off by omentum but has perforated and an abscess will develop in the periappendiceal region. This may be in the right paracolic gutter, the subcaecal area or the pelvis and can be visualised by either ultrasound (**Fig. 9.10**) or CT (**Fig. 9.11**). Unlike with a simple 'appendix mass', the patient is usually systemically unwell with abdominal tenderness. As for all abscesses, drainage is the best treatment, either under radiological control or surgically. There is no doubt that surgical drainage can be associated with significant complications, not least because tissues and organs adjacent to the abscess will be friable and must be handled with great care. The alternative of radiologically guided drainage

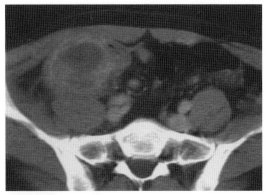

Figure 9.11 • CT scan of the same patient as shown in Fig. 9.10, demonstrating the appendix abscess. With thanks to Dr Paul Allan, Consultant Radiologist, Royal Infirmary, Edinburgh.

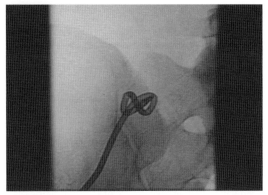

Figure 9.12 • Radiograph of the same patient as shown in Figs 9.10 and 9.11, following percutaneous drainage of the appendix abscess, with drain in situ.

(**Fig. 9.12**) has been reported to produce lower complications and equivalent early operation/re-operation rates.[51,54,55] It would therefore seem reasonable to use the non-operative approach in any patient in whom overt signs of peritonitis are absent. If surgery is required then the residual necrotic appendix should be identified and resected along with the inevitable faecolith, which if left contributes to a protracted recovery.

Chronic appendicitis

As mentioned above, there is certainly a group of patients who suffer from recurrent appendicitis[45] and who benefit from appendicectomy. Similarly, there are some patients who, having recovered from an acute attack of appendicitis, go on to suffer from recurrent less-acute episodes of abdominal pain. These also benefit from appendicectomy, usually as an elective procedure. Assessment in difficult cases can be helped by CT (**Fig. 9.13**), but

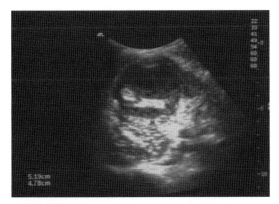

Figure 9.10 • Ultrasound scan demonstrating an appendix abscess. With thanks to Dr Paul Allan, Consultant Radiologist, Royal Infirmary, Edinburgh.

Figure 9.13 • CT image showing an abnormal and thickened tip of appendix without contrast. These findings were confirmed at appendicectomy when a grossly abnormal distal half of appendix was found.

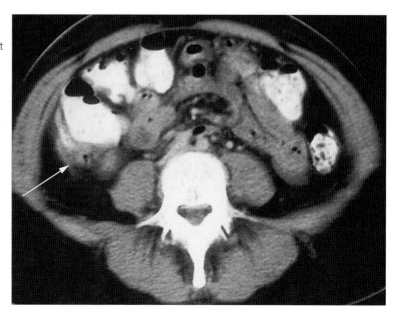

for many patients laparoscopy is the best investigation, at which the appendix can be removed. A small randomised trial has reported improvement in chronic recurrent right lower quadrant pain following laparoscopic appendicectomy compared to laparoscopy alone.[56]

Appendicitis in pregnancy

The rate of appendicitis in pregnancy is similar to that in the non-pregnant female population. The preoperative diagnosis of acute appendicitis can be difficult in pregnancy, and a low threshold for surgical intervention has traditionally been recommended, as complicated appendicitis is associated with a higher rate of foetal loss and increased maternal morbidity. A recent systematic review reported a negative appendicectomy rate of 27%, higher than in the non-pregnant population, and rates of foetal loss of 3.4%, 12.1% and 7.3% in simple, complicated and negative appendicectomy, respectively.[57] Recognition of the risk associated with negative appendicectomy[58] has led to guidelines from the American College of Radiology recommending that 'magnetic resonance imaging can be accurate in excluding appendicitis where the ultrasound exam does not visualise a normal appendix'. Where emergency access to such imaging is possible it is recommended, but it should not delay surgery in patients with a high clinical suspicion of appendicitis.

Many reports have demonstrated laparoscopic appendicectomy to be a safe and effective procedure during pregnancy. With modification of port position the laparoscopic approach has even been reported during the third trimester. One recent large observational study has reported a higher risk for laparoscopy, with an odds ratio of 2.3 for foetal loss compared to conventional surgery,[58] and this has influenced the results of a subsequent systematic review.[57] The result of this single study does not contraindicate laparoscopic appendicectomy in pregnancy, but does indicate a need for further research on the subject. Currently the Society of American Gastrointestinal and Endoscopic Surgeons continues to recommend laparoscopic appendicectomy as the treatment of choice for pregnant patients.[59]

The assessment and decision-making for such patients should involve both senior general and obstetric surgeons. A reasonable approach is to use laparoscopy in the first trimester or when, despite adequate imaging, the diagnosis is in doubt. In later pregnancy open surgery may be preferred when the diagnosis is confirmed but the approach will depend upon surgeon expertise. In all cases there should be a low threshold for conversion to open surgery if difficulties are encountered. If the appendix is found not to be inflamed at laparoscopy then it should not routinely be removed.

Postoperative complications and outcome

Hospital stay

The duration of hospital stay depends on local resources, policies, the patient's general condition and any coexisting disease. It is now clear that laparoscopic appendicectomy is associated with a more rapid return to normal activities[36] than conventional surgery, but this does not necessarily relate to a shorter hospital stay. Much will depend on local factors, and reports of routine early discharge

(24–48 hours) after conventional appendicectomy[60] suggest that full diet and early mobilisation are well tolerated by the majority of patients.

Wound infection

This is the commonest postoperative complication, occurring in around 10–15% of patients following a conventional right iliac fossa incision. In most patients there is superficial inflammation, which responds to antibiotics. In a smaller number there will be dehiscence of the wound and purulent discharge. Occasionally, surgical intervention may be required to drain a collection in the abdominal wall. The current practice of early discharge from hospital results in many wound infections developing once the patient is at home, and the possibility of this complication should always be discussed with the patient. Wound infection appears to be significantly less following laparoscopic appendicectomy.[36]

There is no evidence that wound infiltration with local anaesthetic is associated with any increase in the incidence of wound infection but there is also minimal benefit in reducing postoperative wound pain.[61,62] After open appendicectomy the skin may be closed with interrupted stitches or a continuous suture and this does not appear to affect wound infection rates. Some surgeons leave the skin incision open if there has been gross contamination of the wound in perforated appendicitis. The subsequent cosmetic result of such a scar is usually satisfactory but healing takes several weeks.

Other septic complications

Pericaecal fluid collections are relatively common and are usually indicated by the presence of abdominal discomfort and a low-grade pyrexia. They can usually be diagnosed by ultrasound and treated by antibiotics, especially in children,[63] or occasionally aspiration; formal drainage is rarely necessary. Pelvic abscess is a less common complication that presents with lower abdominal discomfort and swinging pyrexia. The symptoms may be delayed by 10 days or more and a soft tender mass may be palpable on rectal examination, although this is not always the case. Again, ultrasound and often CT is required for diagnosis and, if pus is aspirated, a percutaneous drain should be placed if possible. Occasionally, a pelvic abscess may be difficult to drain percutaneously and in this situation the options are between antibiotics, drainage of the abscess into the rectum or to proceed to surgical drainage through the abdomen. The decision is influenced by the general condition of the patient. Prolonged use of antibiotics should be avoided and further attempts made for drainage if the collection is not resolving on repeated imaging.

In patients who have undergone laparoscopic appendicectomy for perforated appendicitis, signs of generalised peritonitis can develop in the first 48 hours. This may be due to dissemination of infected fluid through the abdominal cavity, possibly by circulation of the carbon dioxide used to create the pneumoperitoneum. The main differential diagnosis in this situation is iatrogenic injury to the intestine and, if in doubt, re-laparoscopy is indicated.

Prognosis

The mortality of appendicitis is associated with the age of the patient and delayed diagnosis (perforated appendix). A report from the Royal College of Surgeons of England showed a mortality of 0.24% and morbidity of 7.7% in 6596 patients undergoing open appendicectomy between 1990 and 1992.[64] A further prognostic consideration is the incidence of subsequent tubal infertility after appendicectomy. Although one report suggested that the increased risk of tubal infertility following perforated appendicitis was 4.8 in nulliparous women and 3.2 in multiparous women,[65] a more recent historical cohort study revealed no long-term consequence on fertility.[66]

Key points

- The main emergency conditions affecting the small bowel are obstruction, haemorrhage and ischaemia.
- Early management requires adequate clinical and radiological assessment, which might include contrast radiology and, increasingly, CT (see also Chapter 5).
- Early appendicectomy for acute appendicitis is better than non-operative treatment with antibiotics because of a high recurrence rate.
- Laparoscopic appendicectomy results in less pain and faster return to normal activities than open appendicectomy but there may be a higher risk of postoperative abscess formation.
- A non-operative approach is indicated in the majority of patients with appendix mass or abscess, with radiological drainage as required. Subsequent interval appendicectomy is only indicated in those patients with recurrent symptoms. Care must be taken to ensure that underlying disease other than appendicitis has been excluded (e.g. caecal carcinoma and Crohn's disease).

References

1. Ellis H, Thompson JN, Parker MC, et al. Adhesion-related hospital re-admissions after abdominal and pelvic surgery: a retrospective study. Lancet 1999;353:1476–9.

2. Tingstedt B, Isaksson J, Andersson R. Long-term follow-up and cost analysis following surgery for small bowel obstruction caused by intra-abdominal adhesions. Br J Surg 2007;94:743–8.

3. Attard AR, Corlett MJ, Kidner NJ, et al. Safety of early pain relief for acute abdominal pain. Br Med J 1992;30:554–6.

4. Zielinski MD, Eiken PW, Bannon MP, et al. Small bowel obstruction-who needs an operation? A multivariate prediction model. World J Surg 2010;34(5):910–9.

5. Branco BC, Barmparas G, Schnüriger B, et al. Systematic review and meta-analysis of the diagnostic and therapeutic role of water-soluble contrast agent in adhesive small bowel obstruction. Br J Surg 2010;97(4):470–8.

6. Catena F, Di Saverio S, Kelly MD, et al. Bologna Guidelines for diagnosis and management of adhesive small bowel obstruction (ASBO): 2010 evidence-based guidelines of the World Society of Emergency Surgery. World J Emerg Surg 2011;6:5.

7. Catena F, Ansaloni L, Di Saverio S, et al. P.O.P.A. study: prevention of postoperative abdominal adhesions by icodextrin 4% solution after laparotomy for adhesive small bowel obstruction. A prospective randomized controlled trial. J Gastrointest Surg 2012;16(2):382–8.

8. Walsh HPJ, Schofield PE. Is laparotomy for small bowel obstruction justified in patients with previously treated malignancy? Br J Surg 1984;71:933–5.

9. Nakane Y, Okumura S, Akehira K, et al. Management of intestinal obstruction after gastrectomy for carcinoma. Br J Surg 1996;83:133.

10. Parker MC, Baines MJ. Intestinal obstruction in patients with advanced malignant disease. Br J Surg 1996;83:12.

11. Sajja SBS, Schein M. Early post-operative small bowel obstruction. Br J Surg 2004;91:683–91.

12. Grafen FC, Neuhaus V, Schöb O, et al. Management of acute small bowel obstruction from intestinal adhesions: indications for laparoscopic surgery in a community teaching hospital. Langenbecks Arch Surg 2010;395(1):57–63.

13. Paterson-Brown S. Emergency laparoscopic surgery. Br J Surg 1993;80:279–83.

14. Thompson-Fawcett MW, Mortensen NJMcC. Crohn's disease. In: Phillips RKS, editor. Colorectal surgery. 5th ed. Edinburgh: Elsevier; in press [chapter 10].

15. Mowat C, Cole A, Windsor A, et al., IBD Section of the British Society of Gastroenterology. Guidelines for the management of inflammatory bowel disease in adults. Gut 2011;60(5):571–607.

16. Newton WB, Sagransky MJ, Andrews JS, et al. Outcomes of revascularized acute mesenteric ischemia in the American College of Surgeons National Surgical Quality Improvement Program database. Am Surg 2011;77(7):832–8.

17. Schoots IG, Koffeman DA, Levi M, et al. Systematic review of survival after acute mesenteric ischaemia according to disease aetiology. Br J Surg 2004;91:17–27.
Data from 45 observational studies including 3692 patients were reviewed. Prognosis after acute mesenteric venous thrombosis is better than for arterial ischaemia, and that for arterial embolism is better than that for arterial thrombosis.

18. Palmer K, Nairn M, Guideline Development Group. Management of acute gastrointestinal blood loss: summary of SIGN guidelines. Br Med J 2008;337:a1832.

19. Dixon JM, Elton RA, Rainey IB, et al. Rectal examination in patients with pain in the right lower quadrant of the abdomen. Br Med J 1991;302:386–8.

20. Rao PM, Rhea JT, Novelline RA, et al. Effect of computed tomography of the appendix on treatment of patients and use of hospital resources. N Engl J Med 1998;338:141–6.

21. Krajewski S, Brown J, Phang PT, et al. Impact of computed tomography of the abdomen on clinical outcomes in patients with acute right lower quadrant pain: a meta-analysis. Can J Surg 2011;54(1):43–53.

22. Moss JG, Barrie JL, Gunn AA. Delay in surgery for acute appendicitis. J R Coll Surg Edinb 1985;30:290–3.

23. Temple CL, Huchcroft SA, Temple WJ. The natural history of appendicitis in adults. A prospective study. Ann Surg 1995;221:278–81.

24. McLean AD, Stonebridge PA, Bradbury AW, et al. Time of presentation, time of operation, and unnecessary appendicectomy. Br Med J 1993;306:307.

25. Surana R, Quinn F, Puri P. Is it necessary to perform appendicectomy in the middle of the night in children? Br Med J 1993;306:1168.

26. Engstrom L, Fenvo G. Appendicectomy: assessment of stump invagination: a prospective, randomised trial. Br J Surg 1985;72:971–2.

27. Andersen BR, Kallehave FL, Andersen HK. Antibiotics versus placebo for prevention of postoperative infection after appendicectomy [update of Cochrane Database Syst Rev 2003;(2):CD001439. Cochrane Database Syst Rev 2005;(3): CD001439.
This systematic review confirmed the advantage of prophylactic antibiotics in reducing wound infection following appendicectomy.

28. SIGN guideline 104. Antibiotic prophylaxis in surgery. Scottish Intercollegiate Guideline Network; July 2008. www.sign.ac.uk.
This guideline demonstrated that prophylactic antibiotics during appendicectomy reduced wound infection with an odds ratio of 0.33 and the number needed to treat to prevent one wound infection being 11.

29. Fraser JD, Aguayo P, Leys CM, et al. A complete course of intravenous antibiotics vs a combination of intravenous and oral antibiotics for perforated appendicitis in children: a prospective, randomized trial. J Pediatr Surg 2010;45(6):1198–202.

30. Cox MR, McCall JL, Toouli J, et al. Prospective randomized comparison of open versus laparoscopic appendectomy in men. World J Surg 1996;20:263–6.

31. Hansen JB, Smithers BM, Schache D, et al. Laparoscopic versus open appendectomy: prospective randomised trial. World J Surg 1996;20:17–21.

32. Reiertsen O, Larsen S, Trondsen E, et al. Randomised controlled trial with sequential design of laparoscopic versus conventional appendicectomy. Br J Surg 1997;84:842–7.

33. Hellberg A, Rudberg C, Kullman E, et al. Prospective randomised multicentre study of laparoscopic versus open appendicectomy. Br J Surg 1999;86:48–53.

34. Katkhouda N, Mason RJ, Towfigh S, et al. Laparoscopic versus open appendectomy: a prospective randomized double-blind study. Ann Surg 2005;242(3):439–48.

35. Kouhia ST, Heiskanen JT, Huttunen R, et al. Long-term follow-up of a randomized clinical trial of open versus laparoscopic appendectomy. Br J Surg 2010;97:1395–400.

36. Sauerland S, Jaschinski T, Neugebauer EA. Laparoscopic versus open surgery for suspected appendicitis. Cochrane Database Syst Rev 2010;(10)CD001546.

37. Paterson HM, Qadan M, de Luca SM, et al. Changing trends in surgery for acute appendicitis. Br J Surg 2008;95:363–8.

38. Milne AA, Bradbury AW. 'Residual' appendicitis following incomplete laparoscopic appendicectomy. Br J Surg 1996;83:217.

39. Andersson REB. Small bowel obstruction after appendicectomy. Br J Surg 2001;88:1387–91.

40. Chang FC, Hogle HH, Welling DR. The fate of the negative appendix. Am J Surg 1973;126:752–4.

41. Deutsch AA, Shani N, Reiss R. Are some appendicectomies unnecessary? J R Coll Surg Edinb 1983;28:35–40.

42. Lau WY, Fan ST, Yiu TF, et al. The clinical significance of routine histopathological study of the resected appendix and safety of appendiceal inversion. Surg Gynecol Obstet 1986;162:256–8.

43. Wang Y, Reen DJ, Puri P. Is a histologically normal appendix following emergency appendicectomy always normal? Lancet 1996;347:1076–9.

44. Champault G, Taffinder N, Ziol M, et al. Recognition of a pathological appendix during laparoscopy: a prospective study of 81 cases. Br J Surg 1997;84:671.

45. Barber MD, McLaren J, Rainey JB. Recurrent appendicitis. Br J Surg 1997;84:110–2.

46. Eriksson S, Granstrom L. Randomised controlled trial of appendicectomy versus antibiotic therapy for acute appendicitis. Br J Surg 1995;82:166–9.

47. Styrud J, Eriksson S, Nilsson I, et al. Appendectomy versus antibiotic treatment in acute appendicitis. A prospective multicentre randomized controlled trial. World J Surg 2006;30:1033–7.

48. Hansson J, Korner U, Khorram-Manesh A, et al. Randomised clinical trial of antibiotic therapy versus appendicectomy as primary treatment of acute appendicitis in unselected patients. Br J Surg 2009;96:473–81.

49. Vons C, Barry C, Maitre S, et al. Amoxicillin plus clavulanic acid versus appendicectomy for treatment of acute uncomplicated appendicitis: an open-label, non-inferiority, randomised controlled trial. Lancet 2011;377(9777):1573–9.

50. Wilms I, de Hoog D, de Visser DC. Appendectomy versus antibiotic treatment for acute appendicitis. Cochrane Database Syst Rev 2011;(11): CD008359.

51. Simillis C, Symeonides P, Shorthouse AJ, et al. A meta-analysis comparing conservative treatment versus acute appendectomy for complicated appendicitis (abscess or phlegmon). Surgery 2010;147(6): 818–29.

52. Bagi P, Dueholm S. Nonoperative management of the ultrasonically evaluated appendiceal mass. Surgery 1987;101:602–5.

53. Deakin DE, Ahmed I. Interval appendicectomy after resolution of adult inflammatory appendix mass – is it necessary? Surgeon 2007;5(1):45–50.
A systematic review confirming that non-operative management will be successful in the majority of patients and recurrence of symptoms is low.

54. Hurme T, Nyalamo E. Conservative versus operative treatment of appendicular abscess. Ann Chir Gynaecol 1995;84:33–6.

55. Oliak D, Yamini D, Udani VM, et al. Initial non-operative management for periappendiceal abscess. Dis Colon Rectum 2001;44:936–41.

56. Roumen RM, Groenendijk RP, Sloots CE, et al. Randomized clinical trial evaluating elective laparoscopic appendicectomy for chronic right lower-quadrant pain. Br J Surg 2008;95(2):169–74.

57. Walsh CA, Tang T, Walsh SR, et al. Laparoscopic versus open appendicectomy in pregnancy: a systematic review. Int J Surg 2008;6:339–44.

58. McGory ML, Zingmond DS, Tillou A, et al. Negative appendectomy in pregnant women is associated with a substantial risk of fetal loss. J Am Coll Surg 2007;205(4):534–40.

59. Guidelines for Diagnosis, Treatment, and Use of Laparoscopy for Surgical Problems during

Pregnancy. Society of American Gastrointestinal and Endoscopic Surgeons (SAGES); January 2011.

60. Salam IMA, Fallouji MA, El Ashaal YI, et al. Early patient discharge following appendicectomy: safety and feasibility. J R Coll Surg Edinb 1995;40:300–2.

61. Dahl IB, Moiniche S, Kehle H. Wound infiltration with local anaesthetics for post-operative pain relief. Acta Anaesthesiol Scand 1994;38:7–14.

62. Turner GA, Chalkiadis G. Comparison of preoperative with postoperative lignocaine infiltration on postoperative analgesic requirements. Br J Anaesth 1994;72:541–3.

63. Okoye BO, Rampersad B, Marantos A, et al. Abscess after appendicectomy in children: the role of conservative management. Br J Surg 1998;85:1111–3.

64. Baigrie RJ, Dehn TCB, Fowler SM, et al. Analysis of 8651 appendicectomies in England and Wales during 1992. Br J Surg 1995;82:933.

65. Mueller BA, Daling JR, Moore DE, et al. Appendectomy and the risk of tubal infertility. N Engl J Med 1986;315:1506–7.

66. Andersson R, Lambe M, Bergstrom R. Fertility patterns after appendicectomy: historical cohort study. Br Med J 1999;318:963–7.

10

Colonic emergencies

David E. Beck

Introduction

Emergency conditions of the large bowel are common and changes in their evaluation and management have continued. Rather than rushing the patient to the operating room after a token resuscitation, current standards suggest that an initial appropriate period of resuscitation along with physiological and radiological evaluation should be undertaken. Many patients with colonic conditions can be managed non-operatively with bowel rest, antibiotics and blood components. Comorbid disease such as cardiac, pulmonary and metabolic conditions are optimised and critically ill patients are monitored in an intensive care setting. If adequate facilities and personnel are not readily available, transfer to a tertiary care facility should be considered if the patient can be readily stabilised.

The operative mortality for emergency colon resections is two to three times that associated with elective resection. As a result, surgeons have investigated ways of stabilising patients in order to convert emergency into more planned, elective procedures. Deciding if and when to operate can be difficult, and active observation and consultation with colleagues is often helpful in the decision-making process. Active participation of the attending/consultant surgeon in both the assessment and operative procedure is essential in this group of very challenging patients.

When emergency surgery is necessary, there has been a clear trend towards single rather than staged procedures for large-bowel disorders. When feasible, this approach reduces the length of hospital stay and avoids the risks of multiple operations. However, in some unfit or acutely septic patients, a staged approach may still be preferable.

Preparation for operation

Patients should be adequately informed of their likely diagnosis and management options. Alternatives and risks as well as the potential need for a stoma should be explained carefully. Patients requiring emergency large-bowel surgery should be marked for potential stoma sites and if possible participation of a stoma therapist arranged.

The risk of postoperative deep vein thrombosis and pulmonary embolus is substantial in this group of patients, and prophylactic measures are essential. Options include intermittent pneumatic calf compression and subcutaneous low-molecular-weight heparin. Prophylactic antibiotic therapy is standard, with broad-spectrum single-dose therapy as effective as multiple-dose regimens. The duration of prophylactic antibiotics should be less than 24 hours. If significant infection or contamination is found intraoperatively, empirical therapeutic antibiotics may be indicated.

Disease process

Colonic emergencies can be divided into ischaemia, obstruction, perforation and bleeding. These categories will be discussed in turn, with attention to their pathophysiology, evaluation and management.

Colonic ischaemia

Although the colon has a generous overlapping blood supply, any interruption in blood flow produces ischaemia. Anatomical locations that have the potential to be vulnerable to ischaemic disease include: Griffith's point at the splenic flexure (junction of the superior mesenteric artery (SMA) and the inferior mesenteric artery (IMA)); Sudeck's critical point at the mid-sigmoid colon (junction of the IMA and hypogastric vasculature); and the caecum (distal distribution of the SMA).

Aetiological factors and pathophysiology

As outlined in Box 10.1, colonic ischaemia can result from a number of conditions.

Interruption of flow in large vessels following aortic surgery varies from 1–2% for elective cases to as high as 60% during emergency aneurysm repair.[1] Sudden occlusion of the IMA can also occur as a result of angiographic trauma with subintimal dissection or as a result of either blunt or penetrating abdominal trauma. Atheromatous narrowing or occlusion of the IMA is not unusual. However, in most cases this occurs gradually, and the collateral circulation from the SMA can compensate for the decrease in flow through collateral circulation via the marginal artery. If the IMA becomes acutely thrombosed or occluded with an embolus and the collateral circulation is inadequate, the clinical picture will be similar to that found after IMA ligation during aortic surgery.

Any of the connective tissue diseases that produce inflammation in the small-intestinal arteries (intrinsic small-vessel disease) can also result in colonic ischaemia.[2] Another variant of ischaemic colitis occurs in patients who are severely ill with conditions that cause hypotension, decreased cardiac output or peripheral vasoconstriction, with a decreased flow to the end organ (low-flow states). This group of patients appears to have a higher incidence of

full-thickness necrosis and right-sided involvement than do those with spontaneous ischaemic colitis who were previously well. The mortality associated with colonic infarction in these patients who are severely ill from another disease process is extremely high. In one report of 17 such patients the mortality rate was 57%.[3] One must therefore have a very high index of suspicion for full-thickness necrosis in this group of patients and be ready to intervene early.

Spontaneous ischaemic colitis may occur without any demonstrable vessel occlusion on angiography.[4] The pathological changes seen in the colon are identical to those caused by vessel occlusion and resulting decreased in blood flow to the colon. The spectrum of disease varies from mild submucosal oedema to frank full-thickness necrosis. Most cases are the milder self-limiting variety that are typically seen in middle-aged or elderly patients, often following episodes of dehydration. In younger patients, who are mostly women, there has been an association between ischaemic colitis and the use of oral contraceptive drugs.[5]

Diagnosis

Colonic ischaemia usually presents in one of two ways. The milder cases are manifest by diffuse and/or bloody diarrhoea. Patients with frank colonic infarction frequently develop acidosis, glucose intolerance, renal failure, obvious sepsis, and abdominal distension or tenderness. The diagnosis of postoperative ischaemia can be made with flexible sigmoidoscopy performed at the bedside. If the symptoms are not explained by flexible sigmoidoscopy, a colonoscopy may occasionally be required to rule out more proximal disease. The endoscopic appearance of colonic ischaemia may range from submucosal oedema with haemorrhage and ulceration to the dusky blue mucosal colour of infarction. Frank gangrene mandates immediate surgery and resection; however, the colon with just mucosal oedema and haemorrhage may be watched closely.

The diagnosis can be made with endoscopy, barium enema or computed tomography (CT). Endoscopy can be performed in the office or at the bedside and the pathological state can be viewed directly (**Fig. 10.1**). CT is rapidly becoming more common and ischaemia presents as thickened bowel wall (**Fig. 10.2**).

There are three possible outcomes of ischaemic colitis:

1. Resolution of the process is the most common clinical course.
2. Progression to full-thickness necrosis is unusual, especially if there is no evidence of gangrenous bowel at the first examination.
3. The condition may evolve to an ulcerative stage, which may eventually result in stricture formation.

Box 10.1 • Classification of ischaemic colitis

I. Interruption of flow in large vessels
  A. Following ligation during aortic surgery
  B. Injury secondary to angiographic, blunt or penetrating trauma
  C. Spontaneous thrombosis of large vessels
II. Intrinsic small-vessel disease
III. Low-flow state in the critically ill
IV. Spontaneous ischaemic colitis without demonstrable vessel occlusion
  A. Self-limiting without sequelae
  B. With subsequent stricture formation
V. Miscellaneous
  A. Secondary to luminal obstruction
  B. Young adults
  C. Renal allograft recipients

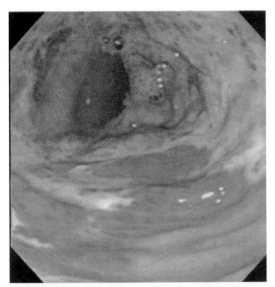

Figure 10.1 • Endoscopic view of colonic ischaemia.

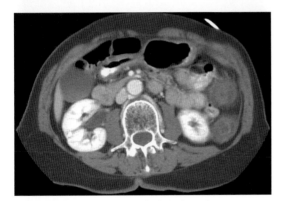

Figure 10.2 • CT scan of colonic ischaemia.

During the ulcerative stage the endoscopic and radiographic findings may mimic Crohn's disease. Occasionally the early phases of this disease will go unnoticed or undiagnosed, and the patient will present with a stricture.

Ischaemic colitis may also be associated with a complete or partial bowel obstruction. In one reported series,[6] 10% of patients with colonic ischaemia had an associated carcinoma and another 10% had some other condition that potentially interfered with colonic motility. When ischaemic colitis occurs in association with tumour, the ischaemic area is usually proximal to the tumour and may or may not be associated with obstruction. The investigators in this study and others speculated that colonic blood flow could be decreased as a consequence of increased intraluminal pressure, hyperperistalsis with increased muscular spasm,

and resultant diminution of blood flow in the colonic wall, or a decrease in aortic blood pressure and vena caval return with straining in obstructive lesions.[7] Knowledge of this association is of obvious importance to avoid using ischaemic bowel for an anastomosis.

Treatment

If the diagnosis of ischaemic colitis is made early, non-operative treatment is warranted in the first instance. Mild cases can be managed on an outpatient basis with a clear liquid diet, close observation and possibly antibiotic therapy. More serious cases require hospitalisation, bowel rest, nasogastric suction (if there are any signs of ileus), and optimisation of blood flow to the mucosa (intravenous hydration and optimisation of cardiac output). If the patient is receiving digitalis, a serum level should be checked because toxic digitalis levels can have a marked vasoconstrictive effect on visceral circulation. Parenteral antibiotics (such as a second- or third-generation cephalosporin) are used by some surgeons because of the suggestion that colonic ischaemia may allow colonic bacterial transmigration, although there are no strong data to support or refute their use. Patients with ischaemia resulting from arteritides may respond to corticosteroid treatment.

Specific indications for surgery include peritonitis, perforation, sepsis and failure of non-operative therapy. At operation a wide resection of non-viable colon is performed. Primary anastomosis is usually unsafe because of the potential for postoperative progression of the ischaemia. A double-barrel stoma or end stoma and separate mucous fistula is safer and allows assessment of the bowel viability in the postoperative period. The mortality rate for ischaemic colitis among renal transplant patients is 70%.[2] Diagnostic manoeuvres should therefore be initiated at the first suspicion of ischaemia in these high-risk patients, and surgery should be aggressive once the diagnosis is made (resection of any compromised bowel with an end stoma). Primary anastomosis after resection is ill advised in these patients.

Colonic obstruction

Colonic volvulus

Volvulus can be defined as a twisting or torsion of bowel around its mesentery and occurs most commonly in the sigmoid colon (76%), but also in the caecum (22%) and the transverse colon (2%).[8] One report suggested that 40–60% of patients have had previous episodes of obstruction.[9] In the USA, volvulus represents a rare cause of intestinal obstruction, encompassing less than 5% of large-bowel obstructions. However, worldwide it may represent more than 50% of the cases in some countries.[10]

Sigmoid volvulus

The sigmoid colon rotates through 180–720° in either a clockwise or anticlockwise direction to produce the volvulus.[11] A narrowed sigmoid mesocolon provides a pedicle for rotation. The condition is occasionally associated with Chagas' disease and Hirschsprung's disease, in which redundancy of the colon is a feature, in addition to non-specific motility disorders of the colon.[12]

A typical patient with a sigmoid volvulus presents with abdominal pain, constipation and feeling bloated. On examination there is marked distension, which is often asymmetrical. Severe pain and tenderness, associated with tachycardia and hypotension, may suggest colonic ischaemia. Patients who develop sigmoid volvulus in the industrialised world tend to be older, and one-third either have mental illness or are institutionalised.[12]

Findings on the plain abdominal radiograph are often characteristic. Massive distension of the sigmoid colon is visible; the bowel loses its haustration and extends in an inverted U from the pelvis to the right upper quadrant of the abdomen (**Fig. 10.3**). Fluid levels are seen in both limbs of the loop on the erect film, commonly at different levels ('pair of scales'). In one-third of patients, the appearances are atypical and a water-soluble contrast enema should be carried out. This may demonstrate narrowing of the contrast column at the point of twisting, which has been described as resembling the beak of a bird of prey.

Volvulus patients often present with significant fluid and electrolyte abnormalities, which require careful correction. **Untwisting and decompression** are the initial treatments of choice as long as the patient lacks clinical features suggestive of colonic strangulation. Untwisting has been described using several techniques, including rigid or flexible sigmoidoscopy, colonoscopy, blind passage of a rectal tube, and instillation of rectal contrast during a barium enema examination.[13–15] The endoscopic method of decompression has the advantage that decompression can be done under vision, increasing the accuracy of insertion through the twisted segment in the sigmoid colon. In addition, the mucosa of the whole sigmoid loop can be visualised directly and the identification of gangrenous mucosal patches is an indication for operative management.

If symptoms and signs suggest ischaemia of the colon, **laparotomy** should be undertaken after the patient has been adequately resuscitated. Likewise, the patient who has unsuccessful non-operative treatment and those who have clinical features suggestive of colonic

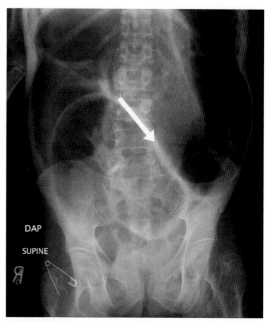

Figure 10.3 • Radiograph of the abdomen demonstrates the characteristic massive dilation of the sigmoid colon arising from the pelvis and extending to the right diaphragm. The arrow points to three lines representing the twisted walls of the sigmoid colon, which converge in the left lower quadrant.

ischaemia at colonoscopy should also undergo emergency laparotomy. Since it is likely that resection will be required, the patient should be placed in the lithotomy/Trendelenburg position on the operating table. If colonic distension makes it difficult to handle the colon, a needle inserted obliquely through a taenia coli attached to a suction apparatus aids decompression. If the colon is gangrenous, it should be resected with as little manipulation as possible; the most widely recommended procedure is a segmental colectomy with an end colostomy and closure of the rectal stump (Hartmann's operation). In a prospective randomised trial from West Africa, Bagarani et al. compared the operative treatment in 31 patients with or without gangrene.[16] When gangrene was present, the mortality for Hartmann's procedure was 12.5% compared with 33.3% when resection and anastomosis were performed.

A small number of surgeons have described resection and primary anastomosis with good results. A study from India reported 197 patients with acute sigmoid volvulus treated by single-stage resection and anastomosis, 23 of whom had gangrene of the bowel.[17] Only two patients had anastomotic leaks, both of which responded to non-operative management. The two mortalities occurred in elderly patients who presented with perforations. A study from Ghana reported 21 patients with acute sigmoid volvulus treated by single-stage resection and anastomosis, 15 of whom had gangrene of the bowel.[18] Only one patient had a minor anastomotic leak, which responded to conservative management. However, it is important to stress that the majority of the patients in these studies were young and these results may not be applicable to the typical Western patient. In contrast, a series from the USA with 228 patients reported a mortality rate of 24% for emergency operations and 6% for elective operations. This study found mortality to correlate with emergency surgery and necrotic colon.[14]

Intraoperative colonic irrigation may facilitate primary anastomosis in patients with sigmoid volvulus who require emergency operation, since faecal loading proximal to the volvulus may increase the risk of anastomotic dehiscence. However, it is still important that only patients who are generally fit and without systemic sepsis and peritoneal contamination are selected for this procedure.

Because the risk of recurrent volvulus after decompression and de-rotation has been reported to be between 40% and 60%,[9] elective surgery to prevent further volvulus should always be considered. The most widely accepted procedure is resection, which is now associated with an operative mortality of 2–3%. The operation may be performed as a laparoscopic-assisted procedure through a small incision under local anaesthesia if required.

A variety of fixation procedures have been described but have been associated with high recurrence rates.[15]

Ileosigmoid knotting

Ileosigmoid knotting is a variant of sigmoid volvulus in which the ileum twists around the base of the mesocolon (**Fig. 10.4**). It is also known as double volvulus. Three factors are responsible for ileosigmoid knotting: (i) a long small-bowel mesentery and freely mobile small bowel; (ii) a long sigmoid colon on a narrow pedicle; and (iii) ingestion of high-bulk diet in the presence of empty small bowel.[19]

The condition is characterised by very acute onset of agonising generalised abdominal pain and repeated vomiting. Gangrene of the ileum and sigmoid colon is common. Generalised peritonitis, sepsis and dehydration are recognised complications, with hypovolaemic shock occurring early. The erect plain abdominal radiograph shows a dilated sigmoid colon and fluid levels in the small bowel.

Initial management consists of resuscitation and administration of antibiotics followed by surgical intervention. Resection and anastomosis of the terminal ileum and a Hartmann procedure is the most commonly performed operation. Recent reports suggest that primary colonic anastomosis can be

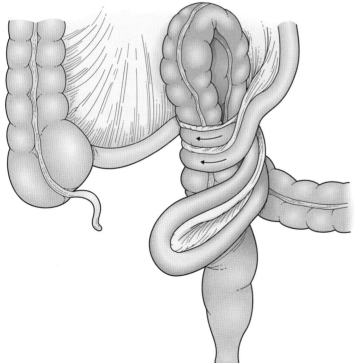

Figure 10.4 • Ileosigmoid knotting.

undertaken safely when there is a short history and the colon is clean and well vascularised. The condition unfortunately carries a very high mortality rate, ranging from 15% to 73%.[20]

Transverse colon volvulus

Volvulus affecting the transverse colon is less common than sigmoid volvulus, accounting for only 2.6% of all cases of colonic volvulus in one series.[21] Predisposing conditions include pregnancy, chronic constipation, distal colonic obstruction and previous gastric surgery. The plain abdominal radiograph usually shows gas-filled loops of large intestine with wide fluid levels. The condition is often mistaken for sigmoid volvulus and the diagnosis is rarely made preoperatively. After the operative diagnosis is confirmed and the transverse colon untwisted, evidence of distal obstruction should be sought. Operative choices include a transverse colectomy or an extended right hemicolectomy.

A primary anastomosis after resection is probably safe. However, in the presence of gangrenous bowel and significant peritoneal contamination, the safest approach may be to resect the affected colon and exteriorise both ends.

Caecal volvulus

Volvulus of the caecum is less common than volvulus of the sigmoid colon, representing 28% of all cases of colonic volvulus reported over a 10-year period in Edinburgh.[22] It is likely that incomplete rotation of the midgut leaves the caecum and ascending colon inadequately fixed to the posterior abdominal wall with a substantial length of mesentery. Conditions that alter the normal anatomy may predispose to caecal volvulus. There is an increased risk of caecal volvulus in pregnancy, and some patients are found to have adhesions from previous surgery. There is also an association with distal colonic obstruction. Volvulus usually takes place in a clockwise direction around the ileocolic vessels and, although the term 'caecal volvulus' is used, the condition also involves the ascending colon and ileum. As it twists, the caecum comes to occupy a position above and to the left of its original position. A similar condition, which is seen very occasionally, is 'caecal bascule'. In this condition, the caecum folds upwards on itself, producing a sharp kink in the ascending colon.

It is difficult to differentiate between caecal volvulus and other forms of proximal large-bowel obstruction on clinical grounds. Some patients will have a previous history of episodes of obstruction that subsequently settled with non-operative treatment. The main presenting symptoms are colicky abdominal pain and vomiting. A tympanitic abdominal swelling will usually be present in the mid-abdomen.

On the supine abdominal radiograph, a 'comma'-shaped caecal shadow in the mid-abdomen or left

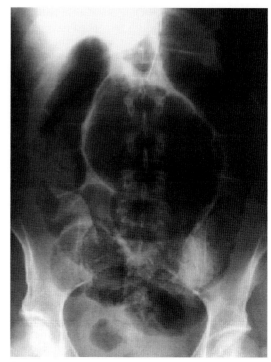

Figure 10.5 • Abdominal radiograph demonstrates a massively dilated caecum folded over into the left upper quadrant with distended small bowel.

upper quadrant with a concavity to the right iliac fossa is diagnostic (**Fig. 10.5**) and there may be small-bowel loops lying to the right side of the caecum. A single, long fluid level on the erect film is characteristic. If doubt persists, a contrast enema will show a beaked appearance in the ascending colon at the site of the volvulus (**Fig. 10.6**).

Management depends on the clinical picture. The patient who is unfit for surgical treatment can be considered for colonoscopy since occasional successes have been reported using this method.[23] However, laparotomy is necessary in most patients. If the right colon is gangrenous at operation, the treatment of choice is a right hemicolectomy. A primary anastomosis should be possible in most cases even in the presence of contamination of the peritoneal cavity. It should be remembered that there is a markedly increased mortality in patients who have caecal gangrene. A report from the Mayo Clinic found a mortality rate of 12% in patients with caecal volvulus with a viable caecum, rising to 33% in the presence of colonic gangrene.[24]

There is more controversy about the procedure of choice in patients who have a viable caecum after reduction of the volvulus. On the one hand untwisting alone is associated with a high recurrence rate, but on the other hand resection, which avoids all risk of recurrence, carries a small risk of anastomotic leak.

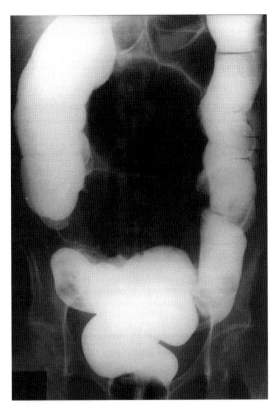

Figure 10.6 • Water-soluble contrast enema demonstrates a beak-like termination at the point of obstruction in the ascending colon with a markedly dilated caecum seen high in the abdomen.

However, in one study of 22 patients there was no mortality and no anastomotic leaks. A 14% morbidity included one abdominal wall abscess, one intra-abdominal abscess and one medical complication.[25] The other two procedures commonly performed for caecal volvulus are caecostomy and caecopexy. Reports on the use of caecostomy demonstrate a wide variation in terms of both recurrence (0–25%) and mortality (0–33%). Some authors express concern over the morbidity of caecostomy and the occasional serious complication of abdominal wall sepsis and fasciitis, in addition to the potential for a persistent fistula.

✅ The treatment of caecal volvulus has been reviewed in a large study comprising 561 published cases.[26] This review showed that caecopexy was associated with a mortality rate of 10% and a recurrence rate of 13%. If all circumstances are favourable, resection appears to be a justifiable procedure with minimal risk of recurrence, accepting that there may be a small number of patients who will have increased bowel frequency. In other circumstances, the minimum procedure compatible with survival becomes the goal.

Acute colonic pseudo-obstruction

Acute colonic pseudo-obstruction (ACPO) is the term used to describe the syndrome in which patients present with symptoms and signs of large-bowel obstruction but in whom no mechanical cause can be demonstrated at contrast radiology. In more than 80% of patients with ACPO, an underlying precipitating condition exists, of which at least 50 have been described.[27] The most common of these associated conditions are metabolic disorders, trauma and cardiorespiratory disease (Box 10.2). The term 'Ogilvie's syndrome' is loosely used in the literature as a synonym for ACPO, although it was actually used first to describe the pseudo-obstruction associated with retroperitoneal malignant infiltration. The mortality rate of ACPO is high, partly as a result of the underlying disorders but also related to failure to recognise the condition, leading to inappropriate operation. The true incidence is hard to ascertain since a number of unrecognised cases are likely to resolve spontaneously and diagnostic criteria are variable. However, it has been estimated that some 200 deaths per annum in the UK may result from ACPO.[28]

Aetiology

The state of colonic motility at any point in time is determined by a balance of the inhibitory influence of the sympathetic nervous supply and the stimulatory effect of the parasympathetic system. It has been suggested that 'neuropraxia' of the sacral parasympathetic nerves may be a factor in the aetiology of ACPO, leading to a failure of propulsion in the left colon. This would also explain the 'cut-off' between dilated and collapsed bowel, which is located on the left side of the large bowel in 82% of patients.[29] Many of the conditions commonly associated with ACPO, such as sepsis, are likely to result from sympathetic overactivity.

Presentation

The clinical features of ACPO are almost identical to those of mechanical large-bowel obstruction, making

---

Box 10.2 • Predisposing conditions in acute colonic pseudo-obstruction

Chest infection
Myocardial infarction
Cerebrovascular accident
Renal failure
Puerperium
Retroperitoneal malignancy (Ogilvie's syndrome)
Orthopaedic trauma
Myxoedema
Electrolyte disturbance

differentiation on clinical grounds alone almost impossible. In a review of 400 patients it was noted that the clinical features of ACPO were abdominal pain (83%), constipation (51%), diarrhoea (41%), fever (37%) and abdominal distension (100%).[29] On examination, the abdomen is generally very distended and tympanitic, but tenderness is often less than expected. The majority of patients will already have had operative procedures or have been hospitalised for some time because of some other disorder, and serum electrolytes are often abnormal.

Investigation (see also Chapter 5)

Plain radiographs of the abdomen in ACPO typically show gross distension of the large bowel with cut-off at the splenic flexure, rectosigmoid junction or, less commonly, the hepatic flexure (**Fig. 10.7**). Gas–fluid levels are less commonly seen on the plain radiograph in patients with ACPO compared with those presenting with mechanical obstruction.[30] It has been suggested that a prone lateral view of the rectum may be useful in making the diagnosis since gaseous filling of the rectum will tend to exclude mechanical obstruction. The caecal diameter should

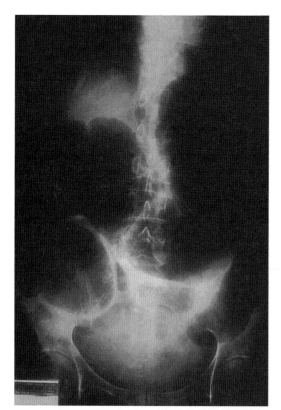

Figure 10.7 • Plain abdominal radiograph of a patient with acute colonic pseudo-obstruction.

be measured on sequential abdominal radiographs since it is believed that the risk of caecal rupture increases greatly with increasing caecal diameter.[30]

> ✓✓ There is overwhelming support for the use of a contrast enema in all patients with suspected ACPO in order to establish the diagnosis, since the differentiation from mechanical obstruction can be extremely difficult. This is well illustrated in a study reported by Koruth et al., who performed a contrast enema on 91 patients with suspected large-bowel obstruction.[31] Of the 79 patients who were thought clinically to have mechanical obstruction, the diagnosis was confirmed in 50. There was free flow of contrast to the caecum in the remaining 29 patients. Of these 29, 11 had non-obstructing colonic pathology such as diverticular disease and ulcerative colitis and 18 patients had pseudo-obstruction. Of the 12 patients who were thought to have pseudo-obstruction before the water-soluble contrast enema, two were shown to have carcinoma of the colon.

Management

The initial management of ACPO is non-operative and the underlying cause is treated if possible. Any medications that cause gut stasis should be discontinued, particularly analgesics. A nasogastric tube is routinely inserted to prevent swallowed air from entering the intestine and the use of enemas and flatus tubes is said to be of value in the treatment of early colonic pseudo-obstruction; in a number of patients even the water-soluble contrast enema used to establish the diagnosis may have a useful therapeutic effect. In most patients, the condition will resolve without intervention. One study found that it took an average of 6.5 days for complete resolution to take place in a group of 26 patients treated medically.[30] Progress should be checked by serial examination of the abdomen and by abdominal radiographs.

It is only when the risk of perforation increases substantially that more active intervention becomes necessary. The risk of perforation is approximately 3% and it has been shown that there is a correlation between perforation and the duration of distension.[32] The mean duration of distension was 6 days in the group of patients who went on to perforate compared with a mean duration of only 2 days in the group that did not progress to perforation.

> ✓✓ In a randomised, double-blind, controlled trial of neostigmine only, 10 of 11 patients who were treated with intravenous neostigmine had prompt passage of flatus or stool, with reduced abdominal distension, compared with none of 10 patients who received placebo injection.[33]

These results were mirrored in a trial of 28 patients, with rapid resolution in 26. Time to pass flatus varied from 30 seconds to 10 minutes. In the two patients who failed to resolve, one was found to have a sigmoid cancer and the other died of multi-organ failure.[34] There is a risk of bradycardia with cholinergic agonists, and it has been suggested that patients with cardiac instability should not be treated with neostigmine. Interestingly, there is anecdotal evidence that the concomitant administration of glycopyrrolate with neostigmine seems to offset the risk of bradycardia and may be considered in patients with cardiac instability.[35] Epidural anaesthesia blocks sympathetic outflow, and improvement has been observed in a number of patients with ACPO who have had this form of treatment.[36]

The use of colonoscopy to decompress the colon in ACPO has become well established and it is successful in 73–90% of patients.[37] The procedure can be difficult and tedious, requiring a skilled colonoscopist, and air insufflation must be kept to a minimum. Frequent small-volume irrigation is required to ensure good visibility in the colon and maintain the patency of the colonoscope suction channel. A further advantage of colonoscopy is that necrotic patches can be identified on the colonic mucosa, allowing pre-emptive surgical treatment before perforation supervenes. The risk of perforation of the colon during colonoscopy for this condition has been estimated at around 3%,[38] and other complications are very unusual. It should be emphasised, however, that radiographs taken after successful clinical response often fail to show complete resolution of caecal distension, and one disadvantage of colonoscopic treatment is the tendency for the condition to recur. The overall rate of recurrence following initial colonoscopic decompression varies from 15% to 29%.[39] There is some difference of opinion about the best method of management of recurrent ACPO, but the safety and efficacy of repeat colonic decompression has now been reported.[27,37,39] A potential means of avoiding recurrence is intubation of the caecum with a long intestinal tube passed alongside the colonoscope.[40]

The indications for surgery include the following:

1. Caecal distension – the extent of distension varies between authors, from 9 to 12 cm,[41] the threshold rising with increasing availability of medical therapy.
2. Continuing caecal distension beyond 48–72 hours despite maximum medical therapy.
3. Pain over the right iliac fossa, i.e. the caecum.
4. Pneumoperitoneum.

There are doctors who recommend percutaneous caecostomies,[42] where a tube is inserted into the caecum using radiological guidance for the purpose of decompression. A trephine caecostomy may be performed under local anaesthesia. To avoid contamination, the caecum can be sutured to the incised external or internal oblique muscles and only opened when the peritoneal cavity is sealed off. Only when perforation of the caecum is suspected should a full laparotomy be performed. If a perforation or necrosis of the caecum has already occurred, a full laparotomy is necessary and a right hemicolectomy is the treatment of choice. When resection of the right colon is required, it is probably safest to bring out an ileostomy and mucous fistula and reanastomose the two ends of bowel at a later date. Primary anastomosis may be feasible if contamination of the peritoneal cavity is not a feature and the remaining colon looks healthy.

Malignant large-bowel obstruction

Approximately 85% of colonic emergencies are due to colon cancer and most of these occur in the elderly patient.[43] However, only 8–29% of colorectal cancer patients present with intestinal obstruction.[44] Approximately half of splenic flexure tumours present with obstruction, compared to 25% of those in the left colon, 6% of rectosigmoid lesions and 8–30% of right-sided carcinomas.[45] Both obstruction and perforation occur together in approximately 1% of all colon cancers, but in patients who have an obstruction caused by cancer, 12–19% will have a perforation.[44] The perforation may either be at the site of the tumour or in the caecum, caused by back pressure from the distal obstructing lesion.

The influence of obstruction on prognosis is controversial. Some studies suggest that the apparent adverse effect of obstruction on prognosis is a consequence of the stage of the disease rather than obstruction itself, as 27% have liver metastasis at the time of operation.[46] Other reports, however, suggest that obstruction is an independent predictor of poor prognosis.[47]

Presentation

Symptoms associated with large-bowel obstruction frequently reflect the site of the tumour. In right-sided obstruction, particularly at the level of the ileocaecal valve, the onset of colicky central abdominal pain may be quite sudden and vomiting a relatively early feature. If the obstruction is at the rectosigmoid junction, there may be a history of a change in bowel habit and of rectal bleeding, with vomiting uncommon.

On examination, abdominal distension is the most notable feature. Peritoneal irritation suggests that perforation is either imminent or may have already occurred. Palpation of an irregular liver edge suggests that liver metastasis may be present and a palpable mass on rectal examination obviously suggests a carcinoma of the rectum.

Investigation

Plain abdominal radiography will usually provide the diagnosis of large-bowel obstruction. The pattern of gas distribution in both the small and large bowel will depend on the site of obstruction and also on whether the ileocaecal valve is competent. However, as already mentioned, differentiation from ACPO requires a contrast enema.

> ✔✔ A water-soluble contrast enema (**Fig. 10.8**) should be carried out in all patients with suspected large-bowel obstruction without evidence of perforation.[31]

A water-soluble contrast enema will exclude other conditions such as volvulus or pseudo-obstruction and, in addition, may go some way to cleansing the colon distal to the obstructing lesion. Sigmoidoscopy or colonoscopy can be useful, particularly if the suspected obstructing lesion is in the distal colon. In addition, either technique can be used to exclude synchronous carcinoma or adenoma below the level of obstruction. CT with intravenous and water-soluble rectal contrast is increasingly used in the emergency setting and this has the added advantage of providing information on the spread of disease preoperatively (**Fig. 10.9**).

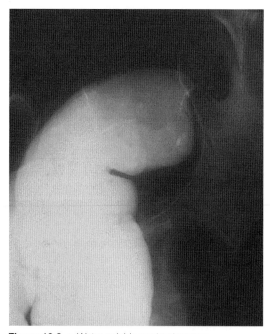

Figure 10.8 • Water-soluble contrast enema demonstrating complete obstruction in the proximal sigmoid colon.

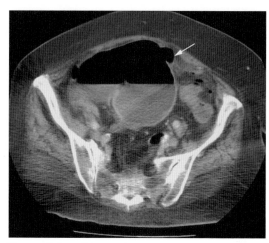

Figure 10.9 • CT scan of a patient with a perforated caecum (perforation indicated by arrow). The scan also revealed an obstructing splenic flexure tumour and extensive liver metastases.

Management

The morbidity and mortality rate associated with emergency procedures for obstruction of the colon is at least twice that for elective surgery. This has encouraged surgeons to develop methods such as the use of expandable intraluminal stents. These can be used to palliate patients or to convert emergency operations into elective procedures. Several colonic stents are currently available and can be placed using radiological or endoscopic assistance. Various models can be deployed over guidewires or through an endoscope.

A review of 54 case series that included 1198 patients[48] found that in 791 palliative patients, technical success was possible in 93% and clinical success (defined as decompression in less than 48 hours) in 91%. Stents also provided successful conversion to elective procedures in 92% of 407 patients. Intraluminal stenting was more successful in shorter, distal lesions and colonic primaries. Technical failure usually results from an inability to pass the guidewire or stent catheter across the lesion. Reported complications include perforation in 3.8%, stent migration in 12% and re-obstruction in 7%.

When surgery is undertaken, patients with right-sided obstruction should be positioned flat on the operating table. Those with left-sided large-bowel obstruction are placed in the lithotomy/Trendelenburg position to allow access to the anus during the procedure for purposes of irrigation of the rectal stump or anal insertion of a surgical stapling instrument. It also allows the surgical assistant the option of standing between the patient's legs. The abdomen is opened through a midline incision.

If the bowel is tense, it should be decompressed: first, to improve visualisation of the rest of the abdomen and, second, to prevent spillage of faecal content. The large bowel can be decompressed by inserting a 16 G intravenous catheter or 18 F nasogastric tube obliquely through the colonic wall, following which suction is applied. This is often enough to make it possible to handle the large bowel without fear of rupture as the distension is mainly gas. After localisation of the primary tumour, synchronous tumours should be excluded. The presence of direct spread to adjacent structures should also be assessed, in addition to any peritoneal seedlings and the presence of liver secondaries. Based on these observations, a decision can be made as to whether the operation is potentially curative or palliative.

When there is a prospect of curative resection, standard techniques of radical cancer therapy should be employed, including wide excision of the lesion en bloc with the appropriate blood vessels and mesentery. If the lesion is adherent to other structures, an attempt should be made to resect the affected part en bloc. High cure rates are possible with locally advanced tumours if a radical resection is performed and clear resection margins obtained. The presence of liver or peritoneal metastases does not preclude resection of the primary carcinoma and gastrointestinal continuity should be restored if at all possible.

If there is a closed loop obstruction because of competence of the ileocaecal valve, the caecum and right colon may be very tense. Decompression can be achieved as a preliminary to resection by making a small enterotomy in the terminal ileum and passing a Foley catheter through the ileocaecal valve into the caecum. This technique is particularly useful in situations where there is splitting of the taenia on the caecum, indicating impending rupture. The range of operations available for treatment of right-sided tumours causing obstruction includes right hemicolectomy with primary anastomosis, right hemicolectomy with exteriorisation of both ends of the large bowel, and ileo-transverse colon bypass. There is general agreement that a right hemicolectomy with primary anastomosis is the treatment of choice in most patients; however, this procedure is by no means free of complications. One report noted an operative mortality rate of 17% in 195 patients who had emergency right hemicolectomy with primary anastomosis for obstructing colonic carcinoma.[49] In addition, a leak rate of 10% was noted in 179 patients who had a right hemicolectomy and primary anastomosis for obstruction. This compares with a leak rate of 6% in 579 patients with right colon cancer who did not have an obstruction.[49] Other studies have shown similar mortality rates, and many of the deaths resulted from anastomotic failure. This suggests that instead of subjecting all patients with obstruction to right hemicolectomy with primary anastomosis, it may be wiser to use a policy of selection, subjecting patients with good risk status to primary anastomosis and managing patients with risk factors for anastomotic failure by resection and exteriorisation of the bowel ends.

The anastomotic technique used will depend on the surgeon's preference. If the obstructed bowel is very thickened and oedematous, care should be taken with the use of stapling instruments since there is a tendency for the instruments to cut through oedematous bowel. On these occasions a sutured anastomosis is preferable. Only on the relatively rare occasion when locally advanced disease is unresectable should the patient be subjected to an ileo-transverse colon bypass procedure. There is almost no place for caecostomy in the current management of right-sided large-bowel obstruction; trephine ileostomy, which can usually be achieved under local anaesthesia, affords better palliation in very sick patients not fit for operation under general anaesthesia.

Most surgeons would advocate an extended right hemicolectomy for patients with transverse colon carcinoma, and decompression of the colon may be necessary to facilitate mobilisation. For the patient who has a large carcinoma obstructing the transverse colon, achieving clearance may be difficult because of involvement of the transverse mesocolon and adjacent organs. The splenic flexure is mobilised to assist with a primary anastomosis between ileum and upper descending colon. In the sick patient who already has a perforated caecum, resection and an ileostomy may be appropriate.

For obstructing left-sided colonic tumours, the two most frequent options are resection and either primary anastomosis, or colostomy and rectal closure (Hartmann's procedure). A three-stage procedure (diverting colostomy, resection and colostomy closure) is now rarely used, and only in critically ill patients. Two-stage procedures became popular during the 1970s and remain the procedure of choice for most surgeons, with an overall mortality around 10%.[44] However, the main disadvantage of this approach, apart from the fact that a second operation is required for reconstruction, is that approximately 40% of patients will be left with a permanent stoma.

The second stage of the two-stage operation may be difficult because of adhesions, although it is facilitated if the rectal stump has been divided above the peritoneal reflection. The timing of the second stage is also important and most surgeons will wait 2–6 months. The second stage of the two-stage procedure is increasingly being performed using laparoscopic techniques. If successful the hospital stay is reduced, but conversion to open surgery may be necessary.

Primary resection and anastomosis is associated with a shorter hospital stay, reduced mortality and morbidity, and the avoidance of a stoma. It is increasingly becoming the operation of choice for colorectal surgeons, with the exact procedure depending on a number of factors. Subtotal colectomy followed by ileosigmoid or ileorectal anastomosis has been reported to have a low operative mortality of 3–11% and a hospital stay of around 15–20 days.[50] Segmental colectomy (left hemicolectomy, sigmoid colectomy or anterior resection of the rectosigmoid) with on-table irrigation followed by primary anastomosis has a reported operative mortality rate around 10%, anastomotic leakage around 4% and hospital stay of approximately 20 days.[51]

A retrospective study of 243 patients who underwent emergency operation for obstructing colorectal cancers showed that primary resection and anastomosis for left-sided malignant obstruction either by segmental resection with on-table lavage or by subtotal colectomy was not more hazardous than primary anastomosis for right-sided obstruction.[52] Single-stage resection with primary anastomosis was possible in 197 patients. Of the 101 patients with left-sided obstruction, segmental resection with on-table colonic lavage was performed in 75 patients and subtotal colectomy in 26. There were no differences in the mortality or leakage rates between patients with right-sided and left-sided lesions (mortality 7.3% vs. 8.9%; leakage 5.2% vs. 6.9%, respectively).

More recent papers have described segmental resection and primary anastomosis without any attempt to clean the bowel. One study reported only one leak and one postoperative death in 58 consecutive patients with left-sided malignant colonic obstruction who underwent bowel decompression without irrigation, followed by resection and primary colocolic anastomosis.[53] The patients in this study had a mean age of 63 (range 54–89) years, the leak occurring in a 61-year-old with a sigmoid carcinoma and the death in an 80-year-old due to myocardial infarction. None of the carcinomas described were rectosigmoid or rectal. A further study of left-sided obstruction in which 40 of 60 patients had carcinoma compared one-stage resection with Hartmann's procedure.[54] There was no significant difference in outcome or time taken to complete the operation, with the only death being in the Hartmann's group. Again, none of the tumours described was more distal than the sigmoid colon.

Circumstances usually dictate the operative choice. In the elderly, segmental resection may be preferable to a more extensive resection, both in terms of operative morbidity and postoperative problems of incontinence. Subtotal colectomy is clearly the procedure of choice when there are synchronous tumours in the colon. When subtotal colectomy with ileorectal anastomosis is selected as the operation of choice, the whole colon is mobilised and the rectum washed out as for elective surgery. After resection of the colon, an ileorectal or ileosigmoid anastomosis is performed using either a sutured or stapled technique. The first randomised trial comparing subtotal versus segmental resection was reported in 1995.[55] This study involved 91 eligible patients recruited by 18 consultant surgeons in 12 centres; 47 were randomised to subtotal colectomy and 44 to on-table irrigation and segmental colectomy. There was no significant difference in operative mortality, hospital stay, anastomotic leakage or wound sepsis between the two groups. There was, however, a significantly higher permanent stoma rate in the subtotal colectomy group compared with the segmental colectomy group (7 vs. 1). The high permanent stoma rate in the subtotal colectomy group was partly accounted for by four patients who were randomised to subtotal colectomy but who underwent Hartmann's procedure because this was thought clinically more appropriate at the time of surgery by the operating surgeon. Two additional patients had the anastomosis taken down at a later date and a stoma formed. At follow-up 4 months after the operation, there was a significantly greater number of patients who had three or more bowel movements a day after subtotal colectomy than after segmental resection (14 of 35 vs. 4 of 35). One patient had 12 bowel movements per day after subtotal colectomy. Nearly one-third of patients randomised to subtotal colectomy had night-time bowel movements during the first few months after operation. In contrast, less than 10% of those who had segmental resection had this problem.

> ✓✓ Segmental resection of the colon, with or without intraoperative irrigation, is the preferred treatment for left-sided malignant colonic obstruction.[55,56]

Although the SCOTIA study[55] addressed the immediate and early results after these two procedures, it did not investigate the long-term implications of either procedure. It has been argued that there are advantages in performing a subtotal colectomy rather than segmental resection because synchronous tumours will be removed along with the obstructing lesion and, since the length of colon left is small, there should be less risk of developing a metachronous tumour. Clearly the operating surgeon needs to take all these factors into account when making the final decision on which procedure is most suitable for the individual patient.

Inflammation and infection

Acute colonic diverticulitis

Colonic diverticula are found with increasing age. It has been estimated that one-third of the population will have colonic diverticula by the age of 50 years and two-thirds after 80 years. Although the vast majority of individuals with colonic diverticula are asymptomatic, most patients who require surgical care do so because of an inflammatory complication. Acute diverticulitis can affect any part of the colon; in Western Europe and North America, the left side is more commonly affected, whereas in Japan and China right-sided diverticulitis is more commonly seen. Symptomatic complications of diverticulitis occur in 10–30% of patients, but the need for surgery in acute diverticulitis is becoming less common.

Presentation

Diverticulitis is thought to result from inspissation of stool in the neck of a diverticulum, with consequent inflammation and possible microperforation. This results in local bacterial proliferation, leading to inflammation in the surrounding colonic wall and mesentery (acute phlegmonous diverticulitis). A collection of pus may form either in the mesentery of the colon or adjacent to the colonic wall. As the collection of pus enlarges, it becomes walled off by loops of small bowel or the peritoneum of the pelvis. Occasionally, free perforation into the peritoneal cavity occurs with consequent purulent or faecal peritonitis. The Hinchey grading system for acute diverticulitis has become fairly widely accepted, allowing more meaningful comparison between outcome studies (Table 10.1).[57]

From time to time other complications also arise. A fistula sometimes develops between bowel and another adjacent organ (ie. the bladder or vaginal cuff). Diverticular disease is responsible for around 10% of all cases of left-sided large-bowel obstruction and is frequently difficult to differentiate from malignant left-sided large-bowel obstruction on clinical grounds. Bleeding also occurs.

There has been controversy regarding the virulence of diverticular disease in younger patients and the possible increase in need for surgical intervention

Table 10.1 • Hinchey classification of peritoneal contamination in diverticulitis

Stage 1	Pericolic or mesenteric abscess
Stage 2	Walled-off pelvic abscess
Stage 3	Generalised purulent peritonitis
Stage 4	Generalised faecal peritonitis

in this group. Recently, Biondo et al. looked at 327 patients treated for acute left colonic diverticulitis and compared those aged 50 or less with those older than 50.[58] No difference was noted regarding severity or recurrence. Another study found that diverticulitis in the young does not follow a particularly aggressive course.[59] In general, there is a trend towards conservative management of acute diverticulitis, with early investigation and confirmation of the diagnosis being a fundamental part of this approach. The mortality and morbidity rates can be high if emergency surgery is necessary.

Investigation

Acute right-sided diverticulitis, a rare condition in the Western world, can be confused with appendicitis as it occurs in a somewhat younger age group than left-sided disease. In the more common left-sided disease, the plain abdominal radiograph may show non-specific abnormalities such as pneumoperitoneum, intestinal obstruction or a soft-tissue mass.

> ✓✓ CT is now the favoured modality for acute investigation of suspected acute colonic diverticultis.[60]

Features of acute diverticulitis include thickening of the bowel wall, increased soft-tissue density within the pericolic fat secondary to inflammation and a soft-tissue mass, which represents either a phlegmon or an abscess. Advantages of CT include the accurate assessment of the extent of pericolonic involvement and the diagnosis of abscess formation or perforation (**Fig. 10.10**). It is also useful for tracking the therapeutic percutaneous drainage of any abscess. When CT is compared with barium enema, CT is no more accurate in terms of diagnosis but undoubtedly provides better definition of the extent

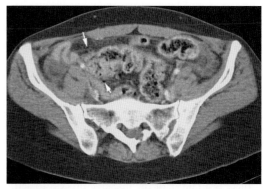

Figure 10.10 • Appearance of perforated sigmoid diverticular disease on CT. The upper arrow shows a small pocket of free air and the lower arrow one of the diverticula.

and severity of the inflammatory process, which is of prognostic value in the short and long term.[61] Ultrasonography has also been used for localised diverticulitis. The main disadvantages of ultrasonography are that assessment of bowel thickening is a non-specific finding and assessment is very operator dependent.

An alternative investigation is contrast enema. Despite the extensive literature on the use of contrast enema in acute diverticulitis, there is no consensus on either the best contrast agent or the optimal timing of the examination. There has been some interest with magnetic resonance imaging in the diagnosis of acute diverticulitis and prospective observational studies have been encouraging, but more formal evaluation is still required.[62]

Management

Right-sided disease may be encountered unexpectedly at surgery or be operated on for a complication diagnosed preoperatively. The treatment options are controversial, ranging from appendicectomy to hemicolectomy. A conservative approach with appendicectomy and antibiotics has resulted in a similar mortality, morbidity and recurrence as for resection of the diverticulum.[63] A right hemicolectomy is the correct operation when it is not possible to rule out the presence of a carcinoma.

A typical patient with localised left-sided diverticulitis will complain of pain in the left iliac fossa and will be febrile. Examination reveals tenderness and sometimes a mass is palpable per abdomen or on rectal examination. In women, a vaginal examination should also be performed to exclude gynaecological pathology. If sigmoidoscopy is performed, it should be done gently with minimal insufflation of air.

In the absence of generalised peritonitis, a non-operative policy is adopted, with antibiotic therapy directed against Gram-negative and anaerobic bacteria. Most clinicians advocate bowel rest initially, and intravenous fluids and antibiotics. If the pain and fever settle within a few days, the patient can go home on oral antibiotics and a barium enema and sigmoidoscopy or colonoscopy can be performed as an outpatient several weeks later to exclude any malignancy.

If the patient continues with fever, pain or enlarging lower abdominal mass, a CT should be obtained. If there is an abscess, it can be drained percutaneously under radiological guidance. In the event of localised abdominal signs becoming more generalised, or if there is a failure of the infective process to settle despite adequate non-operative therapy, operation is indicated. In the small number of patients who require operation for localised diverticulitis, primary resection, with or without on-table irrigation

and primary anastomosis, is becoming increasingly popular among specialist colorectal surgeons.

Pain from perforated sigmoid diverticulitis usually commences in the lower abdomen, mostly on the left side, and gradually spreads throughout the abdomen. In 25% of patients, however, signs and symptoms are predominantly right-sided[63] and in some patients might mimic acute appendicitis. On examination, there are signs of generalised peritonitis including guarding and rebound tenderness. About one-quarter of all patients will have free gas under the diaphragm on plain radiography, and at operation purulent peritonitis is more common than faecal peritonitis.[64] The majority of patients presenting in this way will clearly require operation following adequate resuscitation. Antibiotic therapy should be commenced early to cover both anaerobic organisms and Gram-negative bacteria. Some patients will improve so much with non-operative treatment that it may be appropriate to continue with this therapy for a longer period.

Operative management

The patient is placed in the lithotomy/Trendelenburg position and explored with a midline incision. Pus and faecal material should be removed from the peritoneal cavity and specimens sent for microscopy and both aerobic and anaerobic culture. Intraoperative irrigation of the peritoneal cavity with 6–10 L of warm saline solution is of value, while the addition of topical antibiotics to the solution (e.g. cephradine 1 g in 1 L of 0.9% saline), although logical, remains unproven.

In addition to treating the peritonitis, surgical treatment must minimise continued contamination of the peritoneal cavity. A review of 57 reports[65] on the treatment of acute diverticular disease demonstrated that the operative mortality rates from procedures that involve primary resection (10%) were less than half those from operations that did not include excision of the diseased colon (20%). A further reason for advocating primary resection is the difficulty experienced at the time of operation in deciding whether the lesion is a perforated carcinoma or an area of diverticulitis. At laparotomy, the appearance of both lesions may be similar when the colon is inflamed and oedematous. It has been estimated that as many as 25% of patients with a preoperative diagnosis of perforated diverticulitis may be found to have a perforated carcinoma. If there is reasonable suspicion of carcinoma, a radical resection of the lesion, together with the colonic mesentery, needs to be performed. Examination of the resected specimen at the earliest opportunity is recommended to aid further decision-making.

Failure to take the resection far enough distally beyond the sigmoid colon risks recurrence of diverticular disease. Therefore, Hartmann's resection with complete excision of the sigmoid and closure of the rectum, with formation of a left lower quadrant colostomy, has been the standard procedure advocated by most surgeons. If the operation is exceptionally difficult owing to the colon being very adherent to surrounding structures, making safe mobilisation impossible, it may be reasonable to create a proximal stoma, drain the area and transfer the patient to a tertiary referral centre for more definitive treatment.

There has been an increase in the use of primary anastomosis in selected patients who have operations for acute diverticulitis. The main reasons are: (i) that patients receive one operation rather than two; (ii) after a Hartmann operation many patients are left with a permanent stoma, either because of unwillingness or unfitness to have further surgery; and (iii) reversal operation after Hartmann's resection can be very difficult.

One study reported resection, intraoperative colonic lavage and primary anastomosis in 55 of 124 patients with complicated diverticular disease; 49 of the 55 had diverticulitis, 33 having localised and 16 generalised peritonitis.[66] Faecal peritonitis was considered a contraindication to a one-stage procedure. Four patients died, one from an anastomotic leak. Major complications included two anastomotic leaks (one of which was successfully treated with parenteral nutrition), four re-operations (three for abdominal wound dehiscence and one for anastomotic leak) and four deaths (three of those who died were over 70 years old). The study concluded that one-stage resection is feasible in selected patients.

> ✅✅ One-stage resection for acute complicated diverticultis without faecal peritonitis is feasible and should be considered, depending on patient fitness.[66]

A further study of primary anastomosis in emergency colorectal surgery showed no significant difference in the incidence of complications, even in patients with free peritonitis (21.9% perforation, 17.7% localised sepsis).[67] The necessity for intraoperative colonic lavage has also been challenged. Despite an increasing trend to perform primary anastomosis in patients who have perforated diverticulitis, the number of patients who are suitable for such a procedure will be small.

Laparoscopic techniques continue to be used in an increasing number of diverticular cases with good results,[68] with laparoscopic assessment and lavage also a possibility. A recent review found laparoscopic peritoneal lavage for perforated sigmoid diverticulitis to be a potentially effective and more conservative alternative to a Hartmann procedure.[69] Randomised controlled trials are needed to better evaluate its role.

Neutropenic enterocolitis

Neutropenic enterocolitis, also known as typhlitis, is a potentially life-threatening condition characterised by an inflammatory process that usually involves the caecum and ascending colon. It occurs most often as a complication of chemotherapy and can progress to necrosis and perforation. Although it can affect any part of the small and large intestine, the cause of its predisposition for the right colon is unclear.

Clinical features include nausea, vomiting, abdominal pain, distension and diarrhoea, which can be bloody. Right iliac fossa tenderness and pyrexia are quite common and in later stages peritonitis may be present. CT is the diagnostic modality of choice and may reveal right-sided colon wall thickening, mesenteric stranding, pneumatosis and ascites (**Fig. 10.11**).

Management demands careful evaluation of the patient, with each case treated individually. An initial conservative approach includes fluid and electrolyte replacement, broad-spectrum antibiotics, correction of any attendant coagulopathy and complete bowel rest with parenteral nutrition. The use of recombinant granulocyte colony-stimulating factor to correct chemotherapy-induced neutropenia should be considered. Colonic perforation and generalised peritonitis are clear indications for surgery. The operative procedure of choice is a right hemicolectomy, with either exteriorisation of the bowel ends or a primary anastomosis, depending on the extent of sepsis and peritoneal soiling. In general, most patients can be managed non-operatively.

Toxic colitis

Toxic colitis is a potentially fatal complication of inflammatory bowel disease, particularly

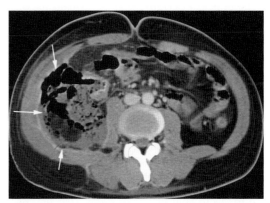

Figure 10.11 • CT scan showing large retroperitoneal collection (indicated by arrows) secondary to acute necrotising enterocolitis with a delayed perforation of the posterior wall of the caecum and ascending colon.

if accompanied by megacolon. While several schemes exist to accurately identify toxic colitis, one reasonably simple system employs a definition that includes a disease flare-up accompanied by two of the following criteria: hypoalbuminaemia (<3.0 g/dL), leucocytosis (>10.5 × 10^{9}cells/L), tachycardia (>100 beats/minute), temperature elevation (>38.6 °C).[70] Use of this relatively objective definition may aid in the diagnosis and care of these patients, whose severe condition can be under-appreciated because of high dosages of steroids, immunomodulators or biological agents.

The initial management is directed at reversing physiological deficits with intravenous hydration, correction of electrolyte imbalances, and blood product transfusions. Free perforation, increasing colonic dilatation, massive haemorrhage, peritonitis and septic shock are indications for emergency operation after the patient has been adequately resuscitated. In the absence of these features, medical therapy is initiated with high dosages of intravenous corticosteroids, immunomodulators and/or biological agents. Broad-spectrum antibiotics directed against intestinal flora are prescribed to minimise the risk of sepsis secondary to transmural inflammation or microperforation. Anticholinergics, antidiarrhoeals and narcotics are avoided as they may worsen already impaired colonic motility or conceal ominous symptoms. Hyperalimentation may be started and the patient is closely observed with serial examinations and abdominal roentgenograms. Any worsening of the clinical course over the ensuing 24–72 hours mandates urgent laparotomy. If the patient improves minimally after 5–7 days of conventional therapy, the medical therapy should be altered or surgery should be advised. Experience with ciclosporin or infliximab in this setting is anecdotal, and should be weighed against operative therapy while understanding that surgery in this setting often relegates the patient to an ileostomy.[71]

The principal operative options in patients with toxic colitis are subtotal colectomy with end ileostomy or loop ileostomy with decompressive blowhole colostomy. The most difficult aspect of a subtotal colectomy is managing the distal bowel stump. The distal limb may be closed with sutures or staples and then delivered to the anterior abdominal wall, where it can lie without tension in the subcutaneous fat of the lower midline wound. If the bowel end is placed above the fascia, dehiscence of the rectal closure during the postoperative period results in a mucous fistula. If the closed stump is left within the peritoneal cavity, staple line dehiscence will produce a pelvic abscess. If the bowel wall is too friable to hold sutures or staples, creation of a mucous fistula is preferred. If there is inadequate residual bowel length to create a mucous fistula, many surgeons will place a catheter through the anus (e.g. Mallencott or Foley) to decompress the rectum and reduce the chance of a stump blowout.

The patient typically improves over the ensuing few days and can be discharged within a week of the operation. An appropriate elective procedure can be considered several months after the patient recovers.

Proctocolectomy with end ileostomy is rarely performed in the severely ill patient with toxic colitis because of the excessive rates of morbidity and mortality.[72] Proctectomy increases the difficulty of the procedure and risks pelvic bleeding as well as autonomic nerve damage. In rare instances of rectal perforation or profuse colorectal haemorrhage, proctocolectomy may be an option. The surgeon must be cautioned, however, that the macroscopic and microscopic differentiation of ulcerative colitis from Crohn's proctocolitis is especially difficult in severe colitis, and primary proctocolectomy would nullify the future option of a restorative procedure in a patient with ulcerative colitis.

The need for loop ileostomy combined with decompression blowhole colostomy has virtually disappeared with improved medical recognition and more sophisticated management of toxic colitis. The operation is still useful in extremely ill patients or those in whom colectomy would be especially hazardous (e.g. contained perforation, high-lying splenic flexure and pregnancy). Contraindications to the procedure include colorectal haemorrhage, free perforation and intra-abdominal abscess. The operation is considered only a temporising procedure, and a definitive operation is commonly performed approximately 6 months later.

Perforation

Stercoral perforation

The word *stercus* means dung or faeces. Perforation of the bowel caused by pressure necrosis from a faecal mass is a rare entity, first reported by Berry at the Pathological Society of London in 1894. Fewer than 100 cases have been reported in the literature, although this may reflect the poor outcome (with mortality rates approaching 50%), an increasing reluctance to publish case reports and ill-defined diagnostic criteria. There appears to be an equal incidence in men and women and the median age for these patients is said to be 60 years.[73]

Reported predisposing factors have included chronic constipation, megacolon, scleroderma, hypercalcaemia, renal failure and renal transplantation. Medications associated with stercoral perforation include narcotics, postoperative analgesia, antacids, calcium channel blockers and antidepressants. Only

11% of cases are accurately diagnosed prior to operation,[74] with investigations frequently non-contributory. Perforations usually occur on the antimesenteric border, with the majority occurring in the sigmoid colon and rectosigmoid region. Multiple perforations are found in about one-fifth of patients, with the remaining patients usually having ulceration extending away from the perforation.

The suggested clinicopathological diagnostic criteria are:

- A round or ovoid colonic perforation exceeding 1 cm in diameter.
- Faecolomas present within the colon.
- Microscopic evidence of pressure necrosis or ulcer and chronic inflammatory reaction around the perforation site.[75] This study, which constitutes one of the largest single-institution reports on stercoral perforation of the colon, defined strict clinical and pathological criteria for its diagnosis. Using these criteria stercoral perforation of the colon would appear to occur more frequently than previously reported in the literature.

Management of these patients is surgical, with the resection margins sufficiently wide to encompass all areas of perforation or impending perforations. The bowel is universally loaded with stool and the tendency towards constipation is not removed by a limited resection. The operation should involve resection of the affected segment and exteriorisation of the bowel for left-sided perforations, with resection and primary anastomosis being reserved for those patients with a right-sided perforation. The risk of recurrent perforation in the proximal colon presents a further problem for those with a left-sided perforation. Milking the stool in an antegrade direction into the resected segment and orthograde colonic irrigation may combine to avoid early re-perforation. However, the fear of recurrent perforation from persistent constipation has led some surgeons to suggest a subtotal colectomy.

Anastomotic dehiscence

Breakdown of an anastomosis is one of the most significant complications after large-bowel surgery. The presentation can be insidious but more commonly the patient becomes acutely ill, particularly if there is generalised peritonitis. If the diagnosis is not made and appropriate treatment undertaken, death is likely to follow. There is no doubt that the presence of anastomotic leakage significantly increases mortality and one study noted a mortality rate of 22% in 191 patients who had leakage after large-bowel anastomosis compared with only 7.2% in 1275 patients without a leak.[76] In the patients who survive this serious complication, morbidity and hospital stay are greatly increased.

Causes

A variety of general and local causative factors of anastomotic dehiscence have been described. General factors listed usually include poor nutritional state, anaemia, uraemia, diabetes, steroid administration and old age, while suggested local factors involved tension, ischaemia or infection of the anastomosis. The risk of anastomotic leakage in low colorectal anastomosis is several times higher than in either ileocolic or colocolic anastomosis. In one report a clinical leak rate for ileocolic and colocolic anastomosis was 0.4%, whereas the leak rate after low colorectal anastomosis was 4.7%.[77] In a review of 477 large-bowel anastomoses, which included 215 colorectal anastomoses, there were eight colorectal and one ileocolic leaks. All nine patients required laparotomy, and seven were salvaged with no mortality. Three colorectal leaks (small posterior defects in stapled anastomoses) were closed with interrupted endoanal sutures and a proximal loop stoma fashioned in two patients who did not already have one. The other two leaks (defect in suture line attributable to a single suture cutting through) were managed by creating a controlled external fistula. None of these patients had further complications and all the stomas were subsequently closed. It is therefore possible to salvage anastomotic leaks with a good outcome in selected patients with appropriate operative treatment.

Another important factor in dehiscence is the oxygen tension at the bowel ends used for the anastomosis. In an elegant study reported in 1987, it was shown that if tissue oxygen tension in the ends of bowel to be anastomosed fell to less than 20 mmHg (2.66 kPa), there was a high likelihood of anastomotic breakdown.[78] However, a significant factor in anastomotic failure is poor surgical technique, irrespective as to whether sutures or staples are used.

Presentation

In general, the clinical features of anastomotic dehiscence will depend on whether the leak is localised or more extensive, causing generalised peritonitis. At one end of the spectrum, when sepsis associated with the leak is localised, the patient may have minimal symptoms and only a few physical signs. There may be 'flu-like' symptoms of feeling vaguely unwell with shivering and nausea. If the anastomosis lies low in the pelvis, there may be some lower abdominal pain and tenderness and on rectal examination a defect can often be felt in the anastomosis. Tachycardia is a common general feature and is often associated with pyrexia. If a drain is still in situ, faecal material or pus may be seen.

At the other end of the spectrum the scenario is associated with a major leak, when faecal material or pus has leaked into the general peritoneal cavity. The effect on the patient is usually profound. Abdominal pain is difficult to control and tachycardia and tachypnoea are common. The temperature is raised and hypotension is often a feature. The patient is distressed and sweaty and on abdominal examination the abdomen is tender with abdominal guarding. Sometimes the features of even an extensive leak can be more insidious, with the patient not making progress as rapidly as expected and suffering abdominal pain that is vague rather than dramatic.

Delay in diagnosis of large-bowel anastomotic leakage is still a major problem and leads to increased morbidity and mortality. It is crucial that surgeons are vigilant about deterioration of any patient who has a large-bowel anastomosis and maintain a low threshold for ordering investigations to identify a leak. It should be remembered that the anastomosis may leak any time during the first 2–3 weeks after operation.

Investigations

Usually the white blood count is elevated, except in patients who have overwhelming sepsis, when it may be either normal or even low. However, the earliest derangement in the white blood count is an increase in the less mature polymorphic neutrophils (e.g. left shift). Erect chest radiograph or abdominal films will sometimes show gas under the diaphragm, but this sign is of debatable significance in the first few days after the original operation because of the presence of intra-abdominal air introduced at the time of operation. The absence of pneumoperitoneum should not discourage the clinician from pursuing investigations to check the integrity of the anastomosis.

Ultrasound examination can be helpful in the patient with a suspected collection of pus related to anastomotic leakage, but the value of this investigation is often impaired by the presence of dilated gas-filled loops of bowel, with dressings and drains on the abdomen further increasing technical difficulties. CT or contrast studies are the investigation of choice.

Water-soluble contrast enema is a simple investigation for assessing anastomotic leakage, particularly on the left side of the large bowel. Another option is a pelvic CT scan with rectal contrast. In addition to demonstrating whether a leak has occurred, assessment of the extent of leakage is of value in deciding the overall management. It is important to be aware of two caveats, however. Occasionally, when the contrast study shows no leak, a later investigation will show one. The corollary of this is also sometimes true. The enema or scan may show a leak that is of no clinical consequence (radiological leak). It is therefore important to look at the overall clinical picture and attempt to assess all the clinical and radiological evidence before coming to a final conclusion about the presence of a clinically significant leak.

Management

Although the literature on colonic anastomotic leak rates is extensive, there is a paucity of information on how to treat the leakage. It is best to consider the management of localised leakage separately from those who present with generalised peritonitis. Most patients with **localised leakage** can be treated non-operatively with bowel rest and antibiotic therapy. If there is a large collection of pus around the anastomosis, it is usual to drain this percutaneously under ultrasound or CT guidance. Patients with **generalised peritonitis** from a large-bowel anastomotic leak are usually dramatically ill and require resuscitation. Assuming that investigations have been performed and the diagnosis confirmed, the next step is to improve the patient's condition before surgical intervention.

Haemodynamic status needs to be assessed and treatment given to improve cardiac and respiratory function. Parenteral antibiotic administration is a priority and inotropic support may be necessary. Adequate pain control is important and these patients are best managed in a high-dependency unit or intensive therapy unit. Anaesthesia is alerted and only when the patient's condition is stabilised is operation undertaken.

The patient is usually placed in the lithotomy/Trendelenburg position. The previous midline incision is reopened and great care is taken not to damage adherent loops of small intestine. Bowel loops are dissected free and the area of anastomosis exposed. Faecal material and pus are removed from the peritoneal cavity and pelvis. Occlusion clamps are gently placed on bowel above and below the leaking anastomosis to limit further contamination. Extensive lavage of the peritoneal cavity is performed with saline or antibiotic solution.

The next steps depend on the size and location of the anastomotic defect. In the majority of cases, the anastomosis is taken apart and the proximal end of bowel is brought out as an end stoma and the distal end as a mucous fistula. If the distal stump is not long enough to be brought out on the abdominal wall, it should be closed carefully using a series of interrupted seromuscular sutures. Some surgeons will place a transanal drain to decompress the bowel. Surgeons must be aware that the more distal the leak, the lower the chances of bowel continuity being restored at a later date.

In selected patients (usually those with a small defect in a low colorectal anastomosis), the anastomosis may be salvaged. A defunctioning ileostomy can be constructed for diversion and the area of the leak can be drained. However, the faecal loading in the colon can lead to continued soiling unless it is removed with transanal irrigation. However, in a patient who has already had an anastomotic leak it is poor practice to risk a further leak and the patient's safety should be the prime objective.

Bowel damage at colonoscopy

The perforation rate at colonoscopy is now generally agreed to be about 1 in 500, varying with the level of intervention employed.

There are three proposed mechanisms for colonoscopic perforation:

1. mechanical perforation directly from the colonoscope or biopsy forceps;
2. barotrauma from overzealous air insufflation;
3. perforations occurring as a result of therapeutic procedures (use of energy sources).

Measurement of forces exerted during colonoscopy has only been reported in one paper from the Royal London Hospital,[79] where an electronic device was used in a research setting. The caecum and right colon are most susceptible to barotrauma, although diverticula can also be directly inflated. The use of carbon dioxide for insufflation may decrease perforation rates and increase levels of patient comfort. Therapeutic interventions such as polyp removal with a hot biopsy or snare and balloon dilatation of strictures are, not surprisingly, associated with a higher risk of perforation.

The most common site of perforation is the sigmoid colon. Signs and symptoms of a perforation are not always obvious at the time of colonosocopy. In retrospective studies, the diagnosis of a perforation is delayed in about 50% of patients.[80] If the endoscopist is worried after an examination has been completed, an erect chest radiograph should be ordered as a screening test and the patient observed until symptoms have settled. In cases where there is a high index of suspicion, a water-soluble enema or CT scan with contrast can be used to confirm the diagnosis.

Non-operative treatment with close observation, intravenous fluids and antibiotics may be possible in selected patients.[81] The authors' approach is presented in **Fig. 10.12**. A large defect or symptoms of peritoneal contamination will usually require operative treatment. If the injury is operated upon early, a direct repair of the defect or small resection and a primary anastomosis is possible. It may also be possible to effect the repair laparoscopically. With delayed diagnosis or clinical deterioration during observation, patients will usually require a temporary defunctioning stoma.

Colonic bleeding

Although upper gastrointestinal and small-bowel bleeding has been covered in Chapters 5 and 7, there remains the problem of patients who bleed from the colon. In approximately 20% of cases, the colon and rectum are the source of acute gastrointestinal haemorrhage. The most common aetiologies of this haemorrhage include diverticulosis, angiodysplasia, ischaemic colitis, inflammatory bowel disease, neoplasms, aorto-enteric fistulas and anorectal diseases such as haemorrhoids.[82] The general principles of management of many of these conditions have already been discussed, but each patient needs to be managed individually. Where possible, management of colonic bleeding is non-operative and usually stops spontaneously, permitting investigation to proceed at

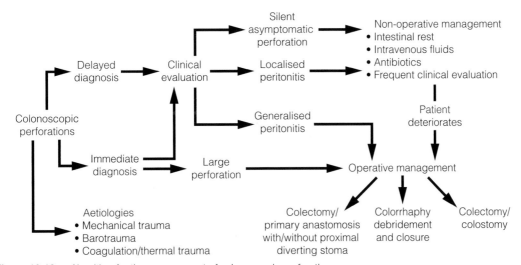

Figure 10.12 • Algorithm for the management of colonoscopic perforation.

a leisurely pace. In some patients, however, the bleeding either does not spontaneously stop or is profuse and urgent investigation, followed occasionally by emergency surgery, is required. In these patients, the source of bleeding is often difficult to identify.

Diagnosis and non-surgical management

Diagnostic tests utilised will vary according to institutional availability, patient characteristics, and the providers' experience and expertise. These investigations are used to localise the site of haemorrhage, cause it to stop or confirm its cessation. Options include radionuclide imaging, colonoscopy, CT angiography and selective angiography.

Radionuclide imaging

Radionuclide imaging with $[^{99m}Tc]$pertechnetate-tagged red cells detects the slowest bleeding rates (0.1–0.5 mL/min) but cannot reliably localise the site of haemorrhage.[83]

The timing of the radionucleotide blush is important. An immediately positive blush (within the first 2 minutes of scanning) is highly predictive of a positive angiogram (60%) and the need for surgery (24%), while a negative scan is highly predictive of a negative angiogram (93%) and the need for surgery falls to 7%.[84] A negative nuclear scan provides objective evidence that the patient is not actively bleeding and may be evaluated by colonoscopy.

Colonoscopy

Many authors believe that colonoscopy has the highest efficacy and should be the first study in patients with major bleeding that appears self-limited.[85] Whether colonoscopy should be undertaken as an 'emergency' depends on the patient's stability. In patients with hypotension and ongoing haemorrhage, it is difficult to safely cleanse the bowel with lavage solutions, and the continued bleeding limits intraluminal visualisation and the ability to utilise therapeutic options. In general, these patients require prompt attention with angiography or surgery.

In stable patients with self-limited haemorrhage, colonoscopy is the preferred diagnostic study. The need for bowel preparation is controversial. Colonoscopy without preparation can be described as 'emergent' while administering a mechanical preparation and then performing colonoscopy within 24 hours of presentation is best termed 'urgent' colonoscopy. The rapid time preferred for mechanical cleansing usually mandates a lavage method.

Proponents of 'emergency colonoscopy' have demonstrated high caecal intubation rates (95%) and a diagnostic accuracy of 72–86%.[86] However, many of the reported series described atypical aetiologies for 'massive haemorrhage', including ischaemic colitis, inflammatory bowel disease and cancer. The usual rate of bleeding in these conditions is more amenable to urgent colonoscopy (within 24 hours) than to emergent colonoscopy. Higher bleeding rates are more common with diverticular or angiodysplastic sources.

The benefit of colonoscopy depends on its ability to provide a definitive localisation of ongoing active bleeding and the potential for therapy. Many landmarks for colonoscopy may be obscured during haemorrhage. Even when pathology is identified, establishing the presence of stigmata of recent haemorrhage is more difficult than in the upper gastrointestinal tract. In addition, colonoscopy is associated with complications such as perforation. Inconclusive findings owing to technically unsatisfactory results are frequent and failure to achieve a firm diagnosis may reflect stricter diagnostic criteria rather than inferior diagnostic skill.

Because of the inability to appreciate all intraluminal landmarks and accurately locate the segment that is bleeding, once the enodoscopist highlights a source of bleeding, the region of the intestine is best marked with a tattoo of India ink. If the haemorrhage continues and the patient fails medical management, a tattoo greatly assists the surgeon in localising the site of bleeding. The endoscopist has many therapeutic options to control the bleeding, including thermal agents (heater probes and bipolar coagulation), monopolar or bipolar diathermy, topical or intramucosal epinephrine injection and endoscopically applied clips.

Angiography

Angiography aids as a diagnostic and therapeutic option in the treatment of intestinal haemorrhage. Acute, major haemorrhage with ongoing bleeding requires emergency angiography, while patients with an early blush during nuclear scintigraphy may benefit from therapeutic angiography. Angiograms may also define a potential source for haemorrhage in occult and recurrent gastrointestinal haemorrhage. In order to appreciate an angiographic blush of contrast, the study requires a bleeding rate of at least 1–1.5 mL/min. Appropriate patient selection increases yields and avoids excessive use of angiograms. Superselective catheterisation of branch arteries and multiple injections of contrast may be required to examine the entire territory. It is important to take late films in the venous phase as they may demonstrate abnormalities that may not be seen in the arterial phase. Major complications of diagnostic arteriography include arterial thrombosis, embolisation and renal failure caused by the contrast material.

The angiographic blush may suggest a specific aetiology, but this finding lacks the accuracy of colonoscopy. Highly accurate localisation also provides for focused therapy. The haemorrhagic site may receive highly selective, intra-arterial vasopressin infusion. This medication produces potent arterial contraction that may reduce or halt the haemorrhage. Infusion rates of vasopressin begin at concentrations of 0.2 U/min and may progress to 0.4 U/min. The systemic effects and cardiac impact of vasopressin may limit maximising the dosage. Vasopressin infusion controls bleeding in as many as 91% of patients, but unfortunately bleeding may recur in up to 50% of patients once the vasopressin is reduced. However, this has been reported as allowing surgery to be performed electively in 57% of patients.[87]

Angiographic technology also allows for arterial embolisation to control haemorrhage. Arterial embolisation of larger vessels produces intestinal ischaemia or infarction in approximately 20% of patients. Much safer superselective mesenteric angiography using microcatheters allows embolisation of the intestinal vasa recta or vessels as small as 1 mm.

✔ The high re-bleeding rate with vasopressin has led to the suggestion that other, more definitive therapeutic manoeuvres should be undertaken during angiography such as superselective embolisation, which is effective in controlling colonic haemorrhage and is associated with a low rate of post-embolisation colonic ischaemia. In a study of 27 patients, all were initially controlled with arterial embolisation although six re-bled, five of whom needed surgical intervention.[88]

Successful embolisation therapy provides immediate arrest of the bleeding. Embolisation agents include gelfoam pledgets, coils and polyvinyl alcohol particles. Success has been better in diverticular bleeds, which are usually fed by one vessel, than with angiodysplasias, which often have multiple feeding vessels.

CT angiography

Advanced CT angiography using thinly sliced, fast image acquisition combined with three-dimensional software packages has revolutionised the imaging of the vascular tree.[89] Vessels smaller than 'named' vessels can be visualised, and use of CT angiography has been reported in chronic conditions such as mesenteric ischaemia and inflammatory bowel disease. Case reports and animal modelling suggest feasibility for gastrointestinal haemorrhage. The sensitivity and specificity of CT angiography in patients with gastrointestinal haemorrhage are unknown and require further research.

Surgical management

Patients require surgical intervention if they continue to bleed profusely and medical, endoscopic and angiographic interventions have failed. Most sources of bleeding spontaneously resolve or are controlled with the therapeutic interventions described previously. Surgical therapy for intestinal bleeding is required infrequently and associated with significant mortality. Patients that are haemodynamically unresponsive to the initial resuscitation obviously require emergency surgery. In other patients the site of haemorrhage may be localised, yet the available therapeutic interventions fail to control the bleeding. Patient mortality increases with transfusion requirements. It has been reported that there is a reduced mortality (7%) for patients requiring less than 10 units of blood, while the mortality increases to 27% for patients receiving in excess of 10 units.[90] Therefore, patients with ongoing haemorrhage who require more than 6–7units of blood during the resuscitation should undergo surgical intervention.

Surgeons should tailor their operative approach based on the preoperative diagnostic evaluations. Surgery starts with a thorough examination of the entire intestine through a large midline open laparotomy incision. The first objective is location of intraluminal blood with the hope of segmentally isolating a possible source of bleeding.

If no source appears obvious after the exploration phase, the surgeon may consider intestinal enteroscopy. The enteroscope or colonoscope exposes the luminal surface and transilluminates the intestinal wall. Transillumination may identify vascular anomalies, small ulcers or tumours. Endoscopic access to the intestine may require a transoral, transgastric, transcolonic or transanal approach, or a combination of these. Intraoperative endoscopy is, however, a technically difficult endeavour. A team approach with two surgeons or the availability of an experienced endoscopist is important in order to identify the elusive lesions causing the haemorrhage.

Once the haemorrhage site is identified, an appropriate segmental resection can be performed. If no source of bleeding is confirmed, but appears to arise from the colon, the surgeon should perform a subtotal or total colectomy. Stable patients will tolerate a primary ileosigmoid or ileorectal anastomosis, while unstable patients are best served with an end ileostomy with closure of the rectal stump or a sigmoid mucous fistula.

Critical issues with operative management include delaying surgery until the haemorrhage reaches a critical point beyond 10 units of blood, with an associated mortality rate between 10% and 35%, and recurrence bleeding rates of 10% due to imprecise localisation of the bleeding.[91] Recurrence rates are higher (e.g. 20%) if a limited right or left colectomy is performed without precise localisation of the haemorrhage.[92] A total colectomy offers the same mortality but with a lower chance of recurrent or persistent bleeding. Therefore, a total colectomy is the preferred option if preoperative localisation is not possible, or a definite site of bleeding cannot be found at laparotomy.

Key points

- There has been a recent swing towards greater emphasis on preoperative investigations, especially CT, and daytime operating by specialist consultant surgeons for most urgent surgery. In cases of colonic emergencies where there is faecal contamination of the peritoneal cavity, emergency surgery may still be life-saving.

Ischaemia

- Mild cases are treated with bowel rest and optimisation of cardiovascular status. Severe cases usually require resection.

Colonic obstruction

- **Volvulus.** Emergency decompression using a proctoscope, a long soft tube such as a chest drain, or a colonoscope should, in most cases, be followed by elective definitive surgery.
- **Acute colonic pseudo-obstruction.** Some patients can be managed conservatively, employing regular review and frequent plain abdominal radiographs to check caecal diameter. As caecal diameter increases, decompression is required. Many patients will respond to a trial of neostigmine. If this treatment is not successful, the colon can be decompressed with the colonoscope. Failure may necessitate caecostomy or resection. If perforation or necrosis is suspected, a full laparotomy is necessary.
- **Malignant disease.** Right hemicolectomy with primary anastomosis is the treatment of choice for most patients with right-sided or transverse colonic obstruction. A subtotal colectomy may be the preferred option for patients who have a lesion at the splenic flexure. Most other patients who have an obstructing carcinoma in the left colon will be best treated by segmental colectomy with primary anastomosis where possible. Patients who are thought to be particularly at risk from lengthy emergency operations are best served by either segmental resection or colostomy.

Inflammation and/or infection

- **Diverticulits.** CT is now the investigation of choice for those patients presenting as emergencies. Abscesses can then be drained percutaneously and perforations requiring surgery diagnosed early. One-stage surgery is ideal; however, in left-sided disease this is not appropriate for the unstable patient or in those with gross faecal contamination.
- **Typhlitis.** There should be a high index of suspicion for this condition in the neutropenic patient. The majority respond to conservative measures including antibiotics and complete bowel rest, but perforation should be actively excluded along the course of the disease, preferably with CT.

Perforation

- **Stercoral perforation.** This rare condition may be difficult to diagnose preoperatively. Awareness of the possibility of postoperative re-perforation, especially where limited resections have been performed, may be the key to a successful outcome.
- **Anastomotic leak.** Postoperative assessment of the abdomen is complex, with many signs being attributable to the surgery itself. In equivocal cases, further investigations should be instigated where there is uncertainty. Active observation should be employed by senior surgical staff. In some instances, transfer to a specialist colorectal unit needs to be considered after initial resuscitation and assessment.
- **Colonoscopic damage.** Signs and symptoms of perforation are not always obvious at the time of colonoscopy. A high index of suspicion, especially following interventional procedures, may allow conservative management or primary repair if surgery is performed early.

Haemorrhage

- The majority of colonic bleeding settles spontaneously, allowing subsequent investigation to take place 'electively'. However, ongoing bleeding should be investigated by CT angiography and then selective angiography, with or without embolisation. Surgery may be required and unless an obvious cause has been identified, subtotal colectomy with stoma formation is probably the safest procedure.

References

1. Hagihara PF, Ernst CB, Griffen Jr WO. Incidence of ischemic colitis following abdominal aortic reconstruction. Surg Gynecol Obstet 1979;149:571–3.

2. Beck DE, Hicks TC. Other conditions: colonic volvulus, ischemia, radiation injury, and trauma. In: Beck DE, editor. Handbook of colorectal surgery. 2nd ed. New York: Marcel Dekker; 2003. p. 483–507.

3. Sakai L, Keltner R, Kaminski D. Spontaneous and shock-associated ischemic colitis. Am J Surg 1980;140:755–60.

4. Marston A, Pheils M, Thomas ML, et al. Ischaemic colitis. Gut 1966;7:1–15.

5. Stamos MJ. Intestinal ischemia and infarction. In: Mazier WP, Levien DH, Luchtefeld MA, et al., editors. Surgery of the colon, rectum and anus. Philadelphia: WB Saunders; 1995. p. 685–718.

6. Boley SJ, Schwartz S, Lash J, et al. Reversible vascular occlusion of the colon. Surg Gynecol Obstet 1963;116:53–60.

7. Boley SJ, Brandt LJ, Veith FJ. Ischemic disorders of the intestines. Curr Probl Surg 1978;15:57–9.

8. Ballantyne GH. Review of sigmoid volvulus: clinical pattern and pathogenesis. Dis Colon Rectum 1982;36:508.

9. Gibney EJ. Volvulus of the sigmoid colon. Surg Gynecol Obstet 1991;173:243–55.

10. Hellinger MD, Steinhagen RM. Colonic volvulus. In: Wolff BG, Fleshman JW, Beck DE, editors. ASCRS textbook of colorectal surgery. New York: Springer; 2007. p. 286–98.

11. Sutcliffe MML. Volvulus of the sigmoid colon. Br J Surg 1968;55:903–10.

12. Sonnenberg A, Tsou VT, Muller AD. The 'institutional colon': a frequent colonic dysmotility in psychiatric and neurologic disease. Am J Gastroenterol 1994;89:62–6.

13. Mangiarte EC, Croce MA, Fabian TC, et al. Sigmoid volvulus, a four decade experience. Am Surg 1989;55:41–4.

14. Grossmann EM, Longo WE, Stratton MD, et al. Sigmoid volvulus in Department of Veterans Affairs Medical Centers. Dis Colon Rectum 2000;43:414–8.

15. Subrahmanyam M. Mesosigmoplasty as a definitive operation for sigmoid volvulus. Br J Surg 1992;79:683–4.

16. Bagarani M, Conde AS, Longo R, et al. Sigmoid volvulus in West Africa: a prospective study on surgical treatments. Dis Colon Rectum 1993;36:186.

17. De U, Ghosh S. Single stage primary anastomosis without colonic lavage for left sided colonic obstruction due to acute sigmoid volvulus: a prospective study of one hundred and ninety seven cases. Aust N Z J Surg 2003;73:390–2.

18. Naeeder SB, Archampong EQ. One-stage resection of acute sigmoid volvulus. Br J Surg 1995;82:1635–6.

19. Akgun Y. Management of ileosigmoid knot. Br J Surg 1997;84:672–3.

20. Miller BJ, Borrowdale RC. Ileosigmoid knotting: a case report and review. Aust N Z J Surg 1992;62:402–4.

21. Anderson JR, Lee D, Taylor TV, et al. Volvulus of the transverse colon. Br J Surg 1981;7:12–8.

22. Anderson JR, Lee D. Acute caecal volvulus. Br J Surg 1980;67:39–41.

23. Anderson MJ, Okike N, Spencer RJ. The colonoscope in cecal volvulus: report of 3 cases. Dis Colon Rectum 1978;21:71–4.

24. Ballantyne GH, Brandner MD, Beart RW, et al. Volvulus of the colon. Ann Surg 1985;202:83–92.

25. Tuech JJ, Pessaux P, Regenet N, et al. Results of resection for volvulus of the right colon. Tech Coloproctol 2002;6:97–9.

26. Rabanovici R, Simansky DA, Kaplan O, et al. Cecal volvulus. Dis Colon Rectum 1990;33:765–9.

27. Dorudi S, Berry AR, Kettewell MGW. Acute colonic pseudo-obstruction. Br J Surg 1992;79:99–103.

28. Datta SN, Stephenson BM, Havard TJ, et al. Acute colonic pseudo-obstruction. Lancet 1993;341:690.

29. Vanek VW, Al-Salti M. Acute pseudo-obstruction of the colon (Ogilvie's syndrome): an analysis of 400 cases. Dis Colon Rectum 1986;29:203–10.

30. Bachulis BL, Smith PE. Pseudo-obstruction of the colon. Am J Surg 1978;136:66–72.

31. Koruth NM, Koruth A, Matheson NA. The place of contrast enema in the management of large bowel obstruction. J R Coll Surg Edinb 1985;30:258–60.
   This paper studied 91 patients with suspected large-bowel obstruction. Of the 79 patients who were thought clinically to have mechanical obstruction, the diagnosis was confirmed in 50 by contrast enema and refuted in 29. Eleven had non-obstructing colonic pathology and 18 patients had pseudo-obstruction. Of the 12 patients who were thought to have pseudo-obstruction before the water-soluble contrast enema, two were shown to have carcinoma of the colon.

32. Johnson CD, Rice RP, Kelvin FM, et al. The radiological evaluation of gross cecal distension. Emphasis on cecal ileus. Am J Radiol 1985;145:1211–7.

33. Ponec RJ, Saunders MD, Kimmey MB. Neostigmine for the treatment of acute colonic pseudo-obstruction. N Engl J Med 1999;341:137–41.
   A randomised study of 21 patients with acute ACPO in which 11 patients were randomised to receive neostigmine and 10 patients received intravenous saline. The study showed that where the conservative treatment of ACPO fails, intravenous injection of 2.0 mg neostigmine results in rapid decompression of the colon.

34. Trevisani GT, Hyman NH, Church JM. Neostigmine. Safe and effective treatment for acute colonic pseudo-obstruction. Dis Colon Rectum 2000;43:599–603.

35. Abbasakoor F, Evans A, Stephenson BM. Neostigmine for acute colonic pseudo-obstruction. N Engl J Med 1999;341:1622–3.

36. Lee JT, Taylor BM, Singleton BC. Epidural anaesthesia for acute pseudo-obstruction of the colon. Dis Colon Rectum 1988;31:686–91.

37. Strodel WE, Brothers T. Colonoscopic decompression of pseudo-obstruction and volvulus. Surg Clin North Am 1989;69:1327–35.

38. Strodel WE, Norstrant TT, Eskhauser FE, et al. Therapeutic and diagnostic colonoscopy in non obstructive colonic dilatation. Ann Surg 1983;197:416–21.

39. Jetmore AB, Timmcke AE, Gathright JB, et al. Ogilvie's syndrome: colonoscopic decompression and analysis of predisposing factors. Dis Colon Rectum 1992;35:1135–42.

40. Stephenson KR, Rodriguez-Bigas MA. Decompression of the large intestine in Ogilvie's syndrome by a colonoscopically placed long intestinal tube. Surg Endosc 1994;8:116–7.

41. Laine L. Management of acute colonic pseudoobstruction. N Engl J Med 1999;341:192–3.

42. Chevallier P, Marcy P, Francois E, et al. Controlled transperitoneal percutaneous cecostomy as a therapy alternative to the endoscopic decompression for Ogilvie's syndrome. Am J Gastroenterol 2002;97:471–4.

43. McKenzie S, Thomson SR, Baker LW. Management options in malignant obstruction of the left colon. Surg Gynecol Obstet 1992;174:337–45.

44. Runkel NS, Schlag P, Schwarz V, et al. Outcome after emergency surgery of the large intestine. Br J Surg 1991;78:183–188.

45. Sjodahl R, Franzen T, Nystrom PO. Primary versus staged resection for acute obstructing colorectal carcinoma. Br J Surg 1992;79:685–8.

46. Phillips RK, Hittinger R, Fry JS, et al. Malignant large bowel obstruction. Br J Surg 1985;72:296–302.

47. Crucitti F, Sofo L, Doglietto GB, et al. Prognostic factors in colorectal cancer: current status and new trends. J SurgOncol 1991;2(Suppl):76–82.

48. Sebastian S, Johnston S, Geoaghegan T, et al. Pooled analysis of the efficacy and safety of self-expanding metal stenting in malignant colorectal obstruction. Am J Gastroenterol 2004;9:2051–7.

49. Dudley H, Phillips R. Intraoperative techniques in large bowel obstruction: methods of management with bowel resection. In: Fielding LP, Welch J, editors. Intestinal obstruction. Edinburgh: Churchill Livingstone; 1987. p. 139–52.

50. Deans GT, Krukowski ZH, Irvin ST. Malignant obstruction of the left colon. Br J Surg 1994;81:1270–6.

51. Murray JJ, Schoetz DJ, Coller JA, et al. Intraoperative colonic lavage and primary anastomosis in non-elective colon resection. Dis Colon Rectum 1991;34:527–31.

52. Lee YM, Law WL, Chu KW, et al. Emergency surgery for obstructing colorectal cancers: a comparison between right-sided and left-sided lesions. J Am Coll Surg 2001;192:719–25.

53. Naraynsingh V, Rampaul R, Maharaj D, et al. Prospective study of primary anastomosis without colonic lavage for patients with an obstructed left colon. Br J Surg 1999;86:1341–3.

54. Turan M, Ok E, Sen M, et al. A simplified operative technique for single-staged resection of left-sided colon obstructions: report of a 9-year experience. Surg Today 2002;32:959–64.

55. The SCOTIA Study Group. Single stage treatment for malignant left sided colonic obstruction: a prospective randomised clinical trial comparing subtotal colectomy with segmental resection following intraoperative irrigation. Br J Surg 1995;82:1622–7.

    A multicentre, prospective, randomised trial comparing subtotal colectomy with segmental resection, intraoperative irrigation and primary anastomosis for left-sided malignant large-bowel obstruction. Although postoperative mortality and length of stay in hospital were similar for both procedures, segmental resection with intraoperative colonic irrigation was superior to subtotal colectomy in terms of stoma rate and bowel function.

56. Hsu TC. Comparison of one-stage resection and anastomosis of acute complete obstruction of left and right colon. Am J Surg 2005;189(4):384–7.

57. Hinchey EJ, Schaal PG, Richards GK. Treatment of perforated diverticular disease of the colon. Adv Surg 1978;12:85–109.

58. Biondo S, Pares D, Marti Rague J, et al. Acute colonic diverticulitis in patients under 50 years of age. Br J Surg 2002;89:1137–41.

59. Reisman Y, Ziv Y, Kravrovitic D, et al. Diverticulitis: the effect of age and location on the course of disease. Int J Colorectal Dis 1999;14:250–4.

60. Ambrosetti P, Becker C, Terrier F. Colonic diverticulitis: impact of imaging on surgical management. A prospective study of 542 patients. Eur Radiol 2002;12:1145–9.

    This study prospectively evaluated 420 patients who underwent both CT and water-soluble contrast enema in the evaluation of acute diverticulitis. The performance of CT was significantly higher than contrast enema both in terms of sensitivity (98% vs. 92%) and in the evaluation of the severity of the inflammation (26% vs. 9%). Furthermore, contrast enema picked up an abscess in 20 patients compared with 69 patients using CT.

61. Hulnick DM, Megibow AJ, Balthazar EJ, et al. Computed tomography in the evaluation of diverticulitis. Radiology 1984;152:491–5.

62. Heverhagen JT, Zielke A, Ishaque N, et al. Acute colonic diverticulitis: visualization in magnetic resonance imaging. Magn Reson Imaging 2001;19:1275–7.

63. Chiu P, Lam C, Lam S, et al. On-table cecoscopy. A novel diagnostic method in acute diverticulitis of the right colon. Dis Colon Rectum 2002;45:611–4.

64. Dawson JL, Hanon I, Roxburgh RA. Diverticulitis coli complicated by diffuse peritonitis. Br J Surg 1965;52:354.

65. Krukowski ZH, Matheson NA. Emergency surgery for diverticular disease complicated by generalised and faecal peritonitis: a review. Br J Surg 1984;71:921–7.

66. Biondo S, Perea M, Ragué J, et al. One-stage procedure in non-elective surgery for diverticular disease complications. Colorectal Dis 2001;3:42–5.

67. Zorcolo L, Covotta L, Carlomagno N, et al. Safety of primary anastomosis in emergency colorectal surgery. Colorectal Dis 2003;5:262–9.

68. Cirocchi R, Farinella E, Trastulli S, et al. Elective sigmoid colectomy for diverticular disease: laparoscopic versus open surgery: a systematic review. Colorectal Dis 2012;14(6):671–83.

69. Afshar S, Kurer MA. Laparoscopic peritoneal lavage for perforated sigmoid diverticulitis. Colorectal Dis 2012;14(2):135–42.

70. Scott SA. Surgery for Crohn's disease. In: Wolff BG, Fleshman JW, Beck DE, et al., editors. ASCRS textbook of colorectal surgery. New York: Springer; 2007. p. 584–600.

71. Yamamoto T, Keighley MR. Long-term outcome of total colectomy and ileostomy for Crohn disease. Scand J Gastroenterol 1999;34:280–6.

72. Binder SC, Miller HH, Deterling Jr RA. Emergency and urgent operations for ulcerative colitis; the procedure of choice. Arch Surg 1975;110:284–9.

73. Dubinsky I. Stercoral perforation of the colon: case report and review of the literature. J Emerg Med 1996;14:323–5.

74. Serpell JW, Nicholls RJ. Stercoral perforation of the colon. Br J Surg 1990;77:1325–9.

75. Maurer CA, Renzulli P, Mazzucchelli L, et al. Use of accurate diagnostic criteria may increase incidence of stercoral perforation of the colon. Dis Colon Rectum 2000;43:991–8.

76. Fielding LP, Stewart Brown S, Blesovsky L, et al. Anastomotic integrity after operation for large bowel cancer: a multicentre study. Br Med J 1980;282:411–4.

77. Watson AJ, Krukoswski ZH, Munro A. Salvage of large bowel anastomotic leaks. Br J Surg 1999;86:499–500.

78. Sheridan WG, Lowndes RH, Young HL. Tissue oxygen measurement as a predictor of colonic anastomotic healing. Dis Colon Rectum 1987;30:867–71.

79. Anderson ML, Pasha TM, Leighton JA. Endoscopic perforation of the colon: lessons from a 10-year study. Am J Gastroenterol 2000;95:3418–22.

80. Damore LJ, Rantis PC, Vernava AM, et al. Colonoscopic perforations. Dis Colon Rectum 1996;39:1308–14.

81. Araghizadeh F, Opelka FG, Hicks TC, et al. Colonoscopic perforations. Dis Colon Rectum 2001;44:713–6.

82. Abbaqsakoor F, Vaizey C. Colonic emergencies. In: Paterson-Brown S, editor. A companion to specialist surgical practice: Core topics in general and emergency surgery. 3rd ed. London: Elsevier; 2006. p. 183–214.

83. Imbembo AL, Bailey RW. Diverticular disease of the colon. In: Sabiston D, editor. Textbook of surgery. Philadelphia: WB Saunders; 1991. p. 910–20.

84. Hammond KL, Beck DE, Hicks TC, et al. Implications of negative technetium 99m-labeled red blood cell scintigraphy in patients presenting with lower gastrointestinal bleeding. Am J Surg 2007;193:404–8.

85. Jensen DM, Machicado GA. Colonoscopy for diagnosis and treatment of severe lower gastrointestinal bleeding. Routine outcomes and cost analysis. Gastrointest Endosc Clin North Am 1997;7(3):477–98.

86. Longstreth GF. Epidemiology and outcome of patients hospitalized with acute lower gastrointestinal hemorrhage: a population-based study. Am J Gastroenterol 1997;92:419–24.

87. Browder W, Cerise EJ, Litwin MS. Impact of emergency angiography in massive lower gastrointestinal bleeding. Ann Surg 1986;204:530–6.

88. DeBarros J, Rosas L, Cohen J, et al. The changing paradigm for the treatment of colonic hemorrhage: superselective angiographic embolisation. Dis Colon Rectum 2002;45:802–8.

89. Horton KM, Fishman EK. CT angiography of the GI tract. Gastrointest Endosc 2002;55:S37–41.

90. Bender JS, Wiencek RG, Bouwman DL. Morbidity and mortality following total abdominal colectomy for massive lower gastrointestinal bleeding. Am Surg 1991;57:536–41.

91. Corman ML. Vascular diseases. In: Corman ML, editor. Colon and rectal surgery. Philadelphia: JB Lippincott; 1993. p. 860–900.

92. Finne III CO. The aggressive management of serious lower gastrointestinal bleeding. Prob Gen Surg 1992;9:597.

11

Anorectal emergencies

Felicity J. Creamer
B. James Mander

Introduction

The emergency presentation of anorectal pathology constitutes a significant proportion of the general surgeon's workload. The problems encountered range from the acute pain of thrombosed haemorrhoids and perianal sepsis to the management of massive bleeding, trauma and foreign bodies. The management of many of these conditions is frequently straightforward; however, the close proximity of pathology to the structures involved in continence does require a degree of care and reflection. It is therefore imperative to ensure that any surgical intervention is appropriate, timely and minimally disruptive.

Anorectal anatomy

Understanding the pathophysiology and rationale for treatment in anorectal disease is impossible without sound knowledge of the anatomy of the anal canal. This is a 3- to 4-cm-long tube running downwards and backwards from the anorectal angle to the anus. It is divided in half by the dentate line, above which the canal is lined with hindgut-derived columnar epithelium and innervated by the autonomic hypogastric nerves, sensitive only to stretch. The section of the canal below the dentate line is lined with stratified squamous epithelium that merges at the anus with the perianal skin, and its nerve supply is derived from the somatic inferior rectal nerve making it sensitive to pain, pressure and temperature.

The canal is surrounded by a funnel of muscle essential in maintaining faecal continence. The inner muscle layer is the involuntary internal sphincter muscle, derived from the circular muscle of the rectum. Beyond this is the voluntary external sphincter, formed from striated muscle, continuous at its superior edge with the levator plate. Between these two muscle layers is the intersphincteric space, which contains mucous-secreting anal glands. Ducts from these glands open into the anal valves at the dentate line.

Three submucosal anal cushions are found, usually at the 3, 7 and 11 o'clock positions within the anal canal and contain fibroelastic tissue and arteriovenous anastamoses. In health they appose to form a tight seal within the canal, which helps to maintain continence, but in some people these can enlarge to form troublesome symptomatic haemorrhoids.

Perianal abscess

Perianal abscesses are defined as any collection of pus in the perianal tissues and are very common, with operative treatment being required in about 1 in 5000 people in Scotland annually.[1] They occur predominantly in adults, with a peak incidence in the third and fourth decades of life, men being affected two to three times more frequently than women. Patients present with signs and symptoms of acute inflammation, with pain being the most common symptom. In approximately one-third of patients they are associated with a persistent fistula-in-ano that, if left untreated, can result in recurrent infections.[2]

Primary perianal abscesses are most commonly caused by infection within the anal glands (the cryptoglandular theory) with the common causative organisms being gut-derived enterococci.[3,4] The resulting suppuration can spread in several directions, resulting in infection in a variety of anatomical spaces (**Fig. 11.1**). The relative frequency with which abscesses occur in the various anatomical locations is shown in Table 11.1.[5] Primary abscesses can also be caused by suppurating skin infections, including carbuncles, furuncles and infected apocrine glands. The responsible bacteria in these cases is almost invariably staphylococcus and as these abscesses do not communicate with the anal canal they are not associated with fistula formation.[6] Studies have shown that taking a swab for culture at the time of abscess drainage can predict whether a fistula is likely to be present and thus guide decision-making regarding future management.[6,7]

> ✅ It is recommended that a swab from the abscess cavity is sent for culture to determine the likelihood of a subsequent fistula.[6,7]

Secondary abscesses are much less common, accounting for just 10% of presentations.[8] They are the manifestation of distinct underlying disease, with inflammatory bowel disease (Crohn's disease in particular), colorectal neoplasia, diabetes mellitus, AIDS and tuberculosis all being potential causes. They can also occur as a complication of haemorrhoid surgery or as a consequence of trauma from foreign bodies.

Clinical features

On examination the abscess can usually be seen as a red, tender, fluctuant swelling near the anal verge; however, ischiorectal abscesses often present as a less distinct brawny swelling on one side of the anus and intersphincteric abscesses cannot usually be seen externally at all. Although this last type of abscess can be felt through the anal wall as a smooth, tender collection, digital rectal examination is usually excruciatingly painful without anaesthesia. This diagnosis should therefore be suspected in patients with severe anal pain and fever. In a few patients (particularly those who are immune-compromised or with diabetes mellitus) the abscess can be associated with cellulitis, which can progress to life-threatening necrotising infection if not treated promptly.[9]

All patients presenting with anorectal sepsis or pain should have an examination of the anorectum, including proctosigmoidoscopy. It is our opinion that this can usually only be performed satisfactorily under general anaesthesia. As the diagnosis is usually obvious, few people would routinely recommend preoperative imaging (although some advocate its use, arguing that by identifying cavities and fistulas there is a reduction in the incidence of recurrence[10]). However, if the diagnosis is unclear (such as in intersphincteric or supralevator abscesses) or in cases of recurrent sepsis, imaging is very useful.

Radiological imaging

Magnetic resonance imaging (MRI) is an accurate method of identifying collections of pus and fistula tracts.[11,12] It is commonly used in investigating complex fistula disease in Crohn's disease but is rarely needed in the acute situation. Endoanal ultrasound is another sensitive method of identifying collections of fluid close to the anal canal and can also be used to identify fistula tracts (**Fig. 11.2**). It remains

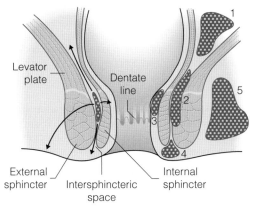

Figure 11.1 • The spread of anal gland infection and common sites of anorectal sepsis. Infection of the anal gland within the intersphincteric space can spread in a variety of directions (see left side of diagram), resulting in abscess in a number of classical sites: 1, supralevator; 2, intersphincteric; 3, submucosal; 4, perianal; 5, ischiorectal. Note also the possibility of circumferential extension of sepsis ('horseshoeing') in the intersphincteric, ischiorectal and supralevator planes.

Table 11.1 • Location of anorectal sepsis by anatomical site

Anatomical site	Number	Percentage
Perianal abscess	437	42.7
Ischiorectal	233	22.8
Intersphincteric	219	21.4
Supralevator	75	7.3
Submucosal	59	5.8

Data from Ramunjam PS, Prasad MI, Abcarian H et al. Perianal abscesses and fistulae: a study of 1023 patients. Dis Colon Rectum 1984; 27:593–7. With kind permission from Wolters Kluwer Health.

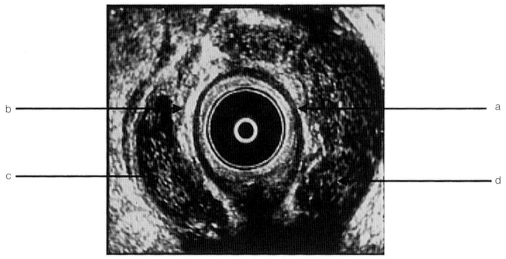

b ⟶ a

c ⟶ d

Figure 11.2 • Endoanal ultrasound examination carried out on a patient under general anaesthesia. This patient presented with severe anal pain and perianal induration but without any specific area of fluctuation. The ultrasound demonstrates an extensive ischiorectal abscess cavity **(c,d)** extending around the anal canal (**a**, internal sphincter; **b**, external sphincter). With thanks to Mr Mike Hulme-Moir, previous Clinical Fellow in Colorectal Surgery, Royal Infirmary, Edinburgh.

a technique practised by only a few specialist surgeons and so is rarely available in the emergency situation. However, it has been shown that in experienced hands it is at least as accurate as MRI and its use is likely to increase.[13,14]

Treatment

Treatment must be aimed at draining the abscess, thereby removing the source of sepsis. This should be done whilst minimising damage to the sphincters, preventing recurrence and minimising hospital stay. In most patients this involves making a linear incision over the cavity, gently breaking down any loculi and then dressing appropriately. There is no role for treatment with antibiotics unless the patient is immune-compromised or there is evidence of florid cellulitis or suspicion of necrotising infection. Although in North America this drainage is commonly undertaken under local anaesthesia, the more thorough examination, drainage and treatment that can be performed under general anaesthesia is, in the opinion of the authors, preferable – and probably prevents a significant proportion of re-operations. A large retrospective case study of 500 patients treated for perianal abscess at the Mayo Clinic was reported in 2001 and revealed a 7.6% re-operation rate.[15] The reasons for re-operation included incomplete drainage of the abscess cavity at the first operation, missed abscesses (most often posterior collections) and postoperative bleeding. There was no association reported between patient

variables (such as age, immune suppression or diabetes) and so it must be concluded that surgical error was the only reason for these findings, emphasising the need for a thorough primary examination.

Historically, it was suggested that thoroughly 'deroofing' the abscess cavity with a wide cruciate incision was beneficial but this does little other than giving the patient a larger wound that will take longer to heal.[16] Similarly, a short-lived enthusiasm for primary wound closure after incision has been abandoned by most surgeons as studies have shown that it offers little immediate benefit in terms of time to wound healing and probably increases the chance of recurrent sepsis.[17]

If the abscess cavity is very large, an alternative to making a huge incision is to insert a de Pezze or Malecott catheter via a smaller skin incision. This was looked at in one study, which showed that of the 91 patients who underwent this treatment compared to the 54 who underwent conventional treatment, hospital stay was shorter (1.4 vs. 4.5 days) and the need for community dressing shorter, with no disadvantages seen at long-term follow-up.[18]

Technical tips

The management of specific abscesses is shown diagrammatically in **Fig. 11.3**. Simple perianal abscesses should be drained and the cavity gently curetted (**Fig. 11.3a**). With ischiorectal abscesses, the cavity is often huge (**Fig. 11.3b**). The cavity should be incised as near to the anal verge as possible to bring the

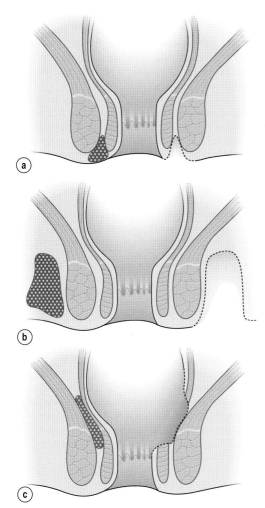

Figure 11.3 • Management of specific abscesses. **(a)** Perianal abscess is treated by excision of a small disc of skin and curettage of the cavity. **(b)** Ischiorectal abscess may require excision of a substantial amount of tissue to facilitate drainage. The alternative is to introduce a drainage catheter through a small stab incision. **(c)** Intersphincteric abscess is treated by excision of the mucosa and internal sphincter overlying the abscess. Such an abscess should not be drained through the perineal skin or a high fistula will result.

external opening of any subsequent fistula close to the anal verge and thus minimise the trauma of subsequent fistulotomy should it be required. A large horseshoe abscess in the ischiorectal space is better drained through multiple short incisions than one large circumferential incision. As mentioned earlier, the size of the drainage wound can be minimised if a drainage catheter is used. Intersphincteric abscesses require drainage into the anorectum, with excision of part of the internal sphincter (**Fig. 11.3c**). Submucosal abscesses, although rare, are drained

into the anal canal. Supralevator or pelvic abscesses must be drained with care and ideally not through the perineum or a high fistula-in-ano will be created. In true pelvic abscesses unrelated to spread from the anal glands, drainage can be achieved into the rectum or vagina. If the abscess is related to pelvic pathology, the primary disease process will need to be excised along with drainage of the pus.

After the abscess has been opened and drained it is common to 'pack' the resulting cavity with absorbent dressing material, which must then be removed and replaced by community nurses. However, there is no good clinical evidence that this practice is beneficial to the patient and indeed, in our opinion, serves only to cause discomfort and inconvenience.[19]

> ✔ Perianal abscesses are best incised under general anaesthesia with the cavity left open. Packing the abscess cavity is clinically unnecessary and unpleasant for the patient.[15,17,19]

Fistula-in-ano

Studies have shown that perianal abscesses are associated with fistulas in about 60% of patients;[7,20] however, only 29–37% of these persist after the acute inflammation has resolved.[2,21,22] A persisting fistula tract increases the chance of a recurrent abscess and can cause perianal discharge, itch and pain even in the absence of an acute infection. However, identifying a fistula when acute inflammation is present can be tricky, especially for the less experienced surgeon. As noted previously, a swab from an abscess cavity that grows gut- rather than skin-derived bacteria would suggest a communication to the bowel.[6,7] These patients can then be reviewed in the clinic after the acute sepsis has resolved and a second-look examination under anaesthesia (EUA) booked if indicated.

However, the cryptoglandular theory of anorectal sepsis would suggest that the presence of intersphincteric pus would definitively predict an underlying fistula tract. This was tested in a 1994 prospective study of 22 patients. A radial drainage incision was made and extended into the intersphincteric space. Careful examination was then made to determine whether there was a fistula tract. It was found that intersphincteric sepsis predicted a fistula with 100% sensitivity and specificity. Patients were followed up for 38 weeks with no adverse outcomes reported. This has the advantage over microbiological analysis of the abscess (which is very sensitive but just 80% specific) in that no second procedure is needed.[23] However, it must be noted that this study was performed by two highly experienced colorectal surgeons and there is no evidence that similar results would be safely obtained by non-specialists.

The probing and opening of tracts within friable, oedematous tissue, with the possibility of creating false passages, may do disproportionate damage to the sphincters and thus continence.

> ✔✔ The majority of anorectal abscesses are adequately treated with incision and drainage alone and if a fistula tract is not obvious it should not be sought.[20,21]

So should synchronous fistulotomy ever be performed? A recent Cochrane review of six randomised control studies from five different centres from 1987 to 2003 looked at concomitant fistula surgery at the time of abscess drainage in terms of recurrence, need for further surgery and postoperative incontinence.[24] However, as would be expected, the eligibility criteria and treatments offered varied considerably between the trials, making definitive recommendations difficult. Three studies also report fistula rates of 83–90%,[20,25,26] which is higher than would be expected, raising questions about whether iatrogenic tracks may have been created.

The majority of the studies included in the review dealt only with the surgical treatment of low fistulas. Of these, one randomised patients *after* the initial abscess drainage, with fistulotomy performed as a second procedure on day 3 of the acute admission.[25] Most studies excluded those with recurrent anorectal sepsis, previous surgery and inflammatory bowel disease (IBD).[24]

All the studies showed that recurrence was less likely after fistula surgery (risk ratio 0.07–0.24), although follow-up times varied. Only two studies looked at short-term incontinence, with one (which included only low fistulas, $n=52$) reporting no clinical incontinence in either group despite anal manometry revealing a transient reduction in the anal resting pressure in the fistulotomy group (76.3 mmHg vs. 91.1 mmHg), which had disappeared by week 12. Squeeze pressures were unaffected.[26] The other group (who had included high trans-sphincteric and suprasphincteric fistulas, which had been treated with cutting setons) reported transient incontinence of flatus in 3/100 of the control and 15/100 of the intervention group. For those who underwent drainage alone this had entirely resolved by 6 months; however, in the fistula surgery group, 6% were still having problems after 1 year.[20]

Long-term continence rates were documented in five studies and were normal in four of them following simple drainage alone at 1 year or later. Of the studies performing low fistulotomy, incontinence of flatus was 0/24,[27] 8/20[25] and 0/24.[26] The study that included high fistulas reported 2/100 incidence of incontinence for flatus and 4/100 for liquid incontinence with urgency.[20] The final study had performed fistulectomy and partial internal sphincterectomy, and

they reported flatus/liquid incontinence in 6/32 of the control and 13/34 of the intervention groups, with four and one patients from each group, respectively, lost to follow-up.[28] All these data combine to give a risk ratio of 2.64 for long-term incontinence following synchronous fistulotomy.[24]

The overall conclusions of the Cochrane meta-analysis were that synchronous fistulotomy is appropriate for low, uncomplicated fistula tracts. It should not be performed for high fistulas or anterior fistulas in women. It should also be avoided for groups where the risk of incontinence is high (e.g. those who have undergone previous anorectal surgery or have IBD).[24]

> ✔✔ Synchronous fistulotomy can be performed with care for low, uncomplicated fistula tracts to reduce the risk of abscess recurrence and further operations.[24]

Management of secondary perianal sepsis

Malignant disease

These abscesses should be drained like any other but definitive treatment will require resection of the malignant lesion. However, it is likely that the presence of anorectal sepsis indicates tumour spread outwith the bowel wall, which has implications for further treatment. Significant malignant fistulas will require a defunctioning stoma as other treatment will not be successful.

Inflammatory bowel disease

All abscesses in patients with IBD should be drained and seton sutures inserted into any fistulous tracts as necessary. MRI is often helpful in demonstrating fistula tracts. Recurrent disease is often very hard to treat and an expert opinion should be sought.

Necrotising infection

This life-threatening condition requires urgent wide debridement of all involved tissue and high-dose antibiotics. A defunctioning stoma may have to be formed to allow healing and several repeat examinations under anaesthetic are often necessary to ensure that only healthy tissue remains. Microbiology advice should be sought for antibiotic choice.

Anorectal sepsis in children

Anorectal sepsis in children is uncommon. One of the largest series in the literature is from Edinburgh, which reported 69 patients in a catchment population of 1 million over a 10-year period.[29] The median age for development of the abscess was 3 years (range 1 month to 12 years), with the male to female ratio 9:1. In total, 24 patients (38%) presented with recurrent sepsis after simple incision and drainage, but in only half of these was a fistula found. The study was unable to relate pus culture to the presence of a fistula. One study has shown that non-operative treatment with needle aspiration and antibiotics was satisfactory in the management of 36 children over 2 years of age, with only four requiring operative incision.[30] However, a recent large study from New Zealand has shown that the risk of recurrence is significantly reduced by incision, drainage and fistulotomy where possible.[31]

Pilonidal abscess

A pilonidal sinus arises from infection within a hair follicle, usually in the natal cleft. It is an acquired condition caused either by an ingrowing hair, which then sets up a local foreign body reaction, or by obstruction of a hair follicle, which then ruptures into the surrounding tissues. It affects twice as many men as women and is more common in the hirsute.[32] In the Second World War it was known as 'Jeep disease' due to its prevalence amongst the drivers in the United States army. The usual emergency presentation of pilonidal disease is with an acutely inflamed tender swelling adjacent to the natal cleft. Midline pits are usually visible. The causative organism is, as with many skin infections, staphylococcus but mixed anaerobes are not infrequently cultured.[33]

In the emergency setting the objective of treatment is to drain the abscess, which usually relieves the acute symptoms and prevents spreading sepsis. Excision for the whole sinus tract at the same time as abscess drainage has been attempted but this has been associated with recurrence rates of up to 60%.[33] In fact, primary drainage alone has a similar recurrence rate of around 50%,[34] but with a much smaller initial wound.

A comparative study from Israel assessed 58 patients with acute pilonidal abscess; 29 patients were treated with incision and drainage, the other 29 with wide excision (without closure). The results are displayed in Table 11.2. The risk of recurrent pilonidal suppuration was similar between the two groups, although those who underwent excision had a longer time off work.[34] It is therefore recommended that excision of the fistula tract is not undertaken synchronously.[35] It is the authors' usual practice only to offer formal excision after the second presentation with a pilonidal abscess and this is always performed as a separate procedure after the acute sepsis has settled. To ensure optimum wound healing it is recommended that the incision is made away from the midline and, as with other abscesses, that packing the wound with dressings is avoided.

> ✔ Fifty per cent of all pilonidal abscesses will be cured with incision and drainage alone.[34] Definitive surgery should be reserved for those who have recurrent disease and performed in the elective setting.[33,35]

Acute anal fissure

A primary anal fissure is a benign, superficial ulcer within the anal canal. Patients present with severe pain on defecation, which is caused by chemical irritation of the ulcer and spasm of the internal sphincter. Some patients will also complain of bright red bleeding caused by irritation of the ulcer bed. Although most patients with anal fissures will be seen in the outpatient clinic, some present acutely with an exacerbation of pain or just out of desperation with their chronic symptoms. It is often an easy diagnosis to make on inspection; gently parting the buttocks will usually reveal the lower edge of the fissure, most commonly in the posterior midline (6 o'clock) position.

The key to treatment is to stop the muscle spasm, which can be achieved by topical administration of smooth muscle relaxants such as glycerine trinitrate (GTN)[36] or diltiazem,[37] which reduce sphincter pressure and aid fissure healing. Diltiazem has a significantly lower side-effects profile than GTN and so

Table 11.2 • Results of treatment for acute pilonidal abscess

	Excision	Incision and drainage	P value
Number	29	29	
Recurrence	12 (41%)	16 (55%)	NS
Hospital stay (days)*	4 (2–8)	3 (0–12)	NS
Time off work (days)*	14 (3–60)	7 (3–30)	0.06
Time to healing (days)*	30 (15–70)	30 (10–60)	NS

NS, non-significant.
*Values expressed as median (range).
Data from Matter I, Kunin J, Schein M et al. Total excision versus non-resectional methods in the treatment of acute and chronic pilonidal disease. Br J Surg 1995; 82:752–3. © British Journal of Surgery Society Ltd. Reproduced with permission. Permission is granted by John Wiley & Sons Ltd on behalf of the BJSS Ltd.

should be used preferentially, if available.[38] These treatments typically take weeks to exert their full effect, but one study has shown that they can be useful in the acute setting – most patients presenting with fissures are too sore to tolerate digital rectal examination but administration of sublingual GTN allowed 13 of the 16 patients to be examined.[39] This allows more sinister pathology to be ruled out without recourse to admission and anaesthesia in some patients.

Medical treatment has excellent short-term results, leading to the healing of 90% of acute fissures without the need for surgery.[40] However, the long-term outlook is less encouraging, with one meta-analysis showing recurrence rates of up to 50%.[41] Lateral internal sphincterotomy (LIS) is much better at reducing recurrence (rates of about 2%) and although some studies have raised concerns about continence disturbance, it has been shown that a well-planned procedure in selected patients has very little effect on continence.[42,43] This, however, has no place in the acute setting and should be reserved for patients with chronic problems. Botox (botulinium toxin) injections into the internal sphincter are something of a middle ground, affecting a temporary sphincterotomy to allow fissure healing. These have again been mostly used for patients with chronic problems but a recent Eygptian randomised control trial has shown good results when used for acute fissures.[44]

It is important not to underestimate the pain caused by anal fissures and if patients are in pain for long periods of the day or unable to sleep at night an EUA should be performed to exclude occult sepsis and botox and local anaesthetic infiltrated into the internal sphincter and under the fissure, respectively, to provide symptomatic relief.

✔✔ Most anal fissures will heal with conservative topical treatment.[36,40] However, an EUA should be performed for those with severe unremitting symptoms. Definitive surgery should be reserved for those with recurrent disease.[41,42]

Haemorrhoids

Haemorrhoidal disease is very common, causing symptoms in approximately 5% of the population.[45] Haemorrhoids can be divided into internal, which originate above the dentate line, and external, which originate below the dentate line and are thus covered in mucosa and sensitive to pain. Although haemorrhoids are associated with symptoms including perianal irritation and small amounts of bleeding, they do not usually cause pain and uncomplicated haemorrhoidal disease is rarely seen as an emergency. However, external haemorrhoids can thrombose spontaneously (this process may be associated with straining to defecate), and internal haemorrhoids may prolapse, strangulate and thrombose. This thrombosis, with associated oedema and sometimes necrosis of the overlying mucosa, combines to cause exquisite tenderness such that patients are often unable to sit, walk or defecate.

Thrombosed haemorrhoids

These tense, tender, purple swellings can be seen by simply parting the buttocks. Although immensely painful they tend to resolve spontaneously after 4–5 days and therefore many surgeons advocate non-surgical management, the mainstays of which are good analgesia, laxatives and topical treatments such as nifedipine.[46] The main argument for this approach is that surgical treatment of haemorrhoids is likely to be painful for about the same amount of time as for natural healing, with little significant advantage in the longer term. However, a review by the American Society of Colon and Rectal Surgeons suggests that although those who present after 72 hours of symptoms are best served by non-operative treatment, those who present before this time would benefit from excision of the external component.[45]

However, definitive emergency surgical treatment can be difficult as swollen, congested tissues distort normal anatomy and restrict views. Although many retrospective and case-controlled studies suggest that outcomes are favourable when emergency haemorrhoidectomy is performed by experienced surgeons,[47,48] the only prospective randomised controlled study to investigate this showed that non-operative treatment was associated with shorter hospital stay and less sphincter damage.[49] If surgery is to be undertaken, several studies have shown that in the acute, as in the elective setting, a stapled procedure is associated with shorter hospital stays, reduced pain and earlier return to work.[50–52] One case–control study from Singapore compared 204 patients who underwent emergency haemorrhoidectomy with 500 who underwent an elective procedure during the same time period. They demonstrated no difference in any of the assessed end-points (haemorrhage, stricture, incontinence and portal pyaemia) between the two groups (see Table 11.3).[53]

✔✔ Thrombosed haemorrhoids will resolve with conservative management but longer remission may be achieved with surgery. If surgery is to be undertaken a stapled haemorrhoidectomy is preferable and has no greater associated risks in the acute situation if undertaken by a suitably experienced surgeon.[49,53]

Table 11.3 • Results from comparative study on emergency and elective haemorrhoidectomy

	Elective surgery (*n*=500)	Emergency surgery (*n*=204)	*P* value
Haemorrhage	27 (5.4)	10 (4.9)	NS
Blood transfusion	10 (2)	4 (2)	NS
Anal stenosis	15 (3)	12 (5.9)	NS
Disturbance of continence	26 (5.2)	9 (4.4)	NS
Sepsis	0	0	NS
Recurrence	38 (7.6)	14 (6.8)	NS

Numbers in parentheses are percentages. NS, non-significant.
Data from Eu KW, Seow Choen F, Goh HS. Comparison of emergency and elective haemorrhoidectomy. Br J Surg 1994; 81:308–10. © British Journal of Surgery Society Ltd. Reproduced with permission. Permission is granted by John Wiley & Sons Ltd on behalf of the BJSS Ltd.

Anorectal haemorrhage

Although per rectal bleeding is a common reason for acute surgical referral, major haemorrhage from an anorectal source is very rare. A series of lower gastrointestinal bleeds in an elderly North American population published in 1979 demonstrated an anorectal cause for massive blood loss in just four out of 98 patients.[54] Bleeding generally comes from a colonic source but rectal cancer, haemorrhoids, proctitis, rectal varices, anal fissures and solitary rectal ulcer syndrome have all been implicated in massive lower gastrointestinal bleeds. The increased use of nicorandil for the treatment of ischaemic heart disease has led to an increased awareness of the rectal ulcers that this drug can cause as a side-effect and a recent case report has been published of a life-threatening bleed secondary to this.[55]

Anorectal trauma

Worldwide the most common cause of anorectal trauma is childbirth, with 0.4% of all vaginal births complicated by a third-degree (into the external sphincter) or fourth-degree (into the rectal wall) tear.[56] One prospective study using endoanal ultrasound to evaluate post-childbirth sphincter function has suggested that as many as 35% of women demonstrate damaged external or internal sphincters following vaginal delivery.[57] These tears are often repaired in the labour suite with interrupted sutures to approximate the sphincters but results from this are poor, with significant levels of faecal urgency and incontinence persisting (up to 50% in one study).[58] In an attempt to improve outcome, a recent randomised controlled study from Norway of 119 women with third- and fourth-degree tears compared this end-to-end approximation with an overlap technique for sphincter repair.[59] Unfortunately, they found no significant difference between the two techniques for reported faecal incontinence at 12 months or on anal manometry.

Anorectal trauma can also occur as a result of penetrating injury, iatrogenic damage or secondary to foreign objects inserted into the anal canal. Injury sustained to the intraperitoneal rectum can sometimes be primarily repaired but if there is significant contamination, large injuries, devascularisation or nearby open fractures, resection and formation of a stoma should be preferred.[60] Damage to the extraperitoneal rectum can also often be repaired primarily but proximal diversion may again be needed if the injuries are extensive.[61] Sigmoidoscopy should always be performed if blood is seen in the rectal lumen or if an extraperitoneal haematoma is seen adjacent to the rectum at laparotomy.

Foreign bodies

Rectally inserted foreign objects and the innovative techniques used to remove them safely are extensively reported in anecdotal case reports in the world literature. These objects are most commonly inserted for sexual gratification and in most circumstances the patient has made an unsuccessful attempt to remove them before presentation. A review of these case reports suggests that in the majority of instances removal is possible under conscious sedation, either digitally for low objects or bimanually for those above the rectosigmoid junction.[62] When this fails, endoscopic extraction with or without fluoroscopic guidance is worth attempting. Some authors have reported success with various obstetric instruments and in one reported case of an irretrievable metallic ball, an electromagnet was employed.[63] If all of these measures fail, or there is radiographic evidence of perforation, laparotomy is usually inevitable. In a series reported from San Diego, this was necessary in five of 64 patients presenting with impacted foreign bodies.[64] It is recommended that all patients undergo sigmoidoscopy after extraction to ensure no damage to the rectal mucosa has been sustained.

Key points

- Anorectal sepsis should be managed by prompt drainage following sound anatomical principles.
- Synchronous fistulotomy can be undertaken with care in low, uncomplicated posterior fistulas but should be avoided in those at high risk of incontinence or when a tract is not easily distinguished.
- Acute pilonidal abscesses should be treated with simple incision and drainage alone.
- Abscess cavities should not be packed following drainage.
- Anal fissures should be managed pharmacologically, with surgery reserved for those that fail to heal.
- Acute thrombosed haemorrhoids should be managed non-operatively. Emergency haemorrhoidectomy is only recommended if carried out within 72 hours of symptom onset by an appropriately skilled surgeon.
- Management of anorectal trauma and retained foreign bodies should be determined by the site of injury and the anorectum should always be re-examined by sigmoidoscopy following removal.

References

1. Information Services Division, NHS Scotland. 2011 (personal communication).

2. Nelson R. Anorectal abscess fistula: what do we know? Surg Clin North Am 2002;82:1139–51.

3. Eisenhammer S. The internal anal sphincter and the anorectal abscess. Surg Gynecol Obstet 1956;103(4):501–6.

4. Parks AG. Pathogenesis and treatment of fistula in ano. Br Med J 1961;1:63–9.

5. Ramanujam PS, Prasad ML, Abcairn H, et al. Perianal abscesses and fistulas. A study of 1023 patients. Dis Colon Rectum 1984;27(9):593–7.

6. Eykyn SJ, Grace RH. The relevance of microbiology in the management of anorectal sepsis. Ann R Coll Surg Engl 1986;68(5):237–9.

7. Toyonaga T, Matsushima M, Tanaka Y, et al. Microbiological analysis and endoanal ultrasonography for diagnosis of anal fistula in acute anorectal sepsis. Int J Colorectal Dis 2007;22(2):209–13.

8. Winslett MC, Allan A, Ambrose NS. Anorectal sepsis as a presentation of occult rectal and systemic disease. Dis Colon Rectum 1988;31(8):597–600.

9. Badrinath K, Jairam N, Ravi HR. Spreading extraperitoneal cellulitis following perirectal sepsis. Br J Surg 1994;81(2):297–8.

10. Halligan S, Stoker J. Imaging in fistula in ano. Radiology 2006;239(1):18–33.

11. Sahni VA, Ahmad R, Burling D. Which method is best for imaging of perianal fistula? Abdom Imaging 2008;33(1):26–30.

12. Lunniss PJ, Barker PG, Sultan AH, et al. Magnetic resonance imaging of fistula-in-ano. Dis Colon Rectum 1994;37(7):708–18.

13. Gustafsson UM, Kanvecloglu B, Anstrom M, et al. Endoanal ultrasound or magnetic resonance imaging for pre-operative assessment of anal fistula: a comparative study. Colorectal Dis 2001;3(3):189–97.

14. Law PJ, Talbot RW, Bartram CJ, et al. Anal endoscopy in the evaluation of perianal sepsis and fistula in ano. Br J Surg 1989;76(7):752–5.

15. Onanca N, Hirshberg J, Adar R. Early reoperation for perianal abscess: a preventable complication. Dis Colon Rectum 2001;44(10):1469–73.

16. Golligher JC. Surgery of the anus, rectum and colon. 3rd ed. London: BalliereTindall; 1975.

17. Mortensen J, Kraglund K, Klaerke M, et al. Primary suture of anorectal abscesses A randomised study comparing treatment with clindamycin vs clindamycin and Gentacoll. Dis Colon Rectum 1995;38(4):398–401.

18. Kyle S, Isbister WH. Management of anorectal abscesses: comparison between traditional incision and packing and de Pezzer catheter drainage. Aust N Z J Surg 1990;60(2):129–31.

19. Tonkin DM, Murphy E, Brooke-Smith M, et al. Perianal abscess: a pilot study comparing packing with non-packing of the abscess cavity. Dis Colon Rectum 2004;47(9):1510–4.

20. Oliver I, Lacueva FJ, Vincente Perez, et al. Randomised clinical trial comparing simple drainage of anorectal abscess with and without fistula track treatment. Int J Colorectal Dis 2003;18(2):107–10.

    A prospective, randomised trial of 200 consecutive patients showed recurrence reduced from 29% to 5% in patients in whom definitive treatment of the fistula track was attempted rather than simple drainage. However, due to the higher risk of incontinence these recommendations were limited to those with low fistulas.

21. Read DR, Abcarian H. A prospective study of 474 patients with anorectal abscess. Dis Colon Rectum 1979;22:566–8.

    A large prospective study showing good results for primary fistulotomy along with drainage.

22. Henrichsen S, Christiansen J. Incidence of fistula in ano complicating anorectal sepsis; a prospective study. Br J Surg 1986;73:371–2.

23. Lunniss PJ, Phillips RK. Surgical assessment of acute anorectal sepsis is a better predictor of fistula than microbiological analysis. Br J Surg 1994;81(3):368–9.

24. Malik AI, Nelson RL, Tou S. Incision and drainage of perianal abscess with or without treatment of anal fistula. Cochrane Database Syst Rev 2010;(7) CD006827.

A review of the current evidence for concurrent fistulotomy at the time of incision and drainage of an acute abscess, showing good results for fistulotomy in low, uncomplicated disease.

25. Hejoborn M, Olson O, Haakansson T, et al. A randomised trial of fistulotomy in perianal abscess. Scand J Gastroenterol 1987;22:174–6.

26. Ho YH, Tan M, Chui CH, et al. Randomised control trial of primary fistulotomy with drainage alone for perianal abscesses. Dis Colon Rectum 1998;40:1435–8.

27. Tang CL, Chew SP, Seow-Choen F. Prospective randomised trial of drainage alone vs. drainage and fistulotomy for acute perianal abscesses with proven internal opening. Dis Colon Rectum 1996;39:1415–7.

28. Schouten WR, Van Vroonhoven TJ. Treatment of anorectal abscess with or without primary fistulectomy: Results of a prospective randomised trial. Dis Colon Rectum 1991;34:60–3.

29. Macdonald A, Wilson-Storey D, Munro F. Treatment of perianal abscess and fistula-in-ano in children. Br J Surg 2003;2:220–1.

30. Serour F, Gorenstein A. Characteristics of perianal abscess and fistula-in-ano in healthy children. World J Surg 2006;30(3):467–72.

31. Buddicom E, Janieson A, Beasley S, et al. Perianal abscess in children: aiming for optimal management. Aust N Z J Surg 2012;82:60–2.

32. Sondenaa K, Nesvik I, Andersen E, et al. Bacteriology and complications of chronic pilonidal sinus treated with excision and primary suture. Int J Colorectal Dis 1995;10(3):161–6.

33. Clothier PR, Haywood IR. The natural history of the post anal (pilonidal) sinus. Ann R Coll Surg Engl 1984;66(3):201–3.

34. Jensen SL, Harling H. Prognosis after simple incision and drainage for a first-episode acute pilonidal abscess. Br J Surg 1988;75(1):60–1.

35. Matter I, Kunin J, Schein M, et al. Total excision versus non-resectional methods in the treatment of acute and chronic pilonidal disease. Br J Surg 1995;82(6):752–3.

36. Lund JN, Scholefield JH. A randomised, prospective, double-blind, placebo-controlled trial of glyceryltrinitrate ointment in treatment of anal fissure. Lancet 1997;349(9044):11–4.

This study of 80 consecutive patients demonstrated rapid relief of symptoms and after 8 weeks of ongoing treatment 68% demonstrated fissure healing compared to 8% in the placebo group.

37. Knight JS, Birks M, Farouk R. Topical diltiazem ointment in the treatment of chronic anal fissure. Br J Surg 2001;88(4):553–6.

38. Kocher HM, Steward M, Leather AJ, et al. Randomized clinical trial assessing the side-effects of glyceryltrinitrate and diltiazem hydrochloride in the treatment of chronic anal fissure. Br J Surg 2002;89(4):413–7.

39. Larpent JL, Dussaud F, Gorce D, et al. The use of glyceryltrinitrate in inexaminable patients with anal fissure. Int J Colorectal Dis 1996;11(6):263.

40. Frezza EE, Sandei F, Leoni G, et al. Conservative and surgical treatment in acute and chronic anal fissure. A study on 308 patients. Int J Colorectal Dis 1992;7(4):188–91.

A large study concluding that the condition is self-limiting in the vast majority of patients.

41. Nelson R. Non surgical therapy for anal fissure. Cochrane Database Syst Rev 2006;4: CD003431.

A review of 53 randomised controlled trials comparing medical and surgical therapy for anal fissure showed some advantage to topical treatments over placebo for acute fissure symptoms but that surgery was by far the best solution for chronic fissure problems.

42. Brown CJ, Dubreuil D, Santoro L, et al. Lateral internal sphincterotomy is superior to topical nitroglycerin for healing chronic anal fissure and does not compromise long-term fecal continence: six-year follow-up of a multicenter, randomized, controlled trial. Dis Colon Rectum 2007;50(4):442–8.

A study of 82 patients with chronic anal fissure randomised to GTN treatment or LIS showed better long-term patient satisfaction in the surgical group with no significant compromise to continence.

43. Ho KS, Ho YH. Randomized clinical trial comparing oral nifedipine with lateral anal sphincterotomy and tailored sphincterotomy in the treatment of chronic anal fissure. Br J Surg 2005;92(4):403–8.

44. Othman I. Bilateral versus posterior injection of botuliniumtoxin in the internal anal sphincter for the treatment of acute anal fissure. S Afr J Surg 2010;48(1):20–2.

45. Cataldo P, Ellis CN, Gregorcyk S, et al. Practice parameters for the management of hemorrhoids (revised). Dis Colon Rectum 2005;48:189–94.

46. Perrotti P, Antropoli C, Molino D, et al. Conservative treatment of acute thrombosed external hemorrhoids with topical nifedipine. Dis Colon Rectum 2001;44(3):405–9.

47. Mazier WP. Emergency hemorrhoidectomy – a worthwhile procedure. Dis Colon Rectum 1973;16(3):200–5.

48. Greenspon J, Williams SB, Young HA, et al. Thrombosed external hemorrhoids: outcome after

conservative or surgical management. Dis Colon Rectum 2004;47(9):1493–8.

49. Allan A, Samad AJ, Mellon A, et al. Prospective randomised study of urgent haemorrhoidectomy compared with non-operative treatment in the management of prolapsed thrombosed internal haemorrhoids. Colorectal Dis 2006;8(1):41–5.
    This study of 50 patients found that conservative treatment was associated with shorter admission duration and less anal sphincter damage as assessed by endoanal ultrasound, with no difference in the number of symptomatic patients at 24-month follow-up.

50. Wong JC, Chung CC, Yau KK, et al. Stapled technique for acute thrombosed hemorrhoids: a randomized, controlled trial with long-term results. Dis Colon Rectum 2008;51(4):397–403.

51. Lai HJ, Jao SW, Su CC, et al. Stapled hemorrhoidectomy versus conventional excision hemorrhoidectomy for acute hemorrhoidal crisis. J Gastrointest Surg 2007;11(12):1654–61.

52. Brown SR, Ballan K, Ho E, et al. Stapled mucosectomy for acute thrombosed circumferentially prolapsed piles: a prospective randomized comparison with conventional haemorrhoidectomy. Colorectal Dis 2001;3(3):175–8.

53. Eu KW, Seow-Choen F, Goh HS. Comparison of emergency and elective haemorrhoidectomy. Br J Surg 1994;81(2):308–10.
    A large case–control study from an expert centre showing that almost identical results can be achieved in acute and elective settings. However, there is no suggestion that this technique should be undertaken without appropriate training in the emergency situation.

54. Boley SJ, DiBiase A, Brandt LJ, et al. Lower intestinal bleeding in the elderly. Am J Surg 1979;137(1):57–64.

55. Mosely F, Bhasin N, Davies JB, et al. Life-threatening haemorrhage secondary to nicorandil-induced severe peri-anal ulceration. Ann R Coll Surg Engl 2010;92(6):W39–40.

56. Sleep J, Grant A, Garcia J, et al. West Berkshire perineal management trial. Br Med J (Clin Res Ed) 1984;289(6445):587–90.

57. Sultan AH, Kamm MA, Hudson CN, et al. Anal sphincter disruption during vaginal delivery. N Engl J Med 1993;329(26):1905–11.

58. Sultan AH, Kamm MA, Hudson CN, et al. Third degree obstetric anal sphincter tears: risk factors and outcome of primary repair. Br Med J 1994;308(6933):887–91.

59. Rygh AB, Korner H. The overlap technique versus end-to-end approximation technique for primary repair of obstetric anal sphincter rupture: a randomized control study. Acta Obstet Gynecol Scand 2010;89(10):1256–62.

60. McGrath V, Fabian TC, Croce MA, et al. Rectal trauma: management based on anatomic distinctions. Am Surg 1998;64(12):1136–41.

61. Weinberg JA, Fabian TC, Magnotti LJ, et al. Penetrating rectal trauma: management by anatomic distinction improves outcome. J Trauma 2006;60(3):508–14.

62. Kornstra JJ, Weersma RK. Management of rectal foreign bodies: description of a new technique and practice guidelines. World J Gastroenterol 2008;14(27):4403–6.

63. Coulson CJ, Brammer RD, Stonelake PS. Extraction of a rectal foreign body using an electromagnet. Int J Colorectal Dis 2005;20:194–5.

64. Cohen JS, Sackier JM. Management of colorectal foreign bodies. J R Coll Surg Edinb 1996;41(5):312–5.

12

Paediatric surgical emergencies

Dafydd A. Davies
Jacob C. Langer

Introduction

While paediatric surgery has increasingly become the domain of the subspecialist paediatric surgeon, adult general surgeons are still often faced with the challenges of assessing and managing children with surgical emergencies. The unique differences between adults and children must be taken into account when addressing every aspect of surgical management, including assessment, diagnosis, resuscitation and operative interventions. Children face a different spectrum of conditions, have different physiological responses to trauma, illness and surgical stress, and have different psychosocial needs.

This chapter will address the common abdominal paediatric surgical emergencies encountered by general surgeons. These will be categorised according to age: (i) Neonates (up to 44 weeks postgestational age), (ii) infants (1 month to 2 years of age) and (iii) children (2 years of age and older).

Neonatal period

Prenatal diagnosis

Routine prenatal ultrasonography has become the standard of care in many parts of the developed world, and has resulted in the detection of many congenital anomalies before birth. Common detectable anomalies relevant to the general surgeon include: abdominal wall defects, congenital diaphragmatic hernia, intestinal obstruction, and intra-abdominal masses.

Whenever possible these patients should be referred for prenatal consultation with obstetrics, neonatology and paediatric general surgery. In most cases, delivery should occur at a hospital with a neonatal intensive care unit and paediatric surgical service. If this is not possible they should be immediately transferred following delivery and resuscitation.

Intestinal obstruction

Intestinal obstruction is the most common abdominal emergency in the neonatal period, and is usually due to a congenital, developmental or genetic anomaly.

Assessment

Assessing neonatal patients for obstruction requires a thorough history, including the nature of any vomiting and the presence or absence of abdominal distention. Since neonates are unable to verbalise, surgeons must gather as many clues as possible from the prenatal, perinatal and family historical details (Table 12.1).

Examination of neonates with suspected intestinal obstruction should start with vital signs and an assessment of the level of resuscitation required. Certain forms of obstruction can cause severe dehydration or sepsis, which will need to be addressed early. Dysmorphic features may give clues to syndromes in which obstruction is common. The abdominal examination should make note of any discoloration, distention and signs of

Table 12.1 • Important considerations in the neonatal history

Prenatal history	• Previous pregnancies (complications and outcomes) • Maternal gestational illnesses (e.g. gestational diabetes, pregnancy induced hypertension) • Screening ultrasonoography (dates and findings) • Other prenatal investigations and outcomes (e.g. maternal alpha-fetoprotein/betaHCG/oestrogen levels, chorionic villous sampling, amniocentesis)
Perinatal history	• Weeks of gestation • Induced or spontaneous labour • Complications of delivery • APGAR scores
Neonatal history	• Complications • Infections • Feeding history (initiation, type, rate achieved) • Passage of meconium in the first 24 hours of life • Other anomalies identified
Family history	• Maternal and paternal health • Previous congenital anomalies • Cystic fibrosis • Consanguinity

peritoneal inflammation, such as guarding and rigidity. It is important to look for an incarcerated inguinal hernia as the cause of obstruction (see later). A thorough evaluation of the perineum must also be carried out to ensure normal location and patency of the anus.

Routine blood tests including electrolytes and full blood count are helpful in assessing the level of dehydration as well as helping determine if electrolyte disturbances or sepsis are contributing to the presentation. It should be kept in mind that serum creatinine in the newborn reflects the mother's levels, and may not be helpful in assessing the neonate's renal function.

Abdominal radiography should be the initial imaging modality for neonates with possible intestinal obstruction. Typically, infants with duodenal obstruction have a 'double-bubble' appearance (**Fig. 12. 1**), whereas those with distal intestinal obstruction will have multiple dilated bowel loops. It is impossible to differentiate distal small-bowel obstruction from colonic obstruction based on the plain abdominal radiograph in neonates, as the haustral markings seen in adults are not visible in this age group.

A contrast study is often required to definitively diagnose the aetiology of intestinal obstruction. If malrotation is suspected, an urgent upper gastrointestinal contrast study should be performed first. Once this diagnosis has been excluded a contrast enema can be done to exclude distal pathology if this is indicated. For those infants with distal obstruction on plain radiograph, a contrast enema will help to differentiate the three most common causes

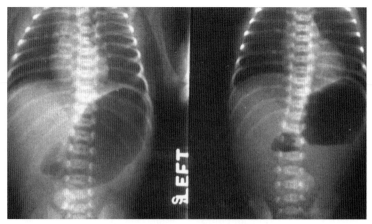

Figure 12.1 • Abdominal radiograph of an infant showing the typical 'double-bubble' appearance resulting from duodenal obstruction.

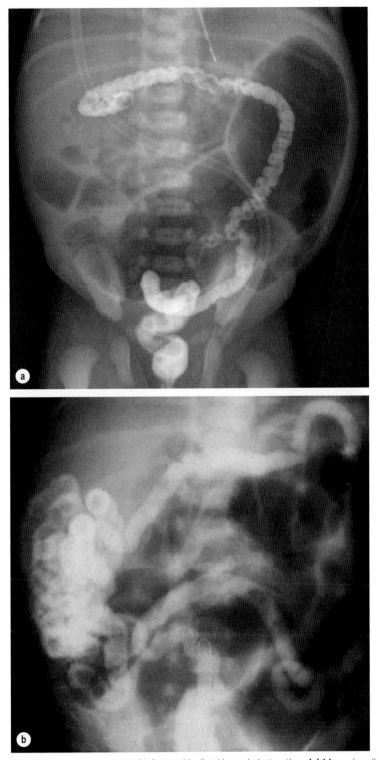

Figure 12.2 • Water-soluble contrast enemas of infants with distal bowel obstruction. **(a)** Meconium ileus, showing a microcolon, dilated proximal small bowel and a soap-bubble appearance in the right lower quadrant. **(b)** Ileal atresia, showing a microcolon, contrast entering the distal small bowel but dilated proximal small bowel without contrast.

(Continued)

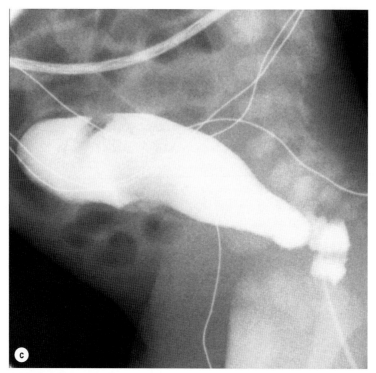

Figure 12.2 • (*cont.*) **(c)** Hirschsprung's disease: lateral film showing a contracted distal rectum with dilated bowel proximally.

of distal obstruction: meconium ileus, jejuno-ileal atresia and Hirschsprung's disease (**Fig. 12.2**). Water-soluble contrast should always be used instead of barium, to avoid the possibility of barium leaking into the abdominal cavity should a perforation occur, and also because water-soluble contrast is more effective in relieving the obstruction in cases of meconium obstruction.

Neonates with suspected intestinal obstruction should be transferred in a temperature-controlled transport isolette to a specialised paediatric surgical unit for evaluation and definitive management. Resuscitation should begin as soon as the patient is assessed and should continue during transport. Nasogastric decompression with a large-calibre nasogastric tube (size 8–10 French) is important to improve ventilation, monitor resuscitation, and limit bowel distention and subsequent ischaemia.

Specific forms of intestinal obstruction

Oesophageal atresia

This anomaly is characterised by a gap in the oesophagus, resulting in a blind-ending proximal pouch. In 90% of cases, the distal oesophagus is connected to the back of the trachea as a tracheo-oesophageal fistula. Oesophageal atresia is usually first suspected when the baby has difficulty swallowing saliva and may have coughing or respiratory distress during the first feed.[1] Intubation may be needed if ventilation or respiration are significantly impaired. The diagnosis is confirmed by the inability to pass a 10–12 French nasogastric tube. This tube should be left in the proximal oesophageal pouch and placed on suction to prevent aspiration of secretions. Operative repair should only be performed by an experienced paediatric surgeon and involves division of the fistula and end-to-end anastamosis of the proximal and distal oesophagus.

Meconium ileus

Cystic fibrosis (CF) is the most common autosomal recessive disorder in Caucasian children.[2] The disease alters the regulation of chloride transport in epithelial cells, resulting in a variety of clinical manifestations. Ten to fifteen per cent of children born with CF will develop meconium ileus, in which the meconium becomes sticky and causes intraluminal obstruction. This can further lead to complications of volvulus, atresia or perforation. In addition, meconium ileus may occasionally occur in children without CF. A diagnostic work-up, including both sweat chloride determination and genetic studies, must therefore be performed on all children with meconium ileus.

Abdominal radiographs may show distal intestinal obstruction with a bubbly appearance in the right lower quadrant due to gas mixing with the viscous meconium (Fig. 12.2a).[2] There may also be intraperitoneal calcification if in-utero perforation has occurred.

Following resuscitation and nasogastric decompression, a water-soluble contrast enema will reveal a microcolon (small calibre) and multiple meconium plugs in the terminal ileum (Fig. 12.2a). In approximately 50% of cases, the contrast enema will relieve the obstruction. If progress is made, but the infant remains obstructed after the initial enema and is otherwise stable, the procedure can be repeated. If the contrast enema is unsuccessful in relieving the obstruction and/or no further progress has been made, a laparotomy must be carried out. If there is no volvulus or perforation, enterotomies are made and mechanical washout is performed. Complications of volvulus, acquired atresia or perforation are managed by intestinal resection with or without a stoma, depending on the condition of the bowel and of the patient.

Intestinal atresia/stenosis

Atresia and stenosis can occur at any point in the alimentary canal. The two prominent aetiological theories are failure of recanalisation of the intestine during foetal development or an ischaemic event in utero.[3] Early resuscitative measures should be initiated and confirmatory diagnosis can usually be made with either upper or lower gastrointestinal contrast studies. The presence of a 'double-bubble' sign on abdominal radiograph is considered diagnostic for duodenal atresia (Fig. 12.1), although this finding associated with distal gas may also be due to stenosis, duodenal web, or malrotation. Trisomy 21 is present in one-third of children with duodenal atresia. Patients with distal atresia will typically have multiple dilated loops of bowel on the plain abdominal radiograph. Although a diagnosis of proximal obstruction can be confidently made based on plain radiography, those with distal obstruction should always undergo water-soluble contrast enema to differentiate atresia from meconium ileus or Hirschsprung's disease.

Since most infants with intestinal atresia are stable once decompressed and resuscitated, they should then be transferred to a facility with paediatric surgical expertise. Most of these anomalies are treated with a primary anastomosis. If there is significant dilatation of the proximal segment, a tapering enteroplasty should be performed as the dilated bowel tends not to have effective peristalsis.

Hirschsprung's disease

Hirschsprung's disease (HD) is a congenital disorder characterised by a lack of ganglion cells in the distal bowel. This results in failure of peristalsis and functional obstruction. The 'transition zone' is usually located in the rectosigmoid region, but HD can affect the entire colon and in rare occurrences the small bowel. HD most often presents in the neonatal period with distal bowel obstruction and failure to pass meconium in the first 24 hours of life. Patients can present later in life with a history of severe constipation. Early identification and management are important to prevent complications of HD such as enterocolitis and nutritional problems.

Water-soluble contrast enema has a sensitivity and specificity of 70% and 83%, respectively, and may therefore be normal, particularly in the newborn.[4] The gold standard for the diagnosis of HD is rectal biopsy, either by a suction technique at the bedside or full-thickness biopsy.

Initial management, after resuscitation and nasogastric decompression, includes digital rectal stimulation and/or rectal irrigations (10 mL/kg normal saline).

✅ Although the historical teaching used to be routine diverting colostomy followed by a 'pull-through' operation several months later, the current standard of care is primary reconstructive surgery without a routine colostomy in most patients.[5]

Preliminary colostomy should be reserved for infants presenting with severe enterocolitis or colonic perforation.

There are a number of options for the surgical correction of HD, including the Swenson, Soave and Duhamel procedures. In recent years, laparoscopic and trans-anal approaches have been described, which have decreased morbidity and shortened hospital stay. It goes without saying that these operations should all be carried out by an experienced paediatric surgeon.

Anorectal malformations

Anorectal malformations can be divided into low and high anomalies. Low anomalies are characterised by rectoperineal or rectovestibular fistulas in female patients. Most males with high malformations have a fistula from the rectum to the bladder neck or urethra. Females with high anomalies usually have a single channel (cloaca) formed by coalescence of the urethra, vagina, and rectum. Less commonly, there may be rectal atresia without a fistula, and some infants present with an anal membrane or anal stenosis.

Infants with these malformations usually present in the first day of life with distal bowel obstruction. Low malformations in girls with large fistulas can permit adequate evacuation of stool, and are occasionally missed. Careful examination of the perineum of all newborns for anal patency and position is therefore important. Many of these patients will suffer from associated anomalies which need to be investigated prior to proceeding with anatomical repair of the anorectal malformation.

The next consideration is to determine if the defect is amenable to primary repair or whether faecal flow should be diverted with a colostomy followed by delayed secondary anatomical repair. Children with a rectoperineal fistula can usually be managed with a local procedure from below, without a colostomy. Children with high anomalies are usually managed with a preliminary colostomy. The use of a colostomy in females with a rectovestibular fistula is controversial. The colostomy can be made using either the transverse or the sigmoid colon, and can be a loop or divided stoma. The authors favour Pena's recommendation for a divided colostomy in the proximal sigmoid colon.[6] Long-term continence in these patients is determined by the level of the rectal fistula, and the presence of an absent or hypoplastic sacrum. Depending on the nature of the anomaly, repair can be carried out using a posterior sagittal approach, a laparoscopic approach, or a combination of posterior and abdominal approaches. Technical expertise is crucial to success, and again these procedures should only be performed by experienced paediatric surgeons.

Malrotation

The process of normal rotation and fixation occurs between the sixth and tenth weeks of development. If no rotation occurs, the patient is left in a position of non-rotation, which has a wide-based mesentery and does not require correction. Classic malrotation occurs when the process is interrupted part way through, leaving the caecum and the duodeno-jejunal junction (ligament of Treitz) close to each other (**Fig. 12.3**). Because this arrangement results in a narrow-based mesentery, the bowel is prone to midgut volvulus around the superior mesenteric vessels, which may lead to intestinal ischaemia. Malrotation with midgut volvulus is one of the true paediatric surgical emergencies and failure to recognise it early can be catastrophic, leading to loss of large portions of bowel and subsequent short-bowel syndrome or death.

Rotation abnormalities are most often asymptomatic. While volvulus can occur at any time, it is most common in the first week of life.[7] The most common presentation of malrotation is bilious vomiting, which may occur for two reasons: midgut volvulus with kinking of the duodenum, or compression of the duodenum by Ladd's bands. Peritonitis and shock from midgut volvulus are late symptoms and are associated with a worse prognosis. Every attempt should be made to diagnose and correct malrotation before this occurs.[8] For this reason, every infant who presents with

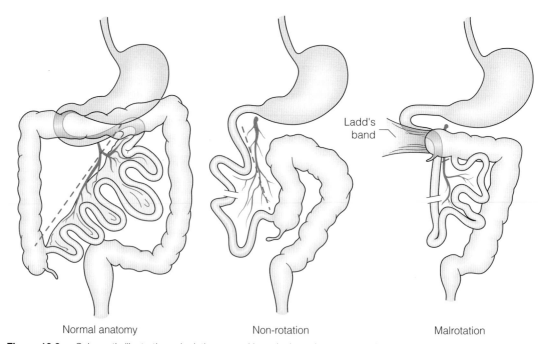

Normal anatomy   Non-rotation   Malrotation

Figure 12.3 • Schematic illustrations depicting normal intestinal rotation, non-rotation and malrotation. Bold dotted lines illustrate the width of the mesenteric base in each situation.

bilious vomiting should be considered to have malrotation with midgut volvulus until proven otherwise.

Any patient with suspected malrotation and volvulus needs urgent imaging and surgical consultation. Abdominal radiograph is often non-diagnostic but may show a dilated stomach, a 'double bubble' with distal gas or a relatively gasless abdomen. Upper gastrointestinal contrast study is the preferred examination. A nasogastric tube placed prior to the exam can not only aid in decompression of the stomach, but also the administration of the water-soluble contrast. The chief radiographic signs of malrotation are: (1) abnormal position of the duodenojejunal junction, (2) a spiral, 'corkscrew' or Z-shaped course of the distal duodenum and proximal jejunum, and (3) location of the proximal jejunum in the right abdomen.[8] Abdominal ultrasound may show abnormal orientation of the superior mesenteric artery and vein, or a 'whirlpool sign'.[9]

The operation to correct malrotation involves a laparotomy, although a laparoscopic approach may be taken for children without evidence of volvulus.[10] If there is volvulus, the bowel is untwisted and checked for viability. If there is ischaemia, the bowel is wrapped with warm towels and re-inspected. Grossly necrotic bowel is resected and the rest is left, with a second-look laparotomy planned for 24–48 hours later. In children who have necrosis of the entire midgut, a palliative approach should be considered.

If the intestine is viable, a Ladd procedure should be performed. This operation consists of five stages: (1) division of Ladd's bands; (2) mobilisation of the colon to the left side of the abdomen; (3) mobilisation and straightening of the duodenum; (4) dissection and widening of the small bowel mesentery; and (5) appendicectomy.

Inflammatory conditions

Assessment

The diagnosis of peritonitis in the neonate is complicated by a number of factors, including the patient's inability to communicate with the surgeon, as well as several anatomical and physiological differences between neonates and older children/adults. The very thin abdominal wall may develop oedema and erythema as a result of underlying inflammation. Neonates breathe primarily with their diaphragms, so peritonitis results in rapid, shallow respiration, and ultimately will cause elevation in pCO_2 and respiratory failure. Localised peritoneal signs can be elicited by palpation, but the examiner must be gentle, since the signs of involuntary guarding

may be very subtle. In addition, the neonate does not have a well-developed omentum, so ability to localise inflammation may be impaired.

Neonates with peritonitis will often develop systemic sepsis, which may differ in its presentation from that in older children and adults. Signs of sepsis in neonates may include lethargy, temperature instability (either fever or hypothermia), increased ventilation requirements, thrombocytopenia, a high or low white blood cell count, and acidosis.

Specific forms of abdominal inflammation

Meconium peritonitis

This condition occurs when there has been prenatal intestinal perforation, resulting in chemical peritonitis. Prenatally there may be evidence of free fluid or calcification within the abdomen. In some cases, the foetus is able to localise and wall off the perforation, which may result in a meconium cyst. The aetiology of the perforation is often distal obstruction, usually from meconium ileus or intestinal atresia, but in some cases the perforation is idiopathic.

Management of meconium peritonitis involves fluid resuscitation, nasogastric drainage and antibiotics. If there is evidence of associated intestinal obstruction, a contrast enema may be helpful preoperatively. Laparotomy should be performed, with resection of the involved bowel and either stomas or primary anastomosis, depending on the condition of the child and the bowel.

Necrotising enterocolitis

Necrotising enterocolitis (NEC) is most commonly seen in low-birth-weight and small-for-gestational-age infants.[11] The aetiology of NEC is unknown, but a combination of bacterial colonisation, intraluminal substrate and intestinal ischaemia/hypoxia all appear to be important.[12]

NEC should be suspected in neonates with sepsis, increased abdominal girth, feeding intolerance, abdominal wall discoloration or bloody stools. Abdominal radiograph may show pneumatosis intestinalis, portal venous gas or free intra-abdominal air (**Fig. 12.4**). It is convenient to classify the severity of NEC using the Bell classification (Table 12.2), which helps to guide treatment and may assist the surgeon in decision-making about operative intervention.[13]

Initial management of NEC includes bowel rest, nasogastric decompression, broad-spectrum antibiotics, parenteral nutrition, and supportive measures to optimise perfusion and oxygenation of the bowel. Persistent clinical deterioration and signs of necrosis or perforation are generally considered indications for operative intervention. Options include bedside peritoneal drainage, or laparotomy

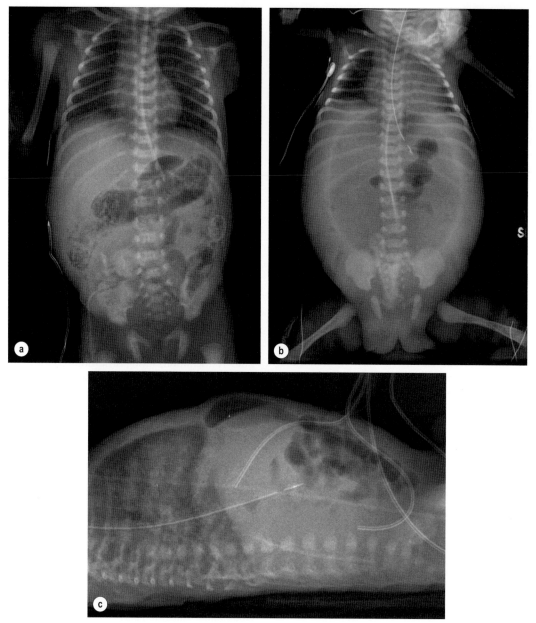

Figure 12.4 • Abdominal radiographs of infants with necrotising enterocolitis. **(a)** Pneumatosis intestinalis. **(b)** 'Football sign' on supine film depicting intra-abdominal free air. **(c)** Free intra-abdominal air on lateral film.

with resection of grossly necrotic bowel and either primary anastomosis or stomas, depending on the status of the child and the bowel.[11,14]

> ✓✓ A recent randomised control trial in neonates less than 1500 g with perforation found no significant difference in outcomes between peritoneal drainage and laparotomy.[15]

Before laparotomy parents should always be informed of the possibility of a long segment of necrosis requiring massive resection that would leave the child with short-bowel syndrome. Palliative management should then be considered in these infants.

Isolated ileal perforation

This condition resembles NEC, in that it primarily affects preterm and small-for-gestational-age

Table 12.2 • Bell stages of necrotising enterocolitis (NEC)

Stage 1 (suspect)	a. Any historical factors producing perinatal stress
	b. Systemic manifestations – temperature instability, lethargy, apnoea, bradycardia
	c. Gastrointestinal manifestations – poor feeding, increased nasogastric tube residuals, emesis (may be bilious or test positive for occult blood), mild abdominal distension, occult blood may be present in stool
Stage 2 (definite)	a. Any historical factors producing perinatal stress
	b. Above signs and symptoms plus persistent occult or gross gastrointestinal bleeding; marked abdominal distension
	c. Abdominal radiographs show significant intestinal distension with ileus; small-bowel separation (oedema in the bowel wall or peritoneal fluid), unchanging or persistent 'rigid' bowel loops, pneumatosis intestinalis, portal vein gas
Stage 3 (advanced)	a. Any historical factors producing perinatal stress
	b. Above signs and symptoms plus deterioration of vital signs, evidence of septic shock or marked gastrointestinal haemorrhage.
	c. Abdominal radiographs may show pneumoperitoneum in addition to the others listed above.

Reprinted from Bell MJ, Ternberg JL, Feigin RD et al. Neonatal necrotizing enterocolitis. Therapeutic decisions based upon clinical staging. Ann Surg 1978; 187(1):1–7. With permission from Wolters Kluwer Health.

infants. However, infants with isolated ileal perforation do not have any abnormalities of the intestine other than localised perforation, usually in the distal ileum. It is unclear whether this represents a very localised form of NEC or a distinct entity. Clinically, these infants present with sudden deterioration, sepsis and free air without any evidence of pneumatosis seen on the abdominal radiograph. In general, the same principles of treatment are applied to ileal perforation and NEC.

Other neonatal conditions

Incarcerated inguinal hernia

Inguinal hernias are very common throughout childhood. Hernias in children almost always arise from persistence of the processus vaginalis. If the processus contains only fluid, it is known as a hydrocele; the hydrocele is communicating if the processus remains open and non-communicating if the processus has become obliterated proximal to the fluid. Communicating hydroceles should be repaired electively if they have not closed by 1 year of age.

In most cases, inguinal hernias are asymptomatic and can be repaired electively. Incarceration of bowel may result in complete bowel obstruction, and represents a surgical emergency since both the bowel and the testis may become ischaemic. The risk of incarceration is greatest in newborns and is approximately 30% in the first 2 years of life. Premature infants are at highest risk.

Neonates and infants presenting with an incarcerated hernia should be resuscitated if necessary, and an immediate attempt should be made to reduce the hernia. In contrast to the adult with an incarcerated hernia, testicular ischaemia is far more common than intestinal ischaemia, and it is appropriate to be aggressive about reducing the hernia. Multiple attempts and the use of sedation may be necessary. Ice should not be applied to the hernia, since it may induce hypothermia. Surgical repair of an incarcerated hernia in an infant is a formidable undertaking. The sac is often thin and oedematous, and the risks of injury to the cord structures and recurrence of the hernia are very high. Therefore, if a general surgeon is unable to reduce the hernia and a paediatric surgeon is accessible, the patient should be referred immediately.

> ✔ If the hernia is reduced, repair should be undertaken 24–48 hours later, allowing some of the oedema to settle, but hopefully before re-incarceration.[16]

Abdominal wall defects

Gastroschisis is characterised by an abdominal wall defect to the right of the umbilicus, through which most of the intestinal tract protrudes.[17] Omphalocele (also called exomphalos) is characterised by herniation of bowel with or without solid organs, into the umbilical cord. Gastroschisis tends to be an isolated anomaly, whereas omphalocele is often associated with chromosomal, cardiac, renal, limb and facial anomalies.

If the diagnosis is made prenatally, delivery should occur at a centre with paediatric surgical support. Resuscitation and nasogastric decompression should begin in the delivery room. The bowel or sac should be wrapped in warm, saline-soaked, sterile gauze and covered with sterile plastic wrap to minimise heat and evaporative fluid loss.

Repair of both conditions should be undertaken by an experienced paediatric surgeon. Options include primary closure, or staged closure using a Silastic® silo that allows the bowel to be reduced gradually into the abdomen over 1–6 days.[18]

Infancy

Hypertrophic pyloric stenosis

Hypertrophic pyloric stenosis (HPS) is an acquired condition in which the pylorus becomes abnormally thickened, causing gastric outlet obstruction. This occurs in infants during the first 2–12 weeks of life and is characterised by projectile, non-bilious vomiting usually occurring after feeds. HPS occurs in approximately 1:400 children, with a significant male predominance.[19]

Diagnosis is suspected based on a history of progressive, forceful, non-bilious vomiting in a child of the appropriate age. Physical examination usually reveals some level of dehydration. The presence of a palpable 'olive' in the epigastrium has a 99% positive predictive value for the disease.[20] Vomiting of gastric contents leads to depletion of sodium, potassium and hydrochloric acid, resulting in the typical hypochloraemic, hypokalaemic metabolic alkalosis. The kidneys attempt to conserve sodium at the expense of hydrogen ions, often leading to paradoxical aciduria.[21] The level of dehydration can be estimated by clinical examination, urine output, and serum chloride and bicarbonate levels. If the pyloric olive is not palpable, the diagnosis can be confirmed by ultrasound (pyloric length >16 mm and single wall thickness >3 mm). If an experienced sonographer is not available, the diagnosis can be made using a barium swallow (**Fig. 12.5**).

Surgery should be deferred until the infant is fully resuscitated. This is accomplished by using normal saline or Ringer's lactate with potassium. Most children should receive a bolus of 20 mL/kg, and then an infusion consisting of 1.5 times the maintenance requirement (i.e. 6 mL/kg/h for this age group) until the urine output and electrolytes have been normalised.

Surgical management of HPS consists of extramucosal longitudinal splitting of the pyloric muscle. The original procedure described by Ramstedt in 1912 was performed through a transverse right upper quadrant incision. This technique has been modified in many institutions to utilise circumumbilical incisions and, more recently, laparoscopic techniques.[22] Following pyloromyotomy, many infants will experience continued vomiting for 24–48 hours, although the majority will eventually tolerate feeds and be discharged. Postoperative complications are rare but include wound infection, duodenal or gastric perforation and incomplete pyloromyotomy.

Intussusception

Intussusception, or 'telescoping of the bowel', occurs when one portion of bowel invaginates into a more distant portion. This results in venous congestion, bowel wall oedema, intestinal obstruction and ultimately full-thickness necrosis of the intussusceptum. The peak incidence of intussusception is seen at 6–9 months of age.[23] The majority are ileocolic with hyperplastic lymphoid tissue in Peyer's patches acting as a lead point.[24] These are often referred to as 'idiopathic'. Asymptomatic small-bowel to small-bowel intussusception may be seen incidentally on abdominal ultrasound, or sometimes may be associated with Henoch–Schonlein purpura or cystic fibrosis. Less than 5% of intussuceptions are due to a pathological lead point such as a Meckel diverticulum, polyp or small-bowel tumour such as lymphoma or leiomyoma. Intussusception occurring outside of the usual age range, or those that recur, should raise suspicion for a pathological lead point.

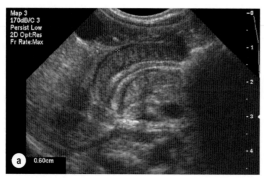 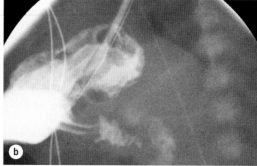

Figure 12.5 • Images of hypertrophic pyloric stenosis. **(a)** Abdominal ultrasound. **(b)** Upper gastrointestinal contrast study.

Few children with ileocolic intussusception will demonstrate the classic triad of intermittent severe abdominal pain with drawing up of the legs, palpable abdominal mass and 'redcurrant jelly' stool. Physicians must therefore have a high index of suspicion due to the variability of symptoms. Patients may present with irritability, lethargy, abdominal pain, vomiting, diarrhoea or constipation, haematochezia, fever, dehydration or shock. Management should initially focus on diagnosis and resuscitation.

Following fluid resuscitation, imaging should be performed to confirm the diagnosis of intussusception. Abdominal radiograph may show air-fluid levels and distention of the small bowel and there may be a characteristic lack of air in the right lower quadrant. Ultrasonography has a high sensitivity and is currently the investigation of choice.[24]

> ✔ Traditionally, the treatment of intussusception has been barium enema. More recently, pneumatic reduction using air or CO_2 has been associated with an 80–95% success rate.[24]

If the intussusception is partially but not completely reduced it is worth trying again a few hours later, since some of the oedema may have been eliminated by the first attempt and a second attempt may be associated with a 50% chance of success.[25] Pneumatic pressures of 60–100 mmHg are recommended.[26]

Surgical intervention is reserved for those patients who fail hydrostatic or pneumatic reduction, or who have signs of infarcted or perforated bowel such as peritonitis or free air on abdominal radiograph at the time of presentation. At laparotomy, the intussusception is manually reduced if possible. If the intussusception is not reducible, the bowel appears necrotic or a pathological lead point is identified, a segmental resection should be performed with primary anastamosis. Recently some authors have documented excellent results using a laparoscopic approach to this condition.[27]

Children

Appendicitis

Appendicitis is the most frequent abdominal surgical emergency in children.[28] As in adults, the classic presentation is mid-abdominal pain moving to the right lower quadrant, anorexia, vomiting, low-grade fever and localised tenderness with peritoneal signs in the right lower quadrant (see also Chapter 9). Presentation in children may be atypical, particularly in those under 5 years of age. Some authors

Table 12.3 • Paediatric Appendicitis Score: a score of 6 or more has been shown to be associated with a high likelihood of the child having acute appendicitis

Paediatric Appendicitis Score	Points
Percussion/hopping/coughing	2
Anorexia	1
Pyrexia	1
Nausea or vomiting	1
RLQ tenderness	2
Leucocytosis (WBC >10 000/μL)	1
Neutrophilia ('left shift')	1
Migration of pain to RLQ	1

RLQ, right lower quadrant; WBC, white blood cell count.
Reprinted from Samuel M. Pediatric Appendicitis Score.
J Pediatr Surg 2002; 37(6):877–81. With permission from Elsevier.

have attempted to quantify the usefulness of specific findings in children using scoring systems. Clinical scoring systems such as the Alvarado Score and the Paediatric Appendicitis Score have been shown to be both sensitive and specific (Table 12.3).[29-31]

In the otherwise well, stable patient with an equivocal presentation, the diagnostic options include observation with serial examinations, or imaging with ultrasound or computed tomography (CT) (**Fig. 12.6**). There is a great deal of controversy as to which technique is more appropriate (see also Chapter 5). Ultrasound is clearly more operator dependent, but recent analyses have suggested that CT scans in childhood may be associated with an increased risk of radiation-induced malignancy later in life.[32] Both have excellent accuracy.

Increasingly, surgeons are using a laparoscopic approach to appendicectomy in children. As in adults, the benefits of the laparoscopic approach include reduced postoperative pain and length of stay, in addition to a decrease in wound infection rate. There is some evidence that the rate of intra-abdominal abscess may be higher after laparoscopic appendicectomy in children with perforated appendicitis.[33] The laparoscopic approach may also be beneficial in children who are muscular or obese, and in adolescent females, where the incidence of ovarian pathology as a cause for the symptoms is higher.

Approximately 40% of children present with perforation, and the incidence is over 65% in those aged 0–4 years old.[28] In contrast to non-perforated appendicitis, these children usually present with prolonged symptoms, higher fever, higher white blood cell count and more diffuse peritoneal signs. Some children present with frank sepsis and diffuse peritoneal contamination; these children benefit

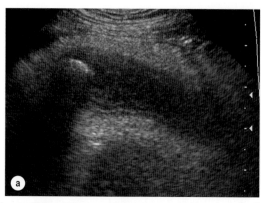 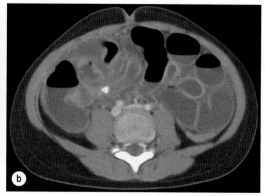

Figure 12.6 • Ultrasound **(a)** and computed tomography **(b)** images of children with acute appendicitis. A faecolith is visible at the base of the inflamed appendix in both images.

from resuscitation, followed by immediate appendicectomy and peritoneal washout. Many children with perforated appendicitis present with a prolonged history and a localised abscess or phlegmon on imaging. This condition can be managed either by early operation or by non-operative management consisting of broad-spectrum antibiotics and image-guided drainage of any purulent collections. As in adults (see also Chapter 9), the need for a subsequent interval appendectomy several months later is controversial. The authors reserve the use of interval appendectomy for those with an appendicolith on imaging, since their risk of recurrent appendicitis is over 50%.[34]

Fluid resuscitation of the child with a surgical emergency

Fluid and electrolyte management in children are made challenging by differences in total body water and compensatory mechanisms, as well as changes in physiology throughout childhood. Total body water is as high as 80% of body weight in neonates, and decreases to the adult level of approximately 60% by 1 year. Degree of dehydration can be estimated from the history and physical examination. Children with mild dehydration (1–5% of body fluid volume) show few clinical signs but frequently have a history of 12–24 hours of vomiting or diarrhoea. Those with moderate dehydration (6–10%) are often lethargic, have low urine output (usually evident as fewer wet nappies/diapers), weight loss, loss of skin turgor, sunken eyes or fontanel, dry mucus membranes and crying without tears. If severe dehydration (11–15%) is reached the child may develop cardiovascular or neurological instability. Children have very active peripheral vasoconstriction, so that blood pressure will be maintained until advanced intravascular volume depletion is

reached with onset of hypotension, irritability or coma. However, tachycardia is an early sign that should be recognised and treated.[21]

The urgency of fluid replacement depends on the degree of dehydration and the cause of the fluid loss. The goals of treatment are the restoration and preservation of cardiovascular, neurological and renal perfusion. In the event of dehydration resulting from an inflammatory condition that will require urgent surgical intervention, such as appendicitis, isotonic fluid (normal saline or Ringer's lactate solution) should be given in 20 mL/kg boluses until signs of cardiovascular compromise subside. For situations in which there is no urgency to do an operation, such as pyloric stenosis, the fluid deficit can be replaced more slowly. This has the advantage of avoiding sudden fluid shifts, and the possibility of cerebral oedema and seizures, which are particularly likely in neonates and infants. The commonly used protocol is to calculate the fluid deficit, and replace half over the first 8 hours and the other half over the subsequent 16 hours.

Paediatric trauma

The principles of trauma management are the same for children as they are for adults (see also Chapter 13). Securing the airway and ensuring adequate ventilation are paramount prior to treating bleeding and circulatory collapse. Fluid resuscitation is based on the patient's size, keeping in mind the differences in physiological response to hypovolaemia mentioned in the previous section. As with adults, two boluses of crystalloid (20 mL/kg) should be given through large-bore intravenous lines as quickly as possible. If there is still suspicion for ongoing bleeding, blood products are administered in 20 mL/kg boluses.

The principles of managing penetrating trauma in children are also the same as in adults (see Chapter 13). However, children sustaining blunt abdominal trauma are more prone to solid-organ injury due to the low-lying nature of these organs with respect to the paediatric ribcage and the relative laxity of the abdominal wall. In general, injuries to the spleen, liver and kidney can be managed non-operatively regardless of the grade of injury and operations are rare for blunt abdominal trauma in children. The indications for laparotomy in a child with blunt abdominal trauma include: evidence of peritonitis on abdominal examination; free intra-abdominal air on imaging; inability to normalise haemodynamic status despite resuscitation efforts; a rapidly expanding abdomen associated with persistent hypotension; and the need for transfusion of more than one-half of a blood volume over 24 hours.

Key points

- Neonatal and complex surgery in children should ideally take place in specialised paediatric surgical units, with subspecialised paediatric surgical, anaesthetic and intensive care unit support.
- Resuscitation is the first step in the management of all children with surgical problems.
- *Beware the child who vomits green!* Bilious vomiting in a neonate or child is usually associated with intestinal obstruction, and every child with bilious vomiting should be assumed to have life-threatening malrotation and midgut volvulus until proven otherwise.
- A high index of suspicion for intussusception should be maintained in children in the high-risk age group (3–12 months of age) presenting with intermittent abdominal pain, vomiting and/or bloody stools.
- Delayed passage of meconium (>24 hours of life) should arouse suspicion of Hirschsprung's disease.
- Incarcerated inguinal hernias should be reduced if possible and repaired within 48 hours of reduction.
- Tachycardia is an important sign of intravascular fluid depletion in children; hypotension is a late finding.

References

1. Spitz L. Oesophageal atresia. Orphanet J Rare Dis 2007;2:24.

2. Chaudry G, Navarro OM, Levine DS, et al. Abdominal manifestations of cystic fibrosis in children. Pediatr Radiol 2006;36(3):233–240.

3. Dalla Vecchia LK, Grosfeld JL, West KW, et al. Intestinal atresia and stenosis: a 25-year experience with 277 cases. Arch Surg 1998;133(5):490–7.

4. de Lorijn F, Kremer LC, Reitsma JB, et al. Diagnostic tests in Hirschsprung disease: a systematic review. J Pediatr Gastroenterol Nutr 2006;42(5):496–505.

5. Nasr A, Langer JC. Evolution of the technique in the transanal pull-through for Hirschsprung's disease: effect on outcome. J Pediatr Surg 2007;42(1):36–40.

6. Pena A, Hong A. Advances in the management of anorectal malformations. Am J Surg 2000;180(5):370–6.

7. Torres AM, Ziegler MM. Malrotation of the intestine. World J Surg 1993;17(3):326–31.

8. Strouse PJ. Disorders of intestinal rotation and fixation ("malrotation"). Pediatr Radiol 2004;34(11):837–51.

9. Orzech N, Navarro OM, Langer JC. Is ultrasonography a good screening test for intestinal malrotation? J Pediatr Surg 2006;41(5):1005–9.

10. Mazziotti MV, Strasberg SM, Langer JC. Intestinal rotation abnormalities without volvulus: the role of laparoscopy. J Am Coll Surg 1997;185(2):172–6.

11. Lee JS, Polin RA. Treatment and prevention of necrotizing enterocolitis. Semin Neonatol 2003;8(6):449–59.

12. Caplan MS, Jilling T. New concepts in necrotizing enterocolitis. Curr Opin Pediatr 2001;13(2):111–5.

13. Bell MJ, Ternberg JL, Feigin RD, et al. Neonatal necrotizing enterocolitis. Therapeutic decisions based upon clinical staging. Ann Surg 1978;187(1):1–7.

14. Pierro A, Hall N. Surgical treatments of infants with necrotizing enterocolitis. Semin Neonatol 2003;8(3):223–32.

15. Moss RL, Dimmitt RA, Barnhart DC, et al. Laparotomy versus peritoneal drainage for necrotizing enterocolitis and perforation. N Engl J Med 2006;354(21):2225–34.
    A randomised trial that did not show any difference between the two modalities.

16. Baguley PE, Fitzgerald PG, Srinathan SK, et al. Emergency room reduction of incarcerated inguinal hernia in infants: is routine hospital admission necessary? Pediatr Surg Int 1992;7:366–7.

17. Langer JC. Abdominal wall defects. World J Surg 2003;27(1):117–24.

18. Langer JC. Gastroschisis and omphalocele. Semin Pediatr Surg 1996;5(2):124–8.

19. To T, Wajja A, Wales PW, et al. Population demographic indicators associated with incidence of pyloric stenosis. Arch Pediatr Adolesc Med 2005;159(6):520–5.

20. White MC, Langer JC, Don S, et al. Sensitivity and cost minimization analysis of radiology versus olive palpation for the diagnosis of hypertrophic pyloric stenosis. J Pediatr Surg 1998;33(6):913–7.

21. Rice HE, Caty MG, Glick PL. Fluid therapy for the pediatric surgical patient. Pediatr Clin North Am 1998;45(4):719–27.

22. van der Bilt JD, Kramer WL, van der Zee DC, et al. Laparoscopic pyloromyotomy for hypertrophic pyloric stenosis: impact of experience on the results in 182 cases. Surg Endosc 2004;18(6):907–9.

23. Huppertz HI, Soriano-Gabarro M, Grimprel E, et al. Intussusception among young children in Europe. Pediatr Infect Dis J 2006;25(1, Suppl.):S22–9.

24. Daneman A, Navarro O. Intussusception. Part 1: a review of diagnostic approaches. Pediatr Radiol 2003;33(2):79–85.

25. Saxton V, Katz M, Phelan E, et al. Intussusception: a repeat delayed gas enema increases the nonoperative reduction rate. J Pediatr Surg 1994;29(5):588–9.

26. Paterson CA, Langer JC, Somers S, et al. Pneumatic reduction of intussusception using carbon dioxide. Pediatr Radiol 1994;24(4):296–7.

27. Bailey KA, Wales PW, Gerstle JT. Laparoscopic versus open reduction of intussusception in children: a single-institution comparative experience. J Pediatr Surg 2007;42(5):845–8.

28. Newman K, Ponsky T, Kittle K, et al. Appendicitis 2000: variability in practice, outcomes, and resource utilization at thirty pediatric hospitals. J Pediatr Surg 2003;38(3):372–9.

29. Owen TD, Williams H, Stiff G, et al. Evaluation of the Alvarado score in acute appendicitis. J R Soc Med 1992;85(2):87–8.

30. Samuel M. Pediatric Appendicitis Score. J Pediatr Surg 2002;37(6):877–81.

31. Goldman RD, Crump S, Stephens D, et al. Prospective validation of the pediatric appendicitis score. J Pediatr Surg 2008;153:178–82.

32. Frush DP, Donnelly LF, Rosen NS. Computed tomography and radiation risks: what pediatric health care providers should know. Pediatrics 2003;112(4):951–7.

33. Sauerland S, Lefering R, Neugebauer EA. Laparoscopic versus open surgery for suspected appendicitis. Cochrane Database Syst Rev 2004;(4):CD001546.

34. Ein SH, Langer JC, Daneman A. Nonoperative management of pediatric ruptured appendix with inflammatory mass or abscess: presence of an appendicolith predicts recurrent appendicitis. J Pediatr Surg 2005;40(10):1612–5.

13

Abdominal trauma

Kenneth D. Boffard

Introduction

In 1988, without organised trauma care, some 20–35% of patients who reached hospital alive in the UK died unnecessarily,[1] and even in a recent study of the NHS, almost 60% of patients received a standard of care that was considered less than good practice.[2] In the now classic study of trauma centres versus non-trauma centres in California published in 1979, West et al. demonstrated that the majority of preventable deaths resulted from unrecognised, and therefore untreated, intra-abdominal haemorrhage.[3]

Approximately 6% of all patients with blunt abdominal trauma will require laparotomy, primarily for haemorrhage from solid-organ injuries. Penetrating torso trauma poses its own problems, especially with regard to whether the peritoneal cavity has actually been penetrated, whether intra-abdominal injury has occurred and, in the presence of competing injuries, the decision-making required for best management.

Risk factors

Mackersie et al., in an evaluation of 3223 patients with blunt trauma, found that the risk of abdominal injury was significantly increased in the presence of an arterial base deficit of 3 mmol/L or more, the presence of major chest trauma, the presence of pelvic fractures or the presence of hypotension.[4]

The current 'gold standard' for assessment of perfusion following injury is measurement of the serum lactate. Elevated lactate levels indicate organ dysfunction and failure in severely injured trauma patients, and therefore reflect inadequate perfusion and oxygenation of ischaemic tissues. Several studies in critically ill intensive care patients have demonstrated that elevated initial or 24-hour lactate levels correlate significantly with mortality and appear to have a more superior predictive value than corresponding base deficit level changes.[5,6] Similarly, prolonged elevation of blood lactate levels has been correlated with increased organ failure and mortality after trauma.[7]

Criteria that identify patients at significant risk for abdominal injury, and therefore requiring objective evaluation, are:

Anatomy

- major mechanism of injury;
- associated major chest injury;
- presence of pelvic fracture;
- presence of haematuria;
- objective physical findings (e.g. tenderness of the abdomen);
- impaired sensorium and consequent inability for objective abdominal examination.

Physiology

- significant rise in the serum lactate or significant base deficit;
- unexplained haemodynamic instability;
- unexplained hypovolaemic shock.

Transport

Helicopter Emergency Medical Services (HEMS) and its possible association with outcomes improvement continues to be a subject of debate.

In an effort to facilitate the academic pursuit of assessment of HEMS utility, in late 2000 the National Association of EMS Physicians (NAEMSP) Air Medical Taskforce reviewed the use of HEMS in both trauma and non-trauma. A more recent literature analysis by Thomas[8] showed, like most HEMS trauma studies, that the crude mortality was much higher in the HEMS patients; however, control for acuity reversed the association and outcomes point estimates favoured HEMS in nine of 10 analyses. Penetrating trauma was the only group for which the non-significant outcome impact was on the side of better outcome with ground EMS. For patients with severe head injuries HEMS response was associated with borderline significant outcome improvement. The authors concluded that HEMS was called for in patients of higher injury acuity with diminished (poorer) vital signs, and that HEMS response resulted in improved outcome for patients with blunt trauma and those with severe head injuries.

In a more recent study of 56 744 inured adults transported to US trauma centres by either ground transport or helicopter, the odds of death were 39% lower in those transported by HEMS, compared to those transported by road, especially in the 18- to 54-year-old age group.[9] A second recent study of 223 475 patients transported by ground and air showed that certain patients transported to level I and II centres by helicopter had an improved odds of survival to hospital discharge.[10]

In summary, therefore, HEMS is associated with a reduction in mortality, particularly in patients under 55 years. However, overall survival, especially in those patients with torso or penetrating injury, and patients who are actively bleeding, is best achieved by early control of bleeding. This implies that the time between injury and successful surgical intervention is the single biggest factor in determining a favourable outcome, and in the urban environment this may imply rapid road transport with limited resuscitation en route. *The right patient by the right transport to the right hospital in the right time.*

Regional trauma systems

Dating from 1979,[3] outcomes have been shown to be improved if a regional trauma system is present, and the importance of transporting a patient to an appropriate centre, capable of managing the injuries (actual and potential) in a timely and comprehensive fashion, is well established. The American College of Surgeons Committee on Trauma provides criteria for classification of trauma centres from level I to level IV and definitions for a level I patient.[11] When one or more of the following criteria are present in the trauma patient, he or she is classified as a level I trauma patient and should be transported to the nearest appropriate centre:

- confirmed blood pressure (BP) less than 90 mmHg at any time;
- respiratory compromise, obstruction and/or intubation;
- patients from other hospitals receiving blood to maintain vital signs;
- emergency physicians' discretion, especially where there is unexplained hypotension, or the expected need for damage control may exist.

Assessment in the emergency department

The entire philosophy of the abdominal injury can be summed up by answering the following questions:

- Is the abdomen involved in an injury process?
- Is a surgical procedure necessary to correct it?
- What additional support does the patient require?

In hypotensive patients, the goal is to stop the bleeding, and this includes the rapid determination of whether the abdomen is the cause of the hypotension. If intra-abdominal bleeding *is* the cause, then emergency measures will be needed to control that bleeding. These include emergency transfusion in order to 'buy time' or emergency thoracotomy in the emergency room to control the descending aorta and therefore control distal bleeding. Transfusion alone is only a means to an end, and for hypotensive patients with penetrating torso injuries, delay in aggressive fluid resuscitation until rapid operative intervention and control has occurred improves outcome.[12] The often quoted paper by Bickell et al. states that this applies primarily to penetrating trauma of the chest and that other injuries, particularly those involving blunt abdominal trauma, should be assessed. Thromboelastography (TEG) has become a further dynamic point-of-care (POC) standard to optimise clotting ability for haemostasis.[13,14]

Haemodynamically stable patients without signs of abdominal irritation may undergo a more extended assessment in order to answer the above questions.

Most conventional texts emphasise the need for a careful history and physical examination of the abdomen. In trauma, it is extremely difficult to assess the abdomen, as the history may not be available and all the available physical signs are misleading. Fresh blood is not a peritoneal irritant! Positive clinical findings may be relevant. Negative ones are not!

The mechanism of injury is critically important in assessing the potential for abdominal injury. This information may be obtained from the patient, relatives, police or emergency care personnel. When assessing the patient who has sustained a penetrating injury, pertinent historical information includes the time of injury, type of weapon, number and direction of (especially) bullet wounds (was it an entrance and an exit wound, or two entry wounds with both bullets retained?).

It is unacceptable to withhold analgesia (see also Chapter 5). Judicious, properly titrated use of intravenous opiates will not significantly affect the clarity of the history, nor will it 'mask' pain, depress cerebration or respiration, or alter the blood pressure. What it will do is make the injury more comfortable for the patient and allow the clinician a much more accurate picture of both the history and the clinical presentation.

Diagnostic modalities in blunt abdominal trauma

The accuracy of physical examination of the abdomen in detecting intra-abdominal injuries is limited. There are many patient factors that contribute to the difficult physical examination, including the presence of other painful distracting injuries, especially if they occur both above and below the abdomen, and an altered level of consciousness as the result of drugs, alcohol or head injury. Recognising these limitations, most trauma surgeons advocate a more objective evaluation of the abdomen in patients at risk for intra-abdominal injury.

Routine screening radiographs

The routine radiographs as laid down by the Advanced Trauma Life Support Programme (ATLS®) of the American College of Surgeons are an anteroposterior (AP) chest film and a pelvic film.[15] Abdominal films are not usually useful. If possible (and it is safe to do so), an erect chest radiograph will provide more information than an erect abdominal film in looking for infradiaphragmatic free air (see also Chapter 5).

In all cases of penetrating trauma, it is important to appreciate that in the *unstable* patient, the radiograph is unlikely to influence management and the patient requires an immediate laparotomy. However, in the stable patient, useful additional information regarding the track of the bullet can be obtained. It is essential in such a situation to make use of bullet markers to show the entry/exit wounds.[16] These can be simply paper clips taped onto the skin. If there are wounds on both front and back, then one of the paper clips can be unfolded. After the clips are applied to all relevant torso wounds, the radiographs are taken and will give an indication of the track of the bullet, which wound is at the front and which is at the back, and also the presence of other fragments.

Special diagnostic studies

The advantages and disadvantages of each of the objective methods of examining the abdomen for injuries are summarised in Table 13.1.

Computed tomography (CT)

With contrast-enhanced CT (CECT), it is possible both to recognise the organ that is injured and to grade the severity of the injury. Intravascular contrast is essential. There is only limited evidence that enteral (via stomach or rectum) contrast is helpful, and its use may delay the examination. Both intraperitoneal and retroperitoneal injuries can be detected with CECT, and the amount of intra-abdominal blood loss can be estimated. Serial scanning can be used to follow the resolution (or progression) of an injury. The disadvantages of CECT include the need to move the patient to the radiology suite and the time required to perform the scan, although with the introduction of 64-slice spiral scanners, the latter factor has become less important. CT is expensive, there is the potential for allergic reaction to the injected contrast material,

Table 13.1 • Comparison of diagnostic methods for abdominal injury

Method	Advantages	Disadvantages
Clinical		
Clinical examination	Quick Non-invasive	Unreliable
Diagnostic		
Computed tomography 'Gold standard'	Organ-specific retroperitoneal information	Patient must be stable Expensive
Ultrasound	Quick Non-invasive	User dependent Unhelpful for hollow viscus injury
Diagnostic peritoneal lavage	Quick Inexpensive	Invasive Too sensitive Limited specificity
Laparoscopy	Organ specific	Painful Anaesthesia required User dependent Patient must be stable
Laparotomy	Highly specific	Complications Expensive

or for aspiration of oral contrast (a rare event), and the danger of the radiation dose administered should not be underestimated.[17] It has been estimated that the danger of CT scan-induced cancer may be as high as 2%.[18]

Although CT is relatively insensitive in the detection of hollow viscus injuries, a bowel injury (and especially a duodenal injury) is suggested by finding a thickened bowel wall, extraluminal air and the presence of intraperitoneal fluid in the absence of a solid-organ injury.[19,20] CT may also miss a pancreatic injury early in its course. The accuracy of CT is generally poor in the detection of diaphragmatic, hollow-organ and mesenteric injuries, and there have been reports of a high incidence of false-negative results.[21] Despite these limitations, however, CT remains the method of choice for objective evaluation of the abdomen in *stable* trauma patients who are likely to have an intra-abdominal injury, and is currently the 'gold standard' of investigation.

Diagnostic ultrasound

The sensitivity of ultrasound for the detection of free intraperitoneal fluid in abdominal blunt trauma has been shown to be 81–99%.[22] The disadvantage of ultrasound is its lack of sensitivity for injuries that do not produce blood or peritoneal fluid and the fact that its accuracy is directly related to the experience of the ultrasonographer. Nonetheless, surgeons can be taught to perform and interpret ultrasound examinations rapidly and accurately, with a sensitivity/specificity and accuracy each over 90%.[23] This diagnostic method has particular appeal in paediatric trauma patients and in the injured gravid patient.

In most centres, ultrasound has replaced diagnostic peritoneal lavage (DPL) for evaluation of the unstable patient following blunt trauma. However, the role of ultrasound in the assessment of penetrating abdominal trauma is still controversial, since the examination will miss small amounts of intraperitoneal fluid.

Diagnostic peritoneal lavage (DPL)

Root et al. introduced DPL as a method of evaluation of the abdomen some 50 years ago,[24] and while it has frequently been superseded by more sophisticated (and potentially more expensive) techniques, it remains the standard against which all other diagnostic examinations are judged. The main advantage of DPL is that it can be performed quickly and with few complications by relatively inexperienced clinicians. DPL is also reproducible, as well as highly sensitive and specific for the detection of abdominal blood (>97%), but it does not identify the organ of injury.

Injuries of the retroperitoneum will be missed by DPL, and the presence of pelvic fractures may lead to a false-positive result.

A DPL is generally considered as positive if:

- red cell count is >100 000 cells/mm^3;
- white cell count is >500/mm^3;
- there is amylase or bowel content in the lavage return.

However, if surgeons are committed to operating on all patients with positive DPL the ability to manage patients non-operatively may be lost. The lavage is therefore regarded as an indicator of the presence of abdominal pathology, but not necessarily an indication for surgery (see section on non-operative management below).

Diagnostic laparoscopy

Laparoscopy has yet to find its role in the evaluation of the patient with blunt abdominal trauma.[25] With few exceptions, laparoscopy requires general anaesthesia, is expensive and has the potential to create a tension pneumothorax[26] or air embolus during insufflation. Laparoscopy in penetrating injury has been reported with the successful repair of injuries of the diaphragm and stomach.[27]

An additional drawback of diagnostic laparoscopy currently is the relative cost compared with other modalities, especially those performed at the bedside, such as ultrasound. The technique should only be used on relatively stable patients, and laparoscopy is still limited in its ability to detect penetrating intestinal injury, especially in the hands of an operator unskilled in the specific techniques required for elucidation of intra-abdominal injury. Currently, laparoscopy is most useful in the patient with penetrating abdominal trauma when there is a question of peritoneal penetration or diaphragmatic injury. The diaphragm is also an area where delay or missed diagnosis dramatically increases the morbidity.[28] Laparoscopy can identify not only clinically unsuspected diaphragm injuries but also other injuries that have been 'missed' by other diagnostic tests.

Diagnostic laparoscopy does not confer any advantages or improvements over other techniques when it comes to investigation of retroperitoneal injuries to organs such as the duodenum and pancreas, and CT remains more accurate in this regard.

Laparotomy

Mandatory laparotomy

While laparotomy remains the most appropriate therapy for an unstable patient with obvious abdominal trauma, a non-therapeutic laparotomy is not necessarily benign. In a prospective study of unnecessary laparotomies performed in 254 trauma

Temporary abdominal closure

The abdomen is only closed to limit heat and fluid loss and to protect viscera. Closure is usually achieved using the 'sandwich technique', first described by Schein et al. in 1986[40] and subsequently popularised by Rotondo et al.[36]

A sheet of self-adhesive incise drape (Opsite®, Steridrape® or Ioban®) is placed flat, sticky side up, and an abdominal swab placed upon it. The plastic edges are trimmed, to produce a sheet with membrane on one side and abdominal swab on the other. If extra firmness is required, a surgical drape can be used instead of the swab. It is worth noting that it is unnecessary to make any perforations in the membrane, and to do so may increase subsequent fistula formation.

The membrane is utilised as an on-lay with the margins 'tucked in' under the edges of the open sheath, the membrane being in contact with the bowel.

The appreciable drainage of serosanguinous fluid that occurs is best dealt with by placing a pair of drainage tubes (e.g. sump-type nasogastric tubes or closed-system suction drains) through separate stab incisions onto the membrane and utilising continuous low-vacuum suction. This arrangement is covered by an occlusive incise drape applied to the skin, thus providing a closed system.

Other techniques, such as the use of towel clips or the so-called 'Bogota bag', are now generally regarded as obsolete. The use of proprietary vacuum suction devices at this stage is not only expensive, but the suction used is often above mean arterial pressure, which increases the risk of subsequent fistula. Such devices should generally only be used at the final stage of closure if definitive closure is not possible.

Stage 2: Transfer to the intensive care unit for ongoing resuscitation

The timing of the transfer of the patient from the operating theatre to the intensive care unit is critical. Early transfer is cost-effective; premature transfer is counter-productive. In addition, once haemostasis has been properly achieved, it may not be necessary to abort the procedure and it may be possible to proceed to definitive surgery. Conversely, there are some patients with severe head injuries where the coagulopathy is induced by severe irreversible cerebral damage, and further surgical energy is futile.

In the operating theatre, efforts must be started to reverse all the associated adjuncts, such as acidosis, hypothermia and hypoxia, and it may be possible to improve the coagulation status through these methods alone. Adequate time should still be allowed for this, following which reassessment of the abdominal injuries should take place, as it is not infrequent to discover further injuries or ongoing bleeding.

Stage 3: Resuscitation in the intensive care unit

Priorities on reaching the intensive care are:

1. The restoration of body temperature using:
   a. passive rewarming with warming blankets, warmed fluids, etc.;
   b. active rewarming using lavage of chest or abdomen.
2. Correction of clotting profiles by blood component repletion. This is best directed by the results of the TEG/RoTEM.[13]
3. Optimisation of oxygen delivery:
   a. volume loading to achieve optimum preload;
   b. haemoglobin optimisation to a value of 9 g/dL;
   c. temperature optimisation (>35 °C).
4. Monitoring of intra-abdominal pressure (IAP) to prevent abdominal compartment syndrome (ACS).

Stage 4: Return to the operating theatre for definitive surgery

The patient is returned to the operating theatre as soon as stage 3 is achieved. The timing is determined by:

- the indication for damage control in the first place;
- the injury pattern;
- the physiological response.

Patients with persistent bleeding despite correction of the other parameters merit early return to control the bleeding.

Every effort must be made to return *all* patients to the operating theatre within 24–48 hours of their initial surgery.

Stage 5: Definitive surgery and abdominal wall reconstruction if required

Once definitive surgery is complete, and no further operations are contemplated, then the abdominal wall can be closed. This is often difficult and methods involved include:

- primary closure;
- closure of the sheath, leaving the skin open;
- grafts with Vicryl® mesh, or other synthetic sheets;
- use of lateral relieving incisions to allow closure of sheath (component separation).

Abdominal compartment syndrome

There have been major developments in our understanding of intra-abdominal pressure (IAP) and intra-abdominal hypertension (IAH). Raised IAP has far-reaching consequences for the physiology of the patient.[41] Clinically, the organ systems most affected include the cardiovascular, renal and pulmonary systems. A sustained IAP≥20 mmHg associated with new organ dysfunction is known as abdominal compartment syndrome (ACS; see Table 13.2). With increasing awareness of the problem, reduced fluid resuscitation and more appropriate damage control, the incidence of ACS in trauma is decreasing. Failure to detect ACS in a timely fashion and treat it aggressively results in high mortality in such patients.

Definition

The first World Congress on ACS was held in 2005 and an internal consensus agreement relating to current definitions[42] is shown in Table 13.2.

> ✅ ACS is defined as a sustained IAP ≥20 mmHg (with or without an abdominal perfusion pressure <60 mmHg) that is associated with new organ dysfunction/failure.

Pathophysiology

The incidence of increased IAP may be 30% of postoperative general surgery patients in intensive care and after emergency surgery the incidence is

even higher. The causes of acutely increased IAP are usually multifactorial (see also Chapter 18). The first clinical reports of postoperative increased IAP were often after aortic surgery, with postoperative haemorrhage from the graft suture line. Peritonitis and intra-abdominal sepsis, tissue oedema and ileus are the predominant cause of increased IAP. Raised IAP in trauma patients is often caused by a combination of blood loss and tissue oedema. Causes of increased intra-abdominal pressure include:

- tissue oedema secondary to insults such as ischaemia, trauma and sepsis;
- paralytic ileus;
- intraperitoneal or retroperitoneal haematoma;
- ascites;
- trauma with hypothermia, coagulopathy and acidosis.

Effect of raised IAP on organ function

Renal function

The most likely direct effect of increased IAP is an increase in the renal vascular resistance, coupled with a moderate reduction in cardiac output.

Table 13.2 • Consensus definitions related to IAP, IAH and ACS

Definition 1	IAP is the pressure concealed within the abdominal cavity
Definition 2	APP = MAP − IAP
Definition 3	FG = GFP − PTP = MAP − 2 × IAP FG, filtration gradient; GFP, glomerular filtration pressure; PTP, proximal tubular pressure
Definition 4	IAP should be expressed in mmHg and measured at end-expiration in the complete supine position after ensuring that abdominal muscle contractions are absent and with the transducer zeroed at the level of the mid-axillary line
Definition 5	The reference standard for intermittent IAP measurement is via the bladder with a maximal instillation volume of 25 mL of sterile saline
Definition 6	Normal IAP is approximately 5–7 mmHg in critically ill adults
Definition 7	IAH is defined by a sustained or repeated pathological elevation of IAP >12 mmHg
Definition 8	IAH is graded as follows: • Grade I: IAP 12–15 mmHg • Grade II: IAP 16–20 mmHg • Grade III: IAP 21–25 mmHg • Grade IV: IAP >25 mmHg
Definition 9	ACS is defined as a sustained IAP ≥20 mmHg (with or without an APP <60 mmHg) that is associated with new organ dysfunction/failure
Definition 10	Primary ACS is a condition associated with injury or disease in the abdomino-pelvic region that frequently requires early surgical or interventional radiological intervention.
Definition 11	Secondary ACS refers to conditions that do not originate from the abdomino-pelvic region
Definition 12	Recurrent ACS refers to the condition in which ACS redevelops following previous surgical or medical treatment of primary or secondary ACS

Reproduced with permission from the World Society for Abdominal Compartment Syndrome.

The absolute value of IAP that is required to cause renal impairment is probably in the region of 20 mmHg. Maintaining adequate cardiovascular filling pressures in the presence of increased IAP also seems to be important.[43]

Cardiac function

Increased IAP reduces cardiac output as well as increasing central venous pressure, systemic vascular resistance, pulmonary artery pressure and pulmonary artery wedge pressure. Cardiac output is affected mainly by a reduction in stroke volume, secondary to a reduction in preload and an increase in afterload. This is further aggravated by hypovolaemia. Paradoxically, in the presence of hypovolaemia, an increase in IAP can be temporarily associated with an increase in cardiac output. Venous stasis occurs in the legs of patients with IAP values above 12 mmHg. In addition, recent studies of patients undergoing laparoscopic cholecystectomy show up to a fourfold increase in renin and aldosterone levels.

Respiratory function

In association with increased IAP, there is diaphragmatic splinting, exerting a restrictive effect on the lungs with reduction in ventilation, decreased lung compliance, increase in airway pressures and reduction in tidal volumes. The mechanism by which increased IAP impairs pulmonary function appears to be purely mechanical. As IAP increases, the diaphragm is forced higher into the chest, thereby compressing the lungs. Adequate ventilation can still be achieved, but only at the cost of increased airway pressures.

In critically ill, ventilated patients the effect on the respiratory system can be significant, resulting in reduced lung volumes, impaired gas exchange and high ventilatory pressures. Hypercarbia can occur and the resulting acidosis can be exacerbated by simultaneous cardiovascular depression as a result of the raised IAP. The effects of raised IAP on the respiratory system in the intensive care setting can sometimes be life threatening, requiring urgent abdominal decompression. Patients with true ACS demonstrate a remarkable improvement in their intraoperative vital signs following abdominal decompression.

Visceral perfusion

Interest in visceral perfusion has increased with increased awareness of gastric tonometry, and there is an association between IAP and visceral perfusion as measured by gastric pH. In a study of 73 patients after laparotomy, it was shown that IAP and gastric pH are strongly associated, suggesting that early decreases in visceral perfusion are related to IAP at levels as low as 12 mmHg.[43] Visceral reperfusion injury is a major consideration after a period of raised IAP, and may of itself have fatal consequences.

Intracranial contents

Raised IAP can have a marked effect on intracranial pathophysiology and cause severe rises in intracranial pressure.

Measurement of IAP

The most common method for measuring IAP uses a urinary catheter.[44] The patient is positioned flat in the bed and a standard Foley catheter is used with a T-piece bladder pressure device attached between the urinary catheter and the drainage tubing. This piece is then connected to a pressure transducer, which is placed in the mid-axillary line and the urinary tubing clamped. Approximately 50 mL of isotonic saline is inserted into the bladder via a three-way stopcock. After zeroing, the pressure on the monitor is recorded.

Pitfalls of IAP pressure measurement

The following factors are important in achieving effective IAP measurements:

- A strict protocol and staff education on the technique and interpretation of IAP is essential.
- Very high pressures (especially unexpected ones) are usually caused by a blocked urinary catheter.
- The size of the urinary catheter does not matter.
- The volume of saline instilled into the bladder is not critical, but it should be enough to overcome the resistance of the contracted bladder; usually, not more than 50 mL is adequate.
- A central venous pressure manometer system can be used but it is more cumbersome than online monitoring.
- Elevation of the urine catheter and measuring the urine column provides a rough guide and is simple to perform.
- If the patient is not lying flat, IAP can be measured from the pubic symphysis.
- IAP is not a static measurement and should be measured continuously. In addition, whether IAP is measured intermittently or continuously, consideration of abdominal perfusion measurement should be given (see below). Real-time continuous monitoring of IAP is effective and shows trends as well as actual pressures.

✓ Intra-abdominal hypertension (IAH) is defined by a sustained or repeated pathological elevation of IAP >12 mmHg.

Abdominal perfusion pressure

Like the concept of cerebral perfusion pressure, calculation of the 'abdominal perfusion pressure' (APP), which is defined as mean arterial pressure (MAP) minus IAP, assesses not only the severity of IAP present, but also the adequacy of the patient's abdominal blood flow. A retrospective trial of surgical and trauma patients with IAH (mean IAP 22 ± 8 mmHg) concluded that an APP >50 mmHg optimised survival based upon receiver operating characteristic curve analysis.[45] APP was also superior to global resuscitation end-points such as arterial pH, base deficit, arterial lactate and hourly urinary output in its ability to predict patient outcome. Three subsequent trials in mixed medical–surgical patients (mean IAP 10 ± 4 mmHg) suggested that 60 mmHg represented an appropriate resuscitation goal.[46–49] Persistence of IAH and failure to maintain an APP ≥ 60 mmHg by day 3 following development of IAH-induced acute renal failure was found to discriminate between survivors and non-survivors.

Management of raised IAP

General support

In general, the best treatment is prevention, both by minimising the causative agents and early appreciation of the potential complications.

There are a number of key principles in the management of patients with potential ACS:

- regular (<8-hourly) monitoring of IAP;
- optimisation of systemic perfusion and organ function in the patient with IAH;
- institution of specific medical procedures to reduce IAP and the end-organ consequences of IAH/ACS;
- early surgical decompression for refractory IAH.

Reversible factors

The second aspect of management is to correct any reversible cause of ACS, such as intra-abdominal bleeding. Maxwell et al. reported on secondary ACS, which can occur without abdominal injury, and stated that, again, early recognition could improve outcome.[50]

Massive retroperitoneal haemorrhage is often associated with a fractured pelvis, and consideration should be given to measures that would control haemorrhage, such as pelvic fixation or vessel embolisation. In some cases, severe gaseous distension or acute colonic pseudo-obstruction can occur in patients in intensive care. This may respond to drugs such as neostigmine but if it is severe, surgical decompression may be necessary (see also Chapter 10). Ileus is a common cause of raised IAP in patients in intensive care. There is little that can be actively done in these circumstances apart from optimising the patient's cardiorespiratory status and serum electrolytes.

Abdominal evaluation for sepsis is a priority and surgery is obviously the mainstay of treatment in patients whose rise in IAP is caused by postoperative bleeding.

Management of IAH and ACS is summarised in **Figs 13.2** and **13.3**.[42,48,49]

Surgery for raised IAP

As yet, there are few guidelines for exactly when surgical decompression is required in the presence of raised IAP. The indications for abdominal decompression are related to correcting pathophysiological abnormalities as much as achieving a precise and optimum IAP. The abdomen is decompressed, and a temporary abdominal closure (TAC) is achieved. The simplest technique is the Opsite® sandwich technique described above.

Every effort must be made towards the reduction of intra-abdominal pressure, allowing early closure of the abdomen. Clinical infection is common in the open abdomen and the infection is usually polymicrobial. Prophylactic antibiotics are not routinely used.

Summary

Patients with raised IAP require close and careful monitoring, aggressive resuscitation and a low index of suspicion for requirement of surgical abdominal decompression.

> ✓✓ The formation of the World Society on ACS has been a major advance, with production of consensus definitions, formation of a research policy with multicentre trials, and the publishing of the consensus guidelines on ACS.[42,48,49]

Organ injury scaling systems

The American Association for the Surgery of Trauma (AAST) has developed an organ injury scaling system for all major injuries in the body.[51–57] These scores not only allow a clear anatomical language when dealing with organ injury but also, since surgical policies are often dictated by the injuries sustained, a degree of consistency in both treatment and prognosis. The scaling system is outlined in the Appendix to this chapter and can be accessed at http://www.aast.org on the Internet.

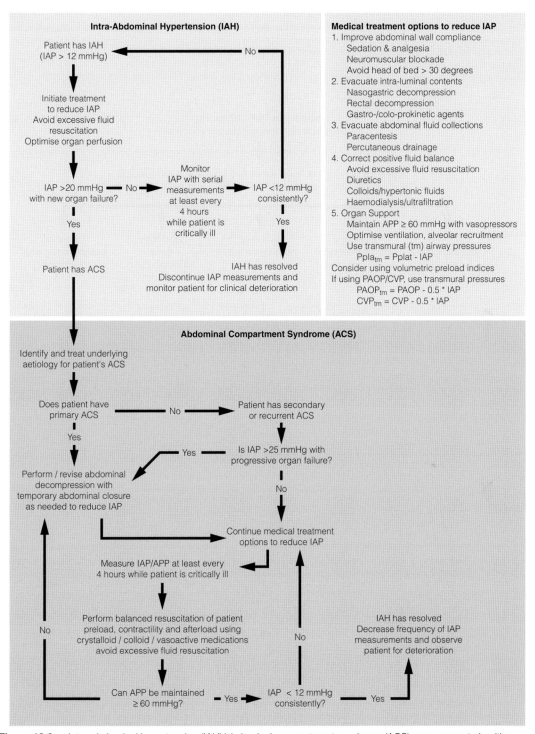

Figure 13.2 • Intra-abdominal hypertension (IAH)/abdominal compartment syndrome (ACS) management algorithm. ACS, abdominal compartment syndrome; APP, abdominal perfusion pressure (MAP−IAP); IAH, intra-abdominal hypertension; IAP, intra-abdominal pressure; Primary ACS, a condition associated with injury or disease in the abdomino-pelvic region that frequently requires early surgical or interventional radiological intervention; Recurrent ACS, the condition in which ACS redevelops following previous surgical or medical treatment of primary ACS; Secondary ACS, ACS due to conditions that do not originate from the abdomino-pelvic region.

- The choice (and success) of the medical management strategies listed below is strongly related to both the aetiology of the patient's IAH / ACS and the patient's clinical situation. The appropriateness of each intervention should always be considered prior to implementing these interventions in any individual patient.
- The interventions should be applied in a stepwise fashion until the patient's intra-abdominal pressure (IAP) decreases.
- If there is no response to a particular intervention, therapy should be escalated to the next step in the algorithm.

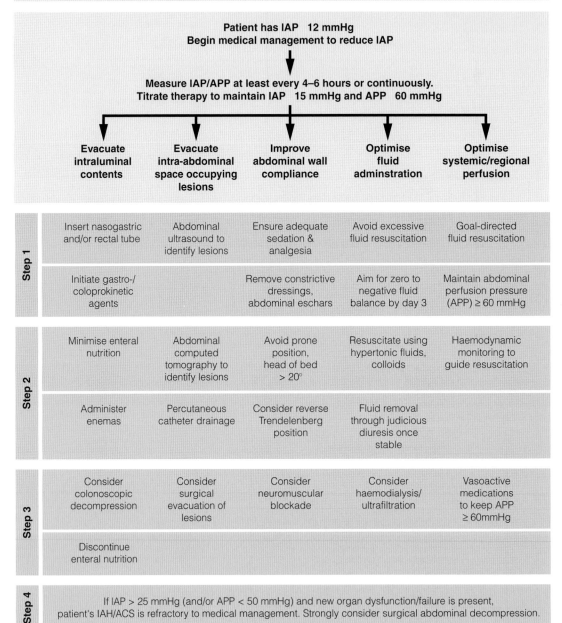

Figure 13.3 • Medical management options to reduce intra-abdominal pressure (IAP). ACS, abdominal compartment syndrome; APP, abdominal perfusion pressure; IAH, intra-abdominal hypertension.

Surgical decision-making in abdominal trauma

Experience in dealing with injury clearly leads to a better outcome:

> Good judgment comes from experience.
>   Unfortunately, experience often comes from bad judgment!

There is limited evidence-based decision-making in trauma, although certain practice guidelines have been developed, primarily by groups working in the Eastern Association for the Surgery of Trauma (www.east.org).[58] Examples of evidence-based practice management guidelines include the following.

Antibiotic prophylaxis in abdominal trauma[58,59]

Guidelines for patient selection and specific antimicrobial regimens are based on good evidence (Box 13.1),[59,60] those regarding high-risk patients and duration of therapy less so (Box 13.2). The trauma surgery setting is fundamentally different to that of elective surgery, especially with regard to prophylactic antibiotics. Antibiotics are given after the peritoneal insult and possible contamination has occurred (Boxes 13.3 and 13.4).

Management of abdominal injury

Abdominal injury is of a blunt or penetrating nature. While it is hard to define precise parameters for the approach to management, the following guidelines are offered.

Hepatic injury

Repair and resection for treatment of hepatic trauma demands a working knowledge of the anatomy of the liver. Segmental anatomical resection has been well documented but usually is not applicable to injury. The three main hepatic veins divide the liver into four sections: right posterior lateral, right anterior medial, left anterior and left posterior. Each of these sectors receives a portal pedicle. The liver is practically divided into eight Couinaud segments (**Fig. 13.4**).

Understanding the anatomy also helps to explain some of the patterns of injury following blunt trauma. There are also differences in tissue elasticity, which determine injury patterns. The forces from blunt injury are usually direct compressive

---

Box 13.1 • Evidence-based guidelines for prophylactic antibiotic administration: summary of recommendations

Strong recommendation

1. Patients with peritoneal contamination due to traumatic bowel injury repaired within 12 hours are not considered to have established intra-abdominal infections, and should be treated with prophylactic antimicrobials for 24 hours or less (**Evidence level I**)

Recommendation based on evidence of effectiveness

2. Systemic antibiotics should be administered as soon as possible after injury for patients with penetrating trauma requiring surgical intervention (**Evidence level II**)
3. A single broad-spectrum agent is at least as safe and effective as a double or triple antibiotic therapeutic regimen (**Evidence level II**)
4. Patients with a fully removable focus of inflammation (e.g. bowel necrosis) should be treated with prophylactic antimicrobials for 24 hours or less (**Evidence level II**)

Recommendation made where there is no adequate evidence as to the most effective practice

5. Patients with more extensive conditions should be treated as having more extensive infections, and given *therapeutic* antimicrobials for more than 24 hours (**Evidence level III**)

Reproduced from Mazuski JE, Sawyer RG, Nathens AB et al. The Surgical Infection Society Guidelines on antimicrobial therapy for intra-abdominal infections: an executive summary. Surg Infect 2002; 3(3):161–73. Cornwell EE IIIrd, Campbell KA. Trauma. In: Gordon TA, Cameron JL (eds) Evidence-based surgery. Hamilton, Ontario: BC Decker, 2000; pp. 415–28. With permission from Mary Ann Liebert Inc./BC Decker Inc.

---

forces or shear forces. The elastic tissue within arterial blood vessels makes them less susceptible to tearing than any other structures within the liver. Venous and biliary ductal tissues are moderately resistant to shear forces, whereas the liver parenchyma is the least resistant of all. Therefore, fractures within the liver parenchyma tend to occur along segmental fissures or directly into the parenchyma. This causes shearing of lateral branches to the major hepatic and portal veins. With severe deceleration injury, the origin of the hepatic veins may be ripped from the inferior vena cava, causing devastating haemorrhage. Similarly, the small branches from the caudate lobe entering directly into the cava are at high risk of shearing with linear tears on the caval surface.

Direct compressive forces usually cause tearing between segmental fissures in an anterior posterior sagittal orientation. Horizontal fracture lines into the parenchyma give the characteristic burst pattern

Box 13.2 • Evidence-based guidelines for duration of antibiotic therapy: summary of recommendations

Recommendation based on evidence of effectiveness

1. High postoperative septic complications can be expected in patients with gunshot injuries to the colon, high Penetrating Abdominal Trauma Index (PATI) scores, major blood loss, and common need for postoperative care. There is no evidence to date that extending prophylactic antibiotic therapy beyond 24 hours decreases that high risk (**Evidence level II**)

2. Antimicrobial therapy of most established intra-abdominal infections should be limited to no more than 5 days (**Evidence level II**)

3. Antimicrobial therapy can be discontinued in patients when they have no clinical evidence of infection such as fever or leucocytosis (**Evidence level II**)

Recommendation made where there is no adequate evidence as to the most effective practice

4. Continued clinical evidence of infection at the end of the time period designated for antimicrobial therapy should prompt appropriate diagnostic investigations rather than prolongation of antimicrobial treatment (**Evidence level III**)

5. If adequate source control cannot be achieved, a longer duration of antimicrobial therapy may be warranted (**Evidence level III**)

Box 13.3 • Evidence-based guidelines for antimicrobial regimens: summary of recommendations

Strong recommendation

1. Antimicrobial regimens for intra-abdominal infections should cover common aerobic and anaerobic enteric flora. No regimen has been demonstrated to be superior to another (**Evidence level I**)

Recommendation based on evidence of effectiveness

2. Once-daily administration of aminoglycoside is the preferred dosing regimen for patients receiving these agents for intra-abdominal infections (**Evidence level II**)

Recommendation made where there is no adequate evidence as to the most effective practice

3. Aminoglycosides should be avoided in the acute trauma patient due to difficulty in reaching adequate MIC levels without toxicity (**Evidence level III**)

For less severely ill patients with community-acquired infections, antimicrobial agents having a narrower spectrum of activity, such as antianaerobic cephalosporins, are preferable to more costly agents having broader coverage of Gram-negative organisms and/or a greater risk of toxicity (**Evidence level III**)

4. The routine use of intraoperative cultures is controversial, and there is no evidence that altering the antimicrobial regimen on the basis of intraoperative culture results improves outcome (**Evidence level III**)

to such liver injuries. If the fracture lines are parallel, these have been dubbed 'bear claw'-type injuries and probably represent where the ribs have been compressed directly into the parenchyma. Occasionally, there will be a single fracture line across the horizontal plane of the liver, usually between the anterior and posterior segments. This can cause massive haemorrhage if there is direct extension or continuity with the peritoneal cavity.

The liver is at risk in any penetrating trauma to the right upper quadrant of the abdomen. CECT has enhanced the diagnosis of significant liver injury in the stable patient. Virtually all penetrating injuries to the abdomen should be explored promptly, especially when they occur in conjunction with hypotension. The surgeon should be aware that penetrating injuries to the right lower chest, presenting with haemothorax, may have penetrated the diaphragm, with the bleeding originating from the liver.

The treatment of severe liver injuries begins with temporary control of haemorrhage. Most catastrophic bleeding from hepatic injury is venous in nature and can therefore be controlled by liver packs. If there is bright red blood pouring from the parenchyma, it is then appropriate to apply a vascular clamp to the porta hepatis (Pringle's manoeuvre), via the gastrohepatic ligament. If this controls the bleeding, the surgeon should be suspicious of hepatic arterial or possible portal venous injury. While control is being obtained, it is important to establish more intravenous access lines and other monitoring devices as needed. (The treatment of bleeding is to stop the bleeding!) Hypothermia should be anticipated and corrective measures taken.

After haemostasis and haemodynamic resuscitation has been achieved, any packs in the two lower abdominal quadrants are removed. If there is abdominal contamination, it is appropriate to control this as rapidly as possible. The packs in the left upper quadrant are then removed. If there is an associated spleen injury a decision must be made either to remove it promptly or to clamp the hilum of the spleen temporarily with a vascular clamp to reduce further bleeding. Finally, the packs are removed in the right upper quadrant and the injury to the liver rapidly assessed.

If there is bleeding from the porta hepatis, careful exploration for a portal vein injury should be carried out, with repair or shunting. Traction on the dome of the liver, which produces a sudden gush of retrohepatic blood, should make the surgeon suspicious of injury to the posterior hepatic veins or inferior vena. The options for hepatic vein and cava injuries include direct compression (packing), extension of the laceration and direct control, atrial–caval shunt, non-shunt isolation (Heaney technique) and veno–veno bypass. Liver packs are increasingly used as definitive treatment, particularly when there is bilobar injury, or they can simply buy time if the patient develops a coagulopathy, hypothermia or there are no blood resources.

Pancreatic trauma

Blunt pancreatic trauma can be subtle and presentation is often that of associated injuries. The pancreas is a retroperitoneal organ and there may be no intraperitoneal signs. History can be helpful, for example if there is a history of epigastric trauma. The physical examination is often misleading. Amylase and blood count are non-specific, and may be normal; CT is 85% accurate, but does not always help with the grading of the injury, and endoscopic retrograde cholangiopancreatography (ERCP) can be helpful in selected stable patients.

Penetrating pancreatic trauma is usually obvious since the patient will almost invariably have been explored for other injuries.[61]

Once the retroperitoneum has been violated it is imperative for the surgeon to do a thorough exploration in the central region. This includes:

- an extended Kocher manoeuvre to examine the entire duodenum;
- a right medial visceral rotation to examine the back of the head of the pancreas;
- division of the ligament of Treitz to examine the front of the pancreas;
- division of the gastrocolic omentum to examine the top of the pancreas;
- a left medial visceral rotation to examine the anterior and posterior surfaces of the tail of the pancreas as it extends towards the splenic hilum.

Injury to the main pancreatic duct appears to increase the pancreatic-specific morbidity and mortality.[62]

Any parenchymal haematoma of the pancreatic head should be thoroughly explored and should include irrigation of the haematoma and adequate drainage with a suction drain (e.g. a Blake® drain).

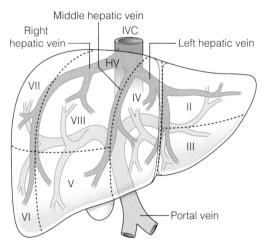

Figure 13.4 • Couinaud's segments of the liver.

Injuries to the tail and body of the pancreas can usually either be drained or, if a strong suspicion for major ductal injury is present (Grade III injury), resection can be carried out as a distal pancreatectomy. In young patients, the duct is not usually visualised following trauma and so cannot specifically be tied off.

The injuries that vex the surgeon most, however, are those to the head of the gland, particularly those with juxtaposed injuries or also involving the duodenum. Resection (Whipple's procedure) is usually reserved for those patients who have destructive injuries or those in whom the blood supply to the duodenum and pancreatic head has been embarrassed. This procedure should only be embarked upon as a planned procedure in the stable patient, with consideration being given to appropriate damage control procedures in all others. The remainder are usually treated with variations of drainage and pyloric exclusion. This would include tube duodenostomy and extensive closed drainage around the injury site. Common duct drainage is not indicated.[63] There are limited guidelines for the management of major pancreatic trauma (Box 13.5).

Aorta and inferior vena cava

Aortic and caval injuries are primarily a problem of access (rapid) and control of haemorrhage. If the surgeon opens the abdomen and there is extensive retroperitoneal bleeding centrally, there are two options. If the bleeding is primarily venous in nature, the right colon should be mobilised to the midline, including the duodenum and head of the pancreas, using a right medial visceral rotation. This will expose the infrarenal cava and infrarenal aorta. It will also facilitate access to the portal vein.

If the bleeding is primarily arterial in nature, it is best to approach the injury from the left. Initial control can be obtained by direct pressure at the oesophageal hiatus or via the lesser sac. Additional exposure can be obtained by simply dividing the left crus of the diaphragm. Exposure includes reflecting the left colon medially and mobilising the pancreas, kidney and spleen to the midline. By approaching the aorta from the left lateral position it is possible to identify the plane of Leriche more rapidly than by approaching it through the lesser sac. The problem is the coeliac and superior mesenteric ganglia, both of which can be quite dense and hinder dissection around the origins of the coeliac and superior mesenteric arteries.

Once isolation of the injury has been achieved, treatment of aortic or caval injuries is usually straightforward, either by direct suture or occasionally grafting. Caval injuries below the renal vein, if extensive, can be ligated, although repair is preferred. Injuries above the renal veins in the cava should be repaired if at all possible. If there is injury to the posterior wall of the vein, it is preferable to isolate the segment and repair it from within the vein using an anterior approach.

Colonic injuries

Many studies have shown primary repair of colonic injuries to be safe in patients at low risk of postoperative complications; however, identification of the high-risk patient in whom avoidance of an intraperitoneal colonic suture line may be beneficial is still controversial. The significant morbidity and financial costs associated with the creation and reversals of colostomy, and the destructive effect of colostomy on the patient's quality of life, have been cited as evidence to support the primary repair of colonic wounds.[60,64–66]

Stone and Fabian excluded patients from primary repair in the presence of shock, major blood loss, more than two organs injured, faecal contamination more than 'minimal', delay to repair of more than 8 hours and wounds of the colon or abdominal wall so destructive as to require resection.[67] Murray et al. reviewed 140 patients with colonic injuries that required resection.[68] They suggested that the majority of patients can safely undergo colonic resection with primary colo-colonic anastomosis, even for severe injuries; however, there is a subgroup of critically injured patients at higher risk of anastomotic leakage who may be best treated by colostomy.

In the 'physiologically challenged' patient, hypoperfusion of splanchnic tissues leads to local tissue hypoxia, and repair or anastomosis under those circumstances is more likely to fail. This high-risk group should be treated by damage control

Box 13.5 • Evidence-based guidelines for diagnosis and management of pancreatic trauma: summary of recommendations

Recommendations made where there is no adequate evidence as to the most effective practice

1. Delay in the recognition of main pancreatic duct injury causes increased morbidity (**Evidence level III**)

2. CT scan is suggestive, but not diagnostic of, pancreatic injury (**Evidence level III**)

3. Amylase/lipase levels are suggestive, but not diagnostic of, pancreatic injury (**Evidence level III**)

4. Grade I and II injuries can be managed by drainage alone (**Evidence level III**)

5. Grade III injuries can be managed with resection and drainage (**Evidence level III**)

6. Closed suction is preferred to sump suction (**Evidence level III**)

techniques with restoration of continuity of the bowel once the physiological insult has been corrected. Outcome is determined by the patient's physiological envelope and not by anatomical integrity[69,70] (Box 13.6).

Complex pelvic fracture

Complex pelvic fractures can be some of the most difficult injuries to treat. Initially, they can cause devastating haemorrhage and subsequently may be associated with overwhelming pelvic sepsis and distant multiple organ failure.

For those patients who present with complex pelvic fractures and who are haemodynamically stable, diagnostic studies should be carried out as rapidly as possible, including plain films of the pelvis, CECT and arteriogram. All haemodynamically unstable patients with such pelvic fractures should be taken to the operating theatre as soon as possible, to allow continuing resuscitation including packing.[71]

The priorities facing the surgeon are to control the pelvic haemorrhage and rule out other intra-abdominal organ injuries with associated haemorrhage. Sometimes it is prudent to perform a rapid laparotomy to rule out additional haemorrhage, but if there is not a strong suspicion of abdominal bleeding, it is best to avoid laparotomy until

the pelvic bleeding has been arrested (Box 13.7). Extrapelvic packing should be considered.

Technique of extraperitoneal packing

The patient is positioned supine and, if necessary, an external fixator or C-clamp is applied. A 5-cm vertical midline suprapubic incision is made and the fascia anterior to the rectus muscle is exposed. The fascia is divided until the symphysis can be palpated directly (the pre-peritoneal plane has been reached). The fascia is divided in the midline, protecting against urinary bladder damage. From the symphysis the pelvic brim is followed laterally and posterior to the sacroiliac (SI) joint (first bony irregularity felt), first on the side of major bleeding (most often the side of SI joint disruption). The fascia is then dissected away from the pelvic brim as far posteriorly as possible at the level of the pelvic brim. The bladder and rectum are then held to the opposite side while the plane is opened bluntly down to the pelvic floor, avoiding injury to vascular and nerve structures in the area. The space is then packed with vascular or abdominal swabs, starting posteriorly and distal to the tip of the sacrum, and building the packs cranially and anteriorly.[72] In an unbroken pelvis with intact pelvic floor, one should be able to accommodate three large abdominal swabs on each side. In severe pelvic fractures,

Box 13.6 • Evidence-based guidelines for management of colon injuries: summary of recommendations

Strong recommendation

1. Primary repair is supported for *non-destructive* (involvement of <50% of the bowel wall without devascularisation) colon wounds in the absence of peritonitis. The risk is not obviated by colostomy, and intra-abdominal sepsis frequently occurs in the absence of suture line disruption. Accordingly, the majority of colon injuries in civilian practice may be managed by primary repair (**Evidence level I**)

Recommendations based on evidence of effectiveness

2. Patients with penetrating colon wounds that are *destructive* can undergo resection and primary anastomosis if they:
   - are haemodynamically stable without evidence of shock
   - have no significant underlying disease
   - have minimal associated injuries (PATI <25, ISS <25)
   - have no peritonitis
     (**Evidence level II**)

3. Given the small number of patients in high-risk categories with destructive colon injuries requiring resection who were randomised to primary repair, there is still room to consider colostomy in the management of these patients (**Evidence level II**)

4. Patients with shock, underlying disease, significant associated injuries or peritonitis should have destructive wounds managed by resection and colostomy (**Evidence level II**)

5. Colostomies performed following colon and rectal trauma can be closed within 2 weeks if contrast enema is performed to confirm distal healing. This recommendation pertains to patients who do not have non-healing bowel injury, unresolved wound sepsis or are unstable (**Evidence level II**)

6. A barium enema should not be performed to rule out colon cancer or polyps prior to colostomy closure for trauma in patients who otherwise have no indications for being at risk (**Evidence level II**)

7. Multiple blood transfusions, shock and a high PATI reliably identify patients at high risk of septic complications following penetrating colon injuries (**Evidence level II**)

Reproduced from Cayten CG, Fabian TC, Garcia VF et al. Patient Management Guidelines for penetrating intraperitoneal injuries. EAST Practice Parameter Working Group; http://www.east.org.

Box 13.7 • Evidence-based guidelines for management of haemorrhage in pelvic fracture: summary of recommendations

Recommendations based on evidence of effectiveness

1. Patients with evidence of unstable fractures of the pelvis associated with hypotension should be considered for some form of pelvic stabilisation (**Evidence level II**)

2. Patients with evidence of unstable pelvic fractures who warrant laparotomy should receive external pelvic stabilisation prior to laparotomy incision (**Evidence level II**)

3. Patients with a major pelvic fracture who have signs of ongoing bleeding after non-pelvic sources of blood loss have been ruled out should be considered for pelvic angiography and possible embolisation (**Evidence level II**)

4. Patients with major pelvic fractures who are found to have bleeding in the pelvis, which cannot be adequately controlled at laparotomy, should be considered for pelvic angiography and possible embolisation (**Evidence level II**)

5. Patients with evidence of arterial extravasation of intravenous contrast in the pelvis by computed tomography should be considered for pelvic angiography and possible embolisation (**Evidence level II**)

6. Patients with hypotension and gross blood in the abdomen or evidence of intestinal perforation warrant emergency laparotomy (**Evidence level II**)

7. The diagnostic peritoneal tap appears to be the most reliable diagnostic test for this purpose. Urgent laparotomy is warranted for patients who demonstrate signs of continued intra-abdominal bleeding after adequate resuscitation or evidence of intestinal perforation (**Evidence level II**)

Recommendation made where there is no adequate evidence as to the most effective practice

8. Patients with evidence of unstable fractures of the pelvis not associated with hypotension but who do require a steady and ongoing resuscitation should be considered for some form of external pelvic stabilisation (**Evidence level III**)

Reproduced from DiGiacomo JC, Bonadies JA, Cole FJ et al. Practice Management Guidelines for haemorrhage in pelvic fracture. EAST Practice Management Guidelines Work Group; http://www.east.org.

efficient packing might require many more (>10 packs is not unusual). The number of packs needed is defined by the available space and the appropriate force applied. The outer fascia is closed with a single running suture and the skin is closed. If laparotomy is required, it should follow the packing procedure.

After a damage control laparotomy with extra-peritoneal pelvic packing, a temporary abdominal closure is appropriate. As in the abdomen, the packs should be removed after 24–48 hours.

Stabilisation of the pelvis is initially by compression (using a knotted sheet or external fixation). External fixation is used for stabilisation of the anterior pelvis but will fail if the posterior pelvis is unstable. These patients may require plating of the SI joint and are best managed by temporary stabilisation using a pelvic binder, and then assessed by CT and arteriography. Based on location of the injury, colostomy may be required in order to prevent contamination of a perineal wound in the post-injury period. In general, all compound injuries involving the perineum and perianal area should have a diverting colostomy (see also Chapter 11).

In patients with associated major perineal injuries, after the initial fixation of the pelvis has been obtained, daily wound examination, debridement and gradual removal of packs should take place. A caveat of pack removal is that the longer they are left in, the greater the risk of pelvic sepsis, and ideally they should be removed within 24–48 hours.

Non-operative approach to abdominal solid-organ injuries

There is a growing body of evidence attesting to the effectiveness and safety of selective non-operative management (SNOM) of abdominal injury, both blunt and penetrating in nature. Most surgeons who practice SNOM regard peritonitis, omental and bowel evisceration, and being unable to evaluate a patient, as a contraindication to attempting non-operative management.[73] Almost all regard CT as essential, and their preparedness to consider SNOM was related to injury extent, as well as the experience of the surgeon concerned.

Liver

In 1990, it was suggested that a number of patients with blunt liver injuries might be candidates for expectant management,[74] and in a multicentre study it was found that, in the hands of experienced trauma surgeons, the success with the non-operative approach to liver injuries was greater than 98%.[75]

Currently, all patients with liver injuries following blunt trauma should be considered candidates for non-operative management, provided that haemodynamic stability can be assured. Unlike the spleen, delayed haemorrhage from the liver is rare. The complications in those patients managed expectantly are frequently related to the biliary system and can usually be managed by endoscopic or interventional techniques. While non-operative management has most frequently been applied to patients with blunt injuries, stable patients with liver injuries as the result of penetrating trauma have also been managed expectantly.[76]

Spleen

In children, the success of non-operative management of the spleen is over 90%, but this has not been the experience in adults. Currently, most surgeons will attempt to manage the injured adult spleen with an AAST grade I–III injury non-operatively; the management of grade IV or V injuries remains controversial. Patients over 55 years of age generally do not do as well and splenectomy continues to be recommended (see Box 13.8).[77]

Box 13.8 • Practice management guidelines for the non-operative management of blunt injury to the liver and spleen: summary of recommendations

Recommendations based on evidence of effectiveness

1. There are class II and mostly class III data to suggest that non-operative management of blunt hepatic and/or splenic injury in a haemodynamically stable patient is reasonable (**Evidence level II**)
2. The severity of hepatic or splenic injury (as suggested by CT grade or degree of haemoperitoneum), neurological status and/or the presence of associated injuries are not contraindications to non-operative management (**Evidence level II**)
3. Abdominal CT is the most reliable method to identify and assess the severity of injury to the spleen or liver (**Evidence level II**)

Recommendations made where there is no adequate evidence as to the most effective practice

4. The clinical status of the patient should dictate the frequency of follow-up scans (**Evidence level III**)
5. Initial CT of the abdomen should be performed with oral and intravenous contrast to facilitate the diagnosis of hollow viscus injuries (**Evidence level III**)
6. Medical clearance to resume normal activity status should be based on evidence of healing (**Evidence level III**)
7. Angiographic embolisation is an adjunct in the non-operative management of the haemodynamically stable patient with hepatic and splenic injuries and evidence of ongoing bleeding (**Evidence level III**)

Reproduced from Alonso M, Brathwaite C, Garcia V et al. Practice Management Guidelines Work Group. Blunt liver and spleen injuries: non-operative management; http://www.east.org/tpg/livspleen.

Penetrating injury

In those patients with penetrating injury to the abdomen, who are haemodynamically unstable, have peritonitis or clear signs of abdominal penetration, there is little debate regarding the need for urgent laparotomy. However, in those patients with penetrating injury where the wounds are tangential, it is clear that if these patients are stable, without peritonitis, some patients may not need surgery despite the penetrating nature of the wound.

In a recent study of gunshot wounds managed non-operatively, clinical examination was a key marker, and all failures occurred within 24 hours of admission, setting a minimum required observation period before discharge.[78]

Laparoscopy may play a role, particularly in the clarification of penetration of the abdominal cavity and of the diaphragm. Current evidence-based guidelines for the management of penetrating trauma are limited, and are perhaps more suited to high-volume centres than those only occasionally dealing with penetrating trauma[79] (see Box 13.9).

Interventional radiology

In a significant number of patients, interventional radiology, with arterial embolisation (AE), stent or stentgraft placement, has become either the first line of treatment or an important adjunct to non-operative management of abdominal and other injuries.[80] Clinical evaluation, however, determines the course of treatment. Patients who are haemodynamically stable should be evaluated with CECT.

Angio-embolisation in liver injuries

Non-operative management (NOM) of blunt liver injuries in haemodynamically stable or stabilised patients has become standard practice. The introduction of AE has been reported to increase the success rate of NOM to well above 80%.[81]

Operative treatment of liver injuries, even in experienced hands, still carries a high mortality and morbidity risk. AE seems to be a valuable adjunct to operative management since most patients are haemodynamically abnormal at the end of a damage control laparotomy, and ongoing arterial bleeding is difficult to rule out clinically.

The indications for AE should include CT evidence of ongoing bleeding with contrast extravasation outside or within the liver, a drop in haemoglobin, tachycardia and haemoperitoneum, as well as for-

Box 13.9 • Selective non-operative management of penetrating injury of the abdomen: summary of recommendations

Strong recommendations

1. Patients who are haemodynamically unstable or who have diffuse abdominal tenderness should be taken for laparotomy as an emergency (**Evidence level I**)

2. Patients who are haemodynamically stable with an unreliable clinical examination (i.e. brain injury, spinal cord injury, intoxication or need for sedation or anaesthesia) should have further diagnostic investigations done for intraperitoneal injury or undergo exploratory laparotomy (**Evidence level I**)

3. Routine laparotomy is not indicated in haemodynamically stable patients and abdominal stab wounds without signs of peritonitis or diffuse abdominal tenderness (away from the wounding site) in centres with surgical expertise (**Evidence level II**)

4. A routine laparotomy is not indicated in haemodynamically stable patients with abdominal gunshot wounds if the wounds are tangential and there are no peritoneal signs (**Evidence level II**)

5. Serial physical examination is reliable in detecting significant injuries after penetrating trauma to the abdomen, if performed by experienced clinicians and preferably by the same team (**Evidence level II**)

6. In patients selected for initial non-operative management, abdomino-pelvic CT should be strongly considered as a diagnostic tool to facilitate initial management decisions (**Evidence level II**)

7. Diagnostic laparoscopy may be considered as a tool to evaluate diaphragmatic lacerations as well as peritoneal penetration (**Evidence level II**)

Recommendations made where there is no adequate evidence as to the most effective practice

8. Patients with penetrating injury isolated to the right upper quadrant of the abdomen may be managed without laparotomy in the presence of stable vital signs, reliable examination and minimal to no abdominal tenderness (**Evidence level III**)

9. The vast majority of patients with penetrating abdominal trauma, managed non-operatively, may be discharged after 24 hours observation, in the presence of a reliable abdominal examination and minimal to no abdominal tenderness (**Evidence level III**)

Reproduced from Como JJ, Bokhari F, Chiu WC et al. Practice Management Guidelines Working Group. Penetrating trauma: selective non-operative management. Eastern Association for the Surgery of Trauma. J Trauma 2010; 68(3):721–33. With permission from Lippincott, Williams & Wilkins.

mation of pseudoaneurysm. The risk of bleeding with NOM in OIS grade 4 and 5 liver injuries is significant, and operative intervention, with packing, followed by AE is preferable.[82]

Angio-embolisation in blunt splenic injuries

Indications for AE include CT evidence of ongoing bleeding with contrast extravasation outside or within the spleen, a drop in haemoglobin, tachycardia and haemoperitoneum, as well as formation of pseudoaneurysm. Selective catheterisation of the splenic artery is performed, followed by superselective catheterisation of the bleeding arteries or feeders to the pseudoaneurysm.[83,84]

Angio-embolisation in severe pelvic fractures

Severe pelvic fractures, particularly with disruption of the sacroiliac joints, are associated with a high risk of severe arterial and venous bleeding. The application of a sheet or external fixation may control the venous bleeding, which constitutes about 85% of all pelvic bleeding. However, arterial bleeding often requires AE, which has become the first line of treatment in patients stable enough to reach angiography.[85] Established indications are CT evidence of ongoing bleeding such as contrast extravasation and pelvic haematoma with bladder compression and ongoing transfusion requirements without evidence of other extrapelvic bleeding sources.

There is also a possibility in this subgroup of patients of severe venous bleeding. The patient in shock refractory to resuscitation should be considered for damage control with (extraperitoneal) pelvic packing before AE.

AE is carried out after performing an abdominal aortography followed by selective catheterisation of the internal iliac arteries. When contrast extravasation is demonstrated, the bleeding vessels are catheterised superselectively and embolised with coils, or a combination of coils and gelfoam particles.

Key points

- In order to avoid missed injuries and preventable deaths, trauma patients who have any of the risk factors for abdominal injury should undergo objective evaluation of the abdomen.
- Delay in surgery is the most common cause of unnecessary ongoing bleeding.
- In patients who are unstable, the preferred objective study is a bedside ultrasound. If an ultrasound examination is unavailable or equivocal, a DPL should be performed.
- In stable patients, abdominal CT with intravenous contrast is the preferred method of objective examination of the abdomen.
- When laparotomy is required, it should be approached in a systematic fashion and the treatment of injuries prioritised.
- In patients who are cold, coagulopathic and acidotic, a damage control operation should be accomplished promptly.

References

1. Anderson ID, Woodford M, de Dombal T, et al. A retrospective study of 1000 deaths from injury in England and Wales. Br Med J 1988;296:1305–8.

2. National Confidential Enquiry into Patient Outcome and Death (NCEPOD). Trauma: Who cares? www.ncepod.org/2007b.htm; [accessed January 2008].

3. West JC, Trunkey DD, Lim RC. System of trauma care: a study of two counties. Arch Surg 1979;114:455–60.

4. Mackersie RC, Tiwary AD, Shackford SR, et al. Intra-abdominal injury following blunt trauma: identifying the high-risk factors. Arch Surg 1989;124:809–13.

5. Nguyen HB, Banta JE, Cho TW, et al. Mortality predictions using current physiologic scoring systems in patients meeting criteria for early goal-directed therapy and the severe sepsis resuscitation bundle. Shock 2008;30(1):23–8.

6. Husain FA, Martin MJ, Mullenix PS, et al. Serum lactate and base deficit as predictors of mortality and morbidity. Am J Surg 2003;185(5):485–91.

7. Manikis P, Jankowski S, Zhang H, et al. Correlation of serial blood lactate levels to organ failure and mortality after trauma. Am J Emerg Med 1995;13(6):619–22.

8. Thomas SH. Helicopter EMS transport outcomes literature: annotated review of articles published 2004–2006. PreHosp Emerg Care 2007;11(4):477–88.

9. Sullivent EE, Faul M, Wald MM. Reduced mortality in injured adults transported by helicopter emergency medical services. PreHosp Emerg Care 2011;15(3):295–302.

10. Galvagno Jr SM, Haut ER, Zafar SN, et al. Association between helicopter vs ground emergency medical services and survival for adults with major trauma. JAMA 2012;307(15):1602–10.

11. Resources for optimal care of the trauma patient. Committee on Trauma of the American College of Surgeons; 2006.
   The definitive manual of standards by which trauma and trauma services are set up and judged.

12. Bickell WH, Wall MJ, Pepe PE, et al. Immediate versus delayed fluid resuscitation for hypotensive patients with penetrating torso injuries. N Engl J Med 1994;331:1105–9.

13. Johansson PI, Ostrowski SR, Secher NH. Management of major blood loss: an update. Acta Anaesthesiol Scand 2010;54(9):1039–49.
   An outstanding review of the current state of knowledge regarding blood administration, massive blood transfusion and goal-directed transfusion therapy.

14. Johannson PI. Emerging treatment strategies for trauma-induced coagulopathy. Br J Surg 2012;99(Suppl. 1):40–50.

15. American College of Surgeons. Advanced Trauma Life Support Programme: Abdominal trauma. Chicago, IL: American College of Surgeons; 2008.

16. Brooks A, Bowley DM, Boffard KD. Bullet markers – a simple technique to assist in the evaluation of penetrating trauma. J R Army Med Corps 2002;148(3):259–61.

17. Smith-Bindman R, Lipson J, Marcus R, et al. Radiation dose associated with common computed tomography examinations and the associated lifetime attributable risk of cancer. Arch Intern Med 2009;169(22):2078–86.

18. Brenner DJ, Hall EJ. Computed tomography: an increasing source of radiation exposure. N Engl J Med 2007;357:2277–84.

19. Donohue JH, Federle MP, Griffiths BG, et al. Computed tomography in the diagnosis of blunt intestinal and mesenteric injuries. J Trauma 1987;27:11–7.

20. Brasel KJ, Olson CH, Stafford R, et al. Incidence and significance of free fluid on abdominal computed tomographic scan in blunt trauma. J Trauma 1998;44:889–92.

21. Sherck JP, Oakes DD. Intestinal injuries missed by computed tomography. J Trauma 1990;30:1–7.

22. McKenney MG, Martin L, Lopez C. 1000 consecutive ultrasounds for blunt abdominal trauma. J Trauma 1996;40:607–12.

23. Rozycki GS, Ochsner MG, Schmidt JA, et al. A prospective study of surgeon-performed ultrasound as the primary adjuvant modality for injured patient assessment. J Trauma 1995;39:492–7.

24. Root HD, Hauser CW, McKinley CR, et al. Diagnostic peritoneal lavage. Surgery 1965;57:633–7.

25. Brooks AJ, Boffard KD. Current technology: laparoscopic surgery in trauma. Trauma 1999;1:53–60.

26. Fabian TC, McCord S. Therapeutic laparoscopy in trauma. Trauma Quart 1993;34:313–5.

27. Zantut LF, Ivatury RR, Smith S. Diagnostic and therapeutic laparoscopy for penetrating abdominal trauma: a multicentre experience. J Trauma 1997;42:825–31.

28. Degiannis E, Levy R, Sofianos C, et al. Diaphragmatic herniation after penetrating trauma. Br J Surg 1996;83:88–91.

29. Renz BM, Feliciano DV. Unnecessary laparotomies for trauma: a prospective study of morbidity. J Trauma 1995;38:350–6.

30. Ross SE, Dragon GM, O'Malley KF, et al. Morbidity of negative celiotomy in trauma. Injury 1995;26:393–4.

31. Muckart DJ, Abdool-Carim AT, King B. Selective conservative management of abdominal gunshot wounds: a prospective study. Br J Surg 1990;77:652–5.

32. Demetriades D, Charalambides D, Lakhoo M, et al. Gunshot wound of the abdomen: role of selective conservative management. Br J Surg 1991;78:220–2.

33. Maggisano R, Nathens A, Alexandrova NA, et al. Traumatic rupture of the thoracic aorta: should one always operate immediately? Ann Vasc Surg 1995;9:44–6.

34. Wisner DH, Victor NS, Holcroft JW. The priorities in the management of multiple trauma: intracranial versus intra-abdominal injury. J Trauma 1993;35:271–8.

35. Archer LP, Rogers RB, Shackford SR. Selective non-operative management of liver and splenic injuries in neurologically impaired adult patients. Arch Surg 1996;131:309–15.

36. Rotondo MF, Schwab CW, McGonigal MD, et al. 'Damage control': an approach for improved survival in exsanguinating penetrating abdominal injury. J Trauma 1993;35:375–82.

37. Loveland JA, Boffard KD. Damage control in the abdomen and beyond. Br J Surg 2004;91(9):1095–101.

38. Hirshberg A, Mattox KL. Planned re-operation for severe trauma. Ann Surg 1995;222:3–8.

39. Garrison JR, Richardson JD, Hilakos A, et al. Predicting the need to pack early for severe intra-abdominal haemorrhage. J Trauma 1996;40:923–9.

40. Schein M, Saadia R, Jamieson JR, et al. The "sandwich technique" in the management of the open abdomen. Br J Surg 1986;73(5):369–70.

41. Burch J, Moore E, Moore F, et al. The abdominal compartment syndrome. Surg Clin North Am 1996;76:833–42.

42. World Society for Abdominal Compartment Syndrome, www.wsacs.org; [accessed February 2012].

43. Sugrue M, Buist MD, Hourihan F, et al. Prospective study of intra-abdominal hypertension and renal function after laparotomy. Br J Surg 1995;82:235–8.

44. Kron IL, Harman PK, Nolan SP. The measurement of intra-abdominal pressure as a criterion for abdominal re-exploration. Ann Surg 1984;199:28–30.

45. Cheatham ML, White MW, Sagraves SG, et al. Abdominal perfusion pressure: a superior parameter in the assessment of intra-abdominal hypertension. J Trauma 2000;49:621–6.

46. Malbrain ML, Chiumello D, Pelosi P, et al. Incidence and prognosis of intraabdominal hypertension in a mixed population of critically ill patients: a multiple-centre epidemiological study. Crit Care Med 2005;33:315–22.

47. Malbrain ML, Chiumello D, Pelosi P, et al. Prevalence of intra-abdominal hypertension in critically ill patients: a multicentre epidemiological study. Intensive Care Med 2004;30:822–9.

48. Malbrain ML, Cheatham ML, Kirkpatrick A, et al. Results from the International Conference of Experts on Intra-abdominal Hypertension and Abdominal Compartment Syndrome. I. Definitions. Intensive Care Med 2006;32(11):1722–32.

49. Cheatham ML, Malbrain ML, Kirkpatrick A, et al. Results from the International Conference of Experts on Intra-abdominal Hypertension and Abdominal Compartment Syndrome. II. Definitions. Intensive Care Med 2007;33(6):951–62.

50. Maxwell RA, Fabian TC, Croce MA, et al. Secondary abdominal compartment syndrome: an underappreciated manifestation of severe haemorrhagic shock. J Trauma 2000;47:995–9.

51. Moore EE, Shackford SR, Pachter HL, et al. Organ Injury Scaling: spleen, liver and kidney. J Trauma 1989;29:1664–6.

52. Moore EE, Cogbill TH, Malangoni MA, et al. Organ Injury Scaling: pancreas, duodenum, small bowel, colon and rectum. J Trauma 1990;30:1427–9.

53. Moore EE, Cogbill TH, Jurkovich GJ, et al. Organ Injury Scaling III: chest wall, abdominal vascular, ureter, bladder and urethra. J Trauma 1992;33:337–8.

54. Moore EE, Malangoni MA, Cogbill TH, et al. Organ Injury Scaling IV: thoracic, vascular, lung, cardiac and diaphragm. J Trauma 1994;36:299–300.

55. Moore EE, Cogbill TH, Jurkovich GJ, et al. Organ Injury Scaling: spleen and liver (1994 revision). J Trauma 1995;38:323–4.

56. Moore EE, Jurkovich GJ, Knudson MM, et al. Organ Injury Scaling VI: extrahepatic biliary, oesophagus, stomach, vulva, vagina, uterus (nonpregnant), uterus (pregnant), fallopian tube, and ovary. J Trauma 1995;39:1069–70.

57. Moore EE, Malangoni MA, Cogbill TH, et al. Organ Injury Scaling VII: cervical vascular, peripheral vascular, adrenal, penis, testis and scrotum. J Trauma 1996;41:523–4.

58. Hoff WS, Holevar M, Nagy KK, et al. Practice Management Guidelines for the evaluation of blunt abdominal trauma. Available at EAST Practice Management Guidelines Work Group; 2001. http://www.east.org; [accessed February 2012].

59. Mazuski JE, Sawyer RG, Nathens AB, et al. The Surgical Infection Society Guidelines on antimicrobial therapy for intra-abdominal infections: an executive summary. Surg Infect 2002;3(3):161–73.

60. Cornwell IIIrd EE, Campbell KA. Trauma. In: Gordon TA, Cameron JL, editors. Evidence-based surgery. Hamilton, Ontario: BC Decker; 2000. p. 415–28.

61. Boffard KD, Brooks AJ. Pancreatic trauma. Eur J Surg 2000;166:4–12.

62. Bradley 3rd EL, Young Jr PR, Chang MC, et al. Diagnosis and intial management of blunt pancreatic trauma: guidelines from a multi-institutional review. Ann Surg 1998;227(6):861–9.

63. Bokhari F, Phelan H, Holevar M, et al. EAST Guidelines for the diagnosis and management of pancreatic trauma. Eastern Association for the Surgery of Trauma: Practice Management Guidelines, http://www.east.org/tpg/pancreas; [accessed February 2012].

64. Brasel KJ, Borgstrom DC, Weigelt JA. Management of penetrating colon trauma: a cost utility analysis. Surgery 1999;125:471–9.

65. Bern JD, Velmahos GC, Chan LS, et al. The high morbidity of colostomy closure after trauma: further support for the primary repair of colon injuries. Surgery 1998;123:157–64.

66. Pachter HL, Hoballah JJ, Corcoran TA, et al. The morbidity and financial impact of colostomy closure in trauma patients. J Trauma 1990;30:1510–4.

67. Stone HH, Fabian TC. Management of perforating colon trauma: randomisation between primary colon closure and exteriorisation. Ann Surg 1979;190:430–6.

68. Murray JA, Demetriades D, Colson M, et al. Colonic resection in trauma, colostomy versus anastomosis. J Trauma 1999;46:250–4.

69. Hirschberg A, Walden R. Damage control for abdominal trauma. Surg Clin North Am 1997;77:813–21.

70. Cayten CG, Fabian TC, Garcia VF, et al. Patient Management Guidelines for penetrating intraperitoneal injuries. EAST Practice Parameter Working Group, http://www.east.org; [accessed February 2012].

71. DiGiacomo JC, Bonadies JA, Cole FJ, et al. Practice Management Guidelines for haemorrhage in pelvic fracture. EAST Practice Management Guidelines Work Group, http://www.east.org; [accessed February 2012].

72. Smith WR, Moore EE, Osborn P, et al. Retroperitoneal packing as a resuscitation technique for haemodynamically unstable patients with pelvic fractures: report of two representative cases and a description of technique. J Trauma 2005;59:1510–4.

73. Jansen JO, Inaba K, Resnick S, et al. Selective non-operative management of abdominal gunshot wounds: survey of practice. Injury 2012;Feb 14. http://dx.doi.org/10.1016/j.injury.2012.01.023. Epub ahead of print

74. Knudson MM, Lim RC, Oakes DD, et al. Nonoperative management of blunt liver injuries in adults: the need for continued surveillance. J Trauma 1990;30:1494–500.

75. Pachter HL, Knudson MM, Esrig B, et al. Status of nonoperative management of blunt hepatic injuries in 1995: a multicenter experience with 404 patients. J Trauma 1996;40:31–8.

76. Renz BM, Feliciano DV. Gunshot wounds to the right thoracoabdomen: a prospective study of nonoperative management. J Trauma 1994;37:737–44.

77. Alonso M, Brathwaite C, Garcia V, et al. Practice Management Guidelines Work Group. Blunt liver and spleen injuries: non-operative management, http://www.east.org/tpg/livspleen; [accessed February 2012].

78. Inaba K, Branco BC, Moe D, et al. Prospective evaluation of selective nonoperative management of torso gunshot wounds: when is it safe to discharge? J Trauma 2012;72(4):884–91.

79. Como JJ, Bokhari F, Chiu WC, et al. Practice Management Guidelines Working Group. Penetrating trauma: selective non-operative management. Eastern Association for the Surgery of Trauma. J Trauma 2010;68(3):721–33.

80. Dondelinger RF, Trotteur G, Ghaye B, et al. Traumatic injuries: radiological hemostatic intervention at admission. Eur Radiol 2002;12(5):979–93.

81. Johnson JW, Gracias VH, Gupta R, et al. Hepatic angiography in patients undergoing damage control laparotomy. J Trauma 2002;52:1102–6.

82. Asensio JA, Roldan G, Petrone P, et al. Operative management and outcomes in 103 AAST-OIS grades

IV and V complex hepatic injuries: trauma surgeons still need to operate, but angioembolization helps. J Trauma 2003;54:647–53.

83. Dent D, Alsabrook G, Erickson BA, et al. Blunt splenic injuries: high nonoperative management rate can be achieved with selective embolization. J Trauma 2004;56(5):1063–7.

84. Haan JM, Biffl W, Knudson MM, et al. Western Trauma Association Multi-institutional Trials Committee. Splenic embolization revisited: a multi-center review. J Trauma 2004;56(3):542–7.

85. Velmahos GC, Toutouzas KG, Vassiliu P, et al. A prospective study on the safety and efficacy of angiographic embolization for pelvic and visceral injuries. J Trauma 2002;53(2):303–8.

Recommended reading

Boffard KD, editor. Manual of definitive surgical trauma care. 3rd ed. London: Hodder Arnold; 2011.

Committee on Trauma of the American College of Surgeons. Resources for optimal care of the trauma patient. Chicago, IL: Committee on Trauma of the American College of Surgeons; 2006.

Peitzman A, Rhodes M, Schwab CW, editors. The trauma manual: Trauma and acute care surgery. Philadelphia, PA: Lippincott, Williams & Wilkins; 2008.

Websites

Organ Injury Scaling of the American Association for the Surgery of Trauma.

www.aast.org.

Eastern Association for the Surgery of Trauma.

Practice Management Guidelines.

www.east.org.

World Society of the Abdominal Compartment Syndrome (WSACS).

www.wsacs.org.

Appendix: Scaling system for organ-specific injuries

Scaling system for organ-specific injuries

Table A1	Cervical vascular organ injury scale	Table A17	Abdominal vascular injury scale
Table A2	Chest wall injury scale	Table A18	Adrenal organ injury scale
Table A3	Heart injury scale	Table A19	Kidney injury scale
Table A4	Lung injury scale	Table A20	Ureter injury scale
Table A5	Thoracic vascular injury scale	Table A21	Bladder injury scale
Table A6	Diaphragm injury scale	Table A22	Urethra injury scale
Table A7	Spleen injury scale	Table A23	Uterus (non-pregnant) injury scale
Table A8	Liver injury scale	Table A24	Uterus (pregnant) injury scale
Table A9	Extrahepatic biliary tree injury scale	Table A25	Fallopian tube injury scale
Table A10	Pancreas injury scale	Table A26	Ovary injury scale
Table A11	Oesophagus injury scale	Table A27	Vagina injury scale
Table A12	Stomach injury scale	Table A28	Vulva injury scale
Table A13	Duodenum injury scale	Table A29	Testis injury scale
Table A14	Small-bowel injury scale	Table A30	Scrotum injury scale
Table A15	Colon injury scale	Table A31	Penis injury scale
Table A16	Rectum injury scale	Table A32	Peripheral vascular organ injury scale

Table A1 • Cervical vascular organ injury scale

Grade*	Description of injury	ICD-9	AIS-90
I	Thyroid vein	900.8	
	Common facial vein	900.8	
	External jugular vein	900.81	1–3
	Non-named arterial/venous branches	900.9	
II	External carotid arterial branches (ascending pharyngeal, superior thyroid, lingual, facial, maxillary, occipital, posterior auricular)	900.8	1–3
	Thyrocervical trunk or primary branches	900.8	1–3
	Internal jugular vein	900.1	1–3
III	External carotid artery	900.02	2–3
	Subclavian vein	901.3	3–4
	Vertebral artery	900.8	2–4
IV	Common carotid artery	900.01	3–5
V	Internal carotid artery (extracranial)	900.03	3–5

*Increase one grade for multiple grade III or IV injuries involving more than 50% vessel circumference. Decrease one grade for less than 25% vessel circumference disruption for grade IV or V.
Reproduced from Moore EE, Malangoni MA, Cogbill TH et al. Organ Injury Scaling VII: Cervical vascular, peripheral vascular, adrenal, penis, testis and scrotum. J Trauma 1996; 41(3):523–4. With permission from Lippincott, Williams & Wilkins.

Table A2 • Chest wall injury scale

Grade*	Injury type	Description of injury	ICD-9	AIS-90
I	Contusion	Any size	911.0/922.1	1
	Laceration	Skin and subcutaneous	875.0	1
	Fracture	<3 ribs, closed	807.01/807.02	1–2
		Non-displaced clavicle closed	810.00/810.03	2
II	Laceration	Skin, subcutaneous and muscle	875.1	2
	Fracture	≥3 adjacent ribs, closed	807.03/807.08	1
		Open or displaced clavicle	810.10/810.13	2–3
		Non-displaced sternum, closed	807.2	2
		Scapular body, open or closed	811.00/811.18	2
III	Laceration	Full thickness including pleural penetration	862.29	2
	Fracture	Open or displaced sternum	807.2	2
		Flail sternum	807.3	2
		Unilateral flail segment (<3 ribs)	807.4	3–4
IV	Laceration	Avulsion of chest wall tissues with underlying rib fractures	807.10/807.18	4
	Fracture	Unilateral flail chest (≥3 ribs)	807.4	3–4
V	Fracture	Bilateral flail chest (≥3 ribs on both sides)	807.4	5

*This scale is confined to the chest wall alone and does not reflect associated internal or abdominal injuries. Therefore, further delineation of upper versus lower or anterior versus posterior chest wall was not considered, and a grade VI was not warranted. Specifically, thoracic crush was not used as a descriptive term; instead, the geography and extent of fractures and soft tissue injury were used to define the grade. Upgrade by one grade for bilateral injuries.
Reproduced from Moore EE, Cogbill TH, Jurkovich GJ. Organ Injury Scaling III: chest wall, abdominal vascular, ureter, bladder and urethra. J Trauma 1992; 33:337–8. With permission from Lippincott, Williams & Wilkins.

Table A3 • Heart injury scale

Grade*	Description of injury	ICD-9	AIS-90
I	Blunt cardiac injury with minor ECG abnormality (non-specific ST or T wave changes, premature arterial or ventricular contraction or persistent sinus tachycardia)	861.01	3
	Blunt or penetrating pericardial wound without cardiac injury, cardiac tamponade, or cardiac herniation	861.01	3
II	Blunt cardiac injury with heart block (right or left bundle branch, left anterior fascicular, or atrioventricular) or ischaemic changes (ST depression or T wave inversion) without cardiac failure	861.12	3
	Penetrating tangential myocardial wound up to, but not extending through endocardium, without tamponade	861.01	3–4
III	Blunt cardiac injury with sustained (>6 beats/min) or multifocal ventricular contractions	861.01	3–4
	Blunt or penetrating cardiac injury with septal rupture, pulmonary or tricuspid valvular incompetence, papillary muscle dysfunction, or distal coronary arterial occlusion without cardiac failure	861.01	3–4
	Blunt pericardial laceration with cardiac herniation	861.12	3
	Blunt cardiac injury with cardiac failure	861.12	3
	Penetrating tangential myocardial wound up to, but extending through, endocardium, with tamponade		
IV	Blunt or penetrating cardiac injury with septal rupture, pulmonary or tricuspid valvular incompetence, papillary muscle dysfunction, or distal coronary arterial occlusion producing cardiac failure	861.03	5
	Blunt or penetrating cardiac injury with aortic mitral valve incompetence	861.03	5
	Blunt or penetrating cardiac injury of the right ventricle, right atrium or left atrium	861.03	5
V	Blunt or penetrating cardiac injury with proximal coronary arterial occlusion	861.03	5
	Blunt or penetrating left ventricular perforation	861.13	5
	Stellate wound with <50% tissue loss of the right ventricle, right atrium or of left atrium	861.03	5
VI	Blunt avulsion of the heart; penetrating wound producing >50% tissue loss of a chamber	861.13	6

*Advance one grade for multiple wounds to a single chamber or multiple chamber involvement.
Reproduced from Moore EE, Malangoni MA, Cogbill TH et al. Organ Injury Scaling IV: thoracic, vascular, lung, cardiac and diaphragm.
J Trauma 1994; 36(3):299–300. With permission from Lippincott, Williams & Wilkins.

Table A4 • Lung injury scale

Grade*	Injury type	Description of injury	ICD-9	AIS-90
I	Contusion	Unilateral, <1 lobe	861.12/861.31	3
II	Contusion	Unilateral, single lobe	861.20/861.30	3
	Laceration	Simple pneumothorax	860.0/1/4/5	3
III	Contusion	Unilateral, >1 lobe	861.20/861.30	3
	Laceration	Persistent (>72 hours) air leak from distal airway	860.0/1/4/5	3–4
	Haematoma	Non-expanding intraparenchymal	862.0/861.30	
IV	Laceration	Major (segmental or lobar) air leak	862.21/861.31	4–5
	Haematoma	Expanding intraparenchymal		
	Vascular	Primary branch intrapulmonary vessel disruption	901.40	3–5
V	Vascular	Hilar vessel disruption	901.41/901.42	4
VI	Vascular	Total uncontained transection of pulmonary hilum	901.41/901.42	4

*Advance one grade for bilateral injuries up to grade III. Haemothorax is scored under thoracic vascular injury scale.
Reproduced from Moore EE, Malangoni MA, Cogbill TH et al. Organ Injury Scaling IV: thoracic, vascular, lung, cardiac and diaphragm.
J Trauma 1994; 36(3):299–300. With permission from Lippincott, Williams & Wilkins.

Table A5 • Thoracic vascular injury scale

Grade*	Description of injury	ICD-9	AIS-90
I	Intercostal artery/vein	901.81	2–3
	Internal mammary artery/vein	901.82	2–3
	Bronchial artery/vein	901.89	2–3
	Oesophageal artery/vein	901.9	2–3
	Hemiazygos vein	901.89	2–3
	Unnamed artery/vein	901.9	2–3
II	Azygos vein	901.89	2–3
	Internal jugular vein	900.1	2–3
	Subclavian vein	901.3	3–4
	Innominate vein	901.3	3–4
III	Carotid artery	900.01	3–5
	Innominate artery	901.1	3–4
	Subclavian artery	901.1	3–4
IV	Thoracic aorta, descending	901.0	4–5
	Inferior vena cava (intrathoracic)	902.10	3–4
	Pulmonary artery, primary intraparenchymal branch	901.41	3
	Pulmonary vein, primary intraparenchymal branch	901.42	3
V	Thoracic aorta, ascending and arch	901.0	5
	Superior vena cava	901.2	3–4
	Pulmonary artery, main trunk	901.41	4
	Pulmonary vein, main trunk	901.42	4
VI	Uncontained total transection of thoracic aorta or pulmonary hilum	901.0 901.41/901.42	5

*Increase one grade for multiple grade III or IV injuries if more than 50% circumference. Decrease one grade for grade IV injuries if less than 25% circumference.
Reproduced from Moore EE, Malangoni MA, Cogbill TH et al. Organ Injury Scaling IV: thoracic, vascular, lung, cardiac and diaphragm. J Trauma 1994; 36(3):299–300. With permission from Lippincott, Williams & Wilkins.

Table A6 • Diaphragm injury scale

Grade*	Description of injury	ICD-9	AIS-90
I	Contusion	862.0	2
II	Laceration <2 cm	862.1	3
III	Laceration 2–10 cm	862.1	3
IV	Laceration >10 cm with tissue loss <25 cm^2	862.1	3
V	Laceration with tissue loss >25 cm^2	862.1	3

*Advance one grade for bilateral injuries up to grade III.
Reproduced from Moore EE, Malangoni MA, Cogbill TH et al. Organ Injury Scaling IV: thoracic, vascular, lung, cardiac and diaphragm. J Trauma 1994; 36(3):299–300. With permission from Lippincott, Williams & Wilkins.

Table A7 • Spleen injury scale (1994 revision)

Grade*	Injury type	Description of injury	ICD-9	AIS-90
I	Haematoma	Subcapsular, <10% surface area	865.01/865.11	2
	Laceration	Capsular tear, <1 cm parenchymal depth	865.02/865.12	2
II	Haematoma	Subcapsular, 10–50% surface area; intraparenchymal, <5 cm in diameter	865.01/865.11	2
	Laceration	Capsular tear, 1–3 cm parenchymal depth that does not involve a trabecular vessel	865.02/865.12	2
III	Haematoma	Subcapsular, >50% surface area or expanding; ruptured subcapsular or parenchymal haematoma; intraparenchymal haematoma >5 cm or expanding	865.03	3
	Laceration	>3 cm parenchymal depth or involving trabecular vessels	865.03	3
IV	Laceration	Laceration involving segmental or hilar vessels producing major devascularisation (>25% of spleen)	865.13	4
V	Laceration	Completely shattered spleen	865.04	5
	Vascular	Hilar vascular injury with devascularised spleen	865.14	5

*Advance one grade for multiple injuries up to grade III.
Reproduced from Moore EE, Cogbill TH, Jurkovich GJ et al. Organ Injury Scaling: spleen and liver (1994 revision). J Trauma 1995; 38(3):323–4. With permission from Lippincott, Williams & Wilkins.

Table A8 • Liver injury scale (1994 revision)

Grade*	Injury type	Description of injury	ICD-9	AIS-90
I	Haematoma	Subcapsular, <10% surface area	864.01/864.11	2
	Laceration	Capsular tear, <1 cm parenchymal depth	864.02/864.12	2
II	Haematoma	Subcapsular, 10–50% surface area; intraparenchymal <10 cm in diameter	864.01/864.11	2
	Laceration	Capsular tear 1–3 cm parenchymal depth, <10 cm in length	864.03/864.13	2
III	Haematoma	Subcapsular, >50% surface area of ruptured subcapsular or parenchymal haematoma; intraparenchymal haematoma >10 cm or expanding	864.04/864.14	3
	Laceration	3 cm parenchymal depth	864.04/864.14	3
IV	Laceration	Parenchymal disruption involving 25–75% hepatic lobe or 1–3 Couinaud segments within a single lobe	864.04/864.14	4
V	Laceration	Parenchymal disruption involving >75% of hepatic lobe or >3 Couinaud segments within a single lobe	864.04/864.14	5
	Vascular	Juxtahepatic venous injuries, i.e. retrohepatic vena cava/central major hepatic veins	864.04/864.14	5
VI	Vascular	Hepatic avulsion	864.04/864.14	5

*Advance one grade for multiple injuries up to grade III.
Reproduced from Moore EE, Cogbill TH, Jurkovich GJ et al. Organ Injury Scaling: spleen and liver (1994 revision). J Trauma 1995; 38(3):323–4. With permission from Lippincott, Williams & Wilkins.

Table A9 • Extrahepatic biliary tree injury scale

Grade*	Description of injury	ICD-9	AIS-90
I	Gallbladder contusion/haematoma	868.02	2
	Portal triad contusion	868.02	2
II	Partial gallbladder avulsion from liver bed; cystic duct intact	868.02	2
	Laceration or perforation of the gallbladder	868.12	2
III	Complete gallbladder avulsion from liver bed	868.02	3
	Cystic duct laceration	868.12	3
IV	Partial or complete right hepatic duct laceration	868.12	3
	Partial or complete left hepatic duct laceration	868.12	3
	Partial common hepatic duct laceration (<50%)	868.12	3
	Partial common bile duct laceration (<50%)	868.12	3
V	>50% transection of common hepatic duct	868.12	3–4
	>50% transection of common bile duct	868.12	3–4
	Combined right and left hepatic duct injuries	868.12	3–4
	Intraduodenal or intrapancreatic bile duct injuries	868.12	3–4

*Advance one grade for multiple injuries up to grade III.
Reproduced from Moore EE, Jurkovich GJ, Knudson MM et al. Organ Injury Scaling VI: extrahepatic biliary, oesophagus, stomach, vulva, vagina, uterus (non-pregnant), uterus (pregnant), Fallopian tube, and ovary. J Trauma 1995; 39(6):1069–70. With permission from Lippincott, Williams & Wilkins.

Table A10 • Pancreas injury scale

Grade*	Injury type	Description of injury	ICD-9	AIS-90
I	Haematoma	Minor contusion without duct injury	863.81/863.84	2
	Laceration	Superficial laceration without duct injury		2
II	Haematoma	Major contusion without duct injury or tissue loss	863.81/863.84	2
	Laceration	Major laceration without duct injury or tissue loss		3
III	Laceration	Distal transection or parenchymal injury with duct injury	863.92/863.94	3
IV	Laceration	Proximal transection or parenchymal injury involving ampulla	863.91	4
V	Laceration	Massive disruption of pancreatic head	863.91	5

*Advance one grade for multiple injuries up to grade III. 863.51, 863.91 – head; 863.99, 862.92 – body; 863.83, 863.93 – tail. Proximal pancreas is to the patient's right of the superior mesenteric vein.
Reproduced from Moore EE, Cogbill TH, Malangoni MA et al. Organ Injury Scaling: pancreas, duodenum, small bowel, colon and rectum. J Trauma 1990; 30(11):1427–9. With permission from Lippincott, Williams & Wilkins.

Table A11 • Oesophagus injury scale

Grade*	Injury type	Description of injury	ICD-9	AIS-90
I	Contusion	Contusion/haematoma	862.22/826.32	2
	Laceration	Partial thickness laceration	862.22/826.32	3
II	Laceration	Laceration <50% circumference	862.22/826.32	4
III	Laceration	Laceration >50% circumference	862.22/826.32	4
IV	Tissue loss	Segmental loss or devascularisation <2 cm	862.22/826.32	5
V	Tissue loss	Segmental loss or devascularisation >2 cm	862.22/826.32	5

*Advance one grade for multiple lesions up to grade III.
Reproduced from Moore EE, Jurkovich GJ, Knudson MM et al. Organ Injury Scaling VI: extrahepatic biliary, oesophagus, stomach, vulva, vagina, uterus (non-pregnant), uterus (pregnant), Fallopian tube, and ovary. J Trauma 1995; 39(6):1069–70. With permission from Lippincott, Williams & Wilkins.

Table A12 • Stomach injury scale

Grade*	Injury type	Description of injury	ICD-9	AIS-90
I	Contusion	Contusion/haematoma	863.0/863.1	2
	Laceration	Partial thickness laceration	863.0/863.1	2
II	Laceration	<2 cm in gastro-oesophageal junction or pylorus	863.0/863.1	3
		<5 cm in proximal one-third stomach	863.0/863.1	3
		<10 cm in distal two-thirds stomach	863.0/863.1	3
III	Laceration	>2 cm in gastro-oesophageal junction or pylorus	863.0/863.1	3
		>5 cm in proximal one-third stomach	863.0/863.1	3
		>10 cm in distal two-thirds stomach	863.0/863.1	3
IV	Tissue loss	Tissue loss or devascularisation<two-thirds stomach	863.0/863.1	4
V	Tissue loss	Tissue loss or devascularisation>two-thirds stomach	863.0/863.1	4

*Advance one grade for multiple lesions up to grade III.
Reproduced from Moore EE, Jurkovich GJ, Knudson MM et al. Organ Injury Scaling VI: extrahepatic biliary, oesophagus, stomach, vulva, vagina, uterus (non-pregnant), uterus (pregnant), Fallopian tube, and ovary. J Trauma 1995; 39(6):1069–70. With permission from Lippincott, Williams & Wilkins.

Table A13 • Duodenum injury scale

Grade*	Injury type	Description of injury[†]	ICD-9	AIS-90
I	Haematoma	Involving single portion of duodenum	863.21	2
	Laceration	Partial thickness, no perforation	863.21	3
II	Haematoma	Involving more than one portion	863.21	2
	Laceration	Disruption <50% of circumference	863.31	4
III	Laceration	Disruption 50–75% of circumference of D2	863.31	4
		Disruption 50–100% of circumference of D1, D3, D4	863.31	4
IV	Laceration	Disruption >75% of circumference of D2	863.31	5
		Involving ampulla or distal common bile duct	863.31	5
V	Laceration	Massive disruption of duodenopancreatic complex	863.31	5
	Vascular	Devascularisation of duodenum	863.31	5

*Advance one grade for multiple injuries up to grade III.
[†]D1, first position of duodenum; D2, second portion of duodenum; D3, third portion of duodenum; D4, fourth portion of duodenum.
Reproduced from Moore EE, Cogbill TH, Malangoni MA et al. Organ Injury Scaling: pancreas, duodenum, small bowel, colon and rectum. J Trauma 1990; 30(11):1427–9. With permission from Lippincott, Williams & Wilkins.

Table A14 • Small-bowel injury scale

Grade*	Injury type	Description of injury	ICD-9	AIS-90
I	Haematoma	Contusion or haematoma without devascularisation	863.20	2
	Laceration	Partial thickness, no perforation	863.20	2
II	Laceration	Laceration <50% of circumference	863.30	3
III	Laceration	Laceration ≥50% of circumference without transection	863.30	3
IV	Laceration	Transection of the small bowel	863.30	4
V	Laceration	Transection of the small bowel with segmental tissue loss	863.30	4
	Vascular	Devascularised segment	863.30	4

*Advance one grade for multiple injuries up to grade III.
Reproduced from Moore EE, Cogbill TH, Malangoni MA et al. Organ Injury Scaling: pancreas, duodenum, small bowel, colon and rectum. J Trauma 1990; 30(11):1427–9. With permission from Lippincott, Williams & Wilkins.

Table A15 • Colon injury scale

Grade*	Injury type	Description of injury	ICD-9†	AIS-90
I	Haematoma	Contusion or haematoma without devascularisation	863.40–863.44	2
	Laceration	Partial thickness, no perforation	863.40–863.44	2
II	Laceration	Laceration <50% of circumference	863.50–863.54	3
III	Laceration	Laceration ≥50% of circumference without transection	863.50–863.54	3
IV	Laceration	Transection of the colon	863.50–863.54	4
V	Laceration	Transection of the colon with segmental tissue loss	863.50–863.54	4

*Advance one grade for multiple injuries up to grade III.
†With ICD-9: 863.40/863.50, non-specific site in colon; 863.41/863.51, ascending; 863.42/863.52, transverse; 863.43/863.53, descending; 863.44/863.54, sigmoid.
Reproduced from Moore EE, Cogbill TH, Malangoni MA et al. Organ Injury Scaling: pancreas, duodenum, small bowel, colon and rectum. J Trauma 1990; 30(11):1427–9. With permission from Lippincott, Williams & Wilkins.

Table A16 • Rectum injury scale

Grade*	Injury type	Description of injury	ICD-9	AIS-90
I	Haematoma	Contusion or haematoma without devascularisation	863.45	2
	Laceration	Partial-thickness laceration	863.45	2
II	Laceration	Laceration <50% of circumference	863.55	3
III	Laceration	Laceration ≥50% of circumference	863.55	4
IV	Laceration	Full-thickness laceration with extension into the perineum	863.55	5
V	Vascular	Devascularised segment	863.55	5

*Advance one grade for multiple injuries up to grade III.
Reproduced from Moore EE, Cogbill TH, Malangoni MA et al. Organ Injury Scaling: pancreas, duodenum, small bowel, colon and rectum. J Trauma 1990; 30(11):1427–9. With permission from Lippincott, Williams & Wilkins.

Table A17 • Abdominal vascular injury scale

Grade*	Description of injury	ICD-9	AIS-90
I	Non-named superior mesenteric artery or superior mesenteric vein branches	902.20/902.39	NS†
	Non-named inferior mesenteric artery or inferior mesenteric vein branches	902.27/902.32	NS
	Phrenic artery or vein	902.89	NS
	Lumbar artery or vein	902.89	NS
	Gonadal artery or vein	902.89	NS
	Ovarian artery or vein	902.81/902.82	NS
	Other non-named small arterial or venous structures requiring ligation	902.80	NS
II	Right, left, or common hepatic artery	902.22	3
	Splenic artery or vein	902.23/902.34	3
	Right or left gastric arteries	902.21	3
	Gastroduodenal artery	902.24	3

(Continued)

Table A17 • (*Cont*). Abdominal vascular injury scale

Grade*	Description of injury	ICD-9	AIS-90
	Inferior mesenteric artery/trunk or inferior mesenteric vein/trunk	902.27/902.32	3
	Primary named branches of mesenteric artery (e.g. ileocolic artery) or mesenteric vein	902.26/902.31	3
	Other named abdominal vessels requiring ligation or repair	902.89	3
III	Superior mesenteric vein, trunk and primary subdivisions	902.31	
	Renal artery or vein	902.41/902.42	3
	Iliac artery or vein	902.53/902.54	3
	Hypogastric artery or vein	902.51/902.52	3
	Vena cava, infrarenal	902.10	4
IV	Superior mesenteric artery, trunk	902.25	3
	Coeliac axis proper	902.24	3
	Vena cava, suprarenal and infrahepatic	902.10	3
	Aorta, infrarenal	902.00	4
V	Portal vein	902.33	3
	Extraparenchymal hepatic vein only	902.11	3
	Extraparenchymal hepatic veins+liver	902.11	5
	Vena cava, retrohepatic or suprahepatic	902.19	5
	Aorta suprarenal, subdiaphragmatic	902.00	4

*This classification system is applicable to extraparenchymal vascular injuries. If the vessel injury is within 2 cm of the organ parenchyma, refer to specific organ injury scale. Increase one grade for multiple grade III or IV injuries involving >50% vessel circumference. Downgrade one grade if <25% vessel circumference laceration for grades IV or V.
†NS, not scored.
Reproduced from Moore EE, Cogbill TH, Jurkovich GJ. Organ Injury Scaling III: chest wall, abdominal vascular, ureter, bladder and urethra. J Trauma 1992; 33:337–8. With permission from Lippincott, Williams & Wilkins.

Table A18 • Adrenal organ injury scale

Grade*	Description of injury	ICD-9	AIS-90
I	Contusion	868.01/868.11	1
II	Laceration involving only cortex (<2 cm)	868.01/868.11	1
III	Laceration extending into medulla (≥2 cm)	868.01/868.11	2
IV	>50% parenchymal destruction	868.01/868.11	2
V	Total parenchymal destruction (including massive intraparenchymal haemorrhage) Avulsion from blood supply	868.01/868.11	3

*Advance one grade for bilateral lesions up to grade V.
Reproduced from Moore EE, Malangoni MA, Cogbill TH et al. Organ Injury Scaling VII: cervical vascular, peripheral vascular, adrenal, penis, testis and scrotum. J Trauma 1996; 41(3):523–4. With permission from Lippincott, Williams & Wilkins.

Table A19 • Kidney injury scale

Grade*	Injury type	Description of injury	ICD-9	AIS-90
I	Contusion	Microscopic or gross haematuria, urological studies normal	866.01	2
	Haematoma	Subcapsular, non-expanding without parenchymal laceration	866.01	2
II	Haematoma	Non-expanding perirenal haematoma confined to renal retroperitoneum	866.01	2
	Laceration	<1.0 cm parenchymal depth of renal cortex without urinary extravasation	866.11	2
III	Laceration	>1.0 cm parenchymal depth of renal cortex without collecting system rupture or urinary extravasation	866.11	3
IV	Laceration	Parenchymal laceration extending through renal cortex, medulla, and collecting system	866.02/866.12	4
	Vascular	Main renal artery or vein injury with contained haemorrhage	866.03/866.13	4
V	Laceration	Completely shattered kidney	866.04/866.14	5
	Vascular	Avulsion of renal hilum that devascularises kidney	866.13	5

*Advance one grade for bilateral injuries up to grade III.
Reproduced from Moore EE, Shackford SR, Pachter HL et al. Organ Injury Scaling: spleen, liver and kidney. J Trauma 1989; 29(12):1664–6. With permission from Lippincott, Williams & Wilkins.

Table A20 • Ureter injury scale

Grade*	Injury type	Description of injury	ICD-9	AIS-90
I	Haematoma	Contusion or haematoma without devascularisation	867.2/867.3	2
II	Laceration	<50% transection	867.2/867.3	2
III	Laceration	≥50% transection	867.2/867.3	3
IV	Laceration	Complete transection with <2 cm devascularisation	867.2/867.3	3
V	Laceration	Avulsion with >2 cm of devascularisation	867.2/867.3	3

*Advance one grade for bilateral up to grade III.
Reproduced from Moore EE, Cogbill TH, Jurkovich GJ. Organ Injury Scaling III: chest wall, abdominal vascular, ureter, bladder and urethra. J Trauma 1992; 33:337–8. With permission from Lippincott, Williams & Wilkins.

Table A21 • Bladder injury scale

Grade*	Injury type	Description of injury	ICD-9	AIS-90
I	Haematoma	Contusion, intramural haematoma	867.0/867.1	2
	Laceration	Partial thickness	867.0/867.1	3
II	Laceration	Extraperitoneal bladder wall laceration <2 cm	867.0/867.1	4
III	Laceration	Extraperitoneal (≥2 cm) or intraperitoneal (<2 cm) bladder wall laceration	867.0/867.1	4
IV	Laceration	Intraperitoneal bladder wall laceration ≥2 cm	867.0/867.1	4
V	Laceration	Intraperitoneal or extraperitoneal bladder wall laceration extending into the bladder neck or ureteral orifice (trigone)	867.0/867.1	4

*Advance one grade for multiple lesions up to grade III.
Reproduced from Moore EE, Cogbill TH, Jurkovich GJ. Organ Injury Scaling III: chest wall, abdominal vascular, ureter, bladder and urethra. J Trauma 1992; 33:337–8. With permission from Lippincott, Williams & Wilkins.

Table A22 • Urethra injury scale

Grade*	Injury type	Description of injury	ICD-9	AIS-90
I	Contusion	Blood at urethral meatus; urethrography normal	867.0/867.1	2
II	Stretch injury	Elongation of urethra without extravasation on urethrography	867.0/867.1	2
III	Partial disruption	Extravasation of urethrography contrast at injury site with visualisation in the bladder	867.0/867.1	2
IV	Complete disruption	Extravasation of urethrography contrast at injury site without visualisation in the bladder; <2 cm of urethra separation	867.0/867.1	3
V	Complete disruption	Complete transaction with ≥2 cm urethral separation, or extension into the prostate or vagina	867.0/867.1	4

*Advance one grade for bilateral injuries up to grade III.
Reproduced from Moore EE, Cogbill TH, Jurkovich GJ. Organ Injury Scaling III: chest wall, abdominal vascular, ureter, bladder and urethra. J Trauma 1992; 33:337–8. With permission from Lippincott, Williams & Wilkins.

Table A23 • Uterus (non-pregnant) injury scale

Grade*	Description of injury	ICD-9	AIS-90
I	Contusion/haematoma	867.4/867.5	2
II	Superficial laceration (<1 cm)	867.4/867.5	2
III	Deep laceration (≥1 cm)	867.4/867.5	3
IV	Laceration involving uterine artery	902.55	3
V	Avulsion/devascularisation	867.4/867.5	3

*Advance one grade for multiple injuries up to grade III.
Reproduced from Moore EE, Jurkovich GJ, Knudson MM et al. Organ Injury Scaling VI: extrahepatic biliary, oesophagus, stomach, vulva, vagina, uterus (non-pregnant), uterus (pregnant), Fallopian tube, and ovary. J Trauma 1995; 39(6):1069–70. With permission from Lippincott, Williams & Wilkins.

Table A24 • Uterus (pregnant) injury scale

Grade*	Description of injury	ICD-9	AIS-90
I	Contusion or haematoma (without placental abruption)	867.4/867.5	2
II	Superficial laceration (<1 cm) or partial placental abruption <25%	867.4/867.5	3
III	Deep laceration (≥1 cm) occurring in second trimester or placental abruption >25% but <50%	867.4/867.5	3
	Deep laceration (≥1 cm) in third trimester	867.4/867.5	4
IV	Laceration involving uterine artery	902.55	4
	Deep laceration (≥1 cm) with >50% placental abruption	867.4/867.5	4
V	Uterine rupture		
	Second trimester	867.4/867.5	4
	Third trimester	867.4/867.5	5
	Complete placental abruption	867.4/867.5	4–5

*Advance one grade for multiple injuries up to grade III.
Reproduced from Moore EE, Jurkovich GJ, Knudson MM et al. Organ Injury Scaling VI: extrahepatic biliary, oesophagus, stomach, vulva, vagina, uterus (non-pregnant), uterus (pregnant), Fallopian tube, and ovary. J Trauma 1995; 39(6):1069–70. With permission from Lippincott, Williams & Wilkins.

Table A25 • Fallopian tube injury scale

Grade*	Description of injury	ICD-9	AIS-90
I	Haematoma or contusion	867.6/867.7	2
II	Laceration <50% circumference	867.6/867.7	2
III	Laceration ≥50% circumference	867.6/867.7	2
IV	Transection	867.6/867.7	2
V	Vascular injury; devascularised segment	902.89	2

*Advance one grade for bilateral injuries up to grade III
Reproduced from Moore EE, Jurkovich GJ, Knudson MM et al. Organ Injury Scaling VI: extrahepatic biliary, oesophagus, stomach, vulva, vagina, uterus (non-pregnant), uterus (pregnant), Fallopian tube, and ovary. J Trauma 1995: 39(6):1069–70. With permission from Lippincott, Williams & Wilkins.

Table A26 • Ovary injury scale

Grade*	Description of injury	ICD-9	AIS-90
I	Contusion or haematoma	867.6/867.7	1
II	Superficial laceration (depth <0.5 cm)	867.6/867.7	2
III	Deep laceration (depth ≥0.5 cm)	867.8/867.7	3
IV	Partial disruption of blood supply	902.81	3
V	Avulsion or complete parenchymal destruction	902.81	3

*Advance one grade for bilateral injuries up to grade III.
Reproduced from Moore EE, Jurkovich GJ, Knudson MM et al. Organ Injury Scaling VI: extrahepatic biliary, oesophagus, stomach, vulva, vagina, uterus (non-pregnant), uterus (pregnant), Fallopian tube, and ovary. J Trauma 1995; 39(6):1069–70. With permission from Lippincott, Williams & Wilkins.

Table A27 • Vagina injury scale

Grade*	Description of injury	ICD-9	AIS-90
I	Contusion or haematoma	922.4	1
II	Laceration, superficial (mucosa only)	878.6	1
III	Laceration, deep into fat or muscle	878.6	2
IV	Laceration, complex, into cervix or peritoneum	868.7	3
V	Injury into adjacent organs (anus, rectum, urethra, bladder)	878.7	3

*Advance one grade for multiple injuries up to grade III.
Reproduced from Moore EE, Jurkovich GJ, Knudson MM et al. Organ Injury Scaling VI: extrahepatic biliary, oesophagus, stomach, vulva, vagina, uterus (non-pregnant), uterus (pregnant), Fallopian tube, and ovary. J Trauma 1995; 39(6):1069–70. With permission from Lippincott, Williams & Wilkins.

Table A28 • Vulva injury scale

Grade*	Description of injury	ICD-9	AIS-90
I	Contusion or haematoma	922.4	1
II	Laceration, superficial (skin only)	878.4	1
III	Laceration, deep (into fat or muscle)	878.4	2
IV	Avulsion; skin, fat or muscle	878.5	3
V	Injury into adjacent organs (anus, rectum, urethra, bladder)	878.5	3

*Advance one grade for multiple injuries up to grade III.
Reproduced from Moore EE, Jurkovich GJ, Knudson MM et al. Organ Injury Scaling VI: extrahepatic biliary, oesophagus, stomach, vulva, vagina, uterus (non-pregnant), uterus (pregnant), Fallopian tube, and ovary. J Trauma 1995; 39(6):1069–70. With permission from Lippincott, Williams & Wilkins.

Table A29 • Testis injury scale

Grade*	Description of injury	ICD-9	AIS-90
I	Contusion/haematoma	911.0–922.4	1
II	Subclinical laceration of tunica albuginea	922.4	1
III	Laceration of tunica albuginea with <50% parenchymal loss	878.2	2
IV	Major laceration of tunica albuginea with ≥50% parenchymal loss	878.3	2
V	Total testicular destruction or avulsion	878.3	2

*Advance one grade for bilateral lesions up to grade V.
Reproduced from Moore EE, Malangoni MA, Cogbill TH et al. Organ Injury Scaling VII: cervical vascular, peripheral vascular, adrenal, penis, testis and scrotum. J Trauma 1996; 41(3):523–4. With permission from Lippincott, Williams & Wilkins.

Table A30 • Scrotum injury scale

Grade	Description of injury	ICD-9	AIS-90
I	Contusion	922.4	1
II	Laceration <25% of scrotal diameter	878.2	1
III	Laceration ≥25% of scrotal diameter	878.3	2
IV	Avulsion <50%	878.3	2
V	Avulsion ≥50%	878.3	2

Reproduced from Moore EE, Malangoni MA, Cogbill TH et al. Organ Injury Scaling VII: cervical vascular, peripheral vascular, adrenal, penis, testis and scrotum. J Trauma 1996; 41(3):523–4. With permission from Lippincott, Williams & Wilkins.

Table A31 • Penis injury scale

Grade*	Description of injury	ICD-9	AIS-90
I	Cutaneous laceration/contusion	911.0/922.4	1
II	Buck's fascia (cavernosum) laceration without tissue loss	878.0	1
III	Cutaneous avulsion	878.1	3
	Laceration through glans/meatus		
	Cavernosal or urethral defect <2 cm		
IV	Partial penectomy	878.1	3
	Cavernosal or urethral defect ≥2 cm		
V	Total penectomy	876.1	3

*Advance one grade for multiple injuries up to grade III.
Reproduced from Moore EE, Malangoni MA, Cogbill TH et al. Organ Injury Scaling VII: cervical vascular, peripheral vascular, adrenal, penis, testis and scrotum. J Trauma 1996; 41(3):523–4. With permission from Lippincott, Williams & Wilkins.

Table A32 • Peripheral vascular organ injury scale

Grade*	Description of injury	ICD-9	AIS-90
I	Digital artery/vein	903.5	1–3
	Palmar artery/vein	903.4	1–3
	Deep palmar artery/vein	904.6	1–3
	Dorsalis pedis artery	904.7	1–3
	Plantar artery/vein	904.5	1–3
	Non-named arterial/venous branches	903.8/904.7	1–3
II	Basilic/cephalic vein	903.8	1–3
	Saphenous vein	904.3	1–3
	Radial artery	903.2	1–3
	Ulnar artery	903.3	1–3
III	Axillary vein	903.02	2–3
	Superficial/deep femoral vein	903.02	2–3
	Popliteal vein	904.42	2–3
	Brachial artery	903.1	2–3
	Anterior tibial artery	904.51/904.52	1–3
	Posterior tibial artery	904.53/904.54	1–3
	Peroneal artery	904.7	1–3
	Tibioperoneal trunk	904.7	2–3
IV	Superficial/deep femoral artery	904.1/904.7	3–4
	Popliteal artery	904.41	2–3
V	Axillary artery	903.01	2–3
	Common femoral artery	904.0	3–4

*Increase one grade for multiple grade III or IV injuries involving >50% vessel circumference. Decrease one grade for <25% vessel circumference disruption for grades IV or V.
Reproduced from Moore EE, Malangoni MA, Cogbill TH et al. Organ Injury Scaling VII: cervical vascular, peripheral vascular, adrenal, penis, testis and scrotum. J Trauma 1996; 41(3):523–4. With permission from Lippincott, Williams & Wilkins.

Venous thromboembolism: prevention, diagnosis and treatment

Rhona M. Maclean

Introduction

Venous thromboembolism (VTE) is the most common cause of preventable death in hospitalised patients, with an estimated 25 000 patients dying from preventable hospital acquired VTE in the UK each year.[1] The two most common manifestations of venous thrombosis are deep vein thrombosis (DVT) and pulmonary embolism (PE), both of which are associated with significant morbidity (post-thrombotic syndrome and chronic thromboembolic pulmonary hypertension respectively). As surgery is associated with a high risk of postoperative VTE, evidence-based thromboprophylaxis strategies should be employed to reduce this risk, and those patients with symptoms and/or signs suggestive of VTE should be thoroughly investigated and managed accordingly.

Epidemiology of VTE

The incidence of a first episode of VTE is estimated at 1–2 per 1000 person-years in white Caucasians, with a lower incidence in Hispanics and Asians.[2,3] The risk of VTE increases progressively with age, with an incidence of >5/1000 person-years in those over the age of 80.[3] The incidence of VTE is approximately equal in men and women; however, it is more frequent in women in the childbearing years, likely due to the use of the hormonal therapies (the combined oral contraceptive pill and hormone replacement therapy) and pregnancy, whereas after the age of 45 incidence rates are generally higher in men. Clinical studies, excluding autopsy data, have consistently shown that the incidence of DVT is approximately twice that of PE.[2,3] It has been estimated that there are over 130 000 cases of VTE in the UK each year, at a cost (direct and indirect) of around £640 million annually.[4]

DVT and PE are the result of the same disease process, VTE; of patients presenting with symptomatic PE, up to 80% will have asymptomatic DVT, and in those presenting with symptomatic DVT, 50–80% can be shown by imaging to have PE.[5]

Approximately half of VTE episodes are idiopathic in nature (defined as having had no recent surgery, trauma, cancer, pregnancy or immobilisation), the remainder presenting after an obvious precipitating event.[2,3] Of patients diagnosed with VTE, the majority (73.7%) present as outpatients and of these a significant proportion have either undergone surgery (23.1%) or been hospitalised (36.8%) in the preceding 3 months.[6] Presentation with VTE after surgery peaks at 21 days postoperatively, with the risk remaining significantly increased for 3 months after surgery.[7]

VTE is associated with a surprisingly high mortality. In a retrospective epidemiological study, the 30-day fatality rate was 4.6% following DVT and 9.7% with PE.[3] Cancer was associated with a worse outcome, with a 30-day fatality rate of 19.1%. Mortality rates associated with PE are high, with approximately 25% of patients dying within a year, many due to malignancy, others from cardiopulmonary disease or recurrent VTE.[7] Overall, pulmonary emboli are thought to be responsible for 10% of hospital inpatient deaths,[8] with many diagnosed for the first time at post-mortem.[9]

Thrombosis in the deep veins damages the deep venous valves, resulting in post-thrombotic scarring, stiffening of the vessel wall, venous insufficiency, reflux and venous hypertension, all of which can result in swelling, pain and heaviness in the affected leg – the post-thrombotic syndrome. In its severe form, this causes marked skin changes – lipodermatosclerosis (varicose eczema and atrophy of the subcutaneous tissues), hyperpigmentation and ulceration – and can be a major cause of morbidity. The incidence of the post-thrombotic syndrome has been reported at approximately 28% after 5 years, with 9% having a severe form.[7] Up to 5% of patients with PE will develop pulmonary hypertension.[7]

Pathophysiology of venous thromboembolism

Thrombus formation

DVTs usually start in the calf veins, and thrombi developing after surgery often originate in the valve cusps of the soleal veins. These thrombi are initially formed of red blood cells caught in a fibrin mesh, which then incorporate platelets and fibrin into the clot, propagating proximally to form a free-floating thrombus, or extending to occlude the vein.[10,11] Many such thrombi start to develop intraoperatively; of these, half will resolve spontaneously within 72 hours and 18% will extend proximally, of which 50% will embolise. Some thromboses, however, begin postoperatively; 20–34% of patients diagnosed as having DVT by screening tests in hospital had been shown to have legs free of thrombosis postoperatively. It has been estimated that 10% of symptomatic PEs cause death within 1 hour of onset (Box 14.1). There is an ongoing debate as to the significance of calf vein thrombosis and whether, if detected, it should be treated. A recent study of isolated symptomatic muscular calf vein thromboses suggested that they are not as innocuous as originally thought; 7% of patients had symptomatic PEs at presentation, and after completing 1–3 months of anticoagulation, 18% had recurrent episodes of VTE within 3 years.[12]

Virchow's triad

In the 1860s, Virchow described three factors implicated in the development of a venous thrombosis: slowing of venous blood flow (stasis), damage to the vessel wall (venous injury), and changes in the blood that increase the propensity to develop thrombosis (hypercoagulability). These are now widely known as Virchow's triad, and this model remains a valid concept today.

Box 14.1 • Natural history of venous thromboembolism

- The majority of deep vein thrombosis (DVT) originates within the calf veins
- About half the episodes of DVT associated with surgery start intraoperatively, of which 50% resolve spontaneously within 72 hours
- Those with persisting risk factors or those with a large initial thrombosis are at highest risk of progression of postoperative DVT
- Symptomatic risk of venous thromboembolic disease is highest within 2 weeks of surgery but patients remain at high risk of VTE for 3 months postoperatively
- Approximately 25% of episodes of untreated symptomatic calf DVT extend to the proximal veins within 1 week of presentation
- Without treatment approximately 50% of patients with symptomatic proximal DVT or pulmonary embolism will have a recurrent thrombosis in 3 months
- The mortality associated with PE is estimated to be 5–25%. The greatest risk of fatal postoperative pulmonary embolism occurs 3–7 days after surgery and 10% of symptomatic DVTs are fatal within 1 hour of first symptoms
- Isolated calf DVT is associated with half the risk of recurrence of proximal DVT or pulmonary embolism
- The risk of recurrence is similar following proximal DVT and pulmonary embolism
- If a first thrombosis was a DVT, it is likely that a recurrence is a DVT. Similarly, if a first VTE was a PE, it is likely that a recurrence will be a PE
- Pulmonary hypertension will develop in approximately 5% of patients with pulmonary embolism

Stasis

Stasis, the slowing of venous return, is associated with an increased risk of VTE (stroke patients have an increased risk of DVT in the paralysed limb[13]). It has been demonstrated that intraoperative paralysis causes 'microtears' in the venous endothelium, exposing circulating blood to procoagulant components in the subendothelium (e.g. collagen, von Willebrand factor, tissue factor).[14] Stasis, in and of itself, is likely to be insufficient to cause VTE, and most patients with significant immobility are likely to have a systemic illness, increasing the risk of VTE by other mechanisms.

Venous injury

Surgery or trauma cause venous injury, which increases the risk of venous thrombosis. Inflammatory cytokines also induce venous injury by down-regulating thrombomodulin, impairing fibrinolysis, stimulating tissue factor expression on monocytes or endothelial cells, and inducing apoptosis of endothelial cells, rendering them thrombogenic.[15]

Hypercoagulability

Hypercoagulability, both inherited and acquired, has been demonstrated to significantly influence the development of VTE. Studies undertaken in families in whom multiple members have presented with VTE have identified a number of inherited thrombophilias.

Risk factors for VTE

Inherited thrombophilias

Antithrombin (AT) is an anticoagulant protein, whose function is predominantly to inactivate thrombin and activated coagulation factor X, thereby limiting ongoing thrombus propagation. **AT deficiency** is found in 1% of consecutive patients presenting with VTE and increases the risk of VTE five- to 50-fold.[16,17] Acquired AT deficiency can occur in a number of different clinical situations, including liver disease, sepsis, acute thrombosis, disseminated intravascular coagulation (DIC) and nephrotic syndrome.

Proteins C and S are both vitamin K-dependent proteins; their activity will be reduced by vitamin K antagonist anticoagulants(such as warfarin and sinthrome). The activated protein C/protein S complex inactivates coagulation factors V and VIII, also limiting ongoing thrombus propagation. **Inherited protein C deficiency** increases the risk of VTE six- to 15-fold and is found in 1–3% of patients presenting with VTE.[16] **Protein S deficiency** is present in 1–3% of patients with VTE. Liver disease, sepsis, DIC and acute thrombosis reduce the levels of proteins C and S, resulting in acquired hypercoagulability.

Factor V Leiden and the prothrombin gene mutation

Factor V Leiden, a mutation of the factor V gene, is the most common inherited thrombophilia, present in 5% of the Caucasian population (and <1% of Africans/South East Asians). It renders activated factor V relatively resistant to inactivation by the activated protein C/protein S complex, and confers an eightfold increased risk of VTE in the heterozygous form (80-fold increased risk in the homozygous form). In Caucasian populations, factor V Leiden is found in >20% of unselected patients presenting with VTE.[16] The prothrombin gene mutation (G20210A) is less prevalent, found in 1% of the general population, and confers a threefold increased risk of VTE. It is found in 5–6% of unselected patients with VTE.[16]

Hyperhomocysteinaemia

Classical homocystinuria causes extremely high levels of plasma homocysteine and is associated with both venous and arterial thrombosis in addition to the other classical disease manifestations (mental retardation, seizures, musculoskeletal abnormalities, eye anomalies including lens dislocation). Neither the common mutation in the methylene tetrahydrofolate reductase gene (*MTHFR C677T*) nor mild elevations in homocysteine levels are associated with thrombosis.[18]

> ✔ Testing for inherited thrombophilia, whilst frequently undertaken, rarely helps in the management of patients with VTE. Such testing should usually only be performed in young individuals with a personal history of VTE who have a history of VTE in a first-degree relative. Testing should not usually be done while a patient is taking anticoagulant therapy.[19]

Other thrombophilias

Elevated factor VIII levels have been demonstrated to increase the risk of developing a first VTE, and also increase the risk of recurrent thrombosis.[16,20]

Association and linkage studies have identified a number of other proteins associated with VTE. This includes high levels of the coagulation factors fibrinogen, prothrombin, IX, XI and von Willebrand factor. There is also an association between VTE and platelet glycoprotein VI, blood group O and deficiencies of proteins associated with fibrinolysis (plasminogen and plasminogen-activated inhibitor-1 (PAI-1)). These proteins are associated with a weak increased risk of thrombosis (1.1- to 2.5-fold).[16,21,22]

Acquired thrombophilias

Antiphospholipid syndrome (APLS)

Diagnosis of the APLS requires the presence of both clinical (arterial or venous thrombosis or recurrent miscarriage) and laboratory (persistent detectable antiphospholipid antibodies such as lupus anticoagulant or anticardiolipin or anti-β2-glycoprotein 1 antibodies) criteria. The mechanism of these antibodies in the development of thrombosis has not been established; however, a number of hypotheses have been suggested, including the interference of antibodies with anticoagulant mechanisms, triggering procoagulant changes in leucocytes, platelets or endothelial cells, or activation of complement triggering an inflammatory reaction.[23] Patients with a diagnosis of APLS who have had a thrombosis should be therapeutically anticoagulated long term (usually with warfarin, target international normalised ratio (INR) 2.5).[23]

Heparin-induced thrombocytopenia (HIT)

HIT is a rare but life-threatening complication of heparin therapy; it confers a high risk of thrombosis (30–75%), and has a significant morbidity and mortality. It occurs more frequently in patients receiving unfractionated heparin (UFH) than low-molecular-weight heparin (LMWH), and the highest risk is in those who have had cardiothoracic surgery. General surgical patients receiving LMWH have a <1% risk of developing HIT. The platelet count characteristically falls by ≥50% from baseline (rarely below 20×10^9/L) between days 5 and 10 of heparin therapy. Less often, if a patient has received heparin within the last 100 days, HIT can present acutely after heparin administration with systemic symptoms (rigors, cardiorespiratory distress). Skin lesions at the site of heparin injections have also been shown to be associated with HIT.[24] Half of patients with HIT will develop thrombosis, and unless heparin is stopped and alternative anticoagulation commenced, there is a considerable risk of further thrombosis developing.[25] HIT is rarely associated with bleeding and so platelet transfusions should not be given due to the risk of thrombosis,[25] unless there is active bleeding.

Patients receiving heparin should have a platelet count checked on the day treatment is started, after 24 hours of therapy (if exposed to heparin within the previous 100 days) and thereafter every 2–4 days until day 14. If the platelet count falls by ≥50% of baseline or the patient develops new venous or arterial thrombosis or skin allergy, then a diagnosis of HIT should be considered and a clinical assessment undertaken; advice should be sought from haematology. If the diagnosis of HIT is thought to be likely, heparin should be stopped (including heparin flushes) and, due to the high risk of thrombosis, an alternative anticoagulant (e.g. danaparoid, argatroban or fondaparinux) should be commenced, pending the results of further investigations. Again, in such circumstances the advice of a haematologist is essential. Warfarin should not be started until the platelet count has fully recovered, and care should be taken to continue an additional anticoagulant until the INR is >2.0 for 2 days.

Other risk factors for VTE

Age

Age is an important risk factor for VTE, with many studies showing an increased risk in patients over 40 years of age and considerably greater in those >70 years of age.[26] It is likely that this is a reflection of medical comorbidities, immobility and coagulation activation.

Obesity

Those with a body mass index (BMI) of over 30 kg/m² have a two- to threefold increased risk of VTE. As with age, it is thought that this might be a reflection of immobility and coagulation activation.[26]

Family history of VTE

A history of VTE in a first-degree family member (aged <50 years) confers an increased risk of developing a VTE.[27]

Medical illness and malignancy

Hospitalisation itself is associated with an eightfold increased risk of VTE, with specific patient groups being at particularly high risk. Congestive cardiac failure, acute infection, central venous access, paralytic stroke, nephrotic syndrome, cancer and chemotherapy are all moderate risk factors for VTE (odds ratio 2–9).[28] It has therefore been proposed that hospitalised medical patients are risk assessed for their level of risk of developing VTE (NICE guideline,[29] SIGN guideline,[30] ACCP guideline[8]).

Cancer is strongly associated with VTE; 15% of patients with VTE have malignancy and 2–3% of patients with VTE are newly diagnosed with malignancy at presentation. Patients with certain cancers (stomach, lung, breast, pancreas, gynaecological, lymphoma) are at particularly high risk of thrombosis, thought to be caused by tissue factor-like substances and microparticles activating the coagulation cascade. Surgery and immobilisation further increase this patient group's risk of thrombosis.

Hormone replacement therapy (HRT) and combined oral contraceptive pill (cOCP)

The risk of VTE is increased two- to fourfold in users of the cOCP.[31] The risk is highest in the first year of use, diminishes thereafter, and is reduced by the use of the lower dose oestrogen preparations. Obese women (BMI >30) have a twofold increased risk of VTE, but a 10-fold increased risk if taking the cOCP. The risk of VTE after surgery in women taking the cOCP is increased 2.5-fold. There is no evidence that the progesterone-only contraceptive increases the risk of VTE. Women with thrombophilia (antithrombin, protein C or S deficiencies, factor V Leiden of the prothrombin gene variant) who take the cOCP are at particularly high risk of VTE.[32] More recently, transdermal contraceptive patches have been introduced containing both oestrogen and progestogen, but the risk of VTE with these preparations appears to be similar to the oral preparations.[33]

HRT is associated with a two-to fourfold increased risk of VTE in women using HRT compared with non-users.[32–34] As with the cOCP, the risk is highest in the first year of HRT,[35] and there is a synergistic effect with the inherited thrombophilias.[36] Unlike the cOCP, there appears to be a lower risk of VTE when the transdermal route is used compared with oral preparations.[37]

Pregnancy and puerperium

VTE is a leading direct cause of maternal death in the UK, primarily due to pulmonary embolism. There is a 10-fold increased risk of VTE in pregnancy and a 25-fold increased risk during the puerperium. Many of these thrombotic events are preventable by the use of appropriate thromboprophylaxis[38] and it therefore follows that all pregnant women, including those in the postpartum period, should be considered 'at risk' of VTE if admitted with an acute illness, and given thromboprophylaxis unless contraindicated. Low-molecular-weight heparins are safe to use in pregnancy as they do not cross the placenta into the foetal circulation.

Travel

Travel of long duration is a relatively weak risk factor for VTE, with risks higher in those with pre-existing risk factors. Studies that have investigated the role of risk factors in travel-related thrombosis have mentioned the role of recent trauma or surgery, in addition to obesity, cancer and hormone therapy. It is important to remember that the risk of developing symptomatic VTE after long-duration travel remains increased in the 8 weeks after the flight.[39–41]

Superficial thrombophlebitis

Superficial thrombophlebitis (STP) of the lower leg is a significant risk factor for VTE and a large prospective epidemiological study found that 3.3% of patients with STP develop symptomatic VTE if untreated. Those with STP >5 cm in length were more likely to have associated DVT if the STP was in the proximal long saphenous vein. STP within a varicose vein was less likely to be associated with DVT.[42]

Surgery

One-third of patients with VTE will have had surgery in the preceding 3 months, with the risk greatest following major abdominal and pelvic surgery (especially if associated with malignancy), and major orthopaedic procedures. Without appropriate thrombosis prevention strategies, 60–80% of such patients will develop venous thrombosis.[8] Major trauma is also associated with a very high risk of VTE. It has been recognised that, in addition to the surgical procedure itself, a number of other factors increase the risk of thrombosis in the surgical

Box 14.2 • Risk factors for venous thromboembolism

Inherited
Antithrombin deficiency
Protein C deficiency
Protein S deficiency
Factor V Leiden
Prothrombin G20210A
Elevated factor VIII levels
Dysfibrinogenaemia

Acquired
Surgery
Trauma
Acute medical illness
Malignancy
Cancer therapies (hormonal, chemotherapy or radiotherapy)
Previous VTE
Antiphospholipid syndrome
Increasing age
Pregnancy and puerperium
Oestrogen-containing oral contraceptives or hormone replacement therapy
Selective oestrogen receptor modulators
Infection/sepsis
Immobility/paresis
Heart or respiratory failure
Inflammatory bowel disease
Nephrotic syndrome
Haemoglobinopathies
Myeloproliferative disease
Paroxysmal nocturnal haemoglobinuria
Paraproteinaemia
Obesity
Smoking
Varicose veins and superficial vein thrombophlebitis
Central venous lines

patient (Box 14.2). It is also now understood that the risk of VTE does not end at the point of discharge as 56% of all VTE episodes within 91 days of surgery occur after discharge.[43,44]

Prevention of venous thromboembolic disease

Guidelines

Over the last few years there has been a proliferation of guidelines for the prevention of VTE, with national guidelines developed in Scotland (SIGN 122)[30] and England and Wales (NICE CG92).[29]

Table 14.2 • Variables used to determine patient pretest probability for pulmonary embolism*

Clinical variable	Score
Clinical signs and symptoms of DVT (minimum of leg swelling and pain with palpation of deep veins)	3
PE as or more likely than an alternative diagnosis	3
Heart rate >100	1.5
Immobilisation or surgery in the previous 4 weeks	1.5
Previous DVT/PE	1.5
Haemoptysis	1
Malignancy (on treatment, treated in the last 6 months or palliative)	1

*Score >4, probability of PE is 'likely'; 4, probability for PE is 'unlikely'. Alternatively, <2 is low probability, 2–6 moderate and >6 high.
Adapted from Wells PS. Integrated strategies for the diagnosis of venous thromboembolism. J Thromb Haemost 2007; 5(Suppl 1):41–50.
With permission from John Wiley and Sons.

Investigation for PE

Chest X-ray (CXR)

Radiographic findings in PE are usually non-specific on a CXR; however, it will exclude other diagnoses (such as infection or pulmonary oedema).

Computed tomography pulmonary angiogram (CTPA)

CTPA is now the gold standard for detecting PE, with multislice scanners reporting sensitivities of 83–100% and specificity of 89–97%. These multislice CTPA scanners allow the entire pulmonary arterial tree to be visualised in less than 10 seconds, and in addition to demonstrating the presence or absence of a PE, an alternative cause for the patient's symptoms may be detected (not possible with V/Q scanning – see below). CTPA also gives an assessment of the right ventricular:left ventricular size, an indicator of the severity of the PE in the acute situation. A good-quality negative CTPA on a multidetector scan effectively excludes PE, and anticoagulation can safely be withheld in such patients.[74]

Ventilation/perfusion (V/Q) scanning

Until recently, V/Q scanning was the imaging investigation of choice for those suspected of having had a PE, but has been largely superseded by CTPA. It is relatively easily performed, is less invasive and cheaper than pulmonary angiography, and can be used as an alternative in patients with contraindications to CTPA. It is of most use in those with normal CXR without underlying lung disease.[74] A normal V/Q scan excludes the diagnosis of PE (1% VTE in follow-up).[75]

Echocardiography

Echocardiography can be particularly useful in unstable patients for whom transport to the radiology department is unfeasible. Right ventricular freewall hypokinesis and increased pulmonary pressures are highly suggestive of PE and can be considered diagnostic if ultrasound evidence of DVT is also seen. It may also allow differentiation between other clinical conditions that can present in a similar fashion, such as aortic dissection, myocardial infarction or pericardial tamponade.[76]

MRI

Currently, the clinical utility of MRI in the diagnosis of PE is low when compared with CTPA. Although preliminary studies suggest contrast-enhanced magnetic resonance angiography (ce-MRA) has a similar sensitivity and specificity to other imaging techniques,[77] there is less access to patients (who may be clinically unstable) whilst in the magnet, the duration of scanning is longer and MRI scanning is generally less easily available. However, MRI scanning has some advantages: firstly, it does not require ionising radiation, which is beneficial for women of childbearing age and/or those who are pregnant; secondly, MRI contrast agents are considered to have fewer side-effects than the iodinated media required for CT; and thirdly, it is possible to carry out a comprehensive protocol of magnetic resonance venography and pulmonary angiography (taking less than 20 minutes in total). As a result, consideration could be given to using MRI in patients with contraindications to contrast media, young women with a low clinical probability of PE, and in pregnancy. However, the other imaging modalities discussed above remain the mainstay of investigation at the present time.

Investigation in pregnancy

Clinical assessment of DVT and PE is especially unreliable in pregnancy and the minority of pregnant women undergoing objective investigation for VTE will have that diagnosis confirmed. It is important, therefore, that the risks of imaging (both to the mother and the foetus) are minimised. The Royal

College of Obstetricians advises that pregnant women suspected of having a PE have a duplex ultrasound performed,[78] with V/Q scanning or CTPA reserved for those with negative ultrasound scans.[30] CTPA has the disadvantage of a high radiation dose to the woman's breasts and an increased lifetime risk of developing breast cancer, with V/Q resulting in a considerably lower radiation dose to the mother.

Summary of diagnostic methods for PE

Patients presenting with symptoms suggestive of PE should have a clinical assessment and pretest probability determined. Those at low risk with D-dimers below the laboratory 'cut-off' for the exclusion of VTE do not usually need further investigation. For those with suspected PE in whom the diagnosis is 'PE likely' or 'PE unlikely but with positive D-dimers', CTPA should be performed; a negative multislice scan can safely exclude the presence of a PE. Hospital inpatients with symptoms/signs of PE should have imaging investigations performed. Pregnant women should have duplex ultrasound of the leg veins performed as the initial investigation.

Management of venous thromboembolic disease

Aims of treatment

The primary aims of the treatment of VTE are to relieve symptoms and to prevent thrombus extension and recurrent thrombotic events, thereby reducing the risks of the long-term complications of VTE (the post-thrombotic syndrome and chronic thromboembolic pulmonary hypertension). Anticoagulation is the mainstay of treatment of VTE for both DVT and PE.

Before starting anticoagulation, assessment should be undertaken to determine whether any disorders predisposing to VTE are present (i.e. malignancy or pregnancy), to assess the safety of proposed anticoagulant therapy and to determine whether appropriate monitoring of anticoagulant therapy is achievable. Thorough clinical history taking and examination will identify factors contributing to the development of VTE and risks for anticoagulant therapy. Baseline blood tests should be undertaken (full blood count, renal function and coagulation screen) to allow safe prescribing of anticoagulant therapy. Heparins are renally excreted, vitamin K antagonists and unfractionated heparin require

coagulation test monitoring, and care should be taken with anticoagulant therapy in anaemia and thrombocytopenia.

Anticoagulation should be started as soon as an objective diagnosis of VTE has been made, of if there are any delays in investigation of patients at high risk of VTE.[29,72] For most patients, this will mean immediate anticoagulation with an injectable anticoagulant (UFH, LMWH or fondaparinux), followed by oral anticoagulation with a vitamin K antagonist. Rivaroxaban, an oral direct Xa antagonist, is now licensed for the treatment of DVT. Some patients (such as those with PE with haemodynamic compromise or DVT associated with phlegmasia caerulea dolens) may benefit from thrombolytic therapy or even surgical intervention.

High-risk PE

Haemodynamically compromised patients with PE should be managed in an appropriate clinical setting – usually a coronary care or high-dependency unit. Haemodyanamic support (inotropes) and oxygen should be administered if required. Intravenous UFH will achieve therapeutic levels faster than LMWH, and the dose can be adjusted if thrombolytic therapy is required; therefore, it should be used in preference to subcutaneous LMWH in shocked patients.

> ✔ Thrombolysis achieves clot lysis more rapidly than anticoagulation alone, accelerating the reduction in pulmonary vascular obstruction, potentially increasing pulmonary perfusion and gas exchange, and should be considered in patients with haemodynamic instability.[72]

Anticoagulation

UFH

UFH is renally excreted, has an unpredictable dose response and a narrow therapeutic window; it therefore needs monitoring. It is an injectable anticoagulant and has a short half-life of 60–90 minutes. It is usually administered by a continuous intravenous infusion after an initial loading dose (loading dose 80 U/kg followed by an infusion of 18 U/kg per hour) with subsequent dose adjustments made to maintain an activated partial thromboplastin time (APTT) ratio of 1.5–2.5. Randomised clinical trials have shown that treatment with intravenous (i.v.) UFH for 5–7 days followed by more prolonged treatment with an oral anticoagulant is as efficacious as longer treatment with i.v. UFH.[79]

Haemorrhage occurs in up to 5% of individuals receiving UFH infusions, the risk being greater in the elderly and those receiving antiplatelet therapies. Care should be taken to monitor for HIT (see earlier). Oral anticoagulation (see below) should be started concurrently with UFH, and the UFH stopped when the INR is therapeutic on two consecutive days.[79] Use of UFH has now largely been superseded by LMWH other than in patients with renal failure, or those at high risk of bleeding.

LMWH

LMWHs are made by chemical or enzymatic depolymerisation of UFH. Their predominant mode of action is to inhibit anti-Xa activity, although all have variable anti-IIa activity. In comparison to UFH, they have more reliable pharmacokinetics and a greater bioavailability and can be given by once or twice daily weight-adjusted subcutaneous administration. A Cochrane review that compared fixed-dose LMWH with UFH for acute PE treatment found an odds ratio of 0.88 (95% confidence interval 0.48–1.63) for risk of recurrent PE in favour of LMWH.[80] LMWH does not, routinely, require monitoring. In certain circumstances, however (e.g. in renal impairment or elderly patients with low body weight), monitoring may be of benefit. Peak anti-Xa levels should be measured 3–4 hours after LMWH injection, the therapeutic range being 1.0–2.0 IU/mL with once-daily injection and 0.5–1.0 IU/mL with twice-daily injections. The risk of bleeding is less with LMWH compared with UFH, as is the risk of HIT.

> ✅✅ Studies have shown that, for the treatment of DVT, outpatient LMWH administration at therapeutic licensed dosages is as safe and efficacious as UFH infusion.[79]

LMWHs have been shown to be as safe and effective as UFH in treating non-massive haemodynamically stable PE, but the optimal dosing schedule (once or twice daily) remains controversial. Prognostic prediction models (such as Pulmonary Embolism Severity Index) are being used to categorise risk of mortality, and patients at low risk are suitable for outpatient management or early discharge.[81]

LMWHs are the treatment of choice for VTE in pregnancy, as warfarin is teratogenic. As the half-life of LMWH in pregnancy is shorter, twice-daily regimens should be utilised for pregnant patients. Furthermore, these patients should be managed in consultation with an obstetrician and a haematologist with an interest in obstetric haematology.[78]

> ✅✅ Studies in cancer patients comparing LMWH to standard warfarin anticoagulation in patients with acute VTE and malignancy demonstrated a significant reduction in the occurrence of recurrent VTE without an increase in bleeding in those receiving LMWH.[82] Although there was no reduction in mortality, LMWH was well tolerated and avoided the necessity of frequent INR checks; it therefore should be offered to patients with malignancy and VTE, especially whilst undergoing chemotherapy, which can cause unstable INRs.

Fondaparinux

Fondaparinux is a pentasaccharide that exerts a selective anti-Xa anticoagulant effect via antithrombin. Once-daily, subcutaneous, fixed-dose fondaparinux (7.5 mg subcutaneously once daily for patients 50–100 kg in weight) has been shown to be as effective and safe as UFH and LMWH for the management of acute symptomatic DVT and PE, and has a licence for these indications. Whilst it is more expensive than UFH and LMWH, it does not need monitoring, nor has it been associated with the development of HIT.[83]

Vitamin K antagonists

Warfarin remains the treatment of choice for the majority of patients with VTE. It has a narrow therapeutic window, there is considerable variability in dose response between subjects, it has numerous drug and food interactions, and requires regular monitoring. All too frequently there are dosing problems due to patient non-adherence or miscommunication between patient and health professional. Warfarin inhibits the metabolism of vitamin K, which is required for the essential post-translational modification (carboxylation) of the vitamin K-dependent coagulation factors (factors II, VII, IX and X). The rate of inhibition of these coagulation factors is dependent on their rate of synthesis; factor VII (with a half-life of 6 h) is rapidly inhibited, whereas it takes considerably longer for the activity of factor II (with a half-life of 72 h) to fall. It usually takes 4–7 days for the activities of these vitamin K-dependent coagulation factors to fall to a level at which the patient is therapeutically anticoagulated.

Warfarin is monitored by the INR (derived from the prothrombin time). 'Bridging' anticoagulation with UFH, LMWH or fondaparinux should be continued for a minimum of 5 days and until the INR is >2. The target INR for a patient with DVT or PE (unless the thrombosis occurred on warfarin) is 2.5. Not surprisingly, the most serious adverse complication of oral anticoagulation is bleeding. The risk is directly related to the intensity of anticoagulation and the length of therapy, and is greatest in the elderly, those with unstable anticoagulation and those with significant concomitant illnesses (including past history of gastrointestinal bleeding, renal or liver failure, anaemia, uncontrolled hypertension). The risk of major bleeding with warfarin anticoagulation is reported to be 0.5–6.5% per year and fatal bleeding 0.1–1.0% per year.[84] For patients newly starting warfarin anticoagulation it is not (yet) possible to predict their dose, and induction algorithms (such as the modified Fennerty algorithm) should be used to guide dosing.[85]

Rivaroxaban

Rivaroxaban, a once-daily, oral, direct Xa inhibitor has now been licensed in the UK and approved by NICE and the Scottish Medicines Consortium for the treatment of DVT and the secondary prevention of VTE. In the management of acute DVT, rivaroxaban was non-inferior when compared to traditional anticoagulation (LMWH and warfarin) in the prevention of symptomatic, recurrent VTE, without an increase in bleeding.[86] Similar findings were seen in the more recently published study in patients presenting with PE,[87] but as yet rivaroxaban is not licensed in the acute management of PE.

There are clear advantages to the use of rivaroxaban in the treatment of patients with DVT; it is an oral medication with a reliable pharmacokinetic profile and therefore does not need monitoring. One disadvantage is that there is no direct antidote, although there is some evidence for the use of prothrombin complex concentrates and novoseven in the management of patients bleeding while taking rivaroxaban.[88] It is expected that as clinical experience with these new anticoagulants grows, they will, in time, largely replace the use of warfarin.

Thrombolysis

Thrombolysis has been used for the treatment of DVT, initially given systemically and more recently by local catheter. Thrombolysis has been demonstrated to produce more rapid early clot lysis and reduced incidence of the post-thrombotic syndrome (PTS), but is associated with a significant risk of bleeding. Patients at low risk of bleeding (predominantly young patients), with extensive iliofemoral DVT, may significantly benefit from this treatment.[89] Local administration of thrombolytic agents, or the use of combined catheter-directed thrombolysis with mechanical thrombectomy, reduces that bleeding risk.[90] Thrombolytic therapy should be considered for patients with recent-onset (within 7–10 days) massive iliofemoral DVT or those with limb-threatening thrombosis.[91]

Inferior vena caval (IVC) filters

There is no evidence to support the routine use of IVC filters where a patient can be anticoaguated. There is only one randomised trial of the use of vena caval filters in the management of VTE in patients who were anticoagulated; this demonstrated a reduction in symptomatic PE, but a higher risk of recurrent DVT without a reduction in mortality in patients with IVC filters.[92]

The remainder of the evidence for IVC filter use comes predominantly from descriptive case series and therefore there is little robust evidence to guide the clinician on their use. Both permanent and retrievable filters are available (some may be retrieved up to a few months after insertion). It is recommended that insertion of an IVC filter be considered to prevent PE in patients with VTE and a contraindication to anticoagulation; this includes patients with recent (within 2 months) VTE who require cessation of anticoagulation for surgery. Anticoagulation should be commenced when the contraindication to its use resolves, and should be considered for all patients with IVC filters in situ (dependent on perceived risks of thrombosis from disease and bleeding associated with anticoagulant therapy). It is also reasonable to consider IVC filter insertion in patients who have PE despite therapeutic anticoagulation. If the indication for the filter is temporary, retrievable filters should be used (and then removed) where possible.

Duration of anticoagulation

There remains uncertainty about the optimal duration of anticoagulation following a VTE. Systematic reviews have considered the duration of anticoagulation after an episode of VTE and have reported that, while the risk of recurrent VTE is low should anticoagulant therapy be continued, the risk of bleeding is increased.[93] Short-term anticoagulation (less than 3 months) is associated with a higher risk of recurrence compared with longer-term treatment.[94] Following cessation of oral anticoagulation after a first episode of VTE, the risk of recurrence is 7–12.9% after 1 year and 21.5–22.8% after 5 years.[9,95]

✔ At least 3 months of anticoagulant therapy is required after a proximal DVT or PE; 3 months is likely sufficient after a first event if it was associated with a transient risk factor, such as surgery. Calf vein thromboses, if diagnosed, should be treated with anticoagulation for 6–12 weeks.[85]

A prospective study followed 570 patients with a first episode of VTE for 2 years after the cessation of oral anticoagulant therapy.[95] The risk of recurrence at 2 years in those who had presented with VTE within 6 weeks of surgery or in pregnancy or post-partum was zero, in contrast to those who had had idiopathic events (19.4%) and those who had had a non-surgical risk factor for VTE (8.8%). Patients with a clear precipitating factor for VTE are at low risk of recurrence once stopping anticoagulation if the underlying risk factor has resolved.

Longer-term anticoagulation after a first idiopathic VTE may be appropriate in patients considered at high risk of recurrent VTE, who are at low risk of bleeding, following an individual assessment of risk factors. As active cancer and anticancer treatment both increase the risk of VTE, consideration should be given to continuing anticoagulation.

Key points

- The risk of developing VTE increases steadily with age, with 1 in 100 individuals over the age of 80 developing a VTE each year.
- Thromboembolism in hospital inpatients is common, developing in over 20% of general surgical patients in the absence of thromboprophylaxis. PE is a well-recognised complication of surgery, and a significant cause of perioperative morbidity and death. There are frequently no signs of DVT prior to the onset of PE.
- Patients can be identified to be at risk of VTE both by surgical (i.e. procedural) and patient (i.e. thrombophilia or medical comorbidity) risk factors. Undertaking a risk assessment and using appropriate thromboprophylaxis will reduce the risk of VTE.
- Thromboprophylaxis with a combination of mechanical and pharmacological agents is effective in preventing VTE in high-risk surgical patients. Further studies to evaluate the efficacy of newer methods (both pharmacological and mechanical) are needed.
- If a diagnosis of VTE is considered, appropriate investigations should be performed. Clinical pretest probability and D-dimer testing are useful in the assessment of outpatients, but have not been validated within the hospital inpatient population. Such patients should have appropriate imaging investigations undertaken. If there is a delay in investigation, therapeutic anticoagulation should be commenced unless the bleeding risks outweigh the potential benefits of anticoagulation.
- Anticoagulation is the mainstay of treatment for DVT and PE. If anticoagulation is contraindicated, IVC filter insertion should be considered.

References

1. House of Commons Health Committee. The prevention of venous thromboembolism in hospitalised patients. London: The Stationery Office; 2005.
2. White RH. The epidemiology of venous thromboembolism. Circulation 2003;107(23, Suppl.):I4–8.
3. Naess IA, Christiansen SC, Romundstad P, et al. Incidence and mortality of venous thrombosis: a population-based study. J Thromb Haemost 2007;5:692–9.
4. Cohen AT, Agnelli G, Anderson FA, et al. Venous thromboembolism in Europe. Thromb Haemost 2007;98:756–64.
5. Buller HR, Sohne M, Middeldorp S. Treatment of venous thromboembolism. J Thromb Haemost 2005;3:1554–60.
6. Spencer FA, Lessard D, Emery C, et al. Venous thromboembolism in the outpatient setting. Arch Intern Med 2007;167(14):1471–5.
7. Kearon C. Natural history of venous thromboembolism. Circulation 2003;107(23):I22–30.
8. Geerts WH, Bergqvist D, Pineo GF, et al. Prevention of venous thromboembolism: the Eighth ACCP Clinical Practice Guidelines. Chest 2008;133(6, Suppl.):318S–453S.
9. Pineda LA, Hatahwar VS, Grant BJ. Clinical suspicion of fatal pulmonary embolism. Chest 2001;120(3):791–5.
10. Thomas DP. Pathogenesis of venous thrombosis. In: Bloom AL, Forbes CD, Tuddenham EGD, editors. Haemostasis and thrombosis. 3rd ed. Edinburgh: Churchill Livingstone; 1994. p. 1327–33.
11. Hamilton G, Platt SA. Deep vein thrombosis. In: Beard JD, Gaines PA, editors. Vascular and endovascular surgery. London: WB Saunders; 1998. p. 351–96.

12. Gillet JL, Perrin MR, Allaert FA. Short-term and mid-term outcome of isolated symptomatic muscular calf vein thrombosis. J Vasc Surg 2007;46(3):513–9.

13. Warlow C, Ogston D, Douglas AS. Deep venous thrombosis of the legs after strokes. Part I: Incidence and predisposing factors. Br Med J 1976;1:1178–81.

14. Comerota AJ, Stewart GJ, Alburger PD, et al. Operative venodilation: a previously unsuspected factor in the cause of postoperative deep vein thrombosis. Surgery 1989;106:301–9.

15. Flynn PD, Byrne CD, Baglin TP, et al. Thrombin generation by apoptotic vascular smooth muscle cells. Blood 1997;89:4378–84.

16. Rosendaal FR. Risk factors for venous thrombotic disease. Thromb Haemost 1999;82(2):610–9.

17. Lane DA, Mannucci PM, Bauer KA, et al. Inherited thrombophilia: part 1. Thromb Haemost 1996;76:651–62.

18. Lijfering WM, Coppens M, Veeger NJ, et al. Hyperhomocysteinemia is not a risk factor for venous and arterial thrombosis, and is associated with elevated factor VIII levels. Thromb Res 2008;123(2):244–50.

19. Baglin T, Gray E, Greaves M, et al. Clinical guidelines for testing for heritable thrombophilia. Br J Haematol 2010;149:209–20.

20. Cristina L, Benilde C, Michela C, et al. High plasma levels of factor VIII and risk of recurrence of venous thromboembolism. Br J Haematol 2004;124(4):504–10.

21. Bolton-Maggs PH, Perry DJ, Chalmers EA, et al. The rare coagulation disorders – review with guidelines for management from the United Kingdom Haemophilia Centre Doctors' Organisation. Haemophilia 2004;10:593–628.

22. Zwicker J, Bauer KA. Thrombophilia. In: Kitchens CS, Alving BA, Kessler CM, editors. Consultative hemostasis and thrombosis. Elsevier Science; 2002. p. 181–96.

23. Rand JH. The antiphospholipid syndrome. Hematology Am Soc Hematol Educ Program 2007;136–42.

24. Linkins LA, Dans AL, Moores LK, et al. Treatment and prevention of HIT: Antithrombotic Therapy and Prevention of Thrombosis, 9th ed: American College of Chest Physicians Evidence-Based Clinical Practice Guidelines. Chest 2012;141:e495S–530S.

25. Keeling D, Davidson S, Watson H. The management of heparin-induced thrombocytopenia. Br J Haematol 2006;133:259–69.

26. Heit JA, Silverstein MD, Mohr DN, et al. The epidemiology of venous thromboembolism in the community. Thromb Haemost 2001;86(1):452–63.

27. Bezemer ID, van der Meer FJ, Eikenboom JC, et al. The value of family history as a risk indicator for venous thrombosis. Arch Intern Med 2009;169(6):610–5.

28. Prandoni P, Samama MM. Risk stratification and venous thromboprophylaxis in hospitalized medical and cancer patients. Br J Haematol 2008;141:587–97.

29. NICE (National Institute for Health and Clinical Excellence). Clinical Guideline 144. Venous thromboembolic diseases: the management of venous thromboembolic diseases and the role of thrombophilia testing. Available at http://publications. nice.org.uk/venous-thromboembolic-diseases-the-management-of-venous-thromboembolic-diseases-and-the-role-of-cg144; 2012 [accessed 06.12.12].

30. SIGN (Scottish Intercollegiate Guidelines Network). Guideline 122. Prevention and management of venous thromboembolism. A national clinical guideline. Available at http://www.sign.ac.uk/pdf/sign122. pdf; 2010 [accessed 06.12.12].

31. Wu O, Robertson L, Langhorne P, et al. Oral contraceptives, hormone replacement therapy, thrombophilias and risk of venous thromboembolism: a systematic review. The Thrombosis: Risk and Economic Assessment of Thrombophilia Screening (TREATS) Study. Thromb Haemost 2005;94(1):17–25.

32. Rosendaal FR, Van Hylckama Vlieg A, Tanis BC, et al. Estrogens, progestogens and thrombosis. J Thromb Haemost 2003;1: 1371–80.

33. Jick S, Kaye JA, Li L, et al. Further results on the risk of non-fatal venous thrombembolism in users of the contraceptive transdermal patch compared to users of oral contraceptives containing norgestimate and 35 μg of ethinyl estradiol. Contraception 2007;76(1):4–7.

34. Daly E, Vessey MP, Hawkins MM, et al. Risk of venous thromboembolism in users of hormone replacement therapy. Lancet 1996;348:977–80.

35. Jick H, Derby LE, Myers MW, et al. Risk of hospital admission for idiopathic venous thromboembolism among users of postmenopausal oestrogens. Lancet 1996;348:981–3.

36. Grodstein F, Stampfer MJ, Goldhaber SZ, et al. Prospective study of exogenous hormones and risk of pulmonary embolism in women. Lancet 1996;348:983–7.

37. Wu O. Postmenopausal hormone replacement therapy and venous thromboembolism. Gend Med 2005;2(Suppl. A):S18–27.

38. Confidential Enquiry into Maternal and Child Health, et al. Saving Mothers' Lives: Reviewing Maternal Deaths to Make Motherhood Safer, 2006–2008. The Eigth Report of the Confidential Enquiries into Maternal Deaths in the United Kingdom. London: CEMACH; 2011. BJOG vol 118; suppl 1, March 2011 http://www.oaa-anaes.ac.uk/assets/_managed/editor/File/Reports/2006-2008%20CEMD.pdf

39. Watson HG, Baglin TP. Guidelines on travel-related venous thrombosis. Br J Haematol 2011;152(1): 31–4.

40. Kuipers S, Cannegieter SC, Middeldorp S, et al. The absolute risk of venous thrombosis after air travel:

a cohort study of 8755 employees of international organizations. PLoS Med 2007;4(9):e290.

41. Cannegieter SC, Doggen CJ, van Houwelingen HC, et al. Travel-related venous thrombosis: results from a large population-based case control study (MEGA study). PLoS Med 2006;3(8):e307.

42. Decousus H, Quere I, Presle E, et al. Superficial vein thrombosis and venous thromboembolism: a large, prospective epidemiological study. Ann Intern Med 2010;152:218–24.

43. Sweetland S, Green J, Liu B, et al. Duration and magnitude of the postoperative risk of venous thromboembolism in middle aged women: prospective cohort study. Br Med J 2009;339:b4583.

44. White RH, Zhou H, Romano PS. Incidence of symptomatic venous thromboembolism after different elective or urgent surgical procedures. Thromb Haemost 2003;90:446–55.

45. Thromboembolic Risk Factors (THRIFT) Consensus Group. Risk of, and prophylaxis for, venous thromboembolism in hospital patients. Br Med J 1992;305:567–74.

46. Sachdeva A, Dalton M, Amaragiri SV, et al. Elastic compression stockings for prevention of deep vein thrombosis. Cochrane Database Syst Rev 2010;(7): CD001484.

47. Wells PS, Lensing AW, Hirsh J. Graduated compression stockings in the prevention of postoperative venous thromboembolism. A meta-analysis. Arch Intern Med 1994;154:67–72.
Graduated compression stockings significantly reduce venous thromboembolic disease in moderate-risk patients (insufficient evidence in high-risk orthopaedic surgery).

48. Amaragiri SV, Lees TA. Elastic compression stocking for prevention of deep vein thrombosis. Cochrane Database Syst Rev 2000;(3):CD001484.
A review of randomised controlled trials that confirms the efficacy of stockings in prevention of venous thromboembolic disease in hospitalised patients.

49. Comerota AJ, Chouhan V, Harada RN, et al. The fibrinolytic effects of intermittent pneumatic compression: mechanism of enhanced fibrinolysis. Ann Surg 1997;226:306–13.

50. Chouhan VD, Comerota AJ, Sun L, et al. Inhibition of tissue factor pathway during intermittent pneumatic compression: a possible mechanism for antithrombotic effect. Arterioscler Thromb Vasc Biol 1999;19:2812–7.

51. Browse NL, Burnand KG, Irvine AT, et al. Deep vein thrombosis: prevention. In: Browse NL, Burnand KG, Irvine AT, editors. Diseases of the veins. 2nd ed. London: Arnold; 1999. p. 359–83.

52. Watson HG, Chee YL. Aspirin and other antiplatelet drugs in the prevention of venous thromboembolism. Blood Rev 2008;22:107–16.

53. Imperiale TF, Speroff T. A meta-analysis of methods to prevent venous thromboembolism following total hip replacement. JAMA 1994;271:1780–5.

54. Antiplatelet Trialists' Collaboration. Collaborative overview of randomized trials of antiplatelet therapy – III: Reduction in venous thrombosis and pulmonary embolism by antiplatelet prophylaxis among surgical and medical patients. Br Med J 1994;308:235–46.

55. Pulmonary Embolism Prevention (PEP) Trial. Prevention of pulmonary embolism and deep vein thrombosis with low dose aspirin. Lancet 2000;355:1295–302.

56. Collins R, Scrimgeour A, Yusuf S, et al. Reduction in fatal pulmonary embolism and venous thrombosis by perioperative administration of subcutaneous heparin. Overview of results of randomized trials in general, orthopaedic and urological surgery. N Engl J Med 1988;318:1162–73.

57. Leizorovicz A, Haugh MC, Chapuis FR, et al. Low molecular weight heparin in prevention of perioperative thrombosis. Br Med J 1992;305:913–20.

58. Nurmohamed MT, Rosendaal FR, Buller HR, et al. Low-molecular-weight heparin versus standard heparin in general and orthopaedic surgery: a meta-analysis. Lancet 1992;340:152–6.

59. Bergqvist D, Burmark US, Flordal PA, et al. Low molecular weight heparin started before surgery as prophylaxis against deep vein thrombosis: 2500 versus 5000 Xai units in 2070 patients. Br J Surg 1995;82:496–501.

60. Agnelli G, Bergqvist D, Cohen AT, et al. Randomized clinical trial of postoperative fondaparinux versus perioperative dalteparin for prevention of venous thromboembolism in high-risk abdominal surgery. Br J Surg 2005;92(10):1212–20.

61. Bergqvist D, Lowe GD, Berstad A, et al. Prevention of venous thromboembolism after surgery: a review of enoxaparin. Br J Surg 1992;79:495–8.

62. Bergqvist D, Agnelli G, Cohen AT, et al. Duration of prophylaxis against venous thromboembolism with enoxaparin after surgery for cancer. N Engl J Med 2002;346(13):975–80.

63. Arumilli BR, Lenin Babu V, Paul AS. Painful swollen leg: think beyond deep vein thrombosis or Baker's cyst. World J Surg Oncol 2008;6:6.

64. Wells PS. Integrated strategies for the diagnosis of venous thromboembolism. J Thromb Haemost 2007;5(Suppl. 1):41–50.

65. Wells PS, Anderson DR, Bormanis J, et al. Value of assessment of pretest probability of deep vein thrombosis in clinical management. Lancet 1997;350:1795–8.

66. Keeling DM, Mackie IJ, Moody A, et al. The Haemostasis and Thrombosis Task Force of the British Committee for Standards in Haematology. The diagnosis of deep vein thrombosis in symptomatic outpatients and the potential for clinical assessment and D-dimer assays to reduce the need for diagnostic imaging. Br J Haematol 2004;124(1):15–25.

67. Ten Cate-Hoek AJ, Prins MH. Management studies using a combination of D-dimer test result and clinical probability to rule out venous thromboembolism: a systematic review. J Thromb Haemost 2005;3(11):2465–70.

68. Kearon C, Julian AJ, Newman TE, et al. Noninvasive diagnosis of deep vein thrombosis. Ann Intern Med 1998;128:663–77.

69. Stevens SM, Elliott CG, Chan KJ, et al. Withholding anticoagulation after a negative result on duplex ultrasonography for suspected symptomatic deep venous thrombosis. Ann Intern Med 2004;140(12):985–91.

70. Cogo A, Lensing AW, Prandoni P, et al. Distribution of thrombosis in patients with symptomatic deep vein thrombosis. Implications for simplifying the diagnostic process with compression ultrasound. Arch Intern Med 1993;153(24):2777–80.

71. Goodacre S, Sampson F, Stevenson M, et al. Measurement of the clinical and cost-effectiveness of non-invasive diagnostic testing strategies for deep vein thrombosis. Health Technol Assess 2006;10(15):1–168, iii–iv.

72. Torbicki A, Perrier A, Konstantinides S, et al. Guidelines on the diagnosis and management of acute pulmonary embolism: the Task Force for the Diagnosis and Management of Acute Pulmonary Embolism of the European Society of Cardiology (ESC). Eur Heart J 2008;29(18):2276–315.

73. Wells PS, Anderson DR, Rodger M, et al. Derivation of a simple clinical model to categorize patients probability of pulmonary embolism: increasing the model's utility with the SimpliRED D-dimer. Thromb Haemost 2000;83:416–20.

74. Anderson DR, Kahn SR, Rodger MA, et al. Computed tomographic pulmonary angiography vs ventilation perfusion lung scanning in patients with suspected pulmonary embolism. JAMA 2007;298(23):2743–53.

75. Van Beek EJR, Brouwers EMJ, Song B, et al. Lung scintigraphy and helical computed tomography for the diagnosis of pulmonary embolism: a meta-analysis. Clin Appl Thromb Hemost 2001;7(2):87–92.

76. Garcia D, Ageno W, Libby E, et al. Update on the diagnosis and management of pulmonary embolism. Br J Haematol 2005;131:301–12.

77. Clemens S, Leeper KV. Newer modalities for detection of pulmonary emboli. Am J Med 2007;120(10, Suppl. 2):S2–12.

78. Royal College of Obstetricians and Gynaecologists. Green Top Guideline No. 28. Thromboembolic disease in pregnancy and the puerperium: acute management.

79. Büller H, Agnelli G, Hull RD, et al. Antithrombotic therapy for venous thromboembolic disease: the Seventh ACCP Conference on Antithrombotic and Thrombolytic Therapy. Chest 2004;126(3, Suppl.):401S–28S.
Evidence-based guideline for the use of anticoagulants for the treatment of VTE recommending that outpatient LMWH is as safe as UFH for the management of DVT (grade I recommendation).

80. van Dongen CJ, van den Belt AG, Prins MH, et al. Fixed dose subcutaneous low molecular weight heparins versus adjusted dose unfractionated heparin for venous thromboembolism. Cochrane Database Syst Rev 2004;(4):CD001100.

81. Sanchez O, Trinquart L, Colombet I, et al. Prognostic value of right ventricular dysfunction in patients with haemodynamically stable pulmonary embolism: a systematic review. Eur Heart J 2008;29(12):1569–77.

82. Lee AY, Levine MN, Baker RI, et al. Low-molecular-weight heparin versus a coumarin for the prevention of recurrent venous thromboembolism in patients with cancer. N Engl J Med 2003;349(2):146–53.
The first study of extended LMWH anticoagulation for VTE. It demonstrated a clear reduction in recurrent thromboses in patients with VTE and cancer compared to adjusted-dose coumarin with no increase in bleeding.

83. Shorr AF, Jackson WL, Moores LK, et al. Minimizing costs for treating deep vein thrombosis: the role for fondaparinux. J Thromb Thrombolysis 2007;23(3):229–36.

84. Makris M, Watson HG. The management of coumarin-induced over-anticoagulation. Br J Haematol 2001;114(2):271–80.

85. Baglin TP, Keeling DM, Watson HG. Guidelines on oral anticoagulation (warfarin): third edition 2005 update. Br J Haematol 2006;132:277–85.

86. The Einstein Investigators. Oral rivaroxaban for symptomatic venous thromboembolism. N Engl J Med 2010;363:2499–510.

87. The Einstein-PE investigators. Oral rivaroxaban for the treatment of symptomatic pulmonary embolism. N Engl J Med 2012;366:1287–97.

88. Schulman S, Crowther MA. How I treat with anticoagulants in 2012: new and old anticoagulants, and when and how to switch. Blood 2012;119(13):3016–23.

89. Watson LI, Armon MP. Thrombolysis for acute deep vein thrombosis. Cochrane Database Syst Rev 2004;(4):CD002783.

90. Alesh I, Kayali F, Stein PD. Catheter-directed thrombolysis (intrathrombus injection) in treatment of deep venous thrombosis: a systematic review. Catheter Cardiovasc Interv 2007;70(1):143–8.

91. Segal JB, Streiff MB, Hofmann LV, et al. Management of venous thromboembolism: a systematic review for a practice guideline. Ann Intern Med 2007;146(3):211–22.

92. The PREPIC Study Group. Eight-year follow-up of patients with permanent vena cava filters in the prevention of pulmonary embolism: the PREPIC (Prevention du Risque d'Embolie Pulmonaire par Interruption Cave) randomized study. Circulation 2005;112:416–22.

93. Hutten BA, Prins MH. Duration of treatment with vitamin K antagonists in symptomatic venous thromboembolism. Cochrane Database Syst Rev 2006;(1):CD001367.

94. Schulman S. The effect of the duration of anticoagulation and other risk factors on the recurrence of venous thromboembolisms. Duration of Anticoagulation Study Group. Wien Med Wochenschr 1999;149(2–4):66–9.

95. Baglin T, Luddington R, Brown K, et al. Incidence of recurrent venous thromboembolism in relation to clinical and thrombophilic risk factors: prospective cohort study. Lancet 2003;362: 523–6.

15

Patient assessment and surgical risk

Chris Deans

Introduction

Surgical risk is an estimation of the likelihood of an adverse event occurring as a consequence of a patient undergoing a particular surgical procedure or intervention. **Patient assessment** is a process that attempts to quantify this risk for an individual patient. The ability to undertake patient assessment to determine surgical risk for a patient is fundamental to modern surgical practice. Appropriate patient assessment and estimation of risk will inform surgical decision-making, assist patient decision-making and facilitate informed consent. It is important to remember that risk is not only associated with undertaking surgical procedures, but may also include other treatments or investigations that may pose a particular risk to the patient, for example performing a colonoscopy or interventional radiological procedure. The risks of not performing a particular procedure or intervention should also be considered and the possible implications for the patient of not undertaking a procedure should be part of any informed consent process (Box 15.1).[1]

Why assess surgical risk?

Estimation of surgical risk is important for several reasons. Firstly, as already stated, determining a

patient's risk will influence surgical decision-making and, in turn, facilitate informed consent. This process will ultimately influence choice of treatment options for individual patients. Secondly, identifying higher risk patients will also allow appropriate pre-emptive measures to be undertaken and target particular areas of concern to optimise the patient in the perioperative period (see also Chapter 16). This process may also help anticipate potential adverse events. A further positive effect of this process is to aid case mix adjustment. There is increasing public release of activity/outcome figures (or 'league tables') in surgery, which may be crude mortality or complication rates. Case mix adjustment allows units with a greater proportion of high-risk patients to compensate for any differences in their figures with respect to national outcomes and allow for meaningful comparison of data against national audits. This will ensure quality assurance for the future (Box 15.2).

How can we assess surgical risk?

Determination of surgical risk is complex and is influenced by many variables. However, the process may be simplified by thinking of the assessment according to two main factors – the patient,

Box 15.1 • GMC definition of risk of investigation/treatment

1. Side-effects
2. Complications
3. Failure of an intervention to achieve the desired aim
4. The potential outcome of taking no action

Box 15.2 • Why assess surgical risk?

1. Allow informed consent
2. Facilitate surgical decision-making
3. To anticipate adverse events
4. To minimise risk to patients, staff and healthcare system
5. To allow for meaningful comparison of outcomes

and those related to the surgical procedure itself. **Procedural-related risks** are generally easier to quantify where national, local and even individual complication rates may be known. The introduction of national and regional audit programmes in some specialities, as well as the improved quality of data collection in local departments, have enabled a better understanding of the more common risks and complications that are associated with many surgical procedures. However, procedural-related risk will also depend on additional factors, such as the urgency and duration of the procedure, volume of blood loss and type of surgery undertaken. The National Institute for Clinical Excellence (NICE) has attempted to stratify surgical procedures into different grades of severity in an effort to provide guidance on the use of preoperative investigations and estimate the likelihood of perioperative risk (Table 15.1).[2]

Patient-related risk factors are less easy to quantify. They may be broadly divided into either subjective or objective factors. *Subjective risk* assessment includes patient history, clinical examination, pattern recognition, accumulated clinical experience and 'the end of the bed test'. *Objective risk* assessment includes formal laboratory results and assessment of comorbidity and physiological function through further investigation. Patient factors will be influenced by the 'fitness' of the patient (functional/performance status), age, comorbid illness, the underlying disease process and nutritional status, as well as many other inter-related variables.

Several **risk prediction models and scoring systems** have been developed in an attempt to help measure surgical risk. In addition, techniques to formally quantify levels of patient fitness (**functional assessment**), such as exercise testing, and measurements of **serum biomarkers** have also been introduced specifically to predict perioperative risk, with variable success. This chapter will discuss some of these scoring systems and functional assessment tools that may be used for patient assessment and estimation of surgical risk. These may be broadly classified into risk prediction models (general and specific), functional assessment tools and novel biomarkers.

Estimation of surgical risk

Clinical assessment

It is the role of the surgeon as a clinician to undertake a thorough clinical assessment of every patient in order to carefully identify individual characteristics of the patient's comorbidity and underlying disease process that may influence surgical risk. Only then may a fully informed decision be made regarding treatment choices for individual patients. Some patient factors may be clearly identifiable, such as the presence of ischaemic heart disease or obesity, whereas others may not yet have been diagnosed. A thorough history and examination should be undertaken and targeted investigations requested, based on the clinical findings. This process may be difficult and more challenging situations should involve consultation with colleagues and other clinicians as part of the wider multidisciplinary team – for example, obtaining a cardiology review or asking for an anaesthetic opinion. In difficult cases a second opinion may be sought from an independent source.

There are in fact data to support the concept that 'gut instinct' or 'surgical intuition' can be more effective than formal risk prediction models in identifying the patient with a poor prognosis in the context of a particular procedure,[3] especially in the elective setting.[4] However, there is also epidemiological evidence suggesting that clinicians often fail to identify patients at high risk of complications and as a result do not allocate them to the appropriate level of perioperative care.[5]

Risk prediction models and scoring systems

Attempts to improve the accuracy of estimation of risk and to provide a more robust quantitative assessment have led to the development of several scoring systems and risk prediction models. Many of these are freely available online.[6] These tools have been developed to objectively estimate morbidity and mortality rates for individual patients prior to the proposed intervention. It should be

Table 15.1 • Examples of surgical procedures by severity grading (NICE)

Grade 1	Grade 2	Grade 3	Grade 4
Upper gastrointestinal endoscopy	Haemorrhoidectomy	Amputation	Gastrectomy
Vasectomy	Varicose vein surgery	Mastectomy	Colectomy
Tooth extraction	Adenoidectomy	Thyroidectomy	Renal transplant
Excision skin lesion	Reduction of dislocated joint	Prostatectomy	Hip replacement

noted that there is no perfect tool, that the models available must not be used to guide decision-making in isolation and that there is no substitute for the combination of objective markers with surgical experience and intuition. Furthermore, the models available pertain to populations rather than individual patients, and therefore have limitations that need to be recognised before using them to inform surgical risk assessment. For example, the mortality rate for a surgical intervention in a particular population may be 5%, but for the individual patient it can only be 0% or 100%.

The scoring systems available usually incorporate physiological and comorbidity data that have been selected using logistical regression techniques in a large database of patients, which may not be similar to the local population. A *coefficient* may be assigned in order to weight the variables and the resulting equation provides a *numerical indication of risk* for the patient, although it is frequently more meaningful to the operating surgeon.

Ideally the patients in the database on which the scoring system is developed and validated should be similar to the individual patient in question. However, publication bias may mean that only the best data are published. While this has inherent flaws, it may also be viewed as an opportunity to benchmark one's own results against those from a centre of excellence.

Finally, the accuracy of predictive models is dynamic and they should be periodically retested against an evolving surgical patient population. When accuracy deteriorates they should be revised and updated.

POSSUM

The Physiological and Operative Severity Score for the enUmeration of Mortality and morbidity (POSSUM) was first described in 1991.[7] It was designed as a scoring system to estimate morbidity and mortality following a surgical procedure and, by including data on the patient's physiological condition, it provides a risk-adjusted prediction of outcome. This facilitates more accurate comparison of hospital or surgeon performance and it can be used as an audit and clinical governance tool. However, the model involves inclusion of operative variables, such as volume of blood loss and the presence of peritoneal soiling, which precludes its use in the preoperative setting to inform the consent process. Despite this, POSSUM is the most widely applied, validated, surgical risk scoring system in the UK and has been modified by several authors to provide speciality-specific information.

The original POSSUM score was developed after initially subjecting 62 parameters to multivariate analysis in order to determine the most powerful

Box 15.3 • Variables used in the calculation of the P-POSSUM score

Physiological variables
Age
Cardiac disease
Respiratory disease
Electrocardiogram (ECG)
Systolic blood pressure
Pulse rate
Haemoglobin concentration
White cell count
Serum urea concentration
Serum sodium concentration
Serum potassium concentration
Glasgow Coma Scale (GCS)
Operative variables
Operation severity class
Number of procedures
Blood loss
Peritoneal contamination
Malignancy status
Urgency
P-POSSUM formula
Ln $R/1-R = -9.065 + (0.1692 \times$ physiological score) $+ (0.1550 \times$ operative severity score)

outcome predictors. Twelve physiological and six operative parameters were identified, and each of these factors were weighted to a value of 1, 2, 4 or 8 to simplify the calculation. It was re-evaluated in 1998 in Portsmouth, UK by Whiteley et al., who reported concerns that it overestimated mortality in their patients, particularly in the lowest risk group.[8] They modified the POSSUM formula and they constructed the Portsmouth predictor equation for mortality (P-POSSUM; Box 15.3). The modified formula fitted well with the observed mortality rate; however, it still overestimates mortality in low-risk groups, the elderly and in certain surgical subspecialities.[9] The latter finding has prompted the development of speciality-specific POSSUM for major elective surgery.

CR-POSSUM (colorectal)

The value of POSSUM and P-POSSUM in predicting in-hospital mortality was examined in patients undergoing colorectal surgery in France. Both POSSUM and P-POSSUM performed well but overestimated postoperative death in elective surgery and the authors concluded that it had not been validated in France in the field of colorectal surgery.[10] The original POSSUM score and P-POSSUM were derived from a heterogeneous population of general surgical patients. Subgroup analysis of high-risk colorectal surgery patients found that the models under-predicted death in the emergency patients.[11] There was also a lack of calibration at the extremes of age in both emergency and elective work. This resulted in remodelling of the POSSUM score for colorectal surgery patients and led to the development of the Colorectal-POSSUM model (CR-POSSUM). The CR-POSSUM model was superior to the P-POSSUM model in predicting operative mortality in a study involving almost 7000 patients undergoing emergency and elective colorectal surgery in the UK.[12]

External validation of CR-POSSUM was derived from three multicentre, UK studies involving a total of 16 006 patients: the original CR-POSSUM study population (n = 6883), the Association of Coloproctology of Great Britain and Ireland (ACPGBI) Colorectal Cancer (CRC) Database (n = 8077) and the ACPGBI Malignant Bowel Obstruction (MBO) Study (n = 1046). Of the different risk models that were tested, CR-POSSUM was superior in predicting postoperative death.[13]

This conflicted to a certain extent with a later study in New Zealand involving 308 patients undergoing major colorectal surgery. In this cohort POSSUM, P-POSSUM and CR-POSSUM were all satisfactory predictive tools for postoperative mortality but the latter tended to be relatively less accurate. However, the authors noted that CR-POSSUM requires fewer individual patient parameters to be calculated and is therefore simpler to use.[14] A more recent systematic review pooled data from 18 studies to compare the accuracy of POSSUM, P-POSSUM and CR-POSSUM in predicting postoperative mortality for patients undergoing colorectal cancer surgery.[15] This study also reported greater predictive accuracy for the P-POSSUM model compared with CR-POSSUM.

CR-POSSUM is not an accurate predictor of disease-specific colorectal mortality. A study from the Netherlands on patients undergoing elective sigmoid resection for either carcinoma or diverticular disease demonstrated that CR-POSSUM over-predicted mortality in the patients with malignant disease and under-predicted it in patients with benign disease. However, in the whole group CR-POSSUM predicted postoperative mortality accurately.[16]

A possible modification to the CR-POSSUM system was suggested following a single-centre UK study in 304 patients. CR-POSSUM proved to be a more accurate predictive model than POSSUM and P-POSSUM and, interestingly, logistic regression demonstrated a significant correlation between albumin and mortality. It may therefore be possible to improve the accuracy of CR-POSSUM further by modifying the equation to include serum albumin.[17]

O-POSSUM (oesophagogastric)

A UK study of 204 patients demonstrated that POSSUM did not accurately predict morbidity and mortality in patients undergoing oesophagectomy.[18] A dedicated oesophagogastric model (O-POSSUM) developed in a study population of 1042 patients was described in 2004. The O-POSSUM model used the following independent factors: age, physiological status, mode of surgery, type of surgery and histological stage. It provided a more accurate risk-adjusted prediction of death from oesophageal and gastric surgery for individual patients than P-POSSUM.[19] However, to date there have been several conflicting studies examining the predictive value and accuracy of O-POSSUM. A Dutch study of 663 patients undergoing potentially curative oesophagectomy in a tertiary referral centre (in-hospital mortality 3.6%) demonstrated that O-POSSUM over-predicted in-hospital mortality threefold and could not identify those patients with an increased risk of death.[20] This was supported in similar studies from both the UK and Hong Kong, which found that P-POSSUM provided the most accurate prediction of in-hospital mortality and O-POSSUM again over-predicted mortality in patients, particularly with low physiological scores and in older patients.[21,22] A recent systematic review comparing P-POSSUM with O-POSSUM, which included data from 10 studies, concluded that P-POSSUM was the most accurate predictor of postoperative mortality and O-POSSUM consistently overestimated postoperative mortality in gastro-oesophageal cancer patients.[23]

In summary, the data reported in the original study to construct O-POSSUM have not been validated in other centres. It may be that individual units have to modify the O-POSSUM model to take account of local factors.

V-POSSUM (vascular)

V-POSSUM was devised for use specifically in patients undergoing arterial surgery. One study examined the records of 1313 patients and added 'extra items' to the original POSSUM dataset, although this did not appear to significantly improve the accuracy of prediction.[24] The model has, however, been used in further studies and has been modified further to only take account of the physiology component of the score, with improved prediction accuracy (V-POSSUM physiology only). However, a current UK study involving almost 11 000 patients undergoing elective abdominal aortic aneurysm repair evaluated the accuracy of five risk prediction models, including V-POSSUM.[25] V-POSSUM performed poorly, with the Medicare and Vascular Governance North West (VGNW) models demonstrating the best discrimination, leaving the authors to conclude that V-POSSUM should not be used for risk prediction for these patients. Neither the V-POSSUM nor P-POSSUM models appear to be accurate in predicting mortality in the context of ruptured aortic aneurysms.[24] The finding that V-POSSUM may be of limited value in the context of emergency arterial surgery was confirmed by a larger and more recent evaluation of the appropriate POSSUM models in the context of ruptured abdominal aortic aneurysms (RAAAs).[26] When the P-POSSUM, RAAA-POSSUM, RAAA-POSSUM (physiology only), V-POSSUM and V-POSSUM (physiology only) models were all compared in 223 patients with RAAA (in-hospital mortality was 32.4%), all except V-POSSUM and P-POSSUM (physiology only) demonstrated no significant lack of fit.

As one may expect, the various POSSUM models are not accurate predictive tools in the context of elective carotid surgery. Both POSSUM and V-POSSUM over-predicted mortality in a large single-centre study ($n = 499$) of patients undergoing carotid endarterectomy.[27] This is not surprising given the nature of the surgery and the reduced surgical insult compared to body cavity procedures.

A recent evaluation of V-POSSUM in New Zealand has indicated that it is a useful tool not only in the assessment of outcome, but of longitudinal surgical performance in major vascular surgery. Major vascular procedures ($n = 454$) were prospectively scored for V-POSSUM over a 10-year period. There was a trend towards improved surgical performance over time, with a drop in the observed to predicted ratios of deaths. This novel role has not yet been tested in the other POSSUM models, but given these data there may be the potential to use them to evaluate surgical training and performance in other surgical subspecialities.[28]

✅ POSSUM is the most widely applied, validated, surgical risk scoring system currently used in the UK. The original POSSUM equation has been modified in an effort to increase its accuracy as a risk prediction tool for in-hospital surgical mortality. Of these, P-POSSUM is the most widely used and validated general modification. Speciality-specific POSSUM has also been developed for use in colorectal, oesophagogastric and vascular patients, with some variable improvement in risk stratification. The available data, however, suggest that the various POSSUM models have a tendency to overestimate mortality rates. Within these limitations, the POSSUM models provide a useful tool for risk assessment, audit, and comparing outcomes between different units and within the same unit over a period of time. However, due to the variables included in the calculation, POSSUM cannot be used in the preoperative setting to inform risk.

ASA

In 1963 the American Society of Anesthesiologists (ASA) adopted a five-point classification system for assessing the physical status of a patient prior to elective surgery. A sixth category was added later (Box 15.4).

The ASA grade is essentially a combination of the subjective opinion of the anaesthetist taken in conjunction with a more objective assessment of the patient's general fitness for surgery, and is used routinely in most centres in the UK. There are a number of studies assessing the utility and accuracy of the ASA grade in determining surgical risk and, as anticipated given the nature of this scoring system, the literature is conflicting.

One study of 113 anaesthetists in the UK demonstrated such marked variation in the inter-individual assessment of 10 hypothetical patients that the authors concluded that the ASA grade should not be used on its own to predict surgical risk.[29] A further study of 97 anaesthetists demonstrated that the agreement for the assessment of each hypothetical patient varied from 31% to 85%. The overall correlation was only *fair*, and the inter-observer inconsistency was similar to that in a study from 20 years previously.[30]

However, the largest study to date is more encouraging.[31] Of 16 227 patients undergoing elective surgery over a 5-year period, 215 died within 4 weeks of operation. There was a significant correlation between perioperative mortality and the ASA grade. The mortality was lowest (0.4%) when the ASA grade was less than or equal to 2 and increased up to 7.3% in ASA grade 4 patients. The authors concluded that perioperative mortality can be predicted using the ASA grade.

✅ The ASA classification remains a quick, simple, widely used and reasonably accurate assessment of surgical risk in both the elective and emergency settings.

Box 15.4 • ASA classification

1. A normal healthy patient
2. A patient with mild systemic disease
3. A patient with severe systemic disease
4. A patient with severe systemic disease that is a constant threat to life
5. A moribund patient who is not expected to survive without the operation
6. A declared brain-dead patient whose organs are being removed for donor purposes

Note: If the surgery is an emergency, the ASA grade is followed by 'E' (for emergency), for example '3E'. Category 5 is always an emergency so should not be written without 'E'.

Surgical mortality probability model

The *surgical mortality probability model* (SMPM) was derived from a retrospective data analysis of almost 300 000 patients using the American College of Surgeons National Surgical Quality Improvement Program Database.[32] The primary outcome was 30-day mortality for patients undergoing non-cardiac surgery. The model identified three risk factors – ASA status; emergency or elective surgery; and surgery risk class – as the main determinants of outcome. Points are allocated in accordance with these three factors and predicted 30-day mortality is calculated from the total score (Table 15.2). Patients with a total risk score less than 5 had a predicted mortality of less than 0.5%, whereas a risk score greater than 6 predicted a mortality of more than 10%. This new model has yet to be fully externally and prospectively validated but may prove to be a useful risk tool for the future.

> ☑ The surgical mortality probability model (SMPM) is a newly devised risk assessment tool to predict 30-day surgical mortality. It has the advantage of using simple data readily available at the bedside. Whether the SMPM becomes widely established as a risk model will depend on the results of future validation studies.

Table 15.2 • The surgical mortality probability model (SMPM)

Risk factor	Points
ASA	
I	0
II	2
III	4
IV	5
V	6
Procedure severity	
Low	0
Intermediate	1
High	2
Urgency	
Elective	0
Emergency	1
Total points	**Mortality risk**
0–4	<0.5%
5–6	1.5–4%
7–9	>10%

The SMPM was developed to predict 30-day mortality for patients undergoing non-cardiac surgery. The model utilises three risk factors (ASA status, severity of procedure and urgency of the procedure). A score is awarded for each variable and the mortality risk is calculated form the total score.

Revised Cardiac Risk Index

The risk models described thus far have been designed to predict general mortality and morbidity for a patient population. Some risk models have been developed with the aim of predicting *specific* complications, such as risk of cardiac or pulmonary complications in the postoperative period. Of these, the *Revised Cardiac Risk Index* (RCRI) is the most commonly used. This model was published in 1999 with the aim to develop an index of risk for cardiac complications in major elective non-cardiac surgery.[33] Six independent predictors of complications were identified and included high-risk type of surgery, history of ischaemic heart disease, history of heart failure, history of stroke, diabetes requiring insulin, and elevated baseline serum creatinine. The risk of myocardial infarction and cardiac death could then be predicted according to the number of risk factors that were present (Table 15.3, **Fig. 15.1**). A recent systematic review was performed to evaluate the current accuracy of the RCRI to predict cardiac complications and death after non-cardiac surgery.[34] The authors concluded that the RCRI discriminated moderately well between patients at low versus high risk for cardiac events, but it did not perform well at predicting cardiac events after vascular surgery or at predicting death within 30 days.

Other risk prediction models

There are many other published risk prediction models that have not been presented here for reasons of brevity. Despite showing initial promise, many of these models have been disappointing when validated against external patient populations. The inability of these models to reproduce initial predictive accuracy has resulted in many failing to gain widespread acceptance. It is fair to say that at present there is no single model that can accurately predict surgical risk for all patient populations.

Functional assessment

Assessment of exercise capacity provides useful information about the functional status of a patient and their response to physiological stress. This information can then be used to inform about how the patient might respond to surgical stress and may therefore be used to predict perioperative risk. Patients with higher exercise tolerance usually have lower risk. Evaluation of exercise capacity may be subjective or objective, where formal exercise testing is performed.

Subjective assessment of exercise tolerance can usually be easily undertaken by asking some simple

Table 15.3 • The Revised Cardiac Risk Index: six risk factors to predict mortality and cardiovascular complications following surgery

Risk factor	Number of risk factors	Risk of death/ myocardial infarction
Major (high risk) surgery	0	0.4%
History of ischaemic heart disease	1	1%
History of heart failure	2	2.4%
History of cerebrovascular disease	3	5.4%
Diabetes requiring insulin treatment		
Serum creatinine concentration >177 μmol/L		

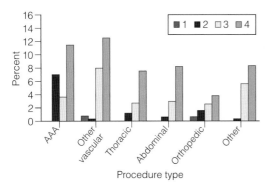

Figure 15.1 • Risk of major cardiac complications predicted by the Revised Cardiac Risk Index according to type of surgical procedure performed. The greater the number of risk factors present, the greater the risk of complications, irrespective of the type of surgery undertaken. Reproduced from Lee TH, Marcantonio ER, Mangione CM et al. Derivation and prospective validation of a simple index for prediction of cardiac risk of major noncardiac surgery. Circulation 1999; 100(10):1043–9. With permission from Wolters Kluwer Health.

Exercise capacity may be more objectively measured. *Metabolic equivalent of tasks* (METs) is a measure of energy expenditure related to physical activity. One MET may be considered as the resting metabolic rate (RMR) and is defined as energy consumption at a rate of 3.5 mL O_2 per kg per minute. Physical activities may be measured as a ratio compared to the RMR. For example, ironing clothes is equivalent to 1.8 METs and climbing two flights of stairs is equivalent to 4 METs. Some further examples are given in Table 15.4. This process may then be used to identify patients with reduced exercise capacity and who may benefit from a more objective assessment of their functional status. A full list of physical activities and the MET equivalents can be found at the web address listed in Ref. 37.

Table 15.4 • Examples of common activities and their metabolic equivalents (METs)

Activity	MET value
Watching television	1
Showering	2
Playing the piano	2.3
Washing the dishes	2.5
Playing snooker	2.5
Walking the dog	3
Slow ballroom dancing	3
Lawn bowls	3
Moderate housework	3.5
Climbing two flights of stairs	4
Golf (using an electric cart)	3.5
Golf (carrying clubs)	4.3
Mowing the lawn	5.5
Moderate swimming	5.8
Jogging	7
Running (10 minute/mile pace)	9.8

questions to assess the functional capacity of the patient. Determination of how many stairs a patient can climb before stopping due to limitation by symptoms, or how far they can walk on the flat without stopping, are commonly employed questions. There is evidence to suggest that these simple assessments of exercise capacity correlate with surgical risk. In a study of 600 patients undergoing major non-cardiac surgery serious postoperative complications, especially cardiac complications, were twice as common for those patients who were unable to climb two flights of stairs preoperatively.[35] Inability to climb two flights of stairs was associated with a positive predictive value of 82% for the development of cardiopulmonary complications in patients undergoing major thoracic and abdominal surgery and stair-climbing ability was inversely related to duration of hospital stay.[36]

Cardiopulmonary exercise testing (CPEX)

Cardiopulmonary exercise testing (CPEX) has been introduced in an attempt to provide a measurable, objective assessment of cardiorespiratory function for the assessment of surgical risk. In 1993 Older et al. performed CPEX testing among a group of elderly patients undergoing major surgery. An anaerobic threshold (AT) of less than 11 O_2 mL/min/kg was associated with a mortality rate of 18% compared with a mortality rate of less than 1% for those patients with an AT greater than 11 O_2 mL/min/kg.[38] Subsequent studies have similarly shown that an AT of less than 11 O_2 mL/min/kg was associated with increased hospital mortality following major elective abdominal and vascular surgery.[39,40] CPEX testing was also predictive of longer-term outcome. In a study of 102 patients undergoing elective abdominal aortic aneurysm repair, CPEX testing was not only predictive of 30-day mortality, but was also predictive of longer-term survival at 30 months.[40] Other studies have identified different values for the optimal discriminatory level for the anaerobic threshold. CPEX testing was undertaken in patients with a low functional capacity (less than 7 METs) who subsequently underwent major surgery. A lower AT value was associated with increased likelihood of postoperative complications and the optimal AT threshold for the study group was identified at 10.1 O_2 mL/min/kg.[41] An AT cut-off of 11 mL/kg/min was also a poor predictor of postoperative cardiopulmonary morbidity for patients undergoing oesophagectomy for cancer.[42] However, this study did demonstrate an association between lower exercise capacity and risk of complications, suggesting that this study was underpowered and/or an alternative AT threshold may be more suitable for this group of patients. The optimal cut-off value for the anaerobic threshold is generally accepted at 11 O_2 mL/min/kg.[43] It is interesting that this value closely relates to 4 METs (14 O_2 mL/min/kg) and, in turn, ability to climb two flights of stairs. This would suggest that patients who are able to climb two flights of stairs would have an anaerobic threshold greater than 11 O_2 mL/min/kg. Stair climbing therefore has the potential to be used as a screening tool for the identification of patients who would benefit from further assessment by CPEX testing. However, it remains unclear whether this is the optimal AT value or indeed if alternative thresholds should be adopted for different patient groups or for different surgical procedures.

Other limitations of CPEX testing relate to the process of conducting the test itself. Patients are required to exercise, usually on a cycle ergometer, and full assessment may be limited by physical ability rather than limitations due to cardiorespiratory function – for example, patients with arthritis or amputees. Another potential limitation of CPEX testing relates to availability and cost. The equipment and expertise to perform the test are not widely available in the UK at present. A survey conducted in England during 2008 found that only 30 (17%) hospitals had a CPEX service, with an additional 12 (7%) in the process of setting one up.[43] Despite these limitations, CPEX testing is becoming an increasingly adopted tool for preoperative assessment of higher risk patients undergoing major surgery.

✔ Cardiopulmonary exercise testing (CPEX) is the 'gold standard' measure of cardiorespiratory function. An anaerobic threshold (AT) less than 11 O_2 mL/min/kg has been associated with increased risk of postoperative complications and mortality, although the exact threshold AT value may need to be modified for different patient groups or different surgical procedures. CPEX testing requires specialist equipment and expertise to perform, and it is not widely available in the UK at present, but it is likely to be increasingly used for assessment of perioperative risk in selected high-risk patient populations.

Other objective measures of exercise capacity

The incremental shuttle walk test (ISWT) requires the patient to walk between two markers placed 10 metres apart within a set time period. This time period becomes progressively shorter, requiring more effort from the patient to make the distance within the shorter time. The test stops when the patient cannot reach the end of the 10-metre course within the given time. The ISWT has been shown to correlate with measured oxygen consumption in patients with cardiac and chronic lung disease.[44] A small study investigated the role of ISWT to predict 30-day mortality following oesophagogastrectomy.[45] No patients with a walk distance greater than 350 metres died in the postoperative period. Patients who managed to walk a distance less than 350 metres had a 50% 30-day mortality. Distance achieved on the shuttle walk test was compared with CPEX measurements in a study of 50 patients undergoing abdominal surgery. All patients who walked in excess of 360 metres had an anaerobic threshold (AT) greater than 11 O_2 mL/min/kg.[46] It was also noted that some patients who walked less than 360 metres may also have had satisfactory CPEX results, suggesting that the ISWT was good at identifying patients with a good AT, but could not accurately identify those who had a poor anaerobic threshold (i.e. a good positive predictive value, but poor negative predictive value). The study was not, however, sufficiently powered to investigate surgical outcomes. These data suggest that the ISWT may be used as a screening tool to identify patients who may then benefit from more formal exercise testing with CPEX (i.e. those who walked less than 350–360 metres).

The 6-minute walk test is another standardised assessment tool for estimation of exercise capacity. The test involves measuring the distance that a patient can cover during a 6-minute period. The patient is instructed to walk as fast as they can to cover the maximum possible distance. The AT determined by CPEX testing was compared with maximum distance achieved during the 6-minute walk test in a study of 110 patients awaiting major general surgery. Patients who completed in excess of 563 metres during the 6-minute test had an AT greater than 11 O_2 mL/min/kg and those who managed less than 427 metres had an AT less than 11 O_2 mL/min/kg.[47] The authors recommended that those patients who completed 563 metres did not require formal exercise testing, whereas those who could not manage more than 427 metres should undergo CPEX assessment. Those patients who walked between 427 and 563 metres belong to a group of 'clinical uncertainty', and other clinical risk factors and magnitude of surgery should be incorporated into the decision-making process.

> ✅ The incremental shuttle walk test (ISWT) and the 6-minute walk test are simple tools to objectively assess exercise capacity. They are indirect tests of oxygen consumption and have been shown to correlate with formal exercise testing values (CPEX). The main value of these tests is to identify higher-risk patient populations who may benefit from formal exercise testing.

Biomarkers to assess risk

There is emerging evidence that estimation of serum concentration of biomarkers in the preoperative period may assist risk stratification for patients undergoing surgery. Brain natriuretic peptide (BNP) and C-reactive protein (CRP) are the most promising biomarkers for risk assessment. BNP is released from cardiac ventricles in response to excessive stretching and elevated serum concentrations are correlated with prognosis in heart failure.[48] Elevated preoperative serum concentration of BNP (> 40 pg/mL) was associated with an increased risk of death and perioperative cardiac events in a study of 204 patients undergoing non-cardiac surgery.[49] A further study of 190 patients undergoing elective non-cardiac surgery also identified elevated serum NT-proBNP (a co-secretory product of BNP) as a predictor of postoperative cardiac complications, which was independently prognostic on multivariate analysis.[50]

A recent meta-analysis examined the predictive value of preoperative serum BNP concentrations for predicting postoperative mortality and cardiac complications following vascular surgery.[51] The authors concluded that elevated BNP concentrations were predictive of adverse outcome, but there was wide variation in the serum concentration of BNP that was chosen as the threshold for discrimination (range 35–100 pg/mL). The optimal discriminatory concentration remains unknown and it is likely that threshold values may vary depending on the patient group under investigation.

CRP is a marker of systemic inflammation and serum concentrations are associated with atherosclerotic disease and adverse outcomes in cancer. A preoperative serum CRP concentration greater than 6.5 mg/L was associated with increased 30-day mortality and postoperative cardiac complication rates in a study involving 592 patients undergoing vascular surgery (odds ratio 2.5; 95% confidence interval 1.5–4.3).[52] Moreover, this association was independent of serum BNP concentration and also established cardiac risk factors. The association between elevated CRP concentration and adverse perioperative outcome may be due, in part, to a correlation between markers of systemic inflammation and exercise capacity. Elevated serum CRP concentrations have been demonstrated to be inversely correlated with VO$_2$ max in male subjects without evidence of coronary heart disease.[53] Further study is required to determine the true value of serum biomarkers in risk assessment for surgical patients.

> ✅ Brain natriuretic peptide (BNP) and C-reactive protein (CRP) are the most promising biomarkers for risk assessment. Elevated preoperative serum concentrations have been associated with increased risk of mortality and cardiac complications in surgical patients; however, the optimal threshold cut-off value remains unknown. The real value of serum biomarkers may lie in the selection of patients into high- or low-risk groups and therefore help identify which patients merit further assessment.

Communicating risk

The use of risk prediction models, scoring systems, exercise tests and serum biomarkers as adjuncts to decision-making is an increasingly important part of surgical practice. This information must then be communicated effectively to the patient to allow fully informed choice. GMC guidance on this issue states that:

Clear, accurate information about the risks of any proposed investigation or treatment, presented in a way patients can understand, can help them make informed decisions. The amount of information about risk that the clinician should share with patients will depend on the individual patient and what they want, or need, to know. Discussions with patients should therefore focus on their individual situation and the risk to them.[1]

In communicating risk there are several techniques to impart the concept of how likely it is that the patient will have a complication of the procedure, or die as a result of it. These broadly fall into using numerical data or descriptive details of risk. As always, this communication must be tailored to the needs and expectations of the individual patient and it is likely that a combination of these techniques will be most appropriate.

Percentages alone are often not well understood, and as they apply to a population rather than an individual patient, they may be misleading. Odds, relative risk and absolute risk may be too complex, but quoting for example 'a 1 in 10 or 1 in 100 chance' may be helpful. Using relativity (comparison with a concept the patient understands) or examples ('of the last 50 patients this has happened to ...') may also clarify the concept of surgical risk to the patient.

Finally, it is worth remembering that the perceived surgical risk that concerns the surgeon is not necessarily what the patient is worried about. Assessing, discussing and communicating risk has the primary aim of allowing patients to understand what may happen to them, and to help them make an informed choice about investigation or therapeutic options. However, as a consequence of this, coupled with careful documentation, it affords the surgeon some protection against litigation.

Key points

- Estimation of surgical risk is vital to enhance treatment decision-making and facilitate informed consent, anticipate potential complications and target aspects of care to optimise the patient, and allow meaningful comparison of clinical outcomes, audit and quality assurance.
- Determination of surgical risk is complex, but may be more simply considered in terms of *patient-related* risks and *procedural-related* risks.
- Patient-related risk factors will be influenced by patient age, comorbidity, the underlying disease process, nutritional status and the performance status of the patient.
- Procedural-related risk factors include the grade of severity of the procedure planned, urgency of the procedure, volume of blood loss and other technical aspects.
- Risk prediction models and scoring systems (such as POSSUM, ASA and the Revised Cardiac Risk Index) have been developed in an attempt to improve risk prediction. These tools work best for patient populations (groups) rather than individual patients, and therefore their main value is for audit purposes and comparing outcomes between different units and within the same units over time. There is no perfect risk prediction model.
- Assessment of functional capacity may be easily undertaken through the use of simple screening questions. More objective measurements may be performed by using standardised walking tests or CPEX testing.
- Serum biomarkers, such as BNP and CRP, may have a future role in identifying high-risk surgical patient groups, who may then benefit from more detailed assessment.
- Estimation of surgical risk should include a thorough clinical assessment, an assessment of the functional capacity of the patient (through simple questions relating to METs) and should take into account the severity of the surgical procedure proposed. If this process identifies the patient to be at high risk, then further testing should be considered – for example, objective exercise testing (CPEX).

References

1. GMC. Consent: patients and doctors making decisions together. General Medical Council; 2008.

2. NICE. The use of routine preoperative tests for elective surgery. National Institute for Clinical Excellence; 2003.

3. Hartley MN, Sagar PM. The surgeon's 'gut feeling' as a predictor of post-operative outcome. Ann R Coll Surg Engl 1994;76(6, Suppl.):277–8.

4. Markus PM, Martell J, Leister I, et al. Predicting postoperative morbidity by clinical assessment. Br J Surg 2005;92(1):101–6.

5. Pearse RM, Holt PJE, Growcott MPW. Managing perioperative risk in patients undergoing elective non-cardiac surgery. Br Med J 2011;343:5759.

6. http://www.riskprediction.org.uk/; [accessed 25.09.12].

7. Copeland GP, Jones D, Walters M. POSSUM: a scoring system for surgical audit. Br J Surg 1991;78(3):355–60.

8. Whiteley MS, Prytherch DR, Higgins B, et al. An evaluation of the POSSUM surgical scoring system. Br J Surg 1996;83(6):812–5.

9. Wakabayashi H, Sano T, Yachida S, et al. Validation of risk assessment scoring systems for an audit of elective surgery for gastrointestinal cancer in elderly patients: an audit. Int J Surg 2007;5(5): 323–7.

10. Slim K, Panis Y, Alves A, et al. Predicting postoperative mortality in patients undergoing colorectal surgery. World J Surg 2006;30(1):100–6.

11. Tekkis PP, Kessaris N, Kocher HM, et al. Evaluation of POSSUM and P-POSSUM scoring systems in patients undergoing colorectal surgery. Br J Surg 2003;90(3):340–5.

12. Tekkis PP, Prytherch DR, Kocher HM, et al. Development of a dedicated risk-adjustment scoring system for colorectal surgery (colorectal POSSUM). Br J Surg 2004;91(9):1174–82.

13. Al-Homoud S, Purkayastha S, Aziz O, et al. Evaluating operative risk in colorectal cancer surgery: ASA and POSSUM-based predictive models. Surg Oncol 2004;13(2–3):83–92.

14. Vather R, Zargar-Shoshtari K, Adegbola S, et al. Comparison of the POSSUM, P-POSSUM and Cr-POSSUM scoring systems as predictors of postoperative mortality in patients undergoing major colorectal surgery. Aust N Z J Surg 2006;76(9):812–6.

15. Richards C, Leith F, Horgan PG, et al. Predicting post-operative mortality in colorectal cancer surgery: a systematic review of the accuracy of POSSUM, P-POSSUM and CR-POSSUM. Gastroenterology 2010;38(5, Suppl. 1):S-853.

16. Oomen JL, Cuesta MA, Engel AF. Comparison of outcome of POSSUM, P-POSSUM, and CR-POSSUM scoring after elective resection of the sigmoid colon for carcinoma or complicated diverticular disease. Scand J Gastroenterol 2007;42(7):841–7.

17. Bromage SJ, Cunliffe WJ. Validation of the CR-POSSUM risk-adjusted scoring system for major colorectal cancer surgery in a single center. Dis Colon Rectum 2007;50(2):192–6.

18. Zafirellis KD, Fountoulakis A, Dolan K, et al. Evaluation of POSSUM in patients with oesophageal cancer undergoing resection. Br J Surg 2002;89(9): 1150–5.

19. Tekkis PP, McCulloch P, Poloniecki JD, et al. Risk-adjusted prediction of operative mortality in oesophagogastric surgery with O-POSSUM. Br J Surg 2004;91(3):288–95.

20. Lagarde SM, Maris AK, de Castro SM, et al. Evaluation of O-POSSUM in predicting in-hospital mortality after resection for oesophageal cancer. Br J Surg 2007;94(12):1521–6.

21. Nagabhushan JS, Srinath S, Weir F, et al. Comparison of P-POSSUM and O-POSSUM in predicting mortality after oesophagogastric resections. Postgrad Med J 2007;83(979):355–8.

22. Lai F, Kwan TL, Yuen WC, et al. Evaluation of various POSSUM models for predicting mortality in patients undergoing elective oesophagectomy for carcinoma. Br J Surg 2007;94(9):1172–8.

23. Dutta S, Horgan PG, McMillan DC. POSSUM and its related models as predictors of postoperative mortality and morbidity in patients undergoing surgery for gastro-oesophageal cancer: a systematic review. World J Surg 2010;34(9):2076–82.

24. Prytherch DR, Sutton GL, Boyle JR. Portsmouth POSSUM models for abdominal aortic aneurysm surgery. Br J Surg 2001;88(7):958–63.

25. Grant SW, Grayson AD, Mitchell DC, et al. Evaluation of five risk prediction models for elective abdominal aortic aneurysm repair using the UK National Vascular Database. Br J Surg 2012;99(5):673–9.

26. Bown MJ, Cooper NJ, Sutton AJ, et al. The postoperative mortality of ruptured abdominal aortic aneurysm repair. Eur J Vasc Endovasc Surg 2004;27(1):65–74.

27. Kuhan G, Abidia AF, Wijesinghe LD, et al. POSSUM and P-POSSUM overpredict mortality for carotid endarterectomy. Eur J Vasc Endovasc Surg 2002;23(3): 209–11.

28. Mosquera D, Chiang N, Gibberd R. Evaluation of surgical performance using V-POSSUM risk-adjusted mortality rates. Aust N Z J Surg 2008;78(7):535–9.

29. Haynes SR, Lawler PG. An assessment of the consistency of ASA physical status classification allocation. Anaesthesia 1995;50(3):195–9.

30. Mak PH, Campbell RC, Irwin MG. The ASA Physical Status Classification: inter-observer consistency. American Society of Anesthesiologists. Anaesth Intensive Care 2002;30(5):633–40.

31. Prause G, Ratzenhofer-Comenda B, Pierer G, et al. Can ASA grade or Goldman's cardiac risk index predict perioperative mortality? A study of 16,227 patients. Anaesthesia 1997;52(3):203–6.

32. Glance LG, Lustik SJ, Hannan EL, et al. The surgical mortality probability model: derivation and validation of a simple risk prediction rule for noncardiac surgery. Ann Surg 2012;255:696–702.

33. Lee TH, Marcantonio ER, Mangione CM, et al. Derivation and prospective validation of a simple index for prediction of cardiac risk for noncardiac surgery. Circulation 1999;100:1043–9.

34. Ford MK, Beattie S, Wijeysundera DN. Systematic review: prediction of perioperative cardiac complications and mortality by the Revised Cardiac Risk Index. Ann Intern Med 2010;152(1):26–35.

35. Reilly DF, McNeely MJ, Doerner D, et al. Self-reported exercise tolerance and the risk of serious perioperative complications. Arch Intern Med 1999;159(18):2185–92.

36. Girish M, Trayney E, Dammann O, et al. Symptom-limited stair climbing as a predictor of postoperative cardiopulmonary complications after high-risk surgery. Chest 2001;120:1147–51.

37. Ainsworth BE, Haskell WL, Herrmann SD, et al. Compendium of physical activities: a second update of codes and MET values. Med Sci Sports Exercise 2011;43(8):1575–81. https://sites.google.com/site/compendiumofphysicalactivities/home; [accessed 25.09.12]

38. Older P, Smith R, Courtney P, et al. Preoperative evaluation of cardiac failure and ischemia in elderly patients by cardiopulmonary exercise testing. Chest 1993;104(3):701–4.

39. Wilson RJ, Davies S, Yates D. Impaired functional capacity is associated with all-cause mortality after major elective abdominal surgery. Br J Anaesth 2010;105:297–303.

40. Thompson AR, Peters N, Lovegrove RE, et al. Cardiopulmonary exercise testing provides a predictive tool for early and late outcomes in abdominal aortic aneurysm patients. Ann R Coll Surg Engl 2011;93(6):474–81.

41. Snowden C, Prentis J, Anderson HL, et al. Submaximal cardiopulmonary exercise testing predicts complications and hospital length of stay in patients undergoing major elective surgery. Ann Surg 2010;251(3):535–41.

42. Forshaw MJ, Strauss DC, Davies AR, et al. Is cardiopulmonary exercise testing a useful test before oesophagectomy? Ann Thorac Surg 2008;85:294–9.

43. Simpson JC, Sutton H, Grocott MP. Cardiopulmonary exercise testing – a survey of current use in England. J Intensive Care Soc 2009;10:275–8.

44. Singh SJ, Morgan MD, Hardman AE, et al. Comparison of oxygen uptake during a conventional treadmill test and the shuttle walking test in chronic airflow limitation. Eur Respir J 1994;7:2016–20.

45. Whiting P, Murray P, Hutchinson S, et al. The role of the shuttle walking test in predicting mortality and morbidity post oesophagogastric surgery. Critical Care 2005;9(Suppl. 1):P43.

46. Struthers R, Erasmus P, Holmes K, et al. Assessing fitness for surgery: a comparison of questionnaire, incremental shuttle walk and cardiopulmonary exercise testing in general surgical patients. Br J Anaesth 2008;101(6):774–80.

47. Sinclair RCF, Batterham AM, Davies S, et al. Validity of the 6 min walk test in prediction of the anaerobic threshold before major non-cardiac surgery. Br J Anaesth 2012;108(1):30–5.

48. Maisel A, Krishnaswamy P, Nowak R, et al. Rapid measurement of B-type natriuretic peptide in the emergency diagnosis of heart failure. N Engl J Med 2002;347(3):161–7.

49. Cuthbertson BH, Amiri AR, Croal BL, et al. The utility of B-type natriuretic peptide in predicting perioperative cardiac events after major non-cardiac surgery. Br J Anaesth 2007;99(2): 170–6.

50. Yeh HM, Lau HP, Lin JM, et al. Preoperative plasma N-terminal pro-brain natriuretic peptide as a marker of cardiac risk in patients undergoing elective non-cardiac surgery. Br J Surg 2005;92: 1041–5.

51. Rodseth RN, Padayachee L, Biccard BM. A meta-analysis of the utility of pre-operative brain natriuretic peptide in predicting early and intermediate-term mortality and major adverse cardiac events in vascular surgical patients. Anaesthesia 2008;63:1226–33.

52. Goei D, Hoeks SE, Boersma E, et al. Incremental value of high-sensitivity C-reactive protein and N-terminal pro-B-type natriuretic peptide for the prediction of postoperative cardiac events in non-cardiac vascular surgery patients. Coron Artery Dis 2009;20:219–24.

53. Kullo IJ, Khaleghi M, Hensrud DD. Markers of inflammation are inversely associated with VO_2 max in asymptomatic men. J Appl Physiol 2007;102:1374–9.

16

Perioperative and intensive care management of the surgical patient

R. Michael Grounds
Andrew Rhodes

Introduction

Over the last 50 years the incidence of death directly attributable to anaesthesia has decreased. In the 1950s a number of studies demonstrated that the postoperative mortality solely associated with anaesthesia was approximately 1 in 2500[1-3] and by 1987, in the *Report of a confidential enquiry into perioperative deaths (CEPOD)*,[4] this cause of death had fallen to 1 in 185000. This chapter deals with the perioperative and intensive care management of these patients with a specific focus on how ensuring that each patient has adequate cardiovascular performance for their needs during the perioperative period can reduce their risk of complications and death.

Postoperative critical care is a key factor to the improvement of outcome in surgical patients, particularly to those patients who are at high risk of postoperative morbidity and mortality. Thus, postoperative critical care admission should always be considered when the preoperative physiological condition of the patient suggests that there is a reasonable probability or risk of postoperative complications and organ dysfunction. In order to provide this postoperative critical care it is obviously necessary to be able to identify these high-risk patients preoperatively.

How big is the problem?

In a recent analysis of over four million surgical procedures in the UK, a subgroup of high-risk patients was identified.[5] The mortality in this high risk group of 513924 patients was 12.3%, compared to the overall mortality rates of 0.44% for elective and 5.4% for emergency surgery. This high-risk group of patients accounted for 83.8% of all deaths but only 12.5% of procedures. For the 31633 patients admitted to an intensive care unit (ICU) electively there was a mortality rate of 10.1% and the 24764 emergency surgical patients carried a mortality of 28.6%. Despite the high mortality rates, fewer than 15% of these patients were admitted to the ICU and the highest mortality rate (39%) was found in patients who required ICU admission following initial care in a ward environment.

Repeated publications by the National Confidential Enquiry into Postoperative Deaths (NCEPOD) have cited inadequate preoperative preparation, inappropriate intraoperative monitoring and poor postoperative care as contributing causes of perioperative mortality. The most recent[6] NCEPOD Report (Knowing the Risk) suggests that patients in the UK often die after surgery because they are not given the level of care they are entitled to or could reasonably expect. In this latest report less than half of the patients actually received the care that the advisors felt was the minimal acceptable standard. Twelve per cent of hospitals had no method for recognising the acutely ill patient and only 22% of patients deemed as being at high risk actually went to any sort of critical care area postoperatively and 48% of high-risk patients who died never went to any sort of critical facility. As far back as 1996, the Department of Health issued guidelines as to which patients should be admitted to critical care units.[7] In particular, they suggested that postoperative patients who needed close monitoring for more than a few hours after surgery should be admitted. However, the great variation in underlying pathology and premorbid physiology of these patients makes it very difficult to provide hard and fast rules as to which patients will benefit from perioperative admission to either ICUs or high-dependency units (HDUs). What is clear from a number of studies is that at present the care of patients before admission to ICU is often suboptimal.[8,9] This situation is partly exacerbated by the paucity of both ICU and HDU beds in the UK[10–12] and the fact that patients were often admitted later and with a worse severity of illness.

Why do patients die after surgery?

Major surgery is associated with a significant stress response[13] that is vital for the body to recover and heal from the surgical trauma. This response manifests in many different ways; however, a common delineating pattern is one of a hyperdynamic circulation with increased oxygen requirements from 110 mL/min per m^2 at rest to 170 mL/min per m^2 postoperatively.[14] If the body is unable to increase the cardiac output in response to the surgical stress, then the increased need for oxygen cannot be met and the patient develops tissue dysoxia and cellular dysfunction. This has been described by some authors as an acquired oxygen debt.[15] If left, this will result in organ failure and death. The important point to recognise is that the normal response to surgery is to increase the cardiac output and the delivery of oxygen to the tissues. Any patient who for whatever reason is unable to develop this response is at higher risk of subsequent complications.

What is a high-risk surgical patient?

The challenge is the early identification of patients who are at high risk of postoperative complications and death, and this is vital in order to ensure that correct care and therapy are initiated at an optimal time in order to reduce the associated morbidity and mortality.[6] On the whole, this patient group is characterised by undergoing major surgery whilst having concurrent medical illnesses that limit their physiological reserve to compensate for the stressful situation (Box 16.1). More sophisticated analyses of these relationships have been described. In particular, elective surgical patients can be assessed by cardiopulmonary exercise testing,[14,16] in which a strong correlation has been demonstrated between anaerobic threshold and perioperative mortality. The anaerobic threshold is the point where aerobic

Box 16.1 • Criteria for identifying high-risk surgical patients developed by Shoemaker[15]

High-risk surgery (intraperitoneal, intrathoracic, or suprainguinal vascular procedures)

Ischaemic heart disease

Previous severe cardiorespiratory illness, including myocardial infarction, stroke, chronic obstructive pulmonary disease, etc., including admission to critical care unit for cardiorespiratory illness

History of congestive heart failure

Late-stage vascular disease

Age >70 years with limited physiological reserve, particularly limited cardiorespiratory reserve

Extensive surgery for carcinoma: oesophagectomy, gastrectomy, cystectomy in patient with limited physiological reserve

Insulin therapy for diabetes

Acute abdominal catastrophe with haemodynamic instability: peritonitis, perforated viscus, pancreatitis

Acute massive blood loss >8 units at time of surgery

Proven septicaemia: positive blood culture or septic focus

Acute respiratory failure: P_aO_2 < 8.0 kPa or F_iO_2 >0.4 or mechanical ventilation > 48 hours

Acute renal failure: urea > 20 mmol/L or creatinine >176 mmol/L

NECPOD reports[6] that the more risk factors or predictors a patient has, the greater the risk of perioperative and postoperative complications and death.

metabolism fails to provide adequate adenosine triphosphate and anaerobic metabolism starts to reduce the resultant deficit. The threshold is determined by monitoring inhaled and exhaled levels of oxygen and carbon dioxide during escalating levels of exercise. This provides an objective measure of physiological reserve. However, it must be remembered that complex cardiopulmonary testing in patients who have established poor cardiorespiratory reserve is only of use if used to target preoperative preparation and these patients must have specific optimisation of their comorbidities prior to surgery whenever possible. This requires that patients booked for elective surgery have all their comorbidities treated and investigated to ensure best possible physiological status prior to surgery. This is also the opportunity to consider if surgical intervention is the best course of action in view of the risk of the potential adverse outcomes. A full and truthful risk assessment should be undertaken and the patient fully involved in the decision to proceed to surgery. A recent report suggested that only 7.5% of patients at high risk of death or severe complications were given any indication of their risks of mortality and morbidity prior to surgery.[6]

Variables associated with postoperative complications and death

Several authors[17,18] have examined the prognostic ability or power of many variables that can be monitored in the postoperative setting. One group[5] found that none of the routinely measured variables such as heart rate, blood pressure, central venous pressure, urine output or any marker of acid–base status was able to predict subsequent postoperative complications. The variables independently associated with subsequent significant complications were the central venous oxygen saturation and the cardiac index. This association between oxygen flux in the perioperative period and subsequent complications is not new and is essentially the same as work published by Shoemaker et al.[15] some 30 years previously, who identified the key variables as being cardiac index, oxygen delivery and oxygen consumption. It was from this body of work that the theories surrounding the targeting of oxygen delivery to values of over 600 mL/min per m^2 in the perioperative period to improve patient outcome originated.

The role of the splanchnic circulation

There is some evidence of the role of the splanchnic circulation in the pathogenesis of postoperative morbidity and mortality. It has been shown that increasing global tissue oxygen delivery will increase splanchnic oxygen delivery.[19–21] It would appear that in the early stages of shock any inadequacy of tissue oxygen delivery predominantly affects the splanchnic circulation.[22] The splanchnic circulation is particularly sensitive to hypoperfusion states, and the reduction in flow to the splanchnic bed is out of proportion to the overall reduction in cardiac output and is usually the last major system blood flow to recover when the hypoperfusion state improves.[23–35] It is thought that this splanchnic hypoperfusion leads to disruption of the enteric mucosal barrier with translocation of endotoxins and micro-organisms into the systemic circulation.[26–29] This translocation initiates a cytokine pathway, increasing the risk of sepsis and organ failure. This risk of splanchnic hypoperfusion and translocation increases with age, the urgency of the surgery and the preoperative presence of bowel obstruction. The translocation of bacteria and endotoxins induces cytokine release by tissue macrophages, activates the complement and coagulation systems, and produces a proinflammatory

state. These cytokines themselves can impair oxygen delivery to the splanchnic circulation, further increasing translocation.

Strategies to improve outcomes

The concept of augmenting cardiac output in the perioperative period to improve the outcome of surgical patients has been described by many authors as 'optimisation' or 'goal-directed therapy'. The main aim of all optimisation strategies for high-risk surgical patients has been to ensure that the circulatory status of the patients is adequate for their needs in the perioperative period. This has been achieved with a number of differing protocols utilising different time periods, resuscitation end-points and pharmacological agents. There are few to no data describing the relative efficacy of the different protocols when compared with each other, as they have nearly all been compared against 'standard' care. Almost all studies where this approach has been used have led to an improved outcome.

Oxygen delivery

In order to understand the rationale behind many of the protocols that have been utilised in the perioperative setting, it is vital to appreciate the important variables that determine oxygen delivery. These variables can be summarised according to the following equations:

$$\text{Oxygen content} = ([1.34 \times \text{Hb} \times (S_aO_2 / 100)] + (0.023 \times P_aO_2))$$

$$\text{Oxygen delivery} = \text{Cardiac output} \times \text{Oxygen content}$$

It therefore becomes clear that in order to ensure that an adequate volume of oxygen is delivered to the body's vital organs, the haemoglobin concentration (Hb), the arterial saturation of haemoglobin with oxygen (S_aO_2) and the cardiac index must all be at a satisfactory level. Maximising all three of these variables to clinically acceptable levels is the aim of resuscitation in any given patient, although not always achievable. The Hb level is governed by the clinical situation as well as the underlying pathophysiological process, but many experts aim to keep the Hb level above 9 g/dL in a stable perioperative setting. The S_aO_2 is usually targeted to be over 95% with increased inspired oxygen and/or continuous positive airways pressure (CPAP) if necessary, so the main variable that can be manipulated is the cardiac output. There is a growing understanding that atelectasis in the postoperative period is not just associated with hypoxaemia but also with a proinflammatory response that potentiates tissue injury. As a result the use of CPAP or other non-invasive positive pressure ventilation (NIPPV) therapy has the potential to improve many physiological parameters without serious side-effects in certain high-risk groups of patients, but whether this leads to improved outcome or reduced hospital stay is not yet clear and requires further investigation.

Cardiac output can be increased with several easy-to-use protocols. The targeting of cardiac index does necessitate the measurement and monitoring of this variable, which nowadays can be done relatively non-invasively. Once measured, if the cardiac output is perceived to be too low, then it is increased with intravenous volume therapy and then, if it has still not improved sufficiently, pharmacologically using appropriate cardiovascular pharmaceutical agents that will improve cardiac output.

Measurement and monitoring of cardiac output

There are a variety of technologies available to monitor cardiac output. Traditionally a pulmonary artery catheter has been used, which enables a thermodilution curve to be constructed across the right ventricle, thus enabling cardiac output to be calculated from the Stewart–Hamilton equation. In recent times this tool has become highly controversial due to a lack of evidence demonstrating a beneficial effect on outcome and the perceived invasiveness of its approach. Many new devices and techniques are now available that can provide the same information in a less invasive fashion. Oesophageal Doppler analysis of the descending aorta has been widely described in the perioperative period, while titrating therapy with pulse power analysis has recently been shown to reduce length of stay and postoperative complications.

Protocol-driven therapy to augment oxygen delivery

Inappropriately low values of cardiac index, oxygen delivery and oxygen consumption result in abnormal microcirculatory blood flow as a result of vasoconstriction in the capillary beds. Unfortunately it is not possible to detect these tissue hypoxic states with traditional monitored variables; therefore, it is necessary to monitor and titrate therapy to cardiac index and oxygen delivery. Shoemaker et al.[30] utilised targets of cardiac index, oxygen delivery and consumption ($4.5 \text{ L/min per m}^2$, $DO_2 > 600 \text{ mL/min per m}^2$ and $VO_2 > 170 \text{ mL/min per m}^2$) that had been previously demonstrated to be the median values for survivors following major surgery, in order to show that the repayment of an incurred oxygen debt within 8 hours resulted in an improved outcome. It has been consistently shown[31–36] that reductions in mortality and morbidity are obtained when these levels of oxygen delivery are achieved and that in conjunction with the decreased complications there is a reduced length of stay. It is worth noting that many patients are unable to achieve adequate levels of oxygen delivery without assistance in this setting. Not all patients will achieve these targets, even with assistance. For these patients an increase in oxygen delivery may still be beneficial, although it is unclear exactly how hard to drive them so that the complications do not override any benefit accrued. Most successful trials have targeted an oxygen delivery of $600 \text{ mL/min per m}^2$. This therefore seems a sensible target to use in this setting. This does not mean, however, that this is the best target as others that may be better may be available but simply have yet to be studied. Other goals or targets are available, for instance maximal stroke volume or central venous saturations and serum lactate. Until they have been proven to be beneficial, however, it would be prudent to continue with the published data.

☑☑ Reductions in mortality, morbidity and hospital stay have consistently been shown to occur with improved tissue levels of oxygen delivery.[30–36]

Fluid resuscitation

It is important to recognise that protocol-driven therapy of this nature is not about giving more intravenous fluid to the patients; it is about giving the right amount at the right time. There is evidence that excessive fluid administration is detrimental in critically ill and postoperative patients (**Fig. 16.1**) and it is likely that inappropriate volume overload has just as many detrimental effects as inadequate volume resuscitation. The 2011 NCEPOD report[6] shows that mortality is related to fluid management, with mortality being only 4.7% in patients receiving adequate preoperative fluids as compared to 20.5% and 33.3%, respectively, in those patients who received either inadequate or excessive preoperative intravenous fluid. This mandates the need to monitor very carefully fluid administration in critically ill or high-risk patients where simple measures or markers of preload status are often inadequate. Defining the end-point at which filling is optimal and the need for inotropic therapy begins is difficult. A plateau in the stroke volume, the flow correction time as determined by oesophageal Doppler and the stroke volume variation (with the pulse pressure analysis) can all be used to define the end-point. The

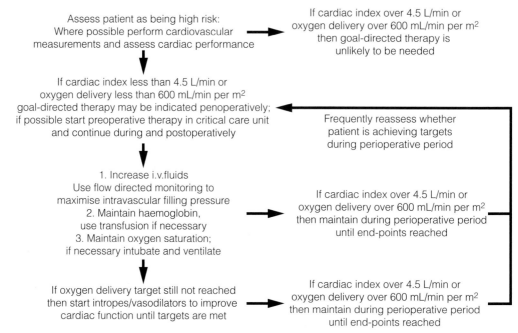

Figure 16.1 • Algorithm for 'protocol-driven therapy'.

British Consensus Guidelines on Intravenous Fluid Therapy for Adult Surgical Patients (GIFTASUP) state that 'in high-risk patients treatment with intravenous fluid and inotropes should be aimed at achieving predetermined goals for cardiac output and oxygen delivery' in order to improve outcome.[37] It is important that the end-points of resuscitation are reached with the minimal amount of volume and inotropic therapy possible.

Timing of protocol-driven therapy

The timing of goal-directed therapy (GDT) is very important in order to achieve the benefits demonstrated in the published studies. Most of the studies that have had significant impact on mortality have been started before surgery and then continued on throughout the perioperative period. Due to resource constraints this is difficult to implement, so many authors have since studied the effects of GDT either only during surgery or during the postoperative period. Although nearly all of these studies have also demonstrated benefit, the effects are not as dramatic as when therapy is started in the preoperative period. Whether this is a real effect or whether it is an artefact of study design is difficult to ascertain. A pragmatic response is to initiate therapy as soon as is practically possible – either during or immediately after surgery. It makes no sense to wait until after problems have developed. In practice this means that

the GDT should be started as early as possible and continue until the patient is stable in the postoperative period (Box 16.2). The duration, timing and setting of therapy will mandate the type of monitoring technology used. For instance, although it has been suggested that intraoperative fluid management can be guided by oesophageal Doppler,[38] this particular monitor is difficult to use in the postoperative phase as awake patients do not readily tolerate the oesophageal Doppler probe.

> ✔ Goal-directed therapy to optimise the patient's circulation and therefore tissue oxygenation should be commenced as soon as possible and continued into the postoperative period.

Box 16.2 • Clinical guidelines for the implementation of goal-directed therapy in high-risk surgical patients

Identify the high-risk patient
See Box 16.1 for Shoemaker criteria
Particularly identify elderly patients with poor cardiorespiratory reserve, ischaemic heart disease with evidence of heart failure

Identify the operation
Operations likely to last longer than 1.5 hours
Lack of postoperative critical care facilities

Box 16.2 • (*cont.*) Clinical guidelines for the implementation of goal-directed therapy in high-risk surgical patients

Emergency surgery, particularly abdominal surgery

Perioperative goal-directed therapy

1. Assess the patient preoperatively: where possible perform cardiovascular measurements to assess cardiac performance. Measure cardiac output and oxygen delivery.
2. If cardiac index > 4.5 L/min per m² and/or oxygen delivery > 600 mL/min per m² (body surface area), then no further goal-directed therapy will be necessary. Patient can proceed to anaesthesia and surgery.
3. If cardiac index < 4.5 L/min per m² and/or oxygen delivery < 600 mL/min per m² (body surface area), then further goal-directed therapy may be Indicated either prior to surgery or, if this is not possible, then Immediately following surgery in a dedicated critical care area.
4. If cardiac index < 4.5 L/min per m² and/or oxygen delivery < 600 mL/min per m² (body surface area):
   (a) Increase intravenous fluids: direct therapy using flow-directed monitoring equipment to maximise intravascular filling pressure.
   (b) Maintain adequate haemoglobin concentration with blood transfusion if necessary.
   (c) Maintain blood oxygen saturation at 95% or greater with supplemental oxygenation or artificial ventilation.
5. If despite these measures cardiac index is <4.5 L/min per m² and/or oxygen delivery <600 mL/min per m² (body surface area), then consider the use of cardiovascular performance-enhancing therapy. Although a number of different inotropic and vasodilator therapies have been used (including adrenaline and dobutamine), the best results seem to have been achieved using dopexamine, which acts mainly as a vasodilator with some positive inotropic effects. Start dopexamine at 0.5 μg/kg per min and increase the rate of infusion incrementally every 10–15 minutes until either the target oxygen delivery has been achieved or there is an increase in heart rate 20% greater than the patient's resting rate or there are signs of ischaemia on the ECG. (If the patient is very tachycardic prior to starting inotropes, it is important to recognise this and not try to increase cardiac output at the expense of increasing the already raised heart rate.) Maintain intravascular filling pressure during this period of inotrope therapy.

Maintain this goal-directed therapy into the postoperative period until there is evidence that the intraoperative oxygen debt is repaid (return of base deficit to normal, blood lactate concentration within normal range).

Conclusions

This overview of the literature relating to the high-risk surgical patient and current improvements associated with goal-directed therapy leads to some inevitable conclusions:

1. There is good evidence to suggest that patients with poor cardiorespiratory reserve have a higher mortality and complication rate when undergoing major surgery. Most of these patients can be identified by simple clinical methods before surgery.
2. It is likely that there are significant numbers of patients undergoing different types of surgery who may be at substantial risk of developing major complications or death.
3. A number of randomised controlled clinical studies have consistently demonstrated the improvement in outcome that can be achieved in these patients by the use of goal-directed therapy aimed at temporarily improving the cardiovascular performance of high-risk patients so that non-survivors have the same cardiorespiratory performance as survivors.
4. Studies have shown that benefit may be obtained in a wide range of surgery, including vascular surgery, colorectal surgery, trauma, orthopaedics, major cancer surgery and cardiac surgery.
5. From the work of Shoemaker and colleagues it would seem that about 8% of the surgical population would fulfil this definition of being at high risk of complications or death following major surgery. It would appear that these patients have a postoperative 30-day mortality of 20–30%, representing 90–95% of all surgical deaths. This number is likely to increase with an ageing population on whom increasingly complex surgery is being performed.
6. Although optimising the circulation produces significant reductions in mortality and postoperative complications in the higher-risk patient, it is now clear that important reductions in complications can be achieved in patients who have a lower mortality risk but for whom a significant complication risk exists.
7. It is also apparent that optimising the circulation can be carried out using several different techniques and at different times (i.e. preoperatively, intraoperatively and postoperatively).

8. The decision to operate on high-risk patients should be made at consultant level and should involve surgeons as well as those who will provide the intra- and postoperative care (anaesthetists and critical care consultants).

9. An assessment of mortality risk should be made explicit to the patient and recorded clearly on the consent form and in the medical notes.

10. Appropriate intraoperative physiological monitoring is required for all high-risk patients and NICE Medical Technology Guidance 3 relating to cardiac output monitoring should be applied.

11. All hospitals undertaking surgery for high-risk patients should have facilities to provide perioperative goal-directed monitoring and therapy and the hospital should analyse the volume of work they undertake to ensure they have sufficient capacity of facilities to be able to accommodate all the patients they treat. This should be assessed annually.[6]

12. The Royal College of Surgeons of England have considered the high-risk surgical patient and have made a series of key suggestions for improvement in care and outcomes.[39] These include recommendations that all hospitals should formalise their pathways for unscheduled adult surgical care. That there should be prompt recognition and treatment of emergencies and complications to improve outcomes and reduce costs. Hospitals should match theatre access to patient needs. Every patient should have his/her expected risk of death estimated and documented. High-risk patients are those at greater risk of death than 5% and all should have active consultant input and be admitted to a critical care area postoperatively for at least 12 hours. Surgical procedures with a risk of death greater than 10% should only be conducted under the direct supervision of a consultant surgeon and consultant anaesthetist.

Key points

- Patients with poor cardiorespiratory reserve undergoing major operations have a high postoperative complication and mortality rate. The mortality rate is much higher if these patients have emergency operations.
- These patients can be identified preoperatively by simple clinical history and examination.
- This high postoperative complication and mortality rate can be significantly reduced by goal-directed therapy aimed at enhancing the cardiorespiratory performance of these patients with poor physiological reserve during the perioperative period.
- Goal-directed therapy aims to ensure that tissue oxygen delivery is enhanced to levels shown to confer survival without postoperative complications.

References

1. Beecher HK, Todd DP. A study of the deaths associated with anaesthesia and surgery. Ann Surg 1954;140:2–5.

2. Edwards G, Morton HJV, Pask EA, et al. Deaths associated with anaesthesia. Anaesthesia 1956;11:194–220.

3. Dornette WHL, Orth OS. Death in the operating room. Anesth Analg 1956;3:545–69.

4. Buck N, Devlin HB, Lunn JN. The report of a confidential enquiry into perioperative deaths. London: Nuffield Provincial Hospitals Trust and the King Edward's Hospital Fund for London; 1987.

5. Pearse RM, Harrison DA, James P, et al. Identification and characterisation of the high-risk surgical population in the United Kingdom. Crit Care 2006;10(3):R81.

6. National Confidential Enquiry into Patient Outcome and Death. Knowing the risk. A review of the perioperative care of surgical patients. 2011.
This report studies the risk of dying and postoperative complications and reports on the deficiencies in the UK NHS hospital system and clearly shows that poor outcome is related to lack of provision of care facilities and the inability of clinicians to grasp the significance that preoperative comorbidities have on patient outcome after surgery.

7. Department of Health. Guidelines on admission to and discharge from intensive care and high dependency units. London: NHS Executive; 1996.

8. McQuillan P, Pilkington S, Allan A, et al. Confidential enquiry into quality of care before admission to intensive care. Br Med J 1998;316(7148):1853–8.

9. Garrard C, Young D. Suboptimal care of patients before admission to intensive care is caused by a failure to appreciate or apply the ABCs of life support. Br Med J 1998;316(7148):1841–2.

10. Purdie JA, Ridley SA, Wallace PG. Effective use of regional intensive therapy units. Br Med J 1990;300(6717):79–81.

11. Henao FJ, Daes JE, Dennis RJ. Risk factors for multi-organ failure: a case control study. J Trauma 1991;31:74–80.

12. Bion J. Rationing intensive care. Br Med J 1995;310(6981):682–3.

13. Desborough JP. The stress response to trauma and surgery. Br J Anaesth 2000;85:109–17.

14. Older P, Hall A, Hader R. Cardiopulmonary exercise testing as a screening test for perioperative management of major surgery in the elderly. Chest 1999;116:355–62.

15. Shoemaker WC, Appel PL, Kram HB. Role of oxygen debt in the development of organ failure, sepsis and death in high-risk surgical patients. Chest 1992;102:208–15.

16. Gibbons RJ, Balady GJ, Timothy Bricker J, et al. ACC/AHA 2002 guideline update for exercise testing: summary article. A report of the American College of Cardiology/American Heart Association Task Force on Practice Guidelines (Committee to Update the 1997 Exercise Testing Guidelines). J Am Coll Cardiol 2002;40:1531–40.

17. Shoemaker WC. Cardiorespiratory patterns of surviving and non-surviving postoperative patients. Surg Gynecol Obstet 1972;134:810–4.

18. Shoemaker WC, Montgomery ES, Kaplan E, et al. Physiologic patterns in surviving and non-surviving shock patients. Use of sequential cardiorespiratory variables in defining criteria for therapeutic goals and early warning of death. Arch Surg 1973;106:630–6.

19. Ruokonen E, Takala J, Kari A. Regional blood flow and oxygen transport in patients with the low cardiac output syndrome after cardiac surgery. Crit Care Med 1993;21:1304–11.

20. Ruokonen E, Takala J, Kari A, et al. Regional blood flow and oxygen transport in septic shock. Crit Care Med 1993;21:1296–303.

21. Uusaro A, Ruokonen E, Takal J. Splanchnic oxygen transport after cardiac surgery: evidence for inadequate tissue perfusion after stabilization of hemodynamics. Intensive Care Med 1996;22:26–33.

22. Gutierrez G, Bismar H, Dantzker DR, et al. Comparison of gastric intramucosal pH with measures of oxygen transport and consumption in critically ill patients. Crit Care Med 1992;20:451–7.

23. Adar R, Franklin A, Spark RF, et al. Effect of dehydration and cardiac tamponade on superior mesenteric artery flow: role of vasoactive substances. Surgery 1976;79:534–43.

24. Bailey RW, Bulkley GB, Hamilton SR, et al. Protection of the small intestine from nonocclusive mesenteric ischemic injury due to cardiogenic shock. Am J Surg 1987;153:108–16.

25. McNeill JR, Stark RD, Greenway CV. Mortality and morbidity in gastro-oesophageal cancer surgery: initial results of ASCOT multi-centre prospective cohort study. Br Med J 2003;327:1192–7.

26. Ohri SK, Somasundaram S, Koak Y, et al. The effect of intestinal hypoperfusion on intestinal absorption and permeability during cardiopulmonary bypass. Gastroenterology 1994;106:318–23.

27. Brooks SG, May J, Sedman P, et al. Translocation of enteric bacteria in humans. Br J Surg 1993;80:901–2.

28. O'Boyle CJ, MacFie J, Mitchell CJ, et al. Microbiology of bacterial translocation in humans. Gut 1998;42:29–35.

29. Deitch EA. Multiple organ failure. Pathophysiology and potential future therapy. Ann Surg 1992;216:117–34.

30. Shoemaker WC, Appel PC, Cram HB, et al. Prospective trial of supranormal values of survivors as therapeutic goals in high risk surgical patients. Chest 1988;94:1176–86.

This study is important because it is the study that introduced the concept of goal-directed therapy for high-risk surgical patients nearly a quarter of a century ago. This year the Royal College of Surgeons of England has finally published guidelines for this group of patients that essentially endorse the findings and recommendations of Shoemaker et al.

31. Boyd O, Grounds RM, Bennett ED. A randomized clinical trial of the effect of deliberate perioperative increase of oxygen delivery on mortality in high risk surgical patients. JAMA 1993;270:2699–708.

This was the first full well-conducted, randomised controlled study of goal-directed therapy for perioperative enhancement of the cardiovascular systems of these high-risk surgical patients. It was stopped before it was completed by the local hospital research ethics committee because the surgeons felt that it was obvious which group their patients were in and felt it was unethical to continue when the benefits were so obvious.

32. Wilson J, Woods I, Fawcett J, et al. Reducing the risk of major elective surgery: randomised controlled trial of preoperative optimization of oxygen delivery. Br Med J 1999;318:1099–103.

This study is important because not only did it have a control group where clinicians not involved with the study were able to decide on the postoperative treatment and send patients back to the ward postoperatively (which is common practice in many hospitals in the UK due to lack of critical care facilities), but it also divided the group admitted to intensive care into two groups for therapeutic intervention and thus showed that there could be a difference in outcome if different drugs were used for goal-directed therapy.

33. Lobo SM, Salgado PF, Castillo VG, et al. Effects of maximizing oxygen delivery on morbidity and mortality in high-risk surgical patients. Crit Care Med 2000;28:3396–404.

34. Bishop MH, Shoemaker WC, Appel PL, et al. Prospective, randomized trial of survivor values of cardiac index, oxygen delivery, and oxygen consumption as resuscitation end points in severe trauma. J Trauma 1995;38:780–7.

35. Polonen P, Rukonen E, Hippelainen M, et al. A prospective, randomized study of goal-orientated hemodynamic therapy in cardiac surgical patients. Anesth Analg 2000;90:1052–9.

36. Pearse R, Dawson D, Fawcett J, et al. Early goal-directed therapy after major surgery reduces complications and duration of hospital stay. A randomized controlled study. Crit Care 2005;9:R687–93

37. British Consensus Guidelines on Intravenous Fluid Therapy for Adult Surgical Patients (GIFTASUP). http://www.bapen.org.uk/pdfs/bapen_pubs/giftasup.pdf.

38. Kuper M, Gold SJ, Callow C, et al. Intraoperative fluid management guided by oesophageal Doppler monitoring. Br Med J 2011;342:d3016. http://dx.doi.org/10.1136/bmj. d3016.

39. The Royal College of Surgeons of England, Department of Health. The higher risk general surgical patient: Towards improved care for a forgotten group. London; 2011.

17

Surgical nutrition

William G. Simpson
Steven D. Heys

Introduction

The importance of nutrition in all fields of clinical practice has become well recognised and none more so than in the management of patients who are undergoing surgery and/or are faced with critical illness. Despite this increasing understanding of the importance of nutrition in health, up to 40% of hospitalised patients can be classified as being malnourished and many of these patients are not recognised clinically as having this problem. In patients undergoing gastrointestinal surgery, for example, the prevalence of 'mild' and 'moderate' malnutrition has been estimated to be approximately 50% and 30%, respectively.

The clinical significance of this is vitally important because when patients are malnourished, disturbances in function at the organ and cellular level can manifest as the following:

- altered partitioning and impairment of normal homeostatic mechanisms;
- muscle wasting and impairment of skeletal muscle function;
- impaired respiratory muscle function;
- impaired cardiac muscle function;
- atrophy of smooth muscle in the gastrointestinal tract;
- impaired immune function;
- impaired healing of wounds and anastomoses.

The key point, therefore, is that as a result of these malnutrition-induced changes, patients have an increased risk of postoperative morbidity and mortality. To further complicate the situation with respect to nutrition, patients undergoing surgery will also be fasted for varying periods of time (preoperatively and/or postoperatively). Moreover, if patients then experience postoperative complications (e.g. sepsis), these effects may be further potentiated and the disturbances of cellular and organ function occurring in malnutrition then made even more complex.

In this chapter the following areas, which are important for surgical practice, will be outlined:

- the principles of the metabolic responses to feeding, trauma and sepsis;
- nutritional requirements for surgical patients;
- identification of patients who are malnourished or are at risk;
- nutritional support principles for surgical practice and modifications in defined common clinical situations;
- modulation of nutritional support with key nutrients – application to clinical practice.

Metabolic response to feeding, trauma and sepsis

In order to maintain the health of cells, tissues and organs, the metabolism must adapt to changes in nutritional intake, trauma and sepsis.While a detailed knowledge of complex biochemical pathways is not necessary, it is important to understand the principles of these metabolic and biochemical changes, and the metabolic response when a patient experiences trauma, undergoes surgery or develops sepsis. This forms the basis for understanding nutrition and nutritional support in critically ill patients.

Trauma

A major advance in understanding occurred more than 80 years ago when Sir David Cuthbertson described the loss of nitrogen from skeletal muscle that occurred following trauma.[1] Cuthbertson concluded that the response to injury could be considered as occurring in two phases (**Fig. 17.1**):

1. the 'ebb' phase, which is a short-lived response associated with hypovolaemic shock, increased sympathetic nervous system activity and reduced metabolic rate;
2. the 'flow' phase, which is associated with a loss of body nitrogen and resultant negative nitrogen balance.

These changes result in the following:

Ebb phase

- decreased resting energy expenditure;
- increased gluconeogenesis;
- increased glycogenolysis.

Flow phase

- increased resting energy expenditure;
- increased heat production, pyrexia;
- increased muscle catabolism and wasting and loss of body nitrogen;
- increased breakdown of fat and reduced fat synthesis;
- increased gluconeogenesis and impairment of glucose tolerance.

If the changes of the 'ebb phase' are not replaced by the 'flow phase', then despite any advances in surgery, anaesthesia and intensive care support, death of the patient is the inevitable outcome.

The central nervous system and the neurohypophyseal axis play key roles in regulating these metabolic changes following trauma, utilising a range of hormones and cytokines. Afferent nerve impulses also stimulate the hypothalamus to secrete hypothalamic releasing factors that, in turn, stimulate the pituitary gland to release prolactin, arginine vasopressin (antidiuretic hormone, ADH), growth hormone and adrenocorticotrophic hormone (ACTH). The changes in hormone levels in plasma following trauma are outlined in Box 17.1, with the stress hormones (adrenaline, cortisol, glucagon) playing pivotal roles.

Protein metabolism

Amino acids are required for:

- synthesis of proteins necessary for growth, function and structural repair;
- energy substrates for gut, lymphocytes and other rapidly proliferating tissues (mostly glutamine), also as fuel in muscle;
- hepatic gluconeogenesis – glucose is produced from alanine, which itself is produced by transamination reactions from other amino acids;
- maintenance of renal acid–base balance (arginine);
- production of proteins with specific roles in repair – immunological, endocrine, etc.

In the well-fed state, proteins are synthesised at a rate exceeding breakdown, whereas in the fasting state breakdown predominates. Following

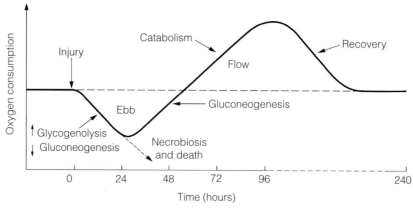

Figure 17.1 • Diagrammatic representation of the ebb and flow phases in the metabolic response to injury. Reproduced from Broom J. Sepsis and trauma. In: Garrow JS, James WPT (eds) Human nutrition and dietetics, 9th edn. Edinburgh: Churchill Livingstone, 1993; pp. 456–64. With permission from Elsevier.

Box 17.1 • Changes in hormone levels in plasma following trauma

Catecholamines

Rapid increases in concentrations of adrenaline and noradrenaline within a few minutes of injury due to increased activity of sympathetic nervous system. Levels return to normal within 24 hours

Glucagon

Rises within a few hours; maximal levels 12–48 hours post-trauma

Insulin

Initially plasma levels are low following trauma, but rise to above normal levels and reach a maximum several days after the injury

Cortisol

Rapid increase in cortisol (due to stimulation by ACTH), returning to normal 24–48 hours later; may remain elevated for up to several days. Has 'permissive' effects with other hormones such as catecholamines

Growth hormone

Levels increased following trauma; usually return to normal levels within 24 hours

Thyroid hormones

Following trauma, the biochemical features of 'sick euthyroid syndrome' may be present: thyroid-stimulating hormone (TSH) levels normal or low, levels of free thyroxine (T_4) and tri-iodothyronine (T_3) normal, whereas the total levels are altered because of changes in binding protein concentration. In addition, reverse T_3 is generally high. These effects may be prolonged for some weeks

Other disturbances of thyroid function may, however, be present, including 'transient hyperthyrotropinaemia of illness' – a transiently raised TSH, not to be confused with hypothyroidism

Renin, aldosterone

Aldosterone levels increased after trauma, returning to normal within 12 hours. Its secretion is stimulated by renin, which in turn is produced in response to reduced renal perfusion

Testosterone

Plasma levels fall after trauma and may remain low for up to 7 days

Vasopressin/antidiuretic hormone

Plasma levels rise following trauma and may remain elevated for several days

Prolactin

Secretion increased following trauma but function in trauma is unknown

Cytokines

Increased secretion of interleukin (IL)-2, IL-6, tumour necrosis factor, etc.; inter-relationship between these changes leads to differential responses seen in trauma and sepsis

prolonged fasting for 1–2 weeks, breakdown still predominates but at a lower rate as the metabolism adapts to starvation. In contrast, following trauma or sepsis, breakdown exceeds synthesis regardless of whether the patient is fed or fasted; this response is, however, impaired if the metabolism is already adapted to starvation.[2] The magnitude of the nitrogen loss is proportional to the degree of operative trauma or the severity of the sepsis, and the major site of protein breakdown is skeletal muscle (contains 80% of the body's amino acid pool, with 60% being glutamine).[3]

Carbohydrate metabolism

Glucose is the main fuel used by many different tissues, being essential for some. In the well-fed state it is available for absorption from the gastrointestinal tract and, mostly driven by insulin, any excess is converted to glycogen (glycogenesis) in both liver and muscle, and to fatty acids (lipogenesis), the latter predominating when glycogen stores are replete. On fasting, insulin levels are lower, with an associated reduction in peripheral utilisation of glucose, and it is endogenously produced from glycogen (glycogenolysis) or other precursors (gluconeogenesis), e.g. amino acids and fatty acids. Initially, glycogenolysis predominates, but after a number of hours (dependent on demands), gluconeogenesis predominates (colloquially referred to as 'getting your second wind'). Following trauma, there is an increase in hepatic glycogenolysis (caused by increased sympathetic activity),[4] with these stores being substantially depleted within 24 hours.[5] Insulin antagonists are also involved in this metabolic response (see Box 17.1), and the insulin resistance is accompanied by a rise in insulin concentration. The circulating insulin level usually reaches a maximum several days after the injury, before returning towards normal levels.

In general, the carbohydrate response is to produce hyperglycaemia both in the immediate 'shock' ('ebb' phase) and later 'flow' phase of the metabolic response. The origin of the increased glucose differs between these two phases – while reduced peripheral utilisation of glucose is common to both phases, the glycogenolysis of the ebb phase must be replaced by gluconeogenesis in the flow phase. In the critically ill patient the advent of hypoglycaemia is an indication of major problems – glycogenolysis has slowed with depletion of glycogen stores, but gluconeogenesis is not yet adequate.

Fat metabolism

In the healthy, resting, fed state, triacylglycerol, being energy dense, is used by the metabolism to efficiently store energy. When fasting, lipolysis of triglyceride releases free fatty acids, which can be used as respiratory fuel for most cells other than brain and red blood cells, and glycerol that can be converted to glucose by hepatic gluconeogenesis.[6] Fatty acids are also metabolised in the liver to form ketone bodies, which are used as a preferential fuel source by many tissues (humans cannot use fatty acids for gluconeogenesis). Lipolysis is stimulated by glucagon during short-term fasting, by ACTH once the metabolism is adapted to starvation, or by adrenaline during exercise and stress. Following trauma, there is therefore an increase in the turnover of fatty acids and glycerol, although raised levels of lactate, for example in hypovolaemic shock, induce re-esterification leading to raised plasma triglyceride levels.

Mineral and micronutrient metabolism

Changes in fluid compartments, minerals and micronutrients (micronutrients are broadly defined as substances required in amounts of <1 g daily) are beyond the scope of this chapter, but it is worth re-emphasising that measured serum concentrations rarely reflect body status, and this is even more pronounced in starvation and illness; for example, hyponatraemia is more often associated with an excess of water than with a deficiency of sodium; hypocalcaemia does not indicate a deficiency of calcium, but can suggest a deficiency of magnesium. It is therefore essential to consider the effect of illness before trying to interpret laboratory results.[7]

Sepsis

The metabolic response to sepsis is also characterised by alterations in protein, carbohydrate and fat metabolism, but the following are key differences:[8]

- The breakdown of skeletal muscle and nitrogen losses can be substantial (more than 15–20 g per day).
- There is increased production of glucose by the liver (both gluconeogenesis and glycogenolysis), resulting in an elevated plasma glucose.
- In contrast to the situation following trauma, there is an increased rate of glucose uptake and oxidation by peripheral tissues.
- Decrease in the peripheral uptake of triacylglycerols and defective ketogenesis in the presence of sepsis (in contrast to the situation occurring after trauma) lead to hypertriglyceridaemia.

A significant abnormality in the patient with sepsis is the disruption of the microstructure of the hepatocyte mitochondria, particularly of the inner membrane. There is a block in energy transduction pathways, with consequent reduction in the aerobic metabolism of both glucose and fatty acids. The body therefore depends on the *anaerobic* metabolism of glucose, which also results in lactate production. It is essential, therefore, that there is an adequate supply of glucose from gluconeogenic pathways. If this is impaired or inadequate, then hypoglycaemia (and death) may ensue. The development of hypoglycaemia during sepsis is an indicator of an extremely poor prognosis and is usually associated with inevitable mortality.

Nutritional requirements

Proteins and amino acids

Protein is required for the maintenance of normal health and cellular function. Proteins have many functions, including being essential components of cellular structure. They are required for the synthesis of a variety of secretory proteins produced by many organs. The average daily intake of protein is approximately 80 g in the UK, with a recommended daily intake of 0.8 g/kg body weight and with nitrogen comprising approximately 16% of its weight. However, more than 50% of the world's population exist on less!

Conventionally, amino acids have been classified as either 'essential' or 'non-essential'. The 'essential' amino acids cannot be synthesised endogenously and are required in the diet. Paradoxically, the so-called 'non-essential' amino acids are actually so metabolically important that humans have retained the ability to synthesise them. Both groups of amino acids are necessary for normal tissue growth and metabolism.

Dietary intake and endogenous synthesis of amino acids in the body maintain the relevant pool of amino acids, replacing those that have been lost by excretion in the urine, losses from the skin and gastrointestinal tract, utilisation as precursors for non-protein synthetic pathways, irreversible modification and irreducible oxidation.

Under certain circumstances (e.g. sepsis, trauma, growth) endogenous synthesis of some amino acids normally considered to be 'non-essential' is inadequate; therefore, these amino acids are described as 'conditionally essential': L-alanine, L-glutamate and L-aspartate, which are produced by a simple transamination reaction. These are the three most important amino acids in times of starvation:

- alanine for hepatic gluconeogenesis;
- glutamate as a fuel source for liver, enterocytes and white blood cells;
- aspartate for maintaining renal acid–base balance.

Energy requirements

Energy transduction is accomplished by the breakdown of carbohydrate, fat and proteins. The energy available from various common nutrients is:

- fat 9.3 kcal/g (38.9 kJ/g);
- glucose 4.1 kcal/g (17.1 kJ/g);
- protein 4.1 kcal/g (17.1 kJ/g);
- alcohol 7.1 kcal/g (29.7 kJ/g).

The principal carbohydrates in the diet are polysaccharides (starch and dietary fibre), dextrins and free sugars (monosaccharides), disaccharides, oligosaccharides and sugar alcohols. Dietary fat includes triacylglycerol, containing long-chain fatty acids (C_{16}–C_{18} triacylglycerols) and medium-chain fatty acids (C_6–C_{12} triacylglycerols) and cholesterol.

If the energy intake of an individual is greater than energy expenditure, extra carbohydrate intake, on reaching the liver via the portal vein, will be channelled into synthesis of glycogen or fat. Glycogenesis dominates until hepatic glycogen stores are replete; thereafter, fat synthesis dominates. Additional fat intake will be stored in adipose tissue as triacylglycerol. In contrast, if there is a negative energy balance, then glycogenolysis dominates until glycogen stores are depleted, then fat and protein will be broken down to provide energy.

Total daily energy expenditure comprises the following:

- resting metabolic expenditure (RME), which is energy required for cardiorespiratory function and synthesis and maintenance of electrochemical gradients across cell membranes;
- activity energy expenditure (depends on type of physical work undertaken);
- diet-induced energy expenditure.

Normally, approximately 25–30 kcal/kg (105–125 kJ/g) are required daily; the magnitudes of changes in requirements in some common conditions are given in Box 17.2.

Box 17.2 • Additional energy requirements in disease states

Trauma: 0.3×RME
Elective surgery: 0.1×RME
Sepsis: up to 0.5×RME
Severe sepsis: up to 0.6×RME
Massive burns: 1×RME

Minerals and micronutrients

A number of specific organic compounds (vitamins) and inorganic elements are essential for tissue growth and repair, and for maintenance of body function, playing key roles in metabolism, including the processing of macronutrients (protein, carbohydrate and fat). For many micronutrients, specific deficiency diseases have been described. Details of individual substances are beyond the scope of this chapter and can be found elsewhere,[9] but some examples are given in Box 17.3.

In general, micronutrients are classified into:

- fat-soluble vitamins (A, D, E and K);
- water-soluble vitamins (C and the B vitamins – folic acid, B_{12}, B_1, B_2, B_3, pantothenic acid, biotin and B_6).
- trace elements (iron, zinc, copper, selenium, etc.).

The exact requirement for micronutrients during trauma and sepsis is unclear and may alter depending on the type of metabolic support provided.

Box 17.3 • Functions of some micronutrients important in surgical practice

Vitamin A
Stabilises epithelial cell membranes; necessary for fibroblast differentiation and collagen secretion
Vitamin D
Role in calcium and phosphate regulation
Vitamin E
Immunostimulant and free radical scavenger
Vitamin K
Required for liver synthesis of clotting factors
Vitamin B_{12}
Important in synthesis of proteins and nucleic acids
Ascorbic acid
Important in hydroxylation (e.g. collagen synthesis) and energy transduction
Thiamine
Necessary for carbohydrate metabolism and ATP synthesis
Iron
Energy transfer
Copper
Collagen synthesis
Selenium
Antioxidant; protection against peroxidation processes occurring in tissue damage and repair
Zinc
Cofactor in numerous enzymes; necessary for wound healing

It should be remembered that micronutrients, if given at high doses, can have toxic effects on tissues. In particular, toxicity can be a problem with excesses of vitamin A, iron, selenium, zinc and copper; vitamin D toxicity is no longer thought to be a significant problem. Care must be taken when these micronutrients are provided for a prolonged period to ensure that toxicity does not occur. It is also unusual to find isolated deficiencies, so identification of one micronutrient deficiency should stimulate consideration of other deficiencies.

Identification of patients who are malnourished

It is important to assess the nutritional status in all patients undergoing surgery and identify those who are malnourished, or who are at risk of becoming so. Measurements used previously in clinical practice include:

- anthropometric – body structure and composition;
- biochemical;
- functional – muscle (skeletal and respiratory) and immunological responses.

Anthropometric measures

Height and weight

Height and weight are two commonly used indices of nutritional status.[10] Body weight on its own takes no account of frame size but body mass index (BMI; weight divided by the square of the height) is a good anthropometric indicator of total body fat in adults.

Loss of body weight has been used as an indicator of nutritional status. This is determined by subtracting current weight from recall weight when the patient was 'well', or from the 'ideal' weight, obtained from published tables. The loss of more than 10% of body weight, or more than 4.5 kg of recall weight, is associated with a significant increase in postoperative mortality. The shorter the period of weight loss, the more significant this is in predicting increased postoperative complications. Malnutrition can be defined as a BMI of less than the 10th percentile with a weight loss of 5% or more.[11]

Body composition

Various techniques for assessing the body's different compartments (e.g. fat, fat-free mass, total body nitrogen and total body mineral contents) have become available but many require specialised equipment and may not be readily applicable to clinical practice. Relatively simple techniques, such as skinfold thickness and bioelectrical impedance, can be used clinically, although even these tend to be used more for research or clinical audits of nutrition and nutritional support.

Subcutaneous fat thickness

Skinfold thickness has been used as an index of total body fat (50% of total body fat is subcutaneous, depending on age, sex and fat pad). Triceps skinfold thickness is most commonly measured but assessment of skinfolds at multiple sites is better and correlates with total body fat. Regression equations for the estimation of total body fat from these measurements are available.[12] However, skinfold thickness measurements are susceptible to intra-observer and inter-observer variability, which limits clinical use.

Bioelectrical impedance

This entails the passage of an alternating electrical current between electrodes attached to the hand and foot. The current passes through the water and electrolyte compartment of lean tissues and the drop in voltage between the electrodes is measured.[13] This change in voltage gives an estimation of total body resistance, which depends principally on total body water and electrolyte content (i.e. lean body mass). This estimate can give an accurate measure of body composition in stable subjects; it becomes less reliable in patients with oedema and electrolyte shifts, and so the value of bioelectrical impedance in critically ill patients remains unclear.[14]

Biochemical measures

Serum proteins

Albumin is the major protein in serum and the relationship between serum proteins and malnutrition was recognised over 150 years ago.[14] Low serum albumin levels are associated with increased risk of complications in patients undergoing surgery.[15] In experimental starvation, however, serum albumin levels may not fall for several weeks[16] because, although synthesis decreases, only 30% of the total exchangeable albumin is in the intravascular space, with the remainder being extravascular. In addition, albumin has a relatively long half-life of approximately 21 days. The flux of albumin between the intravascular and extravascular compartments is about 10 times the rate of albumin synthesis, although this varies greatly depending on capillary permeability.[17]

Importantly, serum albumin acts as a negative marker of the acute-phase response, and so is lowered in malignancy, trauma and sepsis, even in the presence of an adequate intake. Serum albumin should therefore *not* be used as an assessment of nutritional *state*, although low levels point to the increased nutritional *risk* associated with underlying disease, and indeed the implied reduction of gut absorption may indicate that the parenteral route may be preferred for provision of nutrition.

Alternatives to using albumin as a marker of nutritional status by measuring other serum protein concentrations, including transferrin (half-life 7 days), retinol-binding protein (half-life 1–2 hours) and pre-albumin (half-life 2 days), have been suggested. The serum levels of these proteins are, however, also altered in stress, sepsis and cancer, and so, as for albumin, they are not useful for assessing nutritional status in routine clinical practice.

Nitrogen balance

Most of the nitrogen lost from the body is excreted in urine, mainly as urea (approximately 80% of total urinary nitrogen). Urea alone may be measured as an approximate indicator of losses, or total urinary nitrogen may be measured, although this latter technique is not widely available. In addition, there are also losses of nitrogen from the skin and in stool of approximately 2–4 g per day. One equation used for balance studies is:

$$\text{Nitrogen balance (g)} = (\text{dietary protein (g)} \times 0.16) - (\text{urine urea nitrogen (g)} + 2\,\text{g stool} + 2\,\text{g skin})$$

where

$$\text{urine urea nitrogen (g)} = \text{urine urea (mmol)} \times 28.$$

Although nitrogen balance has not been shown to be a prognostic indicator, it is a useful way of assessing a patient's nutritional requirements and the response to provision of nutritional support.

Tests of function

Immune competence

In malnutrition there is a reduction in total circulating lymphocyte count and impairment in immune functions, e.g. decreased skin reactivity to mumps, *Candida* and tuberculin (assuming prior exposure), and reduced lymphocyte responsiveness to mitogens in vitro.[18,19]

A correlation between depressed immune function and postoperative morbidity and mortality has been demonstrated, and depression of total circulating lymphocyte count is associated with a poorer prognosis in surgical patients.[20] However, these alterations in immune function are non-specific and affected by trauma, surgery, anaesthetic and sedative drugs, pain and psychological stress,[21] and are not generally applicable to clinical practice.

Muscle function

Skeletal muscle

Various aspects of skeletal muscle structure and function are deranged in malnutrition. In patients undergoing surgery, handgrip strength (cheap and easy to perform) may predict patients who develop postoperative complications (sensitivity >90%). However, grip strength is influenced by factors such as patients' motivation and cooperation. Furthermore, such tests may be difficult to apply to critically ill patients. Alternatively, stimulation of the ulnar nerve at the wrist with a variable electrical stimulus results in contraction of the adductor pollicis muscle, the force of which reflects nutritional intake.[22]

Respiratory muscle

The function of the respiratory muscles is impaired by malnutrition and can be detected by deterioration in respiratory function tests, in particular vital capacity.[23] Measurements of inspiratory muscle strength have the advantage that they can be performed in patients who are intubated.

Nutrition risk index

A nutrition risk index is an index of nutritional status based on combinations of variables. Although several indices exist, one that is commonly used depends on serum albumin, current weight and the patient's usual weight:

$$\text{Nutrition risk index} = 1.519 \times \text{serum albumin (g/L)} + 0.417 \times (\text{current weight} / \text{usual weight}) \times 100$$

The score obtained is used to categorise nutritional risk: <83.5, 'severe' risk; 83.5–97.5, 'mild' risk; 97.5–100, 'borderline' risk. Note that this is a prognostic index and bears little relationship to the patient's nutritional status.

How should nutritional status be assessed in clinical practice?

Although the various techniques outlined above can help to predict the risks of complications, there is at present no reliable technique for assessing nutritional status. There is, however, increasing support for using the following techniques, which are applicable to clinical practice.

The Malnutrition Universal Screening Tool (MUST)

This simple, yet effective, tool was developed by the British Association for Parenteral and Enteral Nutrition (BAPEN). Details are available from the website, which we recommend you read carefully (www.BAPEN.org.uk). This tool has been endorsed by external organisations and its routine use is recommended for all hospital admissions in the UK. As a minimum standard in clinical practice, the MUST tool should be used to assess nutritional risk. Essentially, MUST consists of a series of five steps:

1. Measure height and weight to obtain BMI (in kg/m^2) – this is then given a numerical score (>20 = 0; 18.5–20 = 1; >18.5 = 2).
2. Note percentage unplanned weight loss in the previous 3–6 months – then give this a numerical score (<5% = 0; 5–10% = 1; >10% = 2).
3. Establish the 'acute disease effect' and also give this a numerical score (if patient is acutely ill and there is or will be no nutritional intake for more than 5 days = 2).
4. Add scores from steps 1, 2 and 3 together to obtain the 'overall risk of malnutrition'.
5. A decision is taken as to what to do depending on the resultant score.

Significance of the resultant score and clinical management

- **Score 0 (low risk)** – repeat the screening process at a future time.
- **Score 1 (medium risk)** – observe by noting the patient's dietary intake for the next 3 days. If this improves then there is little concern. However, if there is no improvement, this is of clinical concern and one should follow the local policies for what to do next, e.g. referral to nutrition support team/dietician.
- **Score 2 or more (high risk)** – these patients should be referred to the nutrition support team/dietician to try to increase their nutritional intake and there should be policies in place for the nutritional support given to these patients.

✔ The MUST tool should be used routinely to assess nutritional risk for all hospital admissions (www.BAPEN.org.uk).

Subjective global assessment

Useful indicators for bedside assessment of nutritional status applicable to clinical practice have been identified,[24] and include estimation of protein and energy balance, assessment of body composition and evaluation of physiological function.

Assessment of protein and energy balance

Protein and energy balance can be assessed either by a dietician or by a clinician, who determines the frequency and size of meals eaten. This information is compared with the patient's rate of loss of body weight and BMI.

Assessment of body composition

Loss of body fat can be determined by observing the physical appearance of the patient (loss of body contours) and feeling the patient's skinfolds between finger and thumb. In particular, if the dermis can be felt on pinching the biceps and triceps skinfolds, then considerable weight loss has occurred.

The stores of protein in the body can be assessed from various muscle groups, including the temporalis, deltoid, suprascapular, infrascapular, biceps and triceps, and the interossei of the hands. When tendons of the muscles are prominent and bony protuberances of the scapula are obvious, greater than 30% of the total body protein stores have been lost.

Assessment of physiological function

Assessments of function are made by observing the patient's activities. Grip strength is determined by asking patients to squeeze the clinician's index and middle fingers for at least 10 seconds, and respiratory function by asking them to blow hard on a strip of paper held 10 cm from the patient's lips. The measurement of metabolic expenditure requires specialised equipment, but additional metabolic stresses on the patient can be determined from clinical examination. Extra metabolic stresses will occur if trauma or surgery has taken place or there is evidence of significant sepsis (elevated temperature and/or white blood cell counts, tachycardia, tachypnoea, positive blood cultures) or active inflammatory bowel disease. In addition, patients should be asked about their ability to heal wounds, changes in exercise tolerance and their 'tiredness'.

Re-feeding syndrome

Once a patient's need for nutritional support has been identified, it is important to consider whether the patient is at risk of re-feeding syndrome. This is described in detail elsewhere, but in essence it is the inability of a patient's metabolism to handle macronutrients. After approximately 10 days without nutritional intake, the metabolism adapts to the state of starvation. Re-feeding with full 'normal' required amounts of macronutrients will induce a sudden reversal of this adaptation, with an anabolic drive that may result in catastrophic depletion of available potassium, phosphate and magnesium. Before re-feeding, the serum biochemistry may appear 'normal', and so the possibility of re-feeding must be anticipated on history alone. The other essential nutrient liable to become depleted in this situation is thiamine, a cofactor of pyruvate kinase, which is required for glucose to undergo oxidative phosphorylation, and without which glucose is metabolised to lactic acid. Thiamine must therefore be replenished before feeding is commenced in the starved patient to prevent development of Wernicke–Korsakoff syndrome. The potential for this is considerably higher in patients with a history of chronic excessive ethanol intake, and so even greater caution is required.

> ✅ Thiamine deficiency must always be considered in patients who have had no nutritional intake for more than 1 week, who have a history of excessive alcohol intake, or in the presence of an unexplained metabolic acidosis.

Nutritional support in surgical practice

Route of nutritional support

The preferred route of administration of nutritional support is through the gastrointestinal tract (enteral), with intravenous (parenteral) nutrient delivery reserved for patients with intestinal failure.

Enteral nutritional support

If there is an intact and functioning gastrointestinal tract, enteral feeding should be used if oral intake is insufficient. Enteral feeding is contraindicated to various degrees in patients with intestinal obstruction, paralytic ileus, vomiting and diarrhoea, high-output intestinal fistulas or in the presence of major intra-abdominal sepsis.

The importance of enteral nutrition

Studies in animals have shown that in the absence of nutrients into the intestinal lumen, changes occur in the intestinal mucosa. There is loss of height of villi, reduction in cellular proliferation and the mucosa becomes atrophic.[25,26] Activities of enzymes found in association with the mucosa are reduced and permeability of the mucosa to macromolecules increased.[27] Stimulation of the intestinal tract by nutrients is important for release of many gut-related hormones, including those responsible for gut motility and stimulation of secretions necessary for normal maintenance of the mucosa. The gut acts as a barrier to bacteria, both physically and by release of chemical and immunological substances. There is evidence to suggest that atrophy of the intestinal mucosa is associated with loss of intercellular adhesion and opening of intercellular channels. This predisposes to increased translocation of bacteria and endotoxin from the gut lumen into portal venous and lymphatic systems.[28] Loss of gut integrity may account for a substantial proportion of septicaemic events in severely ill patients. However, the extent to which it contributes to sepsis in patients is not fully understood.

Routes of access for enteral nutritional support

Nasoenteric tubes

Nasogastric feeding via fine-bore tubes (polyvinyl chloride or polyurethane) may be used in patients who require nutritional support for a short period of time. There has been considerable debate as to whether positioning the feeding tube beyond the pylorus into the duodenum will result in reduction in the risks of regurgitation of gastric contents and pulmonary aspiration (occurs in up to 30% of patients fed this way). This is most likely in patients with impaired gastric motility. In the latter patients, the fine-bore tube can be manipulated through the pylorus into the duodenum, reducing the risk of gastric aspiration. Other complications associated with the use of nasoenteric tubes include:

- pulmonary atelectasis;
- oesophageal necrosis, stricture formation;
- tracheo-oesophageal fistulas;
- sinusitis, postcricoid ulceration.

More recently, double-lumen tubes have been used – one lumen resides in the stomach and is used to aspirate gastric contents, while the distal lumen is placed in the jejunum for feeding, thus reducing risks of aspiration. This can be successful even in patients with relatively high gastric aspirates, previously thought to be a contraindication for feeding via the enteral route.

Gastrostomy tubes

A gastrostomy tube can be placed into the stomach at laparotomy, although percutaneous endoscopic or percutaneous fluoroscopic techniques are preferred. Details of how these are performed can be found in standard texts.

The establishment and use of a gastrostomy has certain disadvantages and there is a recognised morbidity:

- infection of the skin at the puncture site;
- necrotising fasciitis or deeper-sited sepsis;
- damage to adjacent intra-abdominal viscera;
- leakage of gastric contents into the peritoneal cavity;
- haemorrhage from the stomach;
- persistent gastrocutaneous fistula following removal of the feeding tube.

The overall mortality rate for a gastrostomy is 1–2%, with major and minor complications occurring in up to 15% of patients. Mechanical complications associated with the tube include blockage, fracture and displacement. Furthermore, 'dumping' and diarrhoea are more common when the tip of the tube lies in the duodenum or jejunum.[29]

Jejunostomy tubes

A feeding jejunostomy is usually carried out at the time of laparotomy if it is envisaged that a patient will need nutritional support for a longer period. Details of the operative technique are also in standard operative texts and the smaller needle-catheter tubes are to be preferred. Advantages of a feeding jejunostomy compared with a gastrostomy are:

- less stomal leakage;
- gastric and pancreatic secretions are reduced because the stomach is bypassed;
- less nausea, vomiting or bloating;
- reduced risk of pulmonary aspiration.

Nutrient solutions available for enteral nutrition

A range of nutrient solutions are available for use in enteral nutritional support and examples can be found in specialised texts. However, there are four main categories of enteral diet.

Polymeric diets

Polymeric diets are 'nutritionally complete' diets and provided to patients with inadequate oral intake, but whose intestinal function is good. They contain whole protein as the source of nitrogen, and energy is provided as complex carbohydrates and fat. They also contain vitamins, trace elements and electrolytes in standard amounts.

Elemental diets

Elemental diets are required if the patient is unable to produce an adequate amount of digestive enzymes or has a reduced area for absorption (e.g. severe pancreatic insufficiency or short-bowel syndrome). Elemental diets contain nitrogen as oligopeptides (free amino acids are not as easily absorbed as dipeptide and tripeptide mixtures). The energy source is provided as glucose polymers and medium-chain triacylglycerols. Each oligopeptide molecule contributes as much to the osmolarity of the solution as one molecule of intact protein, and it can be difficult to provide complete requirements without producing side-effects associated with an osmotic load, e.g. 'dumping' and diarrhoea.

Special formulations

Special formulations have been developed for patients with particular diseases. Examples of such diets include: (i) those with increased concentrations of branched-chain amino acids and low in aromatic amino acids for patients with hepatic encephalopathy; (ii) those with a higher fat but lower glucose energy content for patients who are artificially ventilated; and (iii) diets containing key nutrients that modulate the immune response (see later).

Modular diets

Modular diets are not commonly used but allow provision of a diet rich in a particular nutrient for specific patients. For example, the diet may be enriched in protein if the patient is protein deficient or in sodium if sodium deficient. These modular diets can be used to supplement other enteral regimens or oral intake.

Enteral nutrition delivery and complications

Previously, when starting an enteral nutrition feeding regimen, patients received either a reduced rate of infusion or a lower strength formula for the first 2 or 3 days to reduce gastrointestinal complications. Recent studies have demonstrated this is not required and nutritional support can commence using full-strength feeds at the desired rate in those not at risk of developing 're-feeding syndrome'. Cyclical feeding (e.g. 16 hours feeding with a post-absorptive period of 8 hours) is optimal and more closely mimics the natural feeding cycle than other types of feeding regimens.[30]

Enteral nutrition should be administered through a volumetric pump. If not available, then it is possible to use a gravity drip flow but care should be taken to reduce the risk of a large bolus being administered. In patients whose conscious level is impaired or confined to bed, the head of the bed should be elevated by 25° to reduce risks of pulmonary aspiration. Some clinicians prefer patients to be sitting upright when receiving enteral nutrition. The stomach contents should be aspirated every 4 hours during feeding and if a residual volume of more than 100 mL is found, enteral nutrition is temporarily discontinued.

The aspirate is checked again after 2 hours, and when satisfactory volumes are aspirated (<100 mL) feeding is re-instituted. If more than 400 mL per 24 hours is aspirated, then feeding is discontinued. Gastric emptying may be improved by the administration of cisapride or erythromycin, which may allow feeding to be continued.

Metabolic disturbances are less likely with enteral feeding. The other complications of enteral nutrition are those associated with the route of access to the gastrointestinal tract (Box 17.4).

Gastrointestinal

Diarrhoea, nausea, vomiting, abdominal discomfort and bloating, regurgitation and aspiration of feed/stomach contents

Mechanical

Dislodgement of the feeding tube, blockage of the tube, leakage of stomach/small intestine contents onto the skin with the use of jejunostomies or gastrostomies

Metabolic

Excess or deficiency of glucose, electrolytes, minerals or trace elements. Some of these will be noted through routine testing protocols, e.g hyperkalaemia, but others such as hypophosphataemia may be missed if not specifically anticipated

Infective

Local effects (e.g. diarrhoea, vomiting) or systemic effects (e.g. pyrexia, malaise)

Parenteral nutritional support

Patients who require nutritional support but with enteral feeding contraindicated will require parenteral nutrition. These include:

- patients with a non-functioning or inaccessible gastrointestinal tract;
- those with high-output enteric fistulas (enteral nutrition may stimulate gastrointestinal secretion – discussed further later);
- those for whom it is not possible to provide sufficient intake of nutrients enterally (e.g. because of a short segment of residual bowel or malabsorption, severe burns, major trauma).

Detailed guidance for parenteral nutrition (PN) in patients has been published by the American Society for Parenteral and Enteral Nutrition (ASPEN).[31] Current ASPEN guidelines are available on their website (www.nutritioncare.org), as are those of the European Society for Clinical Nutrition and Metabolism (www.espen.org/).

Parenteral routes of access

Central venous access

Central venous access is obtained by positioning a catheter into the superior vena cava through subclavian or internal jugular veins. The catheter either emerges through the skin (usually after being tunnelled in the subcutaneous fat) or is connected to a port placed in the subcutaneous fat of the anterior chest wall. A variety of techniques for insertion of central venous lines are used. For example, catheters may be introduced into the internal jugular or subclavian vein directly by 'blind' percutaneous puncture, using small hand-held ultrasound imaging, by 'cut-down' techniques utilising the cephalic vein to access the subclavian vein, or under fluoroscopic control. Details of these techniques, their advantages and disadvantages can be found elsewhere.[32–34] However, it is important that whoever inserts a central venous line is expert, well practised and carries out the procedure under full aseptic techniques.

Technical aspects of feeding lines

Central lines are manufactured from polyurethane or silicone. Both of these materials are tolerated well with low thrombogenic potential. However, polyurethane does have advantages:

- it is stiffer than silicone at room temperature, but at body temperature is pliable;
- it has a higher tensile strength than silicone and is less likely to fracture;
- polyurethane catheters have smaller outside diameters, making cannulation easier, as well as a greater resistance to thrombus development on their surfaces.

Catheter manufacturers have attempted to reduce risks of bacterial colonisation of the line by bonding antiseptics (e.g. chlorhexidene) and antibiotics (e.g. silver sulphadiazine) into the catheter's fabric. Some catheters have an antimicrobial cuff, usually made of Dacron, around their external surface. This acts as a barrier to micro-organisms, which may migrate from subcutaneous tissues along the external aspect of the catheter to its tip. Although studies have suggested that risks of septicaemia are reduced by using a cuff around the catheter, this makes positioning of the catheter more difficult technically. Complications of central venous catheters are shown in Box 17.5.

Catheter-related sepsis: variable, but reported in up to 40% of catheters

Thrombosis of central vein: variable, but reported in up to 20% of catheters

Pleural space damage: pneumothorax (5–10%), haemothorax (2%)

Major arterial damage: subclavian artery (1–2%)

Catheter problems: thrombosis (1–2%), embolism (<1%), air embolism (<1%)

Miscellaneous problems: brachial plexus (<1%), thoracic duct damage (<1%)

Catheter care

Appropriate dressings of the catheter are essential. The dressing should be changed weekly with strict aseptic technique, and the skin exit site cleaned with chlorhexidene. A variety of dressings have been used at the skin exit, but a transparent adherent type of dressing has the advantage of allowing a visible check on the puncture site for inflammation or pus.

Infection of the catheter tip is the most serious type of infection. The patient usually is pyrexial and may have systemic signs of sepsis. This may be diagnosed by blood (at least three cultures 1 hour apart) and catheter cultures.[35] Antibiotic therapy may result in recovery, but in some the feeding line has to be removed to eradicate the infection. However, less serious infection may occur in the skin at the exit site of the catheter. This is recognised by skin erythema, possibly associated with fluid exudate and pus.

Peripheral venous access

Peripheral venous cannulation, using a sterile technique, may be used to supply nutrients intravenously, avoiding complications associated with central venous catheters. Peripheral intravenous nutrition is likely to be used in patients who do not require nutritional support for long enough to justify risks of central vein cannulation or in whom central vein cannulation is contraindicated (e.g. central line insertion sites are traumatised, increased risks of infective complications, thrombosis of the central veins or significant clotting defects).

Problems associated with the delivery of intravenous nutrition using the peripheral route include:

- a limit to nutrient quantity deliverable – this is not the route of choice in those with high requirements for protein or energy;
- a high incidence of complications, particularly phlebitis (occurs in up to 45% of patients), and it is essential to ensure good peripheral venous access.

The lifespan of a peripheral intravenous cannula can be prolonged by treating it as if it is a central line with regard to aseptic care, and by using a narrow-gauge cannula giving better mixing and flow characteristics of the nutrient solution. Risks of phlebitis can be reduced by frequent changes of infusion site, ultrafine-bore catheters or using a vasodilator patch over the cannulation site (e.g. transdermal glyceryl trinitrate). Furthermore, peripheral intravenous nutrition can only be used where fat emulsion is part of the single-phase administration of nutrients to avoid thrombophlebitis.

Nutrients used in parenteral feeding solutions

Various nutrient solutions (amino acids, glucose and fat) are available and a complete list is given in the *British National Formulary* (www.bnf.org/bnf/). There are also available a variety of pre-mixed bags containing various concentrations of amino acids and glucose, with or without fat, which are suitable for different clinical situations. These mixtures do not usually contain vitamins or trace elements, which must be given in addition to avoid development of metabolic complications. Care should be taken that patients receive sufficient electrolytes and minerals to satisfy requirements.

Nitrogen sources

Nitrogen sources are solutions of crystalline L-amino acids containing all essential and a balanced mixture of the non-essential amino acids required. Amino acids that are relatively insoluble (e.g. L-glutamine, L-arginine, L-taurine, L-tyrosine, L-methionine) may be absent or present in inadequate amounts.

Attention has focused on the provision of L-glutamine because of its key roles in metabolism. Despite being one of the most abundant amino acids, its use in PN fluids has been limited by instability. It can, however, be supplied as *N*-acetylglutamine (hydrolysed in the renal tubule to free L-glutamine) or as L-glutamine dipeptides such as alanylglutamine (broken down to release free L-glutamine). Recent evidence, however, questions the need for enrichment of PN with glutamine.[36]

Energy sources

Energy is supplied as a balanced combination of dextrose and fat. Glucose is the primary carbohydrate source and the main form of energy supply to the majority of tissues. During critical illness the body's preferred calorie source is fat (fasted or fed states).[37,38] There are controversies as to the utilisation of fat in sepsis because of defects in energy substrate metabolism at the oxidative level.

Glucose utilisation may be impaired in certain patients and glucose is then metabolised through other pathways. This results in increased production and oxidation of fatty acids, resulting in increased carbon dioxide (excreted through the lungs). In addition, if glucose is the only energy source, patients may develop essential fatty acid (linolenic, linoleic) deficiency.

Fat (e.g. soyabean oil emulsions) provides a more concentrated energy source. Usually, approximately 30–50% of the total calories are given as fat, with non-protein calorie to nitrogen ratio varying from 150:1 to 200:1 (lower in hypercatabolic conditions).

The provision of exogenous lipids has also been associated with problems. Intravenous fat emulsions can impair lung function, inhibit the reticuloendothelial system and modulate neutrophil function; recent interest has also focused on the use of fish oils as a source of fat rich in omega-3 polyunsaturated fatty acids, as this appears to be associated with reduced incidence of hepatic dysfunction.[39,40]

Other nutrients

Commercially available preparations of trace elements (e.g. Additrace®) and vitamins, water soluble (e.g. Solivito®) and fat soluble (e.g. Vitlipid®), supply daily requirements. Larger amounts, particularly of the water-soluble vitamins, may be required initially if recent nutritional intake has been inadequate. Additionally, total fluid volume and amounts of electrolytes can be modified daily to meet particular requirements.

Delivery and administration of PN

In practice, commercially available solutions for parenteral infusion are mixed under sterile conditions in laminar flow facilities. The feeding regimen is made up in an inert 3- to 4-litre bag (ethyl vinyl acetate), comprising all nutrients and stored for up to 1 week, although compatibility between different constituents must be ensured. No additions of drugs should be made as this could make the emulsion unstable, affect the bioavailability of the drug or compromise sterility. Advantages of pre-mixed bags include:

- cost-effectiveness;
- reduced infective risks;
- more uniform administration of a balanced solution over a prolonged period;
- decreased lipid toxicity as a result of the greater dilution of the lipid emulsion and longer duration of infusion;
- ease of delivery and storage and reduced long-term accumulation of triacylglycerols (occurs with glucose-based PN).

Pre-prepared bags are available where the fat emulsion is stored separately from the aqueous solution and is mixed by bag rupture immediately prior to administration, conferring the advantage of a longer shelf life.

Complications of parenteral nutritional support

Instant availability of nutrients provided by the intravenous route can lead to metabolic complications if the composition or flow rate is inappropriate. Rapid infusion of high concentrations of glucose can precipitate hyperglycaemia, which may be further complicated by lactic acidosis. Electrolyte disturbances may present problems, not least because the intravenous feeding regimen is usually prescribed in advance for 24 hours. Prediction of the patient's nutrient requirements must be complemented by frequent monitoring. The provision of nutrients may lead to further electrolyte abnormalities when potassium, magnesium and phosphate enter the intracellular compartment. This is particularly noticeable in patients whose previous nutrient intake was especially poor, as highlighted previously. Others complications of PN are shown in Box 17.6.

Box 17.6 • Metabolic complications of parenteral nutrition

Glucose disturbances

Hyperglycaemia: excessive administration of glucose inadequate insulin, sepsis

Hypoglycaemia: rebound hypoglycaemia occurs if glucose is stopped abruptly but insulin levels remain high

Lipid disturbances

Hyperlipidaemia: directly through excess administration of lipid, or indirectly through excess calories that will be converted to fat or reduced metabolism (e.g. renal failure, liver failure)

Fatty acid deficiency: essential fatty acid deficiency leads to hair loss, dry skin, impaired wound healing

Nitrogen disturbances

Hyperammonaemia: occurs if deficiency of L-arginine, L-ornithine, L-aspartate or L-glutamate in infusion. Also occurs in liver diseases

Metabolic acidosis: caused by excessive amounts of chloride and monochloride amino acids

Electrolyte disturbances

Hyperkalaemia: excessive potassium administration or reduced losses

Hypokalaemia: inadequate potassium administration or excessive loss

Hypocalcaemia: inadequate calcium replacement, losses in pancreatitis, hypoalbuminaemia

Hypophosphataemia: inadequate phosphorus supplementation, also tissue compartment fluxes

Liver disturbances

Elevations in aspartate aminotransferase, alkaline phosphatase and γ-glutamyltransferase may occur because of enzyme induction secondary to amino acid imbalances or deposition of fat and/or glycogen in liver

Ventilatory problems

If excessive amounts of glucose are given, the increased production of CO_2 may precipitate ventilatory failure in non-ventilated patients

Monitoring patients receiving nutritional support

Patients receiving nutritional support should be monitored by accurate recording of fluid balance and daily weighing. Daily intake of calories and nitrogen should be documented. Biochemical assessments include daily measurements of renal and liver function, with twice-weekly checks of phosphate, calcium, magnesium, albumin and protein levels, and haematological indices (haemoglobin, white blood cell count, haematocrit), until the patient is stabilised. Then, weekly or fortnightly measurements are necessary. Patients receiving PN require urinalysis daily initially in case glycosuria occurs, as this induces further fluid and electrolyte losses. If glycosuria occurs, it may be necessary to commence intravenous insulin on a sliding scale with hourly blood glucose monitoring. It is important to note that if the PN fluid is stopped, insulin requirements will reduce immediately; it is safest to discontinue the insulin at the same time as the PN, reviewing the sliding scale with a view to giving intravenous glucose if required.

Routes of access (enteral or parenteral) should be regularly examined to ensure that the catheter is correctly positioned and mechanically satisfactory.

When feeding is prolonged, other assessments, e.g. muscle function, nitrogen balance, measurement of trace elements and vitamins, may be performed regularly to ascertain patient progress (see nutritional assessment section above).

Nutritional support teams

It is clear that for optimal provision of nutritional support, a multidisciplinary nutritional support team is required. This may comprise a clinician with a special interest in nutritional support and understanding of metabolic pathways, a biochemist, a pharmacist, a dietician and a nursing specialist.

> ✓✓ The provision of nutritional support by such a team results in the most cost-effective use of nutritional support and the least risk of infective, metabolic and feeding-line complications.[41]

Nutritional support in defined clinical situations

Nutritional support in the perioperative period

Parenteral nutrition

There is debate as to which patients require preoperative and/or postoperative nutritional support. Many studies have evaluated the effects of nutritional support in the perioperative period; clinical benefit with supplemental nutrition has not been a consistent finding. This may be because the studies were small, with many different end-points (e.g. morbidity, mortality), frequently without proper randomisation or allowance for malnutrition prior to the study commencing.

A meta-analysis has examined 27 randomised controlled trials (almost 3000 patients) of nutritional support in the perioperative period.[42] The results are important and provide a basis for the rational use of nutritional support in this situation. The key findings are detailed in Table 17.1. When PN was given in the preoperative period there was a reduction in complication rates (relative risk 0.52, 95% confidence interval (CI) 0.30–0.91) in malnourished patients but not when nutritional state was adequate. However, there was no difference in mortality. Analysis of patients in the postoperative period indicated no reduction in complications (relative risk 1.08, 95% CI 0.81–1.43) or mortality in patients receiving PN. Subgroup analyses indicated that nutritional support in the preoperative period be considered for:

Table 17.1 • Effect of perioperative nutritional support on morbidity and mortality in surgical patients

	Complications (RR and 95% CI)	Mortality (RR and 95% CI)
Malnourished patients	0.53 (0.30–0.91)	1.13 (0.75–1.71)
Adequate nutrition	0.95 (0.75–1.21)	0.90 (0.66–1.2)
Preoperative TPN	0.70 (0.52–0.95)	0.85 (0.6–1.20)
Postoperative TPN	1.01 (0.70–1.46)	1.08 (0.73–1.58)
Overall effects	0.81 (0.65–1.01)	0.97 (0.76–1.24)

CI, confidence interval; RR, relative risk; TPN, total parenteral nutrition.

- those with a serum albumin <30–32 g/L;
- patients with a weight loss of 15% or more, associated with impairment of physiological function;
- patients with a nutrition (prognostic) risk index <83.5.

✔✔ Nutritional support should be given to malnourished patients for at least 7–10 days preoperatively where possible to reduce postoperative morbidity.[42] Nutritional support in the postoperative period should be considered for:

- patients in whom it is anticipated that normal oral intake is unlikely for 7 days or more after surgery;
- those with severe sepsis or burns;
- those with enterocutaneous fistulas (particularly if high output);
- patients who have lost 15% or more of their usual weight prior to surgery being undertaken.

Enteral nutrition

As discussed, the enteral route is the preferred route except in specific circumstances where not possible (e.g. intestinal obstruction, ileus, intestinal ischaemia, etc.) or used in combination with PN if the nutritional requirements cannot be provided by the enteral route alone. A recent analysis of studies of enteral nutrition given to patients in the perioperative period has been carried out and published as European Society of Parenteral and Enteral Nutrition (ESPEN) guidelines[43] (www.espen.org/Education/documents/ENSurgery.pdf).

Nutritional support in patients with acute pancreatitis (see also Chapter 8)

Severe pancreatitis produces a major catabolic stress with rapid loss of muscle proteins. The daily nitrogen requirements of such patients are high, reaching 1.2–2.0 g protein/kg body weight (0.2–0.3 g of nitrogen/kg). Daily energy requirements also increase with disease severity to be 28–35 kcal/kg. Previously, patients with pancreatitis were fasted in order to avoid pancreatic stimulation. However, views have now changed[44,45] and a recent systematic review[46] has shown that patients with acute severe pancreatitis should commence enteral support early (within 5 days). This resulted in better outcomes with reduced infectious complications and hospital stay, but without effect on mortality.[44–46]

✔✔ Patients with severe acute pancreatitis should commence early enteral nutritional support as this is associated with a better outcome.[46]

Nutritional supplementation in inflammatory bowel disease

A significant number of patients with Crohn's disease and ulcerative colitis become malnourished. The reasons for this include decreased nutrient intake, malabsorption by the small intestine (decreased length, bacterial overgrowth, protein-losing enteropathy) and increased calorie/nitrogen requirements in those with coexistent sepsis. There may be deficiencies of specific vitamins and trace elements.

Nutritional support, therefore, may have different roles: (i) to provide nutritional requirements and correct nutritional deficiencies the patient may have; (ii) the possibility that provision of PN with bowel rest in Crohn's disease may be therapeutically beneficial. The results of studies addressing this latter point are inconclusive,[47,48] suggesting that PN itself does not have a therapeutic effect in inflammatory bowel disease. Furthermore, there is evidence showing that enteral nutrition is as effective as PN in these patients.[49] This has the added benefits of maintaining gut mucosa integrity in addition to stimulating production of gut hormones necessary for function.

✔✔ The ESPEN guidance is summarised as follows.[43] Patients who should receive perioperative nutritional support:

- Those expected not to eat for >7 days perioperatively.
- Those unable to have an oral intake >60% of their recommended intake for >10 days.

Patients who should receive preoperative enteral nutritional support:

- Preoperative nutritional support should be given for 10–14 days to those with 'severe' nutritional risk, which is defined as either a BMI <18.5 kg/m², recent weight loss of 10–15% in the previous 6 months or serum albumin <30 g/L (with no evidence of renal or hepatic failure). For such patients it is recommended that surgery should be delayed if possible to allow nutritional support.

Patients who should receive postoperative nutritional support:

- Early enteral nutritional feeding (i.e. <24 hours after surgery) is recommended for patients who have undergone upper gastrointestinal anastomosis with the tip of a feeding tube placed distal to the anastomosis.

> ✓ While systematic reviews have shown some potential for enteral nutrition in this regard, further studies are required to clarify the use of nutrition in this way.[50,51]

Nutritional support in enterocutaneous fistulas

Nutritional support has an important role to play in management of patients with enterocutaneous fistulas as up to 50% are malnourished. The importance of adequate nutritional support was demonstrated by Chapman et al.,[52] who found that if patients with fistulas received nutritional support with PN and enteral feeding (>3000 kcal (12.6 MJ) daily), spontaneous fistula healing with a reduced mortality occurred compared with patients with fistulas receiving less than 1000 kcal (4.1 MJ) daily. The management of such patients commences with correction of fluid and electrolyte deficits and elimination of septic foci. Nutritional support is required to correct any nutritional deficits and provides maintenance requirements when the patient is stabilised. Whether PN or enteral nutrition is more effective is unknown. Other techniques for providing nutritional support have included collecting the intestinal output from the proximal end of the fistula and re-infusing it into the distal part of the small intestine or by giving enteral nutrition via the fistula. If the fistula output is low, enteral nutritional support should be considered because of the benefits.[53]

> ✓ Enteral nutrition has theoretical benefits due to its effects on gut mucosa and case series have suggested that healing rates with enteral nutrition are comparable to those of parenteral nutrition.[53]

Nutritional support in patients with burns

Major burns induce severe hypermetabolic and hypercatabolic states. There is increased skeletal muscle breakdown, nitrogen losses of 15 g daily or more, and up to a doubling of metabolic rate. In patients with burns of greater than 20% of their body surface area, nutritional support is required, orally or by nasoenteric feeding. There may be clinical benefits by introducing feeding early, and with glutamine supplementation.[54,55] This appears to be associated with reduced infectious complications

> ✓ Glutamine supplementation should be given to patients with substantial burns to reduce their complications and improve healing. If enteral nutritional support is not possible, e.g. with gastric stasis, ileus or other coexistent injuries, parenteral nutrition is required.

and better wound healing, and is recommended by the ESPEN guidelines.[56]

Several formulae exist for calculating the protein and calorie requirements.[57] However, up to 20–25 g of nitrogen per day may be required initially, with a non-protein calorie to nitrogen ratio of 100–200. Energy is provided as carbohydrate and lipids, with the calorie requirement being 35–50% as lipid.

Nutritional supplementation with key nutrients: application to clinical practice

Certain nutrients can have effects on cellular and tissue function. Some of these nutrients modulate immune and inflammatory responses if given in excess of normal intake or requirements. The use of nutrients ('nutriceuticals') in this way has been termed 'nutritional pharmacology'. Examples and specific effects include:

- L-arginine – stimulates aspects of immune function, improves nitrogen retention after surgery, enhances wound healing;[58,59]
- L-glutamine – stimulates immune function, reduces nitrogen loss postoperatively, may be important in maintaining gut-barrier function;[60]
- branched-chain amino acids – may control protein synthesis in muscle and stimulate whole-body protein synthesis, especially in severely traumatised patients;[61]
- essential fatty acids – stimulation or inhibition of immune function, anti-inflammatory effects;[62,63]
- polyribonucleotides and ribonucleic acid – stimulate immune function;
- vitamins, trace elements – stimulation of immune function, antioxidant effects, wound healing;
- selenium – stimulation of immune function, prevention of tissue damage, anti-inflammatory effects;[64]
- omega-3 fatty acids – immunomodulatory effect and avoidance of hepatic dysfunction.[65]

The clinical benefits of supplementation with key nutrients have, however, been difficult to demonstrate.

Combinations of these nutrients and their place in practice

Several studies have evaluated the use of combinations of key nutrients in clinical practice in patients with critical illnesses (trauma, surgery for malignant disease, burns), but particularly in upper gastrointestinal cancer. A combination of L-arginine, n-3 essential fatty acids and ribonucleic acid is commercially available (Impact; Sandoz Nutrition, Minneapolis, MN, USA) and has been used in many trials. The supplemented nutrition has been given in the postoperative period (nasoenteric tube or feeding jejunostomy), starting within 12–48 hours of the critical events and continued for several days.

The first meta-analysis of the studies that have compared supplemented nutritional versus standard nutritional diets (**Figs 17.2** and **17.3**) showed that supplemented nutrition had clinical benefits:[66]

- reduction in infectious complications (wound infections, intra-abdominal abscesses, septicaemia), with an odds ratio of 0.47 (95% CI 0.32–0.70);
- reduction in length of hospital stay, with a weighted mean difference of −2.4 days (95% CI −4 to −1).

However, there was no significant difference in mortality. A subsequent meta-analysis of 17 trials has confirmed this benefit.[67]

Many of these studies had methodological limitations but, nevertheless, the role of immunonutrition in critically ill patients was further investigated by ESPEN[56] (www.espen.org/Education/documents/ENICU.pdf). The conclusion drawn from the consensus based on the available evidence was that an

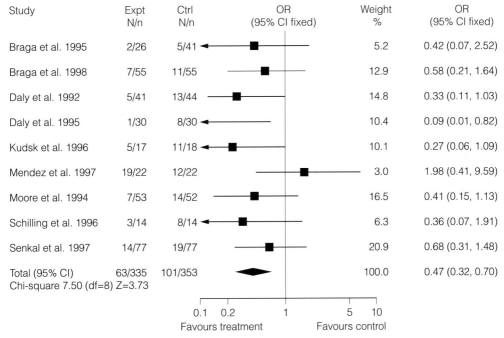

Figure 17.2 • Effect of immune-enhancing diets on the incidence of major infective complications (wound infections, intra-abdominal abscesses, pneumonia, septicaemia). Expt, patients receiving immune-enhancing diets; Ctrl, patients receiving standard nutrition; n, number of events; N, number of patients in each group on an intention-to-treat basis; OR, odds ratio; CI, confidence interval. (Study sources are given in Heys et al.[60]). Reproduced from Heys SD, Walker LG, Smith IC et al. Enteral nutritional supplementation with key nutrients in patients with critical illness and cancer. A meta-analysis of randomised controlled clinical trials. Ann Surg 1999; 229:467–77. With permission from Wolter Kluwers Health.

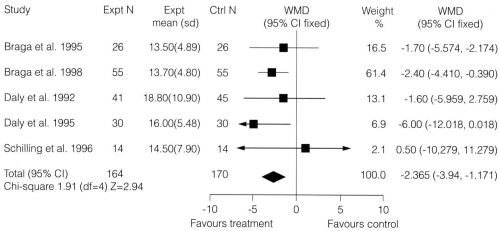

Study	Expt N	Expt mean (sd)	Ctrl N	WMD (95% CI fixed)	Weight %	WMD (95% CI fixed)
Braga et al. 1995	26	13.50(4.89)	26		16.5	-1.70 (-5.574, -2.174)
Braga et al. 1998	55	13.70(4.80)	55		61.4	-2.40 (-4.410, -0.390)
Daly et al. 1992	41	18.80(10.90)	45		13.1	-1.60 (-5.959, 2.759)
Daly et al. 1995	30	16.00(5.48)	30		6.9	-6.00 (-12.018, 0.018)
Schilling et al. 1996	14	14.50(7.90)	14		2.1	0.50 (-10,279, 11.279)
Total (95% CI)	164		170		100.0	-2.365 (-3.94, -1.171)

Chi-square 1.91 (df=4) Z=2.94

-10 -5 0 5 10
Favours treatment   Favours control

Figure 17.3 • Effect of immune-enhancing diets on the length of hospital stay. WMD, weighted mean difference; CI, confidence interval. (Study sources are given in Heys et al.[66]) Reproduced from Heys SD, Walker LG, Smith IC et al. Enteral nutritional supplementation with key nutrients in patients with critical illness and cancer. A meta-analysis of randomised controlled clinical trials. Ann Surg 1999; 229:467–77. With permission from Wolter Kluwers Health.

immune-modulating nutrition (enriched with arginine, nucleotides and omega-3 fatty acids) was beneficial and recommended for the following:

- patients with mild sepsis (APACHE II score <15);
- patients undergoing elective major intra-abdominal surgery for cancer to receive 5–7 days of immune-enhancing nutrition (arginine, omega-3 fatty acids and polyribonucleotides);
- patients with acute respiratory distress syndrome (ARDS) should receive enteral nutrition supplemented with omega-3 fatty acids and antioxidants.

In addition, there were situations identified where immunonutrition should not be given due to potentially adverse effects:

- patients with severe sepsis;
- patients unable to tolerate more than 700 mL/ day of immunonutrition.

✔✔ Immune-modulating nutrition is associated with a reduction in septic complications and a reduced hospital stay. It should be considered in patients with mild sepsis (APACHE II score <15), patients undergoing elective major intra-abdominal surgery for cancer and in patients with ARDS.[56,66,67]

Key points

- Malnutrition is associated with loss of body weight and impairments in organ function.
- The metabolic changes that occur in patients undergoing surgery or in those who have experienced trauma and sepsis can be compounded by inadequate nutritional support.
- Nutritional requirements must take into consideration the underlying pathophysiological changes.
- An assessment of nutritional status should be made in all patients.
- If nutritional support is considered necessary, the route and composition of this support should be considered carefully.
- Remember re-feeding syndrome and possible thiamine deficiency.
- The role of certain key nutrients and their effects, either individually or in combination, on aspects of organ and immune function should be taken into consideration when planning nutritional interventions.
- There is now emerging evidence to indicate that manipulating the composition of nutritional support can affect patient outcome.
- Careful monitoring of patients receiving nutritional support and the role of the multidisciplinary team is essential for all patients.

References

1. Cuthbertson DP. Observations on the disturbances of metabolism produced by injury to the limbs. Q J Med 1932;1:233–46.

2. O'Keefe SJD, Sender PM, James WPT. Catabolic loss of body nitrogen in response to surgery. Lancet 1974;ii:1035–8.

3. Bergstrom J, Furst P, Noree L-O, et al. Intracellular free amino acid concentration in human muscle tissue. J Appl Physiol 1973;36:693–8.

4. Stoner HB. Studies on the mechanism of shock. The quantitative aspects of glycogen metabolism after limb ischaemia in the rat. Br J Exp Pathol 1958;39:635–51.

5. Allsop JR, Wolfe RR, Burke JF. Glucose kinetics and responsiveness to insulin in the rat injured by burn. Surg Gynecol Obstet 1978;147:565–73.

6. Nordenstrom J, Carpentier YA, Askanazi J, et al. Free fatty acid mobilisation and oxidation during total parenteral nutrition in trauma and infection. Ann Surg 1983;198:725–35.

7. Galloway P, McMillan D, Sattar N. Effect of the inflammatory response on trace element and vitamin status. Ann Clin Biochem 2000;37:289–97.

8. Broom J. Sepsis and trauma. In: Garrow JS, James WPT, editors. editors. Human nutrition and dietetics. 9th ed. Edinburgh: Churchill Livingstone; 1993. p. 456–64.

9. Ayling R, Marshall W. Nutrition and laboratory medicine. ACB Venture Publications; 2007.

10. Metropolitan Life Assurance Company. Statist Bull 1959;40:1.

11. Pettigrew RA. Assessment of malnourished patients. In: Burns HG, editor. Clinical gastroenterology. London: BaillièreTindall; 1988. p. 729–49.

12. Durnin J.V.G.A., Womersley J. Body-fat assessed from total body density and its estimation from skin-fold thickness: measurements on 481 men and women aged from 16 to 72 years. Br J Nutr 1987;32:77–97.

13. Lukaski HC. Methods for the assessment of human body composition. Am J Clin Nutr 1987;46:537–56.

14. Kushner RE, Kunigk A, Alspaugh M, et al. Validation of bioelectrical-impedance analysis as a measurement of change in body composition in obesity. Am J Clin Nutr 1990;52:219–23.

15. Ryan JA, Taft DA. Preoperative nutritional assessment does not predict morbidity and mortality in abdominal operations. Surg Forum 1980;31:96–8.

16. Rothschild MA, Oratz M, Schreiber SS. Albumin metabolism. Gastroenterology 1973;64:324–37.

17. Fleck A, Raines G, Hawker F, et al. Increased vascular permeability: a major cause of hypoalbuminaemia in disease and injury. Lancet 1985;i:781–4.

18. Eremin O, Broom J. Nutrition and the immune response. In: Eremin O, Sewell HF, editors. The immunological basis of surgical science and practice. Oxford: Oxford University Press; 1992. p. 133–44.

19. Bistrian BR, Blackburn GL, Scrimshaw NJ, et al. Cellular immunity in semistarved hospitalized adults. Am J Clin Nutr 1975;28:1148–55.

20. Seltzer MH, Bastidas JA, Cooper DM, et al. Instant nutritional assessment. J Parenteral Enteral Nutr 1979;3:157–9.

21. Heys SD, Khan AL, Eremin O. Immune suppression in surgery. Postgrad Surg 1995;5:62–7.

22. Lopes J, Russke DM, Whitwell J, et al. Skeletal muscle function in malnutrition. Am J Clin Nutr 1982;36:602–10.

23. Daley BJ, Bistrian BR. Nutritional assessment. In: Zaloga GP, editor. Nutrition in critical care. St Louis: Mosby Year Book; 1994. p. 28.

24. Hill G, Windsor JA. Nutritional assessment in clinical practice. Nutrition 1995;11(Suppl.):198–201.

25. Johnson LR, Copeland EM, Dudrick SJ, et al. Structural and hormonal alterations in the gastrointestinal tract of parenterally fed rats. Gastroenterology 1975;68:1177–83.

26. Levine GM, Deren JJ, Steiger E, et al. Role of oral intake in maintenance of gut mass and disaccharide activity. Gastroenterology 1974;67:975–82.

27. Wilmore D, Smith R, O'Dwyer S, et al. The gut: a central organ after sepsis. Surgery 1988;104:917–23.

28. Fong Y, Marano MA, Barber A, et al. Total parenteral nutrition and bowel rest modify the metabolic response to endotoxin in humans. Ann Surg 1989;210:449–56.

29. Grimble GK, Payne-James JJ, Rees RGP, et al. Nutrition support. London: Medical Tribune UK; 1989. p. 32–51.

30. Gayle D, Pinchcofsky-Devlin RD, Kaminski MV. Visceral protein increase associated with interrupted versus continuous enteral hyperalimentation. J Parenteral Enteral Nutr 1985;9:474–6.

31. ASPEN Board of Directors The Clinical Guidelines Task Force. Guidelines for the use of parenteral and enteral nutrition in adult and pediatric patients. J Parenter Enteral Nutr 2002;26S:1SA–138SA.

32. Adam A. Insertion of long term central venous catheters: time for a new look. Br Med J 1995;311:341–2.

33. Robertson LJ, Mauro MA, Jaques PF. Radiologic placement of Hickman catheters. Radiology 1989;170:1007.

34. Lameris JS, Post PJM, Zonderland HM, et al. Percutaneous placement of Hickman catheters: comparison of sonographically guided and blinded techniques. Am J Roentgenol 1990;155:1097–9.

35. Maki DG, Ringer M. Evaluation of dressing regimens for prevention of infection with peripheral intravenous catheters. JAMA 1987;258:2396–403.

36. Andrews PJD, Avenell A, Noble DW, et al. Randomised trial of glutamine and selenium supplemented parenteral nutrition for critically ill patients. Br Med J 2011;342:695.

37. Levinson MR, Groeger JS, Jeevanandam M, et al. Free fatty acid turnover and lipolysis in septic mechanically ventilated cancer-bearing humans. Metabolism 1988;37:618–25.

38. Shaw JHF, Woolfe RR. Energy and protein metabolism in sepsis and trauma. Aust N Z J Surg 1987;57:41–7.

39. Venus B, Patel CB, Mathru M, et al. Pulmonary effects of lipid infusion in patients with acute respiratory failure (abstract). Crit Care Med 1984;12:293.

40. Seidner DL, Mascioli EA, Istfan NW, et al. Effects of long chain triacylglycerol emulsions on reticuloendothelial system function in humans. J Parenteral Enteral Nutr 1989;13:614–9.

41. www.nice.org.uk/CG32 [accessed 12.01.13].
NICE guidance on nutrition support in adults: oral nutrition support, enteral tube feeding and parenteral nutrition, including guidelines for the role and function of multidisciplinary nutritional support teams.

42. Heyland DK, Montalvo M, MacDonald S, et al. Total parenteral nutrition in the surgical patient: a meta-analysis. Can J Surg 2001;44:102–11.
A meta-analysis of randomised controlled trials of parenteral nutritional support that attempts to draw together the evidence as to which patients benefit from TPN.

43. Weimann A, Braga M, Harsanyi L, et al. ESPEN Guidelines on Enteral Nutrition: surgery including organ transplantation. Clin Nutr 2006;25(2):224–44.
Evidence-based guidelines summarising the current evidence and making recommendations for clinical practice in patients during the perioperative period.

44. Croad NR. The management of acute severe pancreatitis. Br J Intensive Care 1999;2:38–45.

45. Kanwar A, Windsor ACJ, Li A, et al. Benefits of early enteral nutrition in acute pancreatitis. Br J Surg 1997;84:875.

46. McClave SA, Chang WK, Dhaliwal R, et al. Nutrition support in acute pancreatitis: a systematic review of the literature. J Parenter Enteral Nutr 2006;30:143–56.
Current updated position evaluating evidence for clinical nutritional support in patients with acute pancreatitis.

47. Dickinson RJ, Ashton MG, Axon ATR, et al. Controlled trial of intravenous hyperalimentation as an adjunct to the routine therapy of acute colitis. Gastroenterology 1980;79:1199–204.

48. Muller JM, Keller HW, Erasmi H, et al. Total parenteral nutrition as sole therapy in Crohn's disease: a prospective study. Br J Surg 1983;70:40–3.

49. Jones VA. Comparison of total parenteral nutrition and enteral diet in induction of remission in Crohn's disease: long term maintenance of remission by personalised food exclusion. Dig Dis Sci 1987;32 (Suppl.):1005–75.

50. Zachos M, Tondeur M, Griffiths AM. Enteral nutrition therapy for induction of remission in Crohn's disease. Cochrane Database Syst Rev 2001:CD000542.

51. Akobeng AK, Thomas AG. Enteral nutrition for maintenance of remission in Crohn's disease. Cochrane Database Syst Rev 2007:CD005984.

52. Chapman R, Foran R, Dunphey JE. Management of intestinal fistulas. Am J Surg 1964;108:157–64.

53. Lloyd DA, Gabe SM, Windsor AC. Nutrition and management of enterocutaneous fistula. Br J Surg 2006;93:1045–55.

54. Windle EM. Glutamine supplementation in critical illness: evidence, recommendations, and implications for clinical practice in burns care. J Burn Care Res 2006;27:764–72.

55. Wasiak J, Cleland H, Jeffery R. Early versus late enteral nutrition in adults with burn injury: a systematic review. J Hum Nutr Rev 2007;20:75–83.

56. Kreymann KG, Berger MM, Deutz NEP, et al. ESPEN Guidelines on Enteral Nutrition: intensive care. Clin Nutr 2006;25:210–23.
Evidence-based guidelines summarising the current evidence and making recommendations for clinical practice.

57. Chiarelli A, Siliprandi L. Burns. In: Zagola GP, editor. Nutrition in critical care. St Louis: Mosby Year Book; 1994. p. 587–97.

58. Brittenden J, Park KGM, Heys SD, et al. 1-Arginine stimulates host defences in patients with breast cancer. Surgery 1994;115:205–12.

59. Brittenden J, Heys SD, Ross JA, et al. Nutritional pharmacology: effects of L-arginine on host defences, responses to trauma and tumour growth. Clin Sci 1994;86:123–32.

60. Heys SD, Park KGM, Garlick PJ, et al. Nutrition and malignancy: implications for surgical practice. Br J Surg 1992;79:614–23.

61. Heys SD, Gough DB, Kahn AL, et al. Nutritional pharmacology and malignant disease: a therapeutic modality in patients with cancer? Br J Surg 1996;83:608–19.

62. Purasiri P, Murray A, Richardson S, et al. Modulation of cytokine production in vivo by dietary essential fatty acids in patients with colorectal cancer. ClinSci 1994;87:711–7.

63. Purasiri P, McKechnie A, Heys SD, et al. Modulation in vitro of human natural cytotoxicity, lymphocyte proliferative response to mitogens and cytokine production by essential fatty acids. Immunology 1997;92:166–72.

64. Avenell A, Noble DW, Barr J, et al. Selenium supplementation for critically ill adults. Cochrane Database Syst Rev 2004;4:CD003703.

65. Chen WJ, Yeh SL. Effects of fish oil in parenteral nutrition. Nutrition 2003;19:275–9.

66. Heys SD, Walker LG, Smith IC, et al. Enteral nutritional supplementation with key nutrients in patients with critical illness and cancer. A meta-analysis of randomised controlled clinical trials. Ann Surg 1999;229:467–77.

This is the first meta-analysis that indicated that immunonutrition could result in clinically important benefits for patients in terms of reduction in infectious complications postoperatively.

67. Heyland DK, Novak F, Drover JW, et al. Should immunonutrition become routine in critically ill patients? JAMA 2001;286:944–53.

This is an updated meta-analysis of randomised controlled trials that confirms the previous meta-analysis and extends it further by examining different subgroups of patients in an attempt to try to understand further which patients are the most likely to benefit from immunonutrition.

18

Abdominal sepsis and abdominal compartment syndrome

Emma Barrow
Iain D. Anderson

Introduction

Abdominal sepsis accounts for many of the serious and all too often fatal emergency conditions that the general surgeon is called upon to treat. It may arise primarily from conditions as seemingly simple and routine as appendicitis, to more complicated and serious conditions such as diverticulitis and perforated peptic ulcer disease. Alternatively it may arise as a consequence of complications of surgery, particularly intestinal anastomotic leakage. While, with experience and a few basic principles, even complex cases of abdominal sepsis can be relatively straightforward to manage, not infrequently the diagnosis is obscured and delayed. As a consequence treatment is often complicated and prolonged. Some 80–90% of general surgical deaths follow emergency admission,[1] and much of this morbidity and mortality expresses itself through the processes of abdominal sepsis. Delay to operation is the single most common reason for adverse outcomes and anastomotic leak the single commonest cited complication in fatal cases. These will be recurring themes in this chapter as even with optimal treatment of abdominal sepsis, multiple organ failure (MOF) may ensue. MOF is more likely and often fatal when treatment is slow or suboptimal. In the intensive care unit (ICU), abdominal sepsis constitutes a substantial proportion of the patients with MOF. Given its frequency and severity, a sound understanding of abdominal sepsis must be integral to every general surgeon's professional armamentarium.

This chapter will address the diagnosis and management of abdominal sepsis, including the complex patient in the ICU, where sequelae such as abdominal compartment syndrome, management of the open abdomen and intestinal fistulation can create particular difficulties. The reader is referred to Chapter 16 for a description of the intensive care management of the surgical patient, Chapters 6, 8, 9, 10 and 13 for more detail on specific causal conditions, and to Chapter 17 for surgical nutrition.

Pathophysiology of sepsis

The systemic inflammatory response syndrome (SIRS) is a clinically defined response (Box 18.1) to a variety of insults including trauma, burns, pancreatitis, tissue ischaemia and inflammatory bowel disease. When the cause of SIRS is a proven or suspected infection, it is termed sepsis. The normal response to infection serves to localise and control bacterial invasion. This occurs through the chemotaxis of neutrophils and macrophages, which in turn release inflammatory mediators. When this inflammatory response becomes generalised, sepsis results. This is characterised by systemic vasodilation and resultant hypotension, increased vascular permeability leading to fluid exudate, and microcirculatory dysfunction with decreased capillary flow. These factors ultimately result in tissue hypoxia. Once triggered, the downward spiral of severe sepsis is believed to be independent of the precipitating infectious insult.

The theory that sepsis is due to an exaggerated, uncontrolled inflammatory response has now been shown to be overly simplistic. There is no

Box 18.1 • Sepsis definitions[13]

Systemic inflammatory response syndrome (SIRS)

SIRS is defined by the presence of two or more of the following clinical findings:

- Body temperature >38 °C or >36 °C
- Heart rate >90 per minute
- Respiratory rate >20 per minute or $PaCO_2$ <4.3 kPa
- White cell count >12×10^9/L or <4×10^9/L

Sepsis

SIRS plus a documented or suspected infection

Severe sepsis

Sepsis plus clinical evidence of organ dysfunction:

- Hypoxia
- Oliguria
- Hypotension
- Confusion
- Disturbances to coagulation
- Disturbances to liver synthetic function

Septic shock

Sepsis with acute circulatory failure, despite adequate volume resuscitation in the absence of other causes of hypotension

- SBP <90 mmHg
- MAP <60 mmHg

Multiple organ dysfunction syndrome (MODS)

- Altered organ function in an acutely ill patient such that homeostasis cannot be maintained without intervention
- Potentially reversible
- Affects two or more organ systems

single mediator, system or pathway that drives the pathophysiology of SIRS and sepsis. The predominant theories can be summarised as follows:

1. **Uncontrolled systemic cytokine release.**
   Uncontrolled release of cytokines from macrophages in response to cellular injury is proposed to initiate other mediator cascades and activate neutrophils and platelets. The particular candidate mediators are tumour necrosis factor (TNF) α, interleukin (IL)-1 and IL-6.[2] However, circulating levels of cytokines are highly variable between different studies and indeed within study populations.[3] Numerous trials have been conducted on agents that block the inflammatory cascade: corticosteroids, TNFα antagonists and anticytokine monoclonal antibodies. These have failed to demonstrate a survival

advantage.[3] Individual randomised trials in the clinical effectiveness of activated protein C in severe sepsis showed promising results,[3] but a recent Cochrane review concluded no survival advantage[4] and it has now been withdrawn.

2. **Disturbances to coagulation.** During sepsis, significant alterations occur within both the coagulation and fibrinolytic systems. Activation of vascular endothelial cells by inflammatory mediators leads to a prothrombotic state, which can result in disseminated intravascular coagulation (DIC). This leads to reduced end perfusion, and the subsequent consumption of platelets and clotting factors results in prolonged clotting times.[3,5]

3. **Immunosuppression.** Another emerging theory implicates immunosuppression rather than immunostimulation in the aetiology of sepsis. Patients with sepsis display features of immunosuppression, such as an inability to clear infection and predisposition towards nosocomial pathogens.[3] A proposed mechanism is a shift from T helper cell secretion of inflammatory cytokines such as TNFα, IL-1 and IL-6 to the anti-inflammatory cytokines IL-4 and IL-10.[3,5] This pattern of cytokine release has been observed in septic patients in an intensive care setting.[6,7] Lymphocyte apoptosis is another postulated pathway.[3]

The slippery slope of sepsis

SIRS and sepsis occur commonly amongst surgical patients on the ward, although they are usually resolved by appropriate treatment of the underlying problem. Sometimes the physiological derangement persists and, particularly when it does so beyond 48 hours, outcome is worsened as progression to organ dysfunction is much more likely. Organ dysfunction denotes severe sepsis and the next step is organ failure, which typically carries a mortality of the order of 40%. Mortality, in general, increases with the number of organ systems affected and with the severity of physiological disturbance at onset.[8] While the onset of SIRS does not accurately predict development of sepsis or the multiple organ dysfunction syndrome (MODS), the progression from SIRS to severe sepsis is associated with increasing risk of multiple organ failure.[9] Approximately 30% of septic patients develop at least one organ dysfunction.[10] Therefore, timely recognition of SIRS, particularly if persistent, alerts the clinician to a potentially deteriorating situation at a time when prompt intervention may yet avert catastrophe. By the time the patient with abdominal sepsis has developed shock, the mortality increases from less than 10% to greater than 50%.[11,12]

The identification and active management of SIRS and early organ dysfunction is therefore an important first step as, once organ dysfunction is under way, the patient is on a slippery slope that can lead them rapidly downwards despite the best treatment. It is essential that the surgeon appreciates that these processes often start insidiously on the ward and that early detection is vital, as management is most successful at this stage. While there are objective criteria that define organ dysfunction, clinical findings are useful pointers. Hypoxia, oliguria, hypotension, deranged liver function tests or clotting, thrombocytopenia, acidosis and confusion are some of the plethora of signs that indicate that a severe systemic derangement is in process.

✔✔ The importance of detecting the often subtle signs of abdominal sepsis at the earliest stage cannot be overemphasised and while the rate with which organ dysfunction develops in individual patients will vary, the requirement for rapid identification and treatment remains key.[9]

Treatment strategies in sepsis

SIRS, sepsis and their sequelae are recognised and defined according to a number of clinical criteria;[13] these are summarised in Box 18.1. Whilst these specific criteria are not intended as a substitute for clinical acumen, their use facilitates early identification and appropriate treatment of sepsis by even the most junior member of the surgical team. SIRS and sepsis can be adequately managed on the ward, providing there is response to treatment. However, the deteriorating patient or those with severe sepsis are more appropriately transferred to a critical care environment, where invasive arterial and central venous pressure monitoring will guide resuscitation. The benefits of managing such high-risk surgical patients with early critical care input are well recognised.[14,15]

The Surviving Sepsis Campaign

In 2008, informed by the results of a number of clinical trials, an international campaign was launched,[16] with the intention of improving outcomes in severe sepsis and septic shock by standardising care. The emphasis of the campaign was timely identification and treatment of patients with severe sepsis,

Box 18.2 • Surviving Sepsis Campaign bundles[16]

Sepsis resuscitation bundle

To be accomplished within the first 6 hours of identification of severe sepsis:

1. Measure serum lactate
2. Obtain blood cultures prior to antibiotic administration
3. Administer broad-spectrum antibiotic, within 3 hours of A&E admission and within 1 hour for current inpatients
4. In the event of hypotension and/or a serum lactate >4 mmol/L:
   a. Deliver an initial minimum of 20 mL/kg of crystalloid or an equivalent
   b. Apply vasopressors for hypotension not responding to initial fluid resuscitation to maintain mean arterial pressure (MAP) >65 mmHg
5. In the event of persistent hypotension despite fluid resuscitation (septic shock) and/or lactate >4 mmol/L:
   a. Achieve a central venous pressure (CVP) of >8 mmHg
   b. Achieve a central venous oxygen saturation (ScvO$_2$) >70% or mixed venous oxygen saturation (SvO$_2$) >65%

Sepsis management bundle

To be accomplished within the first 24 hours of identification of severe sepsis:

1. Administer low-dose steroids for septic shock in accordance with a standardised ICU policy
2. Maintain glucose control >70 but <150 mg/dL
3. Maintain a median inspiratory plateau pressure (IPP) <30 cm H$_2$O for mechanically ventilated patients

using goal-directed strategies (the rationale for this is detailed in Chapter 16). Evidence-based guidelines were published in 2004, split into 'bundles' of care to be accomplished within certain time frames (Box 18.2). A total of 165 sites participated in the campaign, submitting bundle compliance and outcome data on 15 022 patients with severe sepsis. Despite incomplete compliance, a significant reduction in unadjusted hospital mortality (37% to 31% over the 2-year study period) was identified in those centres participating in the campaign.[17]

✔✔ The goal-directed treatment bundles developed by the Surviving Sepsis Campaign are to be recommended as a standard of care. Their use in the timely identification and management of patients with severe sepsis has been shown to reduce mortality.[17]

Systematic assessment

Although effective management of patients with severe sepsis may entail complex investigations and procedures, the results of these manoeuvres are often suboptimal or even lethal without adequate prior resuscitation. A systematic approach such as that described in the *Care of the Critically Ill Surgical Patient* (CCrISP) course[18] has much to recommend it, as it provides a common management structure for problems of any type or severity (**Fig. 18.1**). Having a structured approach in times of crisis facilitates speed and may also be important in reducing the likelihood of management errors. It certainly provides a common language and transparency that lets other health professionals understand interventions more easily. With complex abdominal sepsis, a team approach is required: firstly, because help will often be needed from radiology, anaesthesia and intensive care; and secondly, because the illness will often run a prolonged time course of days or weeks and hence many doctors will be involved.

Patients with abdominal sepsis will present with some degree of instability and CCrISP advocates rapid **immediate management** following ABC principles of assessment with simultaneous correction of life-threatening conditions and initiation of high-flow oxygen therapy, fluid resuscitation and

basic monitoring as required. Although some patients will deteriorate catastrophically and require immediate intensive care support, simple resuscitation will more commonly buy sufficient time for a more thorough **full assessment** to be carried out. This aims to determine the cause and severity of any problem and to exclude other conditions that would prove deleterious if left untreated. It also includes a thorough appraisal of the patient's notes and charts.

As the clinical manifestations of abdominal sepsis can be subtle and varied (Box 18.3), a high index of suspicion, combined with anticipation of potential complications, is essential. Complications can usually be anticipated from the surgical condition in question, any operation recently carried out and knowledge of comorbid conditions. Frequently, the range of possible diagnoses is large (Box 18.4) and the initial diagnostic net must be cast wide before drawing it in rapidly with the assistance of selective investigations. Reaching a provisional diagnosis and management plan rapidly is important as outcome worsens with delay and deterioration.

Patients should improve after clinical interventions. Failure to progress, or signs of deterioration, suggest a new problem or an unresolved one. The same systematic CCrISP approach forms the basis of ongoing assessment of the critically ill or at-risk patient on the critical care unit or ward. As repeated complications and setbacks are likely in complex cases, the surgeon must be prepared for a long campaign as compared to a single battle, and be prepared to take a leading role in ongoing management.

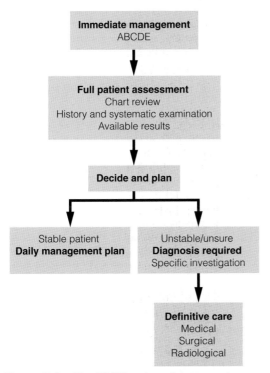

Figure 18.1 • The CCrISP system of assessment. Reproduced from Anderson ID. Assessing the critically ill surgical patient. In: Anderson ID (ed.) Care of the critically ill surgical patient. London: Arnold, 1999; pp. 7–15. © Hodder Arnold. Reproduced by permission of Hodder Education.

Box 18.3 • General manifestations of abdominal sepsis in the ward or HDU patient

Pyrexia or hypothermia
Tachycardia
Tachypnoea
Confusion
Oedema
Metabolic acidosis
Hypoalbuminaemia
Thrombocytopenia
Ileus
Poor peripheral perfusion
Hypotension
Hypoxia
Lethargy
Oliguria
Raised lactate
Hyponatraemia
Leucocytosis or neutropenia

Box 18.4 • Some possible differential diagnoses in patients presenting with abdominal sepsis on the ward (this depends on presenting features)

Sepsis of other origin (urine, line, chest, etc.)
Cardiac (ischaemia, infarction, dysrhythmias, failure)
Cerebral (toxic confusion, ischaemia)
Pulmonary (atelectasis, collapse, infection, pulmonary embolism)
Fluid imbalance
Other non-septic abdominal complications (e.g. ileus, bleeding)

✔✔ When severe sepsis is identified, blood cultures should be taken, and broad-spectrum antibiotics administered within 1 hour. As part of a management strategy in severe sepsis and septic shock, this has been shown to reduce mortality.[17]

✔✔ Combination antibiotic therapy should be used in preference to monotherapy in severe sepsis and septic shock, as it is associated with a reduction in mortality.[21]

Antimicrobial therapy in abdominal sepsis

Definitive management of sepsis requires eradication of the source of infection. However, the role of antimicrobial therapy is also vital.[19] When sepsis is suspected, blood cultures, urine, wound swabs and sputum should be submitted for urgent Gram staining and culture, with all sources of sepsis considered. Cultures from the main source of sepsis are several times more likely to be positive (75% vs. 18%)[20] than blood cultures, but both are important in the critically ill patient. Once cultures are taken, best-guess antibiotic therapy should begin immediately as delay may influence outcome.[17] The role of cultures is to enable the antibiotics to be changed successfully if the patient fails to respond. The choice of antibiotic will be influenced by the clinical circumstances to cover the expected range of infecting organisms. Early combination antibiotic therapy yields significantly improved survival compared with single-agent use in septic shock.[21] The route of administration must ensure adequate plasma levels and the drugs should penetrate adequately into the tissues. Intravenous infusion is usually necessary. Whenever there is doubt concerning the optimal choice of antibiotics, the advice of a medical microbiologist should be urgently sought. For most abdominal sepsis, coverage of Gram-negative and anaerobic bacteria will be necessary. With biliary sepsis, approximately 15% of cases will involve streptococci species that are resistant to cephalosporins, so the addition of a modern penicillin is a common approach. With postoperative hospital acquired infection, cover against a broader and more resistant spectrum of organisms will be needed.[19] Fungal infection (usually *Candida* species) is not uncommon in complex abdominal sepsis requiring ICU care and often antifungal therapy will be required.

Imaging in abdominal sepsis

Various imaging techniques may be employed to localise an infective focus (see also Chapter 5). Computed tomography (CT), usually with gastrointestinal and/or intravenous contrast enhancement, can provide excellent information in thoracic, abdominal and pelvic sepsis. Most surgical patients can be stabilised sufficiently for safe scanning to take place and the assistance that CT gives in terms of accurate diagnosis and selective therapeutic intervention should not be underestimated. CT is excellent at primary diagnosis and at least as useful in the complex or postoperative patient where clinical examination is more difficult.[22] Contrast can be usefully inserted up drains or down stomas when needed. Comparison with previous scans is important and the input of a senior, specialist radiologist will increase the accuracy of the report. In emergency cases, the surgeon should ideally be present at the scan so that decisions about any interventional radiological procedure can be made jointly.

It should not be considered that CT or any other diagnostic test is perfect. Interference from infusions, drains and metallic prostheses may reduce image quality. Intravenous contrast use is often contraindicated in acute renal failure, although gastrointestinal contrast can still be used to advantage. Even in expert hands, there is a small but significant rate of missed diagnoses. When emergency scans are interpreted by trainees, the rate is probably higher.

The chest radiograph remains an integral part of patient assessment and ultrasound has the advantages of being portable, harmless and repeatable. The greatest utility of ultrasound probably lies with the assessment of biliary and renal pathology and the monitoring of identified collections. However, it is limited by operator dependency, and a negative scan will offer little reassurance when the clinical picture is concerning. When a focus of subacute sepsis cannot be identified radiologically, isotopic methods such as labelled white cell scanning using indium-111 may help.

Early source control in abdominal sepsis

Source control describes the physical measures taken to control an infective focus. This includes the drainage of collections, debridement of necrotic tissue and definitive surgical procedures to correct the anatomical abnormality. Whilst it is intuitive that early source control will improve outcomes in abdominal sepsis, there is a relative paucity of data to support this, and obvious ethical considerations in performing prospective randomised trials. Delay to source control significantly increases mortality in septic shock,[23] and there are clear advantages of expedient source control before progression to septic shock occurs.[17,24]

In a complex system such as a hospital, it is all too easy for multiple small delays to add up. Managing the multidisciplinary team to achieve prompt and timely intervention is a considerable skill, which requires active and continued leadership from the surgeon. The Royal College of Surgeons of England and the Department of Health have issued timelines regarding the urgency of source control in sepsis (Box 18.5), which are advocated as a standard of care.

> ✅ Expedient control of the septic focus is of utmost importance in the management of severe sepsis. Neither overly prolonged resuscitation nor observation should delay this.[14]

Aims of treatment in abdominal sepsis

The management of abdominal sepsis in the emergency surgical admission is that of the underlying disease, as covered elsewhere in this book. The aim is to deal not only with the sepsis, but also to deal

Box 18.5 • Timelines for source control in sepsis[14]

Patients with sepsis require immediate broad-spectrum antibiotics with fluid resuscitation and source control.

Septic shock

Control of the source of sepsis by surgery or other means should be immediate and under way **within 3 hours**

Severe sepsis

Control of the source of sepsis should be performed **within 6 hours** of the onset of deterioration

Sepsis

Control of the source of sepsis should be performed **within 18 hours**

definitively with the underlying disease process or cause. In all patients, pus must be drained and dead tissue removed with specimens submitted for urgent microbiology. While localised collections can be drained percutaneously, generalised peritonitis remains an indication for laparotomy. Exceptions to this rule include primary spontaneous bacterial peritonitis and acute pancreatitis. There is an increasing use of laparoscopy in the management of specific surgical conditions causing abdominal sepsis (discussed further in Chapters 6, 8, 9 and 10). However, it must be remembered that a laparoscopic approach may not allow sufficient access to adequately debride and drain the septic focus, and that the physiological sequelae of a pneumoperitoneum may be poorly tolerated in those with septic shock.

Whether treatment is radiological or surgical, adequate preparation is essential (see also Chapter 16). Coagulopathy must be excluded or corrected beforehand and blood for transfusion should be available. Although drainage may be an essential prerequisite to resolution of sepsis, it is not infrequent for bacteraemia, as a consequence of the intervention, to cause a temporary deterioration in the patient's condition. Indeed, a bacteraemia may represent the 'second hit' that precipitates MODS. Such circumstances should be anticipated and an appropriate level of post-procedure care arranged beforehand.

With more complex cases and with older and sicker patients, treatment may need to be tempered in order to be survivable. However, there is a balance to be struck as inadequate treatment will condemn the patient to recurrent sepsis and likely death. The opinion of senior colleagues and specialist centres can be invaluable.

Image-guided percutanous drainage of both spontaneous and postoperative intra-abdominal collections has reported success rates of 70–90%.[25,26] The importance of adequate systemic support for the patient having imaging or image-guided intervention should nowadays be self-evident. Surgeons have a role to play in this, which may involve the assistance of anaesthetists. Percutaneous procedures may be less invasive than open surgery but will only be effective if good drainage is achieved. Many percutaneous drains are narrow and inadequate when infected fluid is viscous or contains necrotic tissue. Larger or multiple drains may be more effective and daily flushing can help. When radiological drains are placed for abdominal sepsis, the responsibility lies with the surgical team to ensure that the patient's condition improves as expected. Failure to respond to radiological intervention is another indication for laparotomy.

When open surgery is performed for sepsis, the procedure will vary according to the underlying pathology. Nonetheless, general principles apply in that the most straightforward adequate procedure is often preferable to a complex and time-consuming operation. The aim is to improve the patient's condition sufficiently without risking further complication. There is a current trend towards primary bowel resection and anastomosis in the acute setting, but this should be avoided in unstable patients, the presence of significant comorbidity, or heavy contamination. Generous saline lavage is recommended on completion of the procedure but there is nothing to be gained either by removing fibrinous debris piecemeal or by postoperative lavage.[19] Delayed skin wound closure may be preferable to primary suture, or wounds may be left to close by secondary intention if sepsis is substantial.

Obtaining informed consent for treatment will involve both patient and relatives. The potential severity of the situation should not be underestimated and the possibility of death, stoma creation, the need for intensive care treatment and further surgery will usually need to be discussed explicitly. The average mortality for an emergency laparotomy is around 15%, and increases with age and physiological disturbance.[14] Complementing clinical assessment with an objective determinant of risk from a scoring system (such as P-Possum) is valuable to help focus efforts.[14,27] See also Chapter 15.

Often the early phase of postoperative care will be delivered on the surgical high-dependency unit (HDU) or ICU. Although we, as surgeons, may sometimes feel uncomfortable on ICU, there is a range of skills that we are usually best placed to deliver, and close cooperation between surgeon and intensivist is essential (Box 18.6).

> ✔ Intraperitoneal abscesses with safe access routes should be drained percutaneously. This intervention carries high success and low recurrence rates.[26]

Box 18.6 • Surgeon's role on the ICU

Daily surgical input to:
- Wound and stoma care
- Tubes and drains
- Nutrition
- Ongoing management of sepsis
- Further operations
- Compartment syndrome
- Postoperative bleeding
- Preparation for HDU/ward
- Treatment/advice regarding the underlying surgical disease

Abdominal sepsis on the ICU

Not infrequently, the surgeon is also involved with the assessment and management of patients already on the ICU who develop recurrent abdominal sepsis. The outcome of patients with abdominal sepsis who require ICU treatment depends on age, comorbidities, source of sepsis and organ dysfunction. Control of the source of sepsis is essential for survival among patients with MOF. When sepsis is eradicated successfully from these patients by surgery over 60% survive, whereas survival is close to zero if significant abdominal sepsis continues.[28]

The principal causes of recurrent abdominal sepsis in the ICU are shown in Box 18.7. The reader is referred to Chapters 6, 8, 9 and 10 for the management of each organ-specific condition. Leaking anastomosis remains the commonest single cause and should be actively suspected in all 'at-risk patients' who are critically ill or deteriorating. Enterotomy during difficult surgery is not uncommon, occurring in up to 20% of patients,[29] and these can also leak in the postoperative period. Gastrostomy or other tubes inserted into the gut occasionally leak as well and this is more likely when tissue healing is poor.

Postoperative small-bowel ileus usually resolves within days, regardless of the extent of bowel handling.[30] Drugs, especially opiates, or electrolyte abnormalities (hypokalaemia, uraemia) may delay resolution, but failure to progress may also indicate ongoing retroperitoneal or abdominal pathology. Ileus may be difficult to distinguish from adhesive obstruction, and contrast studies may clarify the situation (see also Chapter 5). Adhesive obstruction frequently resolves but refractory cases occasionally require laparotomy. However, in a hostile abdomen, such as found in abdominal sepsis, considerable caution should be exercised in subjecting the patient to further surgery.[31] Whereas a 5- to 7-day period of non-operative treatment might be acceptable in the presence of straightforward adhesion

Box 18.7 • The principal causes of recurrent abdominal sepsis in the ICU

Leaked anastomosis or enterotomy
Leaking gastrostomies and other tubes
Abscesses or collections
Dead or ischaemic gut
Acalculous cholecystitis
Clostridium difficile-associated pseudomembranous colitis
Acute massive gastric dilatation
Neutropenic enterocolits
Continuing sepsis from 'common' peritonitis (perforation of peptic stress ulcer or diverticulum)

obstruction (and on occasions perhaps even longer if nutrition is supported), one should be prepared to wait for considerably longer when faced with a hostile abdomen, provided specific indications for surgery are not present. These indications include a known point of unrelieved complete obstruction or where there is a known septic focus.

Assessment on the ICU

Assessing patients on the ICU is difficult for several reasons. Firstly, the patients are often complex yet unfamiliar, perhaps having been treated previously by other surgeons. Secondly, sedated, postoperative patients in organ failure show their abdominal sepsis in different ways to a new emergency admission with peritonitis. Abdominal signs are unlikely to be evident unless gross (e.g. flank cellulitis, bowel contents in a drain, necrotic stoma), and the diagnosis of recurrent abdominal sepsis is often made from deterioration in vital organ function (see Chapter 16) and suspicion based on previous treatment and imaging. Again, contrast-enhanced CT is the gold-standard investigation and of great value, but occasionally patients will be too unwell to travel to the scanner. For them, exploratory laparotomy may still occasionally be necessary. Interpreting CT images in the recently operated abdomen is not easy. With expert help, the CT will not only confirm the diagnosis but can also potentially identify areas where there is no evidence of inflammation. In a difficult re-operative procedure with adhesions, that knowledge can save time and reduce the risk of surgical damage to other organs. Percutaneous drainage has a similar role here as in primary inflammation and the same caveats apply.

The importance of surgeons making their own thorough assessment cannot be overestimated as the stakes are high. The surgeon should be satisfied that the diagnosis is secure and that surgery is the best course of action. Part of that process will be engaging in detailed discussion with the intensivist to weigh up alternative diagnoses and sources of sepsis, and the risks and benefits of intervention at this point in time. Often this is not clear-cut as patients may have multiple potential sources (e.g. simultaneous pneumonia and abdominal sepsis) or other complicating factors, usually revolving around comorbid diseases or other ICU treatments. That said, any significant abdominal sepsis will require treatment.

Whilst the risks of surgery in the ICU population are often self-evident, these patients can sometimes be described as being 'too sick *not* to have an operation'. Clear indications for life-saving surgery include generalised peritonitis, multiple collections and presence of dead tissue. Patients with deteriorating organ function and a strong suspicion

of abdominal pathology also remain a significant group in whom laparotomy may be necessary. In some patients it will be clear that there is no realistic prospect of survival, either of the required operation or, more commonly, of the inevitably prolonged ICU course thereafter. It is important that both intensivist and surgeon counsel the family if care is to be limited.

Re-operating in abdominal sepsis

Re-operating in abdominal sepsis is always difficult: the timing of the most recent operation will influence the degree of difficulty and hence the risk of future complications. Beyond 72 hours adhesions will make surgery increasingly difficult and the risk of bowel damage increases: often the adhesions are stronger than the bowel. Entry to the abdomen can be difficult and an extension of the previous midline incision may help. Adhesions are generally most dense around any site of inflammation, as well as a recent incision. Here, having a preoperative CT scan comes into its own, guiding the surgeon as to the relative necessity to dissect in any difficult area. While a full laparotomy is ideal, prolonged dissection of adhesions in an area not thought from CT to contain inflammation or a collection may not be merited.

The surgeon must deal with the sepsis as thoroughly as possible but also simply and quickly. Prolonged and complex procedures will likely lead to a systemic deterioration in the patient and the prospect of bowel anastomoses healing under these adverse circumstances is not as high as one would like. The ability of the patient to withstand further surgery for further complications is very much lower next time around,[28] and the surgeon should see the present operation as the best opportunity for salvaging the patient. Intestinal reconstruction can be attempted when the patient is well and recovered, some months later.

Hence, in general terms the simplest and safest procedure will be best. This holds true especially in the patient who already has incipient or established organ failure: drain sepsis, debride any necrotic tissue and exteriorise any leaking bowel or anastomoses as stomas. Most controversy relates to the management of enteric and colorectal anastomotic leaks. While in a well patient, with a small leak and minimal contamination, preservation of a repaired anastomosis with proximal defunctioning and local drainage may be appropriate, it is all too often foolhardy in the critically ill. Preserving the anastomosis might work but there is a significant risk of further peritonitis and likely death as further acute surgery will seldom be successful. A first salvage operation in an ICU patient will successfully eradicate sepsis over 40% of the time but a second operation carries a success rate of only 25% and a third operation only 7%.[28] This is reflected in the rate of survival.

In difficult cases, the surgeon must be ready to employ alternative strategies, although it remains essential to drain significant collections of pus or enteric content and to debride any necrotic tissue. In the multiply operated septic abdomen, it may not be possible to take down and exteriorise the prime source of sepsis because of dense adhesions or the anatomical location (oesophagus, duodenum). For inaccessible pelvic sepsis arising from distal small bowel or colon, it may be possible to identify and exteriorise a proximal loop of jejunum without entering and damaging the matted pelvic loops other than to achieve necessary drainage. This will usually relieve the sepsis but at the price of a high-output stoma and prolonged intravenous feeding. For oesophagogastric or duodenal sepsis, all that may be possible is to drain collections and leave large tube or sump drains beside the leaking anastomosis or other septic focus. Placing a second tube in the hole to create a controlled fistula is also of merit. Proximal intestinal contents or secretions can sometimes be diverted away by tube gastrostomy or other techniques, although each has its complications. A further option in difficult situations or resistant cases is to gain entry to locules of pus or enteric content, then to leave the abdomen open as a laparostomy (**Fig. 18.2**). Further pus or enteric content will usually find its way to the surface, assisted by subsequent manual lavage on the ICU or in theatre as necessary.

In addition to their role in draining proximal gut secretions, gastrostomy and enterostomy tubes can be usefully placed to facilitate future, and often prolonged, enteral feeding. The same tube can serve both roles: drainage initially, then feeding as intestinal function returns, provided there is no persisting distal bowel leak. These laparotomies are often oozy and contaminated, and many surgeons would leave large drains (24Ch tube or sump) in the subphrenic spaces and pelvis at the end of the procedure. This is particularly so for certain deep cavities (e.g. psoas abscess) or when further leakage is likely or inevitable. Large Foley catheters can be used to intubate inaccessible bowel to create a controlled fistula (typically the duodenum) and it is often advisable to place an additional large drain just outside the bowel. There is a particular role for local lavage in pancreatic necrosis (see Chapter 8) but, otherwise, continuing lavage down abdominal drains in the postoperative period is of no proven benefit.

Outcome from surgery for abdominal sepsis in the ICU patient depends on many factors. Age and eradication of sepsis have been discussed but numbers of failed organs, comorbid conditions and the underlying surgical disease are also important. Overall, 30–40% will survive,[28] but a further factor that is associated with survival is the early response to the first operation in the ICU. If the patient has improved clinically within 48 hours then survival is much better (80%) than if the patient does not improve in this time frame (10%). Given the cost of intensive care, attempts have been made using a variety of scoring systems to define numerically those patients with negligible chance of survival (see Chapter 15). However, due to the heterogeneity of the patient group and the nature of scoring systems in general, it is not possible to use them for decision-making in individual patients. Clinical judgment is most important and the scoring systems remain primarily tools for audit and research.

Damage control laparotomy

Damage control laparotomy (DCL) is a concept that has expanded from its initial role in trauma surgery (see also Chapter 13). Trauma patients become hypothermic, acidotic and coagulopathic, and surgery becomes unsurvivable. Rapid, immediately life-saving surgery ('staple, pack and go') is carried out and the patient returned to ICU for warming and resuscitation, with more definitive surgery deferred for 24–48 hours once coagulopathy has been corrected and homeostasis returned towards normal. In abdominal sepsis it holds true that the first laparotomy carries the best chance for salvage.[28] However, in severely unstable patients it can be better to make an active decision to quickly drain pus, remove dead tissue, stop bleeding by packing and close overtly leaking bowel with staples (without resection) before terminating the operation.

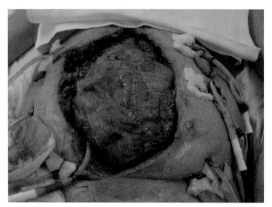

Figure 18.2 • Laparostomy with polyglactin mesh, gastrostomy, jejunostomy, cholecystostomy and drains.

Indications for this include haemodynamic instability, massive haemorrhage, coagulopathy, abdominal compartment syndrome and acute mesenteric ischaemia.[32] Packs should generally be removed as early as possible once clotting is restored and usually the next day. The small bowel becomes adherent remarkably quickly and can be damaged as packs are removed. Packs should be removed cautiously under direct vision with saline irrigation and gentle finger separation.

Second-look or planned re-laparotomy

This term refers to the planned re-exploration of the abdomen, planned at the previous procedure in order to re-operate before any clinical deterioration occurs. The term distinguishes it from 'laparotomy on demand', which is now the more common approach and where the abdomen is only explored when a new problem is diagnosed. After DCL, a second look is obviously required to complete the necessary definitive procedures, but the term is more commonly applied to 'looking again' after laparotomy for intestinal ischaemia. The extent of intestinal ischaemia may not be fully evident at the first operation and, particularly if the bowel has been re-anastomosed, looking again at 48–72 hours, depending on progress, can identify further ischaemia before the patient deteriorates. In some cases of intestinal ischaemia where there may be doubt as to the extent, it may be preferable to resect and staple off the bowel ends, forcing the surgeon to re-explore 48 hours or so later, rather than gamble on anastomosing bowel that might be subclinically ischaemic and subsequently break down at a later date.

Repeated planned re-laparotomies have been used aggressively for abdominal sepsis with MOF in both Europe and North America for some years. In this method of treatment, the abdomen is typically re-operated upon every 24–48 hours for several days to wash out the peritoneal cavity and remove any ongoing sepsis. However, a recent randomised trial has shown that this approach is associated with significantly more laparotomies and prolonged ICU stay compared to a 're-laparotomy on demand' approach.[33] Although on occasions there may be a case for a single planned second-look laparotomy in patients with severe faecal peritonitis, even this is debatable. This should not, however, divert the surgeon from maintaining a

---

✔✔ In patients undergoing surgery for severe secondary peritonitis, re-laparotomy on demand is preferable to 'planned re-laparotomy'.[33]

---

low threshold for early laparotomy on demand when indicated, as delaying necessary surgery worsens outcome.[28]

Leaving the abdomen open (laparostomy)

In adverse circumstances, the abdomen is occasionally left open as a last resort in allowing pus and enteric contents to drain. More often it is left open in preference to closing it with undue tension. Abdominal compartment syndrome (see below) may also lead to an open abdomen. Leaving the abdomen open in appropriate circumstances can avoid or reduce septic, enteric and wound complications. It also allows improved systemic function, faster weaning from the ventilator and can facilitate early enteral nutrition. However, it is deforming, increases evaporative losses, and exposes the bowel to risk of damage and fistulation. The open abdomen is particularly challenging to nurse, and comfortable, secure, wound care may be difficult to achieve.[34] Prolonged healing is usually required with a risk of late herniation. These deleterious effects are significant enough to make one caution against unnecessary use of laparostomy.[19] It is undoubtedly a valuable and life-saving technique when needed but it is also a significant future burden to the patient in its own right.

In closing the abdomen during laparotomy for abdominal sepsis, the surgeon should close the fascia conventionally but avoid tension. Tension sutures have little to recommend them and their continued use is not supported. If bowel distension, oedema, haemorrhage (or packing) combine to make closure impossible, then there are several options open to the surgeon, depending on a number of factors, including the likely time course of recovery. In general, each end of the wound is closed conventionally to the point of reasonable tension and the central defect left open. For short-lived oedema (e.g. after aortic aneurysm repair or traumatic haemorrhage) the defect can be covered with abdominal packing, which is changed daily until such time as the defect can be closed or a longer-term solution implemented (see below). Early dressing changes should be carried out by the surgical team. The small bowel will become adherent to any gauze dressings, and gentle separation will be required to avoid injury.

A double-sandwich dressing of semipermeable adhesive dressing with moist gauze between the layers of dressing protects the bowel with less adhesion formation than with standard gauze packs. There are various commercial plastic sheets that can be used. Alternatively, a version of the Bogota bag can be used (**Fig. 18.3**). In this technique, a sterile 3-litre intravenous fluid bag is slit open and sutured to the

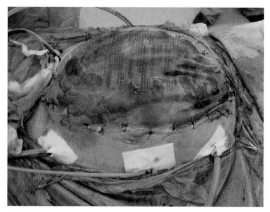

Figure 18.3 • Bogota bag.

fascia, covering and protecting the bowel and providing it with a clean, moist environment. Again, as the oedema subsides, usually within 72 hours or so, the Bogota bag or double-sandwich dressing can be removed and the abdomen either closed or a longer-term technique instituted.

In recurrent sepsis, where recovery is likely to be slow, prosthetic mesh can be used to restrain the viscera. In abdominal sepsis, absorbable polyglactin meshes are preferred to non-absorbable polypropylene meshes, as there is less likelihood of chronic mesh infection and fistulation to underlying bowel.[35] Caution is also required in the use of bioprosthetic collagen meshes on account of complications and cost.[35]

Whichever technique is employed to close the abdomen, the later development of an incisional hernia is almost inevitable, but might be less so with the non-absorbable mesh. If the contamination is particularly severe such that a further laparotomy and lavage is planned in 24–48 hours, then mesh placement can be deferred until then. Likewise if oozing requires gauze packing then mesh placement can be effected when the gauze is removed. The mesh and bowels must still be kept moist and protected, and a double-sandwich dressing achieves this admirably. If there is a lot of effluent or tissue fluid, then use of low-grade suction can help provide control. As the wound shrinks, these bulky dressings can be changed to a large fistula bag, even if there is no fistula, as again it provides a non-adherent moist environment.

Use of commercial vacuum dressings has become widespread as they make wound management considerably easier, and provide a ready-made technique for the non-expert unit. Early cohort studies suggested that vacuum-assisted closure was well tolerated in the open abdomen, with intestinal fistulation rates of 5%.[36] However, these findings have not been borne out by the only randomised trial on vacuum-assisted closure in the open abdomen,

which compared it to polyglactin absorbable mesh. Whilst not statistically significant, the rate of fistulation in the vacuum-assisted closure arm was 21%.[37] Controversy regarding the rate of intestinal fistulation continues,[34,38] while the results of a national audit coordinated by the National Instititute of Health and Clinical Excellence (NICE) are awaited. Until the intestinal fistulation rate has been clarified, particular caution is required on the use of vacuum dressings in the presence of suture or staple lines, repaired serosal tears or enterotomies.

Abdominal compartment syndrome

Normally, intra-abdominal pressure is low (<10 mmHg), but it is increasingly recognised that it can be raised in abdominal sepsis (and other acute abdominal conditions, including trauma and pancreatitis) to the significant detriment of the patient. The condition is recognised with increasing frequency and is probably not as uncommon in our practice as previously thought.[39] As abdominal pressure rises, venous return is impaired and with it cardiac output. The tense abdomen can cause pulmonary compromise, oliguria, mesenteric ischaemia and even raised intracranial pressure. These features constitute the abdominal compartment syndrome (ACS) – similar in some ways to a tension pneumothorax, within the abdomen.[40]

ACS is caused by multiple factors that exist after certain operations, typically those for peritonitis, abdominal aneurysm and abdominal trauma. Tissue oedema results from the combined effects of tissue injury, intravenous fluid infusion and leaky capillaries, while bowel distension and haematomas also contribute. ACS is seen most commonly after fascial closure but it can also occur in the abdomen that has been left open and packed, especially if there is ongoing haemorrhage. Operations likely to cause ACS include those involving significant haemorrhage, retroperitoneal or intestinal oedema, bowel distension, aortic clamping, hypothermia, massive transfusion or prolonged surgery. These circumstances should heighten the surgeon's awareness of ACS as a potential complication. ACS is not restricted to emergency surgery and prolonged elective surgery with a scarred and rigid abdominal wall may also lead to this condition. The anaesthetist may signal an unacceptable rise in the ventilatory pressure as the abdomen is closed but more commonly ACS develops on the critical care unit, some 12–30 hours after surgery. Oligo/anuria and raised ventilatory pressures are the usual presenting features.

Intra-abdominal pressure (IAP) is measured via the bladder following instillation of 25 mL of normal

Box 18.8 • Definitions of abdominal compartment syndrome[41]

Intra-abdominal pressure (IAP)
Steady-state pressure in the abdominal cavity
Between 5 and 7 mmHg in critically unwell adults
Abdominal perfusion pressure (APP)
APP = MAP − IAP
Intra-abdominal hypertension (IAH)
Sustained or repeated pathological elevation in
IAP ≥ 12 mmHg
Abdominal compartment syndrome (ACS)
Sustained IAP > 20 mmHg (with or without an APP < 60 mmHg) that is associated with new organ dysfunction or failure

saline. The IAP is measured through the aspiration port of the catheter tubing using a transducer. The transducer should be zeroed at the level of the mid axillary line, and IAP measured in the supine position at end expiration.[41] Standardised definitions for ACS were developed in 2006 by an international consensus group[41] (Box 18.8).

In intra-abdominal hypertension (IAH) and ACS, a number of medical treatment options are of benefit in reducing IAP.[42] Abdominal wall compliance can be improved with adequate sedation, analgesia and neuromuscular blockade. Intraluminal contents should be evacuated with nasogastric and rectal decompression and the use of prokinetic agents. Abdominal fluid collections should be aspirated. Positive fluid balance can be corrected with fluid restriction, diuretics or dialysis/ultra-filtration. However, if pressures above 20 mmHg persist despite these measures, or organ dysfunction worsens, then the abdomen will need to be decompressed and left open using the techniques discussed above.

Intestinal fistulas

Intestinal fistulas pose their own particular problems and can greatly complicate patient management. They contribute to sepsis, malnutrition, fluid and electrolyte imbalances, difficulties in wound care, as well as posing an enormous psychological challenge to the patient.

A fistula is defined as an abnormal communication between two epithelial lined surfaces. There are many types and exhaustive description is beyond the remit of this chapter. The great majority of those seen within the context of severe abdominal sepsis follow surgery and result from anastomotic leakage or an inadvertent enterotomy, either overlooked or unsuccessfully repaired.

An intestinal fistula, from somewhere in the intestinal tract to the laparotomy wound, will occur occasionally in every gastrointestinal surgeon's practice, arising most commonly as a result of anastomotic leakage or bowel damage. While a few will show signs of severe sepsis, more often than not there is a period of apparent ileus, wound infection and clinical stagnation. When the wound ruptures or is opened to treat the infection, the enteric or faecal nature of the contents will become apparent. This may not be convincing to begin with as the enteric flow is usually preceded by a volume of pus and blood, as with most postoperative wound infections. Postoperative fistulas may also occur through drains or along recent drain sites, to the vaginal vault (especially in those who have undergone previous hysterectomy) and occasionally to the rectum or other parts of the gut.

However, fistulas are more likely to occur after emergency surgery, usually carried out for another postoperative complication, commonly sepsis, obstruction or bleeding. In these operations, the inherent difficulty of the procedure, brought about by adhesions, bowel distension and softened tissues, makes further bowel damage a real possibility. If that damage is not, or cannot, be repaired effectively, if there is persisting obstruction of the intestine postoperatively, a postoperative phlegmon or an open abdomen, then the likelihood of fistulation escalates considerably. Postoperatively, the combination of small-bowel obstruction and an undrained abscess is also likely to result in a fistula as the obstructed bowel eventually softens and gives way at, or into, the collection. Thus it will be evident that repairing a leaking anastomosis once the patient is septic and local tissues oedematous and friable is all too often doomed to failure. Bowel exposed in an open abdomen will also invariably be subject to some degree of trauma unless the dressings or appliances are handled and changed expertly. Again, if there is distal obstruction, a local and exposed suture line or local trauma, a fistula will often occur. Perhaps 10–20% of 'laparostomies' will fistulate and this sometimes happens even with expert care.

A significant number of intestinal fistulas heal spontaneously, although they will cause misery and morbidity while they do so. The factors that contribute to persistence of a fistula are shown in Box 18.9.

The best-known approach to fistula care is that described at the specialist fistula unit in Salford (UK), and known by the acronym SNAP (Sepsis, Nutrition, Anatomy, Procedure). The most pressing effects of a fistula relate to intra-abdominal sepsis. There can also be wound sepsis, usually in the form of cellulitis, although occasionally local necrosis can occur. Once the necessary resuscitation is in hand, an early priority is CT of the abdomen, preferably with both gut and intravenous contrast.

Box 18.9 • Factors contributing to the occurrence and persistence of postoperative fistulas

Occurrence

Repaired anastomosis

Inadvertent enterotomy (repaired or missed)

New anastomosis in unfavourable circumstances

Persisting abscess or phlegmon causing obstruction

Fistulating disease

Open abdomen

Persistence

Distal obstruction (including constipation)

Open abdomen

Disconnected bowel ends

Local abscess

High output from fistula

Complex fistula

Mucocutaneous continuity

The frequency of intra-abdominal abscess formation is high, in the region of 66%,[43] and often these are not evident clinically. Without diagnosis and control of the sepsis, the prognosis is bleak. Management strategies follow the principles outlined above.

An integral part of early management is wound care and control of the fistula effluent. When there is a small fistula orifice in a drain site or through part of a wound, the effluent can be controlled with a stoma bag. At the other extreme, when bowel contents are leaking into a laparostomy, management may be very difficult. Large fistula bags are available; the largest may be needed for a new laparostomy. The author's unit often uses a sandwich dressing initially, as described above, with low-grade suction attached to soft rubber catheters placed near the fistula site. The same suction technique can be placed inside a fistula bag when appropriate in order to reduce the frequency of bag leakage.

Important ancillary techniques include reducing fistula output by avoiding enteral feeding and reducing gastric acid output with proton-pump inhibitors. Codeine and loperamide can subsequently be used to contribute to this control of gut secretions. Octreotide will also reduce gut secretion in some patients but, in the author's experience, its effect is inferior to the steps already described. It is perhaps most useful in pancreatic fistulas and upper small-bowel fistulas.

Immediate fluid management will have been considered as the patient was resuscitated but attention will have to turn rapidly to the optimal means of nutrition. The deleterious effect that enteral nutrition often has on output and wound care, particularly in the early stages, has been noted above.

Additionally, enteral feeding may also 'feed' the abdominal sepsis, if there is complexity to the fistula with a further unrecognised proximal hole in the bowel. There is often partial obstruction associated with the sepsis and with most fistulas it is often better and more reliable to resort to parenteral nutrition while the patient stabilises and the situations with regard to sepsis, wound care and fistula anatomy each become clearer. Indeed, it is often better to see parenteral nutrition as the ongoing mainstay of nutritional support in intestinal fistulation with abdominal sepsis. In some circumstances, enteral nutrition can take over some, or even all, of the role, but this will usually take time and is only possible in selected patients.

Fistulas can be categorised as high or low output (high >500 mL per 24 hours). This cut-off represents a level above which the fistula is likely to have a significant effect on fluid balance and nutrition. Some proximal fistulas have outputs of one or more litres per day and fluid balance will be challenging in its own right. Senior surgical staff will need to commit to adequate supervision of the recording of the various inputs and outputs, particularly in the initial unstable and complicated phase of care. Fistula output will often reduce with time and, when possible, some healing begins to occur. A typical anastomotic wound fistula will be a side hole and if there is free distal flow, no sepsis, no bowel disease and no distal obstruction (or constipation), then healing may occur. It is unknown whether restricted oral intake helps, but it is intuitive to minimise the flow through the hole to encourage healing. As healing occurs, usually after 2–4 weeks, oral intake can be increased. If there is no healing by 6 weeks and no apparently reversible factor (e.g. abscess, constipation), then many would assume the fistula will not heal and allow more liberal oral intake.

In the ICU setting, once sepsis is excluded or controlled and the open abdomen, if present, is starting to granulate, oral or enteral feeding can begin cautiously, maintaining a careful watch for recurrent sepsis. The nutritional effect of this will depend on the length and condition of gut available for absorption and it will often take time for enteral feeding to be tolerated. During this phase, combined enteral and parenteral feeding is used.

It will be clear from the above that further surgery is usually only advocated to deal with abdominal sepsis. Further operations at this stage to try and correct the fistula often cause more harm than good through loss of bowel (risking short-bowel syndrome) or the creation of yet more fistulas. If surgery is undertaken then the approach follows that described above for abdominal sepsis. Surgery for fistulas is best deferred until the patient is well physically, nutritionally and emotionally, and only after the anatomy has been defined radiologically. This is often some months later and in complex cases is a highly specialist undertaking.

Chronic abdominal sepsis

Intestinal fistulas often settle down and can run a course of chronic abdominal sepsis where there is low-grade inflammation but no organ failure. This can be punctuated with further acute episodes and it may be difficult to be certain if the sepsis comes from the feeding line, urinary catheter, chest, wounds or abdomen. Unusual bacteria or fungi can be involved and occasionally less common sites become infected (e.g. myocardium or heart valves secondary to feeding lines). During this period there is a continuing requirement for close daily monitoring with senior surgical input, often for several months, if the patient is to recover. Ongoing parenteral nutrition is often integral to this and, again, the help of a specialist unit can be invaluable. In these units, the support of specialist nursing staff in maintaining sepsis-free nutrition and providing expert fistula care is fundamental to success. The overall recovery or otherwise of the patient will be indicated by the clinical and biochemical picture combined. A falling white count and C-reactive protein with a steady rise in the serum albumin, together with increasing general well-being, are all good signs. Further surgery should probably be deferred for at least 6 months after the last laparotomy in order to allow the abdomen to become less hostile, and prolapse of stomas or fistulas is a useful indicator that re-peritonealisation has occurred. Restorative surgery is still usually prolonged and difficult, and reconstructing the abdominal wall after laparostomy has its own difficulties, which may benefit from help from a plastic surgeon.

Key points

- Abdominal sepsis is a leading cause of death in acute surgical practice and cases still carry a high mortality.
- A systematic approach, based on a sound understanding of pathophysiology, is fundamental to successful sepsis management. Adequate resuscitation, safe, timely diagnosis, rapid definitive treatment, and accurate and ongoing reassessment are essential if the progression to organ dysfunction and failure is to be avoided.
- Identifying and rapidly treating the underlying cause of sepsis ('the septic focus') is fundamental to a successful outcome.
- Radiological intervention for localised sepsis is growing in importance.
- Indications for laparotomy include generalised peritonitis, necrotic tissue, multifocal abscesses and failure of radiological intervention.
- Re-laparotomy is often difficult and advanced techniques may be required.
- Intra-abdominal hypertension and abdominal compartment syndrome are probably under-recognised. Medical management has a role, but in refractory cases surgical abdominal decompression will be required.
- Intestinal fistulas can occur following any abdominal intervention, but are more common after emergency surgery. Prompt eradication of sepsis and attention to nutrition is key. Definitive surgery to correct the fistula should be deferred until the patient is well and the anatomy has been clearly defined.
- Abdominal sepsis often runs a prolonged course in which the surgeon will have to play an ongoing role.

References

1. Scottish Audit of Surgical Mortality 2010. http://www.sasm.org.uk/Publications/SASM_Annual_Report_2010.pdf.

2. Bone RC. Toward a theory regarding the pathogenesis of the systemic inflammatory response syndrome: what we do and do not know about cytokine regulation. Crit Care Med 1996;24(1):163–72.

3. Hotchkiss RS, Karl IE. The pathophysiology and treatment of sepsis. N Engl J Med 2003;348(2):138–50.

4. Marti-Carvajal AJ, Sola I, Lathyris D, et al. Human recombinant activated protein C for severe sepsis. Cochrane Database Syst Rev 2011;(4):CD004388.

5. Remick DG. Pathophysiology of sepsis. Am J Pathol 2007;170(5):1435–44.

6. Opal SM, DePalo VA. Anti-inflammatory cytokines. Chest 2000;117(4):1162–72.

7. O'Sullivan ST, Lederer JA, Horgan AF, et al. Major injury leads to predominance of the T helper-2 lymphocyte phenotype and diminished interleukin-12 production associated with decreased resistance to infection. Ann Surg 1995;222(4):482–92.

8. Zimmerman JE, Knaus WA, Wagner DP, et al. A comparison of risks and outcomes for patients with organ system failure: 1982–1990. Crit Care Med 1996;24(10):1633–41.

9. Rangel-Frausto MS, Pittet D, Costigan M, et al. The natural history of the systemic inflammatory response syndrome (SIRS). A prospective study. JAMA 1995;273(2):117–23.
   This prospective epidemiological study of SIRS and related conditions provides evidence of a clinical progression from SIRS to sepsis to severe sepsis and septic shock.

10. Pinsky MR, Vincent JL, Deviere J, et al. Serum cytokine levels in human septic shock. Relation to multiple-system organ failure and mortality. Chest 1993;103(2):565–75.

11. American College of Chest Physicians/Society of Critical Care Medicine Consensus Conference. Definitions for sepsis and organ failure and guidelines for the use of innovative therapies in sepsis. Crit Care Med 1992;20(6):864–74.

12. McLauchlan GJ, Anderson ID, Grant IS, et al. Outcome of patients with abdominal sepsis treated in an intensive care unit. Br J Surg 1995;82(4):524–9.

13. Levy MM, Fink MP, Marshall JC, et al. SCCM/ESICM/ ACCP/ATS/SIS International Sepsis Definitions Conference. Intensive Care Med 2003 2001;29 (4):530–8.

14. The Royal College of Surgeons of England and Department of Health Working Group on Perioperative Care of the Higher Risk General Surgical Patient. The higher risk general surgical patient: towards improved care of a forgotten group. The Royal College of Surgeons of England and Department of Health; 2011.

15. National Institute for Health and Clinical Excellence. NICE clinical guidline 50: Acutely ill patients in hospital. 2007.

16. Dellinger RP, Levy MM, Carlet JM, et al. Surviving Sepsis Campaign: international guidelines for management of severe sepsis and septic shock: 2008. Crit Care Med 2008;36(1):296–327.

17. Levy MM, Dellinger RP, Townsend SR, et al. The Surviving Sepsis Campaign: results of an international guideline-based performance improvement program targeting severe sepsis. Crit Care Med 2010;38(2):367–74.
   Outcome data on 15 022 patients who were managed according to the Surviving Sepsis Campaign initiative. Despite incomplete compliance with every aspect of the care bundles, a significant reduction in hospital mortality was associated with participation in the initiative.

18. Anderson ID. Assessing the critically ill surgical patient. In: Anderson ID, editor. Care of the critically ill surgical patient. London: Arnold; 1999. p. 7–15.

19. Boermeester MA. Surgical approaches to peritonitis. Br J Surg 2007;94(11):1317–8.

20. Goldie AS, Fearon KC, Ross JA, et al. Natural cytokine antagonists and endogenous antiendotoxin core antibodies in sepsis syndrome. The Sepsis Intervention Group. JAMA 1995;274(2): 172–7.

21. Kumar A, Zarychanski R, Light B, et al. Early combination antibiotic therapy yields improved survival compared with monotherapy in septic shock: a propensity-matched analysis. Crit Care Med 2010;38(9):1773–85.
   A retrospective multicentre cohort study of 4662 culture positive cases of bacterial septic shock showed that combination antibiotic therapy was associated with significantly decreased 28-day mortality compared to monotherapy.

22. Go HL, Baarslag HJ, Vermeulen H, et al. A comparative study to validate the use of ultrasonography and computed tomography in patients with post-operative intra-abdominal sepsis. Eur J Radiol 2005;54(3):383–7.

23. Kumar A, Kazmi M, Ronald J, et al. Rapidity of source control implementation following onset of hypotension is a major determinant of survival in human septic shock. Crit Care Med 2004;32(12):A158.

24. Angus DC, Linde-Zwirble WT, Lidicker J, et al. Epidemiology of severe sepsis in the United States: analysis of incidence, outcome, and associated costs of care. Crit Care Med 2001;29(7):1303–10.

25. Cinat ME, Wilson SE, Din AM. Determinants for successful percutaneous image-guided drainage of intra-abdominal abscess. Arch Surg 2002;137(7):845–9.

26. Akinci D, Akhan O, Ozmen MN, et al. Percutaneous drainage of 300 intraperitoneal abscesses with long-term follow-up. Cardiovasc Intervent Radiol 2005;28(6):744–50.

27. Prytherch DR, Whiteley MS, Higgins B, et al. POSSUM and Portsmouth POSSUM for predicting mortality. Physiological and Operative Severity Score for the enUmeration of Mortality and morbidity. Br J Surg 1998;85(9):1217–20.

28. Anderson ID, Fearon KC, Grant IS. Laparotomy for abdominal sepsis in the critically ill. Br J Surg 1996;83(4):535–9.

29. van Goor H. Consequences and complications of peritoneal adhesions. Colorectal Dis 2007;9(Suppl. 2):25–34.

30. Condon RE, Frantzides CT, Cowles VE, et al. Resolution of postoperative ileus in humans. Ann Surg 1986;203(5):574–81.

31. Sajja SB, Schein M. Early postoperative small bowel obstruction. Br J Surg 2004;91(6):683–91.

32. Jansen JO, Loudon MA. Damage control surgery in a non-trauma setting. Br J Surg 2007;94(7):789–90.

33. van Ruler O, Mahler CW, Boer KR, et al. Comparison of on-demand vs planned relaparotomy strategy in patients with severe peritonitis: a randomized trial. JAMA 2007;298(8):865–72.

34. Carlson GL, Dark P. Acute intestinal failure. Curr Opin Crit Care 2010;16(4):347–52.

35. Connolly PT, Teubner A, Lees NP, et al. Outcome of reconstructive surgery for intestinal fistula in the open abdomen. Ann Surg 2008;247(3):440–4.

36. Barker DE, Green JM, Maxwell RA, et al. Experience with vacuum-pack temporary abdominal wound closure in 258 trauma and general and vascular surgical patients. J Am Coll Surg 2007;204(5):784–93.

37. Bee TK, Croce MA, Magnotti LJ, et al. Temporary abdominal closure techniques: a prospective randomized trial comparing polyglactin 910 mesh and vacuum-assisted closure. J Trauma 2008;65(2):337–44.

38. Teubner A, Anderson ID, Scott NA, et al. Intra-abdominal hypertension and the abdominal compartment syndrome (Br J Surg 2004; 91:1102–1110). Br J Surg 2004;91(11):1527.

39. Moore AF, Hargest R, Martin M, et al. Intra-abdominal hypertension and the abdominal compartment syndrome. Br J Surg 2004;91(9): 1102–10.

40. Hong JJ, Cohn SM, Perez JM, et al. Prospective study of the incidence and outcome of intra-abdominal hypertension and the abdominal compartment syndrome. Br J Surg 2002;89(5):591–6.

41. Malbrain ML, Cheatham ML, Kirkpatrick A, et al. Results from the International Conference of Experts on Intra-abdominal Hypertension and Abdominal Compartment Syndrome. I. Definitions. Intensive Care Med 2006;32(11):1722–32.

42. Cheatham ML, Malbrain ML, Kirkpatrick A, et al. Results from the International Conference of Experts on Intra-abdominal Hypertension and Abdominal Compartment Syndrome. II. Recommendations. Intensive Care Med 2007;33(6):951–62.

43. Harris C, Nicholson DA, Anderson ID. Computed tomography: a vital adjunct in the management of complex postoperative sepsis. Br J Surg 1998;85:861–2.

19

Complications of bariatric surgery presenting to the general surgeon

Bruce R. Tulloh
Andrew C. de Beaux

Introduction

Trends in the UK and many other parts of the developed world show a steady increase in obesity over the last 30 years and there are no signs that this is decreasing. Obesity places an enormous health burden on our society because of the medical comorbidities that are associated with it, such as type II diabetes, hypertension, dyslipidaemia, steatohepatitis, obstructive sleep apnoea, arthritis of the weight-bearing joints, gastro-oesophageal reflux, depression and infertility. In general, these medical problems improve or even resolve in parallel with weight loss. Surgery specifically aimed at weight loss ('bariatric' surgery, from the Greek word *baros* = weight, *iatrikos* = medical) has been developing since the 1950s but it is only in the last 20 years, in the wake of advances in laparoscopy, that surgery has become increasingly popular.

Over the past decade, following the publication of several long-term outcome studies that showed a significant improvement in cardiovascular risk and mortality after bariatric surgery,[1-3] the number of bariatric procedures being carried out annually in the UK has grown exponentially. Surgery remains the only way to produce significant, sustainable weight loss and resolution of comorbidities. Nevertheless, relatively few surgeons have developed an interest in this field. Most bariatric surgery is now performed in centres staffed by surgeons with a bariatric interest, usually as part of a multidisciplinary team.

> ✔✔ Bariatric surgery is the only method of producing long-term, reliable and significant weight loss with resolution of the associated morbidities of morbid obesity.[2]

Although the number of hospitals providing a bariatric service in the UK is undoubtedly growing, many patients still have to travel long distances for their surgery – some even go overseas. Procedures are generally performed using laparoscopic and/or endoscopic techniques and lengths of stay are short. In the event of postoperative complications, patients can therefore present back at their local hospital or clinic, where there may be no specialised knowledge or expertise in the field. The aim of this chapter is to inform general surgeons on the disease process of obesity and the current bariatric procedures that are commonly performed, to outline the common complications that may arise and to provide management guidance for those patients that present in an emergency setting. Several articles have been written on the topic recently,[4-6] which reflects its current level of interest.

Causes of obesity

While obesity is the result of a chronic energy imbalance when food (calorie) intake exceeds energy expenditure, such an explanation on its own is too simplistic. Obesity should be considered a multifactorial socio-psycho-endocrine disease process.

It is now clear that there is a complex physiological adipostatic system in place that works to maintain a constant body weight in the face of daily fluctuations in energy balance.[7] The hypothalamus is an important control centre for this process, integrating a variety of both short-term and long-term energy flux signals. The gastrointestinal (GI) tract produces a number of hormones including ghrelin, glucagon-like peptides (GLP)-1 and 2, peptide tyrosine, insulin and cholecystokinin, which not only influence gut motility and exocrine secretions but also exert positive and negative feedback on the hypothalamus to regulate appetite. Ghrelin, the 'hunger hormone', is released from the gastric body and promotes appetite, while leptin, a hormone that circulates in proportion to the body's fat mass, has a negative feedback on the hypothalamus to promote negative energy balance. Neural pathways are also involved via vagally innervated stretch receptors in the stomach wall, which induce satiety (and even nausea) in response to gastric distension.

There are also social and psychological drivers to eat. Eating is a pleasurable activity and, for many, meals are the hub of family and social events. Eating may also provide comfort to address fear, loneliness or anxiety. There is now evidence that such negative emotions increase food consumption and that obese people eat in response to emotions more than normal-weight people.[8]

Dieting is known to be difficult and, for many, is not successful in the long term. Modern human beings have evolved from nomadic hunter-gatherers and our physiology defaults to energy storing in periods of food shortage. Thus dieting induces a physiological adaptation to starvation. This stimulates appetite, induces the bowel to absorb a greater proportion of food eaten, reduces energy loss by a subtle lowering of body temperature and promotes fat storage.

Surgery is the most effective treatment for severe and complex obesity because it alters the physiological processes at the heart of weight homeostasis. Different procedures do this in different ways.

Mechanisms of weight loss surgery

Traditionally, weight loss operations have been described as either restrictive or malabsorptive, influencing either the volume of food that can be ingested or the absorption of food at the mucosal level, respectively (or both). However, it is more likely that surgery interacts in a beneficial way with the complex adipostatic system outlined above. Gastric band patients, for example, who are restricted in their oral intake by the constricting ring around their upper stomach, do not show the normal hormonal adaptation to starving. Part of the band's action appears to be through feedback to the adipostat, possibly via vagal afferents. Similarly, patients undergoing a so-called malabsorptive operation, such as gastric bypass, do not suffer chronic diarrhoea; their weight loss is mediated by a series of gut hormonal changes that influence appetite, food choices and gut motility, amongst other things.

Even so, iatrogenic manipulations of the adipostat are not the full story. In order to achieve the best outcomes, patients still need to make a series of healthy dietary and lifestyle changes along the lines of eating sensibly and being physically active. Authorities agree that postoperative weight maintenance is improved by the ongoing encouragement, advice and support obtained from long-term follow-up in a bariatric clinic.[9-11]

While weight control is a complex process, the mechanisms behind the postoperative resolution of obesity-related comorbidities are also complex and, even now, not fully understood. Control of type II diabetes mellitus, for example, is known to improve in parallel with the gradual weight loss that follows gastric band surgery.[12] However, the gastric bypass and duodenal switch operations can normalise glucose tolerance much more quickly, even before there has been any appreciable weight loss.[13,14] Such changes are mediated by gut hormones that are stimulated either by a lack of nutrients in the foregut or by the rapid post-prandial delivery of food to the hindgut, with a resultant improvement in pancreatic function and a reduction in peripheral insulin resistance. These processes are well explained elsewhere[7,13,15] and will not be expanded upon here.

Bariatric operations

The commonest weight loss procedures performed around the world at present are the gastric band, the gastric bypass and the sleeve gastrectomy. In very obese patients, an alternative operation is the duodenal switch, while the new ileal transposition procedure represents one of the few purely metabolic operations designed specifically for the treatment of type II diabetes. Older operations such as vertical banded gastroplasty and jejuno-ileal bypass are now obsolete, although patients who have undergone such procedures in the distant past may still present to hospital with complications. The main endoscopic option at present is insertion of a gastric balloon, with newer procedures like the endoscopic duodenojejunal barrier and gastric plication on the horizon. Implantable neuroregulatory devices (gastric 'pacemakers') represent a new direction for surgical weight control by harnessing neural feedback signals to help control eating.

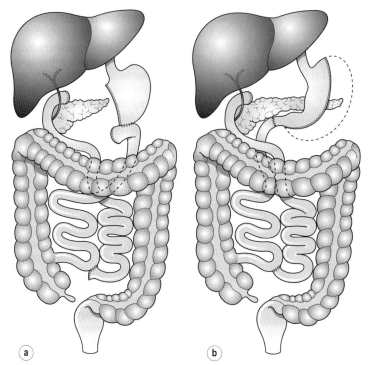

Figure 19.5 • Diagram of bilio-pancreatic diversion (BPD) **(a)** and duodenal switch **(b)**. The common channel is approximately 100 cm long.

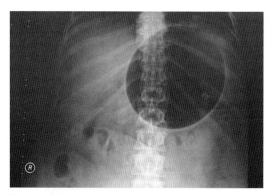

Figure 19.6 • Abdominal X-ray of a patient with a gastric balloon in situ.

in significant protein malabsorption and vitamin/mineral deficiency, the long blind jejunal limb commonly led to bacterial overgrowth, and patients were prone to liver failure as a result of both protein malnutrition and toxaemia from bacterial overgrowth in the blind loop.[9] The majority of patients, if still alive, have had their operations reversed.

Vertical banded gastroplasty (VBG)

This operation gained popularity in the 1980s and early 1990s but its high failure rate, and the advent of

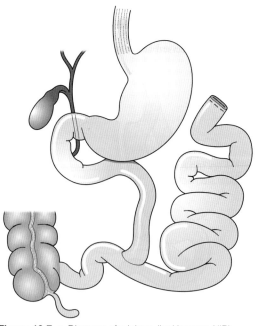

Figure 19.7 • Diagram of a jejuno-ileal bypass (JIB) procedure. Note the long blind loop of jejunum.

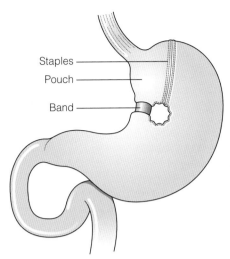

Figure 19.8 • Diagram of the vertical banded gastroplasty (VBG) procedure.

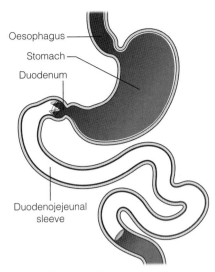

Figure 19.9 • Diagram of the duodenojejunal scene

better procedures, has resulted in it being abandoned. Just above the incisura, a short distance in from the lesser curve, the anterior and posterior walls of the stomach were stapled together with a circular stapler. Through the resultant hole made by the stapler, a linear stapler could be applied vertically towards the angle of His. This staple line fixed the anterior and posterior gastric walls together but did not divide the stomach. The outlet of the small gastric pouch thus created was then 'banded' with a 360° ring of tape to prevent dilatation (**Fig. 19.8**). The high failure rate resulted from pouch outlet stenosis and/or pouch dilatation (usually caused by overeating), and this was often followed by disruption of the vertical staple line with the consequent loss of restriction to eating.

Newer procedures

Ileal transposition

This operation is still experimental although it may have an emerging role in patients with diabetes who have a lower body mass index (BMI) than would traditionally be offered weight loss surgery, or in those with no more than truncal obesity (sometimes termed 'normal-weight obesity'). In essence, a short segment of terminal ileum is excised with preservation of its mesentery, and then re-implanted in an isoperistaltic fashion into the proximal jejunum. This brings endocrine receptors from the hindgut mucosa into the foregut environment, with dramatic effects on the insulin/glucagon axis, pancreatic function and GI tract motility.[21]

Endoscopic duodenojejunal sleeve

This endoscopically inserted tube of thin, impervious plastic material has its proximal end secured to the mucosa of the first part of the duodenum with small barbs and then runs distally, effectively lining the duodenum and upper small bowel, preventing ingested food from making contact with the mucosa until the proximal jejunum is reached (**Fig. 19.9**). Its effect on the gut hormone milieu mimics that of the gastric bypass and early clinical results have shown a similar improvement in type II diabetes control, along with modest weight loss. At present it is suggested that such barriers be removed at around 1 year. As yet, however, no long-term follow-up information is available regarding the extent of weight regain or the return of glucose intolerance after the barrier is removed.

Gastric plication

Reducing the size of the stomach either endoscopically or laparoscopically has been described where the greater curve of the stomach at the fundus is invaginated to reduce gastric volume.[22] Infolding the gastric wall in this way may also provide stimulation of mural stretch receptors to reduce hunger. Endoscopically this can be performed by firing a series of staples or clips that 'gather' the stomach wall from the inside.[23] Outcomes are not yet known, but the same technology has been described previously for plicating the gastro-oesophageal junction for treating reflux where, despite early successes, long-term results have been disappointing.

Implantable neuroregulators (gastric 'pacemakers')

A number of laparoscopically implantable devices are now undergoing trials. They register the presence of food in the stomach and are designed to mediate satiety by vagal feedback. Lack of outcome data in addition to concerns about battery life and cost are currently a block to their more widespread use.

Complications of bariatric surgery

There are *general* complications such as might follow any abdominal operation, and *specific* complications that relate to the procedure performed.

General complications

It should be within the capability of any abdominal surgeon to manage the general complications of bariatric surgery, which include pulmonary atelectasis/pneumonia, intra-abdominal bleeding, anastomotic or staple-line leak with or without abscess formation, deep vein thrombosis (DVT)/pulmonary embolus and superficial wound infections. Patients may be expected to present with malaise, pallor, features of sepsis or obvious wound problems. However, clinical features may be difficult to recognise owing to body habitus. Abdominal distension, tenderness and guarding may be impossible to determine clinically due to the patient's obesity. Pallor is non-specific. Fever and leucocytosis may be absent. Wound collections may be very deep. These complications in a bariatric patient should be actively sought with appropriate investigations. In particular, it is vital for life-threatening complications such as bleeding, sepsis and bowel obstruction to be recognised promptly and treated appropriately. A persistent tachycardia may be the only sign heralding significant complications and should always be taken seriously.[24]

It is useful to classify complications as 'early', 'medium' and 'late' because, from the receiving clinician's point of view, the differential diagnosis will differ accordingly (Table 19.1). Early complications usually arise within the first few days of surgery but, with ever-advancing laparoscopic surgery and shorter lengths of stay, these may still present to the non-bariatric surgeon after the patient has left the specialist centre.

Specific complications

These relate to the procedure performed. Again, they may be grouped into 'early', 'medium' and 'late', although the 'early' complications overlap with the general complications mentioned above. Medium-term complications are likely to arise while the patient is still overweight and thus may be difficult to diagnose. Late complications may

Table 19.1 • General complications following bariatric surgery (similar to those that may arise following any GI operation)

Early	Medium or late
Bleeding: Intraluminal (staple/suture line) Intraperitoneal (staple/suture line, mesentery, omentum, liver/spleen injury) Subcutaneous (trocar site) Staple/suture line leak Inadvertent GI tract perforation Port-site haematoma/ infection DVT/pulmonary embolism Anaesthetic drug reaction, etc. Chest infection/atelectasis Port-site hernia with or without bowel obstruction	Chest infection DVT/pulmonary embolism Haematoma or abscess Incisional or port-site hernia

develop many years later. Patients at this stage may be of normal weight, and therefore a link to their previous bariatric surgery may not be obvious (Table 19.2).

Clinical presentation

Once the receiving clinician understands the operation that has been performed and the specific complications to look out for, the next step is the interpretation of the presenting clinical features and formulation of a management plan.

Gastric band patients

Vomiting and/or dysphagia

These are very common and not surprising symptoms, considering that the band works by causing a constriction ring around the upper stomach. Band patients are accustomed to a degree of dysphagia and occasional vomiting, so for them to present for medical attention implies that it is 'worse than usual'. These symptoms indicate a degree of obstruction at the level of the band and there are three main causes.

Band too tight

Has the patient had an adjustment recently? Perhaps they have a food bolus obstruction. Once the patient begins to vomit the gastric wall becomes

Table 19.2 • Specific complications of bariatric surgery: early, medium and late

Procedure	Early	Medium	Late
Band	Gastric perforation Liver/spleen injury with bleeding	Slippage (with or without gastric necrosis) Injection-port migration or infection	Slippage Erosion Injection-port problems Mega-oesophagus
Sleeve	Reflux oesophagitis Staple-line bleed or leak Splenic infarct Omental necrosis	Intra-abdominal abscess or haematoma	Fistula Stenosis of sleeve
Bypass/duodenal switch/BPD	Anastomosis/staple-line bleed or leak Small-bowel enterotomy Early small-bowel obstruction	Intra-abdominal abscess or haematoma Roux limb obstruction Biliopancreatic (blind) loop obstruction	SBO (internal hernia, volvulus, adhesions) Anastomotic ulcer Anastomotic stricture Dumping syndrome Micronutrient malnutrition Gastro-gastric fistula Hypoglycaemia
Mini-gastric bypass	As above	As above	As above plus bile reflux
Intragastric balloon	Nausea/vomiting Gastric ulceration Gastric or oesophageal perforation	Dehydration and electrolyte imbalance Reflux oesophagitis	Bowel obstruction from deflated balloon
VBG		Stomal stenosis	Staple-line disruption
JIB		Bowel obstruction (internal hernia, adhesions)	Malnutrition Blind loop syndrome Liver failure
Duodenal barrier	Duodenal bleeding Duodenal perforation	Dumping syndrome Food bolus obstruction Migration of the device with mechanical bowel obstruction	Unknown
Gastric plication	Bleeding Splenic or liver injury	–	–
Gastric pacing	Nausea/vomiting Infection of subcutaneous implant	–	–

oedematous within the confines of the band and the apparent obstruction becomes worse. The treatment is urgent band decompression using the subcutaneous injection port (see Box 19.1 and **Fig. 19.10**). Once the patient can drink freely they can be discharged, with arrangement for follow-up by their bariatric specialist team.

Acute band 'slippage'

This is the term commonly used to describe what is really a process of gastric prolapse upwards through the band. It typically occurs months or years after the original operation and is possibly more common when no gastro-gastric tunnelling sutures are used to secure the band in place. The patient usually presents with vomiting, often in association with being able to eat a sizeable meal, as the food accumulates in the large gastric pouch above the band before eventually being regurgitated. Urgent decompression often provides relief but if not, then an urgent contrast swallow should be ordered. Slippage is often evident on a plain abdominal or chest radiograph, with the band lying at an unusual angle (see **Fig. 19.11**), although a contrast swallow provides more conclusive information. The most serious complication of band slippage is ischaemic necrosis of the prolapsed fundus, secondary to distension and/or occlusion of the blood supply to the

The subcutaneous injection port should be palpable beneath the skin on the abdominal wall, usually close to one of the longer laparoscopic scars. Some surgeons place it over the lower sternum. The patient usually knows where it is. Using a strict aseptic technique, the port is steadied between the fingers of one hand while the other holds an empty 10-mL syringe with needle attached. Ideally a non-coring 'Huber' or spinal needle is used so as not to damage the port, but in an emergency a conventional 23-gauge hypodermic needle works well (although it may not be long enough). Entering at right angles to the skin, the rubber diaphragm of the port is punctured. The needle hits the metal base-plate with a 'clunk' and aspiration can begin. The reservoir is aspirated to dryness; it may contain up to 14 mL. The needle is simply withdrawn when finished and a small dressing applied.

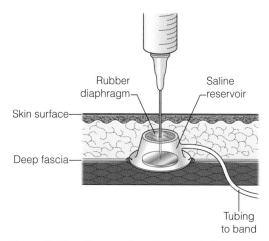

Figure 19.10 • Diagram of needle access to the subcutaneous injection port. Strict aseptic technique is important and a non-coring Huber needle should be used.

proximal stomach as it passes through the band. Failure of the symptoms to resolve with percutaneous band decompression is an indication for urgent surgical intervention.

The operation to remove the band is generally by laparoscopy. The tight band must be released. Unclipping it may be difficult, especially laparoscopically, but if possible – and if the stomach is viable – then it may be left in situ for an experienced bariatric surgeon to re-position at a later date. An alternative to unclipping the band is simply to cut it in half, after which it should be removed. Once local adhesions have been divided the band should just slide out. If there is gastric necrosis then laparotomy and some form of gastrectomy will be required along with complete removal of the band, tubing and injection port.

Band erosion

This is not usually an acute problem but presentation may be precipitated by an aggravation of dysphagia with or without pain and sepsis. Symptoms will not improve after percutaneous band decompression. An urgent contrast swallow may also demonstrate band erosion with leakage of contrast around the band (see **Fig. 19.12**) but the most definitive test for erosion is gastroscopy, where a portion of the white silicone band will be visible from within the lumen.

Abdominal pain

This is uncommon in band patients (as a result of the band) and so should alert the clinician to a serious problem such as visceral distension from acute slippage (see above), inflammation related to band erosion (see above), peritonitis from gastric necrosis with or without perforation or postoperative haematoma. If the symptoms are of recent onset (hours) and pain is a prominent feature, necrosis

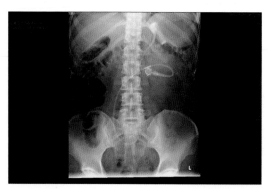

Figure 19.11 • Abdominal X-ray of an acute band slip. The band lies 90° out of alignment (compare with Fig. 19.1).

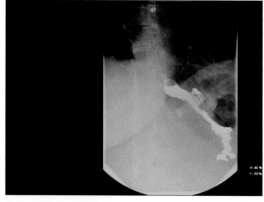

Figure 19.12 • Barium swallow demonstrating band erosion. Note the barium leaking out around the band (arrow). Compare with Fig. 19.1.

and/or perforation should be suspected and urgent imaging is required, followed by laparoscopy with or without laparotomy if necessary. Peritonitis is an unlikely consequence of band erosion but may occur with gastric necrosis (acute band slippage) or perhaps foreign body perforation of the gastric pouch.

Chest pain

This is a common reason for anyone to present to the hospital emergency department and cardiac causes need to be excluded. In patients with a gastric band, the possibility of band slippage, erosion and reflux oesophagitis (secondary to a tight band) needs to be considered.

Mega-oesophagus

This is the result of long-standing, excessive restriction and usually follows either a period of excessive band tightness, or chronic malpositioning due to band slippage. It is recognised on a contrast swallow. It usually improves over a period of several weeks following band decompression but may necessitate band removal to prevent recurrence.

Port problems

Migration

The subcutaneous injection port may move about within its subcutaneous pocket, depending on how well it has been fixed in position. This makes it difficult to access for percutaneous needle aspiration and if it has flipped over completely, the band will be impossible to decompress.

Leakage

Repeated attempts to needle the subcutaneous reservoir should be avoided as damage to the rubber diaphragm or perforation/rupture of the tubing can produce a slow leak.

Infection

The injection port may become infected through breach of sterile technique; this may present as abdominal wall cellulitis or an abscess. An infected port will need to be removed but can be replaced at a later date when the sepsis has completely cleared. Sometimes an infected subcutaneous port may be the first manifestation of band erosion (see above), as the tubing effectively acts as a conduit to convey infected material from the eroded band to the skin surface.

Skin erosion

The port may also erode through the skin surface (**Fig. 19.13**). While not an emergency, this situation may present to the general surgeon. Again, plans will need to be made for removal, then later replacement, of the injection port.

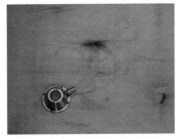

Figure 19.13 • Port erosion through the skin.

Sleeve gastrectomy patients

Early postoperative reflux/vomiting and dysphagia are common as the narrow and oedematous gastric sleeve tends to empty poorly at first. Some degree of reflux oesophagitis is common. Patients are usually discharged from hospital on proton-pump inhibitor (PPI) medication with instructions to adhere to a fluid diet, gradually thickening their intake over several weeks. However, if the problem is severe or associated with early signs of dehydration, then specific complications should be sought.

Staple-line leak or bleed

Any disruption of the staple line along the narrow sleeve of remaining stomach is likely to cause luminal compression, either from oedema or direct pressure such as from a collection or haematoma. A contrast swallow or computed tomography (CT) should demonstrate this, although both imaging modalities may be falsely negative. Furthermore, some obese patients may be too large for the scanner or X-ray table. If there is reasonable clinical concern of a staple-line leak or bleed, perhaps because of grumbling sepsis or worsening anaemia, laparoscopy should be arranged as this is likely to both confirm the diagnosis and allow repair/control/drainage as necessary.

Splenic infarction

As the greater omentum is separated from the fundus of the stomach it is possible to take one or more apical splenic vessels, leading to segmental infarction. This will present as left upper quadrant pain with or without some features of sepsis. A contrast CT should demonstrate this. Conservative management is likely to be successful.

Omental necrosis

The blood supply to the omentum may be compromised if the gastro-epiploic arcade is damaged as it is separated from the stomach. Ischaemic necrosis may be the result, presenting with abdominal pain and features of sepsis. Surgical debridement of the necrotic tissue is likely to be required, either laparoscopically or by open surgery.

Sleeve stenosis

This is usually a late complication of a staple-line problem but may be evident within the first week postoperatively if an intense local inflammatory reaction is established, usually following an otherwise undetected leak. After imaging as above, rehydration and possibly nutritional support are all that is required initially. At a later date, once any evidence of active perforation or leak has settled, endoscopic dilatation may help, although this brings its own risk of causing further disruption/perforation. Completion gastrectomy with conversion to a Roux-en-Y bypass may ultimately be required.

Gastric bypass/BPD/duodenal switch patients

Staple-line leak

These operations have several staple lines to consider: the gastric pouch, the gastro-jejunal anastomosis, the gastric remnant (in a gastric bypass) and the more distal jejuno-jejunostomy. Only the first two of these can be imaged on a contrast swallow. CT may show the others but the receiving surgeon should have a low threshold for returning the patient to theatre for laparoscopy if a leak is suspected. It should be remembered that a tachycardia or elevated C-reactive protein (CRP) may be the only evidence of such a problem in obese patients. If more than 48–72 hours have elapsed since the initial operation, then laparoscopic repair is less likely to be feasible and laparotomy may be required. Surgical treatment should address drainage of sepsis, control of any ongoing leakage and the provision of nutrition (Box 19.2).

Staple-line bleed

Patients may bleed into the GI tract or into the peritoneal cavity. A bleed into the 'blind' gastric remnant after a bypass will only be evident on CT, or by

early return to the operating theatre (see Box 19.3). Treatment involves establishing drainage of the collection of the haematoma by gastrotomy and controlling the bleeding point, usually by oversewing the staple line. Placement of a transcutaneous gastrostomy tube is wise, not only to decompress the stomach but also to use for later nutritional support if required. Angiographic embolisation of the bleeding point may be an alternative but the surgeon must not allow the inherent delays of such intervention to postpone what might be life-saving re-operative surgery.

Small-bowel enterotomy

Full-thickness injury to the small bowel can easily be incurred as a result of handling with instruments, and perforations may occur 'off-camera', out of the laparoscopic field of view. Missed enterotomies may take several days to become apparent, usually presenting with increasing abdominal pain, tachycardia and fever. Enteric fluid may leak out from one or more of the laparoscopic port sites. CT may demonstrate free intraperitoneal fluid and even intraperitoneal gas, but these findings are non-specific. Return to theatre for laparoscopy or laparotomy and drainage/repair is required.

Early small-bowel obstruction

Early postoperative small-bowel obstruction is uncommon after laparoscopic surgery and should not immediately be attributed to a paralytic ileus. Port-site bowel herniation, often of the Richter type, is always a possibility but after operations involving Roux-en-Y reconstruction one should always consider internal herniation, small-bowel volvulus and iatrogenic jejuno-jejunal anastomotic stricture or distortion. Vomiting will be absent if the blind gastroduodenal limb is obstructed and abdominal X-rays may be unreliable, especially in a morbidly obese patient. CT is indicated (**Fig. 19.14**). The treating surgeon should not delay operating to correct an established obstruction.

Late small-bowel obstruction

Small-bowel obstruction arising months or years after laparoscopic gastric bypass is a well-recognised problem. The most frequent cause is internal herniation, occurring in up to 7% of cases if the

Box 19.2 • Nutritional support in the bariatric patient

> It is a mistake to assume that obese patients are well nourished: although their diets may have been high in calories, they have often been deficient in protein, vitamins and other micronutrients. As for any patient with an upper GI anastomotic leak, consideration should be given to commencing enteral feeding or total parenteral nutrition. When re-operating on a bariatric patient for complications, it is sensible to place a feeding gastrostomy or jejunostomy at the same time.

Box 19.3 • Early recognition of complications is essential

> Many of the early complications after gastric bypass and duodenal switch are potentially life threatening. Prompt recognition is important. CT scanning is useful but delay in the diagnosis will worsen a perilous situation so urgent return to theatre is often a better strategy.

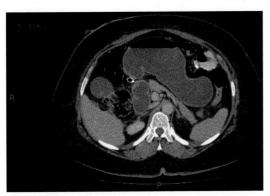

Figure 19.14 • CT scan showing 'blind' gastroduodenal biliopancreatic limb obstruction. Note the dilated, fluid-filled stomach and duodenum (large arrows) and the oral contrast in the non-distended alimentary limb (small arrow).

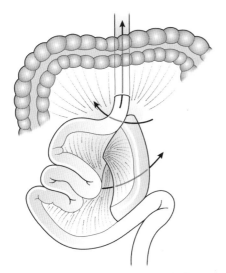

Figure 19.15 • The three common sites for internal hernia after Roux-en-Y reconstruction: the mesocolic defect (green arrow), Petersen's space (blue arrow) and the jejunal mesenteric window (red arrow).

mesenteric defects are not closed.[25,26] Hernias typically develop through the mesocolic defect if the retrocolic route is used, the jejunal mesenteric defect at the site of jejuno-jejunostomy, and Petersen's space between the alimentary limb and the transverse colon (see **Fig. 19.15**). For many patients the presentation is insidious, with post-prandial pain and/or bloating. Imaging may not reveal significant small bowel dilatation. Laparoscopy is the investigation and treatment of choice, where chyle within the abdominal cavity is a clue to the diagnosis. The ileocaecal junction is identified first and then the small bowel is carefully 'walked' back until the point of internal herniation is seen and reduced. The defect is then closed with non-absorbable material to prevent recurrence.

Gastro-gastric fistula

This is a consideration in the medium to long term if a patient develops weight regain. It may also present with dysphagia or pain on eating. It is often associated with stomal ulcers in the gastric pouch, which prove resistant to acid suppression medication, and likely arises following a staple-line leak with abscess formation that discharges into the gastric remnant. The treatment is surgical to divide the fistula and resect some of the distal stomach. This may be achievable laparoscopically.

Dumping syndrome

A recognised complication of gastric resectional surgery, this syndrome comprises post-prandial cramping abdominal pain, nausea, sweating, light-headedness and sleepiness. It reflects hyper-insulinaemic hypoglycaemia, usually precipitated by a high carbohydrate load in the jejunum from rapid gastric emptying,[27] although it is also described after Nissen fundoplication where vagal injury is the likely cause.[28] Mild forms are common and it is rarely severe enough to present as a surgical emergency, but surgeons should nevertheless be aware of it as a cause of post-bypass malaise. Dietary regulation, medication to slow gut motility and/or somatostatin analogues generally provide relief.

Mini-gastric bypass patients

A similar spectrum of complications can be expected as might follow a Roux-en-Y bypass, BPD or duodenal switch. However, because of the loop gastro-jejunostomy, bile reflux can be a problem – especially if the efferent limb takes a long time to function. Prolonged nasogastric drainage and nutritional support may be required, with or without the addition of somatostatin analogues or other agents to reduce secretions. If the problem is intractable, conversion to a Roux-en-Y configuration may be necessary.

Gastric balloon patients

Nausea and vomiting are almost universal symptoms after balloon insertion but usually subside by the end of the first week. Patients may need intravenous hydration, PPI medication and parenteral anti-emetics over this time. A small minority of patients cannot tolerate oral intake even after several weeks and, in this group, early balloon removal should be offered and will provide instant relief. Although a special kit is produced for balloon removal, it can easily be performed by using a standard endoscopic injection needle (to puncture and empty the balloon) and some strong grasping forceps, or a snare, to remove the deflated balloon.

Abdominal or chest pain is uncommon and should raise the possibility of reflux oesophagitis, gastric ulceration or even gastric/oesophageal perforation. If relief is not obtained with hydration, PPI and anti-emetic medication, then gastroscopy is warranted – though urgent CT is the preferred investigation if perforation is a serious consideration.

Duodenojejunal barrier patients

There is little information about the long-term outcomes of this new procedure. Epigastric discomfort, attributable either to the transmucosal barbs that fix the collar of the device into the first part of the duodenum, or simply to the foreign body sensation itself, is common and usually settles within a week or two with PPI medication and analgesics. However, several specific complications have been reported.

Migration
The device may fail to fix adequately in the duodenal cap and shift out of position. This may cause pain, nausea, bleeding or a degree of gastric outflow obstruction. Abdominal X-ray and/or gastroscopy should diagnose the problem, and endoscopic removal is likely to be required. A special kit is needed and so either the original bariatric surgeon, or alternatively the manufacturers, should be contacted.

Duodenal bleeding
This may be minor or catastrophic. Diagnosis and management would be along the lines of any upper GI bleed, although removal of the device is likely to be required if simple endoscopic means do not control the bleeding.

Bowel obstruction
This may occur with a food bolus if the patient does not eat slowly and chew well, but may also arise if the device migrates distally into the small bowel. The wire frame of the collar of the device will be visible on abdominal X-ray but, without some knowledge of the endoscopic procedure done, these appearances may be difficult to interpret. Because of the metal barbs, simply waiting for the device to pass spontaneously is risky and as a result laparotomy is likely to be required.

Gastric plication patients

Whether this is done laparoscopically or endoscopically, the procedure-specific risks include gastric trauma (bleeding or perforation), liver/spleen trauma incurred by traction, direct pressure or injury and perforation of the stomach.[18]

Patients with older, now obsolete operations

As patients will have had their operations many years earlier, only late complications will arise. These include exacerbations of long-standing problems such as blind loop syndrome following a JIB and pouch outlet stenosis after a VBG. Nutritional deficiencies, which may manifest in many ways, are also possible complications (see below).

Other postoperative problems

Gallstones

Dramatic weight loss from any cause promotes gallstone formation owing to mobilisation of cholesterol from peripheral fat stores and changes to the enterohepatic cycle. Patients may present with biliary colic, cholecystitis, pancreatitis or obstructive jaundice and should be managed according to established protocols. Laparoscopic cholecystectomy is generally no more difficult after a bariatric surgical operation than otherwise, but the management of common bile duct stones can be problematic because endoscopic retrograde cholangiopancreatography (ERCP) may be impossible if there has been a previous bypass or duodenal switch/BPD. Intraoperative cholangiography is therefore recommended at the time of cholecystectomy, with concurrent surgical duct exploration as required.

Nutritional deficiencies

The common nutritional deficiencies seen in the bariatric surgery population concern thiamine, iron, zinc, vitamin D and vitamin B_{12}. These may have been present preoperatively, in which case replenishment can be difficult, especially if a malabsorptive-type operation has been done. The clinical features of various deficiency syndromes are well documented but, like the neurological manifestations of thiamine deficiency presenting as Wernicke–Korsakoff's syndrome, may not be readily recognised by general surgeons. If one deficiency is diagnosed then others should be sought. These are of particular importance if re-operative surgery is planned because of the possible detrimental effects that nutritional deficiencies might have on wound healing.

Failure to lose weight

Even the best operations do not work for everyone. While most patients do well in the first few months after surgery, and for many the weight loss is maintained indefinitely as they adopt a new and healthy lifestyle, some degree of late weight regain is very common. This rarely means that the operation has been done incorrectly or failed in some way, although this should be excluded first: bands may become too loose, gastric pouches may stretch, staple lines may disrupt, bypassed bowel may adapt. More usually, however, weight regain reflects a re-emergence of underlying poor eating behaviours – in other words, patients tend to slip back into their old eating habits.[29] Ongoing follow-up with the multidisciplinary bariatric team is important to both prevent and manage postoperative weight regain.[9-11]

Key points

- Weight loss operations are becoming more common and complications are increasingly likely to present to the general surgeon on call.
- Knowledge of the operation performed will help the receiving surgeon anticipate any problems that might arise.
- It is wise to contact the original bariatric surgical team as they may provide useful advice but, as for all emergency admissions, the prime clinical responsibility for the patient rests initially with the receiving surgeon.
- Physical examination may be difficult and X-rays may be hard to interpret. Look carefully for clinical and biochemical features of dehydration and sepsis.
- Beware the acute band slippage in a gastric band patient. Percutaneous band decompression may provide short-term relief but definitive operative release/removal/resection may be required.
- Urgent CT to demonstrate a bleed, leak or obstruction in a patient who is unwell following a gastric bypass or duodenal switch procedure can help to make the diagnosis but immediate return to theatre may be a better strategy.
- Incessant vomiting after gastric balloon insertion may respond to inpatient gut rest and anti-emetic medication but instant and permanent relief will be obtained by removal of the balloon.
- Tachycardia should never be disregarded as it may be the only clue to an intra-abdominal catastrophe.
- Because complications may arise some years after bariatric surgery, patients may no longer be overweight and thus the link to the initial procedure may not be obvious.

References

1. Adams TD, Gress RE, Smith SC, et al. Long-term mortality after gastric bypass surgery. N Engl J Med 2007;8:753–61.

2. Sjöström L, Narbro K, Sjöström CD, et al. Swedish Obese Subjects Study. Effects of bariatric surgery on mortality in Swedish obese subjects. N Engl J Med 2007;357:741–52.
   A classic study and the first to show conclusively that bariatric surgery produced lasting health benefits.

3. Pories WJ, Swanson MS, MacDonald KG, et al. Who would have thought it? An operation proves to be the most effective therapy for adult-onset diabetes mellitus. Ann Surg 1995;222:339–52.

4. Monkhouse SJW, Morgan JDT, Norton SA. Complications of bariatric surgery: presentation and emergency management: a review. Ann R Coll Surg Engl 2009;91:280–6.

5. Kirshtein B, Lantsberg L, Mizrahi S, et al. Bariatric emergencies for non-bariatric surgeons: complications of laparoscopic banding. Obes Surg 2010;20:1468–78.

6. Hamdan K, Somers S, Chand M. Management of late post-operative complications of bariatric surgery. Br J Surg 2011;98:1345–55.

7. Tadross JA, le Roux CW. The mechanisms of weight loss after bariatric surgery. Int J Obes (Lond) 2009;33(Suppl. 1):S28–32.

8. Canetti L, Bachar E, Berry EM. Food and emotion. Behav Processes 2002;60:1–10.

9. Lim RB, Blackburn GL, Jones DB. Benchmarking best practices in weight loss surgery. Curr Probl Surg 2010;47:79–174.

10. Keren D, Matter I, Rainis T, et al. Getting the most from the sleeve: the importance of post-operative follow-up. Obes Surg 2011;21:1887–93.

11. Franco JVA, Ruiz PA, Palermo M, et al. A review of studies comparing three laparoscopic procedures in bariatric surgery: sleeve gastrectomy, Roux-en-Y gastric bypass and adjustable gastric banding. Obes Surg 2011;21:1458–68.

    A good review of several series comparing the outcomes of these three popular operations.

12. Dixon JB, O'Brien PE, Playfair J, et al. Adjustable gastric banding and conventional therapy for type 2 diabetes: a randomised controlled trial. JAMA 2008;299:316–23.

13. Mingrone G, Castagneto-Gissey L. Mechanisms of early improvement/resolution of type 2 diabetes after bariatric surgery. Diabetes Metab 2009;35:518–23.

14. Vetter ML, Cardillo S, Rickels MR, et al. Narrative review: effect of bariatric surgery on type 2 diabetes mellitus. Ann Intern Med 2009;150:94–103.

15. le Roux CW, Welbourn R, Werling M, et al. Gut hormones as mediators of appetite and weight loss after Roux-en-Y gastric bypass. Ann Surg 2007;246:780–5.

16. Tice JA, Karliner L, Walsh J, et al. Gastric banding or bypass? A systematic review comparing the two most popular bariatric procedures. Am J Med 2008;121:885–93.

17. Nocca D, Krawczykowsky D, Bomans B, et al. A prospective multicenter study of 163 sleeve gastrectomies: results at 1 and 2 years. Obes Surg 2008;18:560–5.

18. Kueper MA, Kramer KM, Kirschniak A, et al. Laparoscopic sleeve gastrectomy: standardized technique of a potential stand-alone bariatric procedure in morbidly obese patients. World J Surg 2008;32(7):1462–5.

19. Sudan R, Jacobs DO. Biliopancreatic diversion with duodenal switch. Surg Clin North Am 2011;91:1281–93.

20. Scopinaro N, Marinari GM, Camerini G. Laparoscopic standard biliopancreatic diversion: technique and preliminary results. Obes Surg 2002;12:241–4.

21. Zhang GY, Wang TT, Cheng ZQ, et al. Resolution of diabetes mellitus by ileal transposition compared with biliopancreatic diversion in a non-obese animal model of type 2 diabetes. Can J Surg 2011;54:243–51.

22. Skrekas G, Antiochos K, Stafyla VK. Laparoscopic gastric greater curve plication: results and complications in a series of 135 patients. Obes Surg 2011;21:1657–63.

23. Mikami D, Needleman B, Narula V, et al. Natural orifice surgery: initial US experience utilizing the StomaphyX device to reduce gastric pouches after Roux-en-Y gastric bypass. Surg Endosc 2010;24(1):223–8.

24. Abdemur A, Sucandy I, Szomstein S, et al. Understanding the significance, reasons and patterns of abnormal vital signs after gastric bypass for morbid obesity. Obes Surg 2011;21:707–13.

25. Abasbassi M, Pottel H, Deylgat B, et al. Small bowel obstruction after antecolic antegastric laparoscopic Roux-en-Y gastric bypass without division of small bowel mesentery: a single-centre, 7-year review. Obes Surg 2011;21:1822–7.

26. Bauman RW, Pirrello JR. Internal hernia at Petersen's space after laparoscopic Roux-en-Y gastric bypass: 6.2% incidence without closure – a single surgeon series of 1047 cases. Surg Obes Relat Dis 2009;5:565–70.

27. Tack J, Arts J, Caenepeel P, et al. Pathophysiology, diagnosis and management of postoperative dumping syndrome. Nat Rev Gastroenterol Hepatol 2009;6:583–90.

28. Hejazi RA, Patil H, McCallum RW. Dumping syndrome: establishing criteria for diagnosis and identifying new etiologies. Dig Dis Sci 2010;55:117–23.

29. Niego SH, Kofman MD, Weiss JJ, et al. Binge eating in the bariatric surgery population: a review of the literature. Int J Eating Disorders 2007;40(3):349–59.

Index

NB: Page numbers followed by *f* indicate figures, *t* indicate tables and *b* indicate boxes.